Developmental Origins of Health and Disease

This landmark publication provides the first definitive account of how and why subtle influences on the fetus and during early life can have such profound consequences for adult health and diseases. Although the epidemiological evidence for this link has long proved compelling, it is only much more recently that the scientific basis for this has begun to be studied in depth and fully understood. This compilation, written by many of the world's leading experts in this exciting field, summarises these basic and clinical advances. The link between early development and the onset of many chronic diseases such as coronary heart disease, diabetes and osteoporosis also raises important public health issues. Another fascinating theme in the book concerns evolutionary developmental biology and how the 'evo-devo' debate can cast light on these concepts. Clinicians and basic scientists alike will find this an authoritative book about this exciting and emerging field.

Peter D. Gluckman is Professor of Paediatric and Perinatal Biology, Director of the Liggins Institute (for Medical Research) and Director of the National Research Centre for Growth and Development, at the University of Auckland.

Mark A. Hanson is Director of the Developmental Origins of Health & Disease Research Division at the University of Southampton Medical School, and British Heart Foundation Professor of Cardiovascular Science.

Developmental Origins of Health and Disease

Edited by

Peter Gluckman

University of Auckland, New Zealand

Mark Hanson

University of Southampton, UK

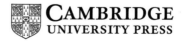

CAMBRIDGE UNIVERSITY PRESS
Cambridge, New York, Melbourne, Madrid, Cape Town, Singapore, São Paulo

Cambridge University Press
The Edinburgh Building, Cambridge CB2 8RU, UK

Published in the United States of America by Cambridge University Press, New York

www.cambridge.org
Information on this title: www.cambridge.org/9780521847438

First published 2006
Reprinted 2007

Printed in the United Kingdom at the University Press, Cambridge

A catalogue record for this publication is available from the British Library

ISBN 978-0-521-84743-8 hardback

Contents

Contributors

Dr Avan Aihie Sayer, MSc, PhD, FRCP
MRC Clinical Scientist & Honorary Senior Lecturer in Geriatric
    Medicine
MRC Epidemiology Resource Centre
University of Southampton
Southampton General Hospital
Southampton S016 6YD, UK

Dr James A. Armitage, BOptom, MOptom, PhD
Postdoctoral Research Fellow
Maternal and Fetal Research Unit
Division of Reproductive Health
Endocrinology and Development
King's College London
St Thomas' Hospital
London SE1 7EH, UK

Dr Janis Baird, MBBS, PhD, MFPH
Research Fellow
MRC Epidemiology Resource Centre
University of Southampton
Southampton General Hospital
Southampton S016 6YD, UK

Professor David Barker, PhD, FRCP, FRS
Professor of Clinical Epidemiology
Developmental Origins of Health & Disease Centre
University of Southampton
Princess Anne Hospital
Southampton S016 5YA, UK
and Professor, Department of Medicine
Oregon Health and Science University
Portland, OR 97239, USA

Dr Chiara Botti, BiolD
Department of General Pathology
II University of Naples
80131 Naples, Italy

Associate Professor Berni Breier, MSc, PhD
Associate Director
Liggins Institute
University of Auckland
Private Bag 92019
Auckland, New Zealand

Dr Graham Burdge, BSc, PhD
Senior Research Fellow
Institute of Human Nutrition
University of Southampton
Bassett Crescent East
Southampton S016 7PX, UK

Professor Christopher D. Byrne, FRCP, FRCPath, PhD
Professor of Endocrinology & Metabolism
University of Southampton
Southampton General Hospital
Southampton S016 6YD, UK

Professor Philip C. Calder, BSc, PhD, DPhil
Professor of Nutritional Immunology
Institute of Human Nutrition
University of Southampton
Bassett Crescent East
Southampton S016 7PX, UK

Professor John R. G. Challis, PhD, DSc, FIBiol, FRCOG, FRSC
Vice-President, Research & Associate Provost
Professor of Physiology, Obstetrics, Gynaecology and
    Medicine
University of Toronto
27 King's College Circle
Toronto M5S 1A8, Canada

Dr Megan L. Cock, PhD
Senior Research Officer
Department of Physiology
Monash University, Clayton
VIC 3800, Australia

Professor Cyrus Cooper, DM, FRCP, FMedSci
Professor of Rheumatology and Director
MRC Epidemiology Resource Centre
University of Southampton
Southampton General Hospital
Southampton S016 6YD, UK

Associate Professor Wayne Cutfield, MBChB, MD, FRACP
Director of Endocrinology
Starship Children's Hospital
Director, Paykel Clinical Research Unit
Liggins Institute
Associate Director, Liggins Institute
University of Auckland
Private Bag 92019
Auckland, New Zealand

Professor Michael Davison, PhD, DSc, FRSNZ
Professor of Psychology
Director, Experimental Analysis of Behaviour Research Unit
University of Auckland
Private Bag 92019
Auckland, New Zealand

Professor Filomena de Nigris, BiolD, PhD
Assistant Professor
Department of General Pathology
II University of Naples, 80131 Naples, Italy
and Department of Pharmacological Sciences
University of Salerno, Italy

Dr Elaine Dennison, MA, MRCP, PhD
Senior Research Fellow/Honorary Consultant in Rheumatology
MRC Epidemiology Resource Centre
University of Southampton
Southampton General Hospital
Southampton S016 6YD, UK

Dr Miodrag Dodic, MD, PhD
Honorary Senior Research Fellow
Department of Physiology
Monash University
Clayton, VIC 3800, Australia

Professor Anders Ekbom, MD, PhD
Department of Medicine
Karolinska Institutet
171 76 Stockholm, Sweden

Professor Mostafa A. El-Haddad, MD, FRCOG
Assistant Professor in Perinatal Medicine
Harbor–UCLA Medical Center
University of California
Los Angeles, 1000 W. Carson Street
Torrance, CA 90502, USA

Adjunct Professor Johan G. Eriksson, MD, PhD
Head of Unit
National Public Health Institute
Department of Epidemiology and Health Promotion
Diabetes and Genetic Epidemiology Unit
Mannerheimintie 166, 00300 Helsinki, Finland

Dr Caroline H. D. Fall, MBChB, DM, FRCPCH
Reader in Epidemiology and Honorary Consultant in Child
   Health
MRC Epidemiology Resource Centre
University of Southampton
Southampton General Hospital
Southampton S016 6YD, UK

Professor Tom Fleming, BSc, PhD
Professor of Developmental Biology
School of Biological Sciences
University of Southampton
Bassett Crescent East
Southampton S016 7PX, UK

Dr Alison J. Forhead, BSc, PhD
University Lecturer
Department of Physiology
University of Cambridge
Downing Street
Cambridge CB2 3EG, UK

Professor Terrence Forrester, DM, FRCP, PhD
Director, Tropical Medicine Research Institute
Tropical Medicine Research Institute
University of the West Indies
Mona, Kingston 7, Jamaica

Professor Abigail L. Fowden, BA, PhD, ScD
Professor of Perinatal Physiology
Department of Physiology
University of Cambridge
Downing Street
Cambridge CB2 3EG, UK

Dr David Gardner, BSc, PhD, RNut
British Heart Foundation Lecturer
Centre for Reproduction and Early Life
School of Human Development
Academic Division of Child Health
Queen's Medical Centre
Nottingham NG7 2UH, UK

Dr David Garrick, BSc, MA, PhD
MRC Molecular Haematology Unit
Weatherall Institute of Molecular Medicine
Oxford University
Oxford OX3 9DS, UK

Dr Dino A. Giussani, BSc, MA, PhD
Reader in Developmental Cardiovascular Physiology &
   Medicine
Department of Physiology
University of Cambridge
Downing Street, Cambridge CB2 3EG, UK

Professor Peter Gluckman, DSc, FRSNZ, FRS
University Distinguished Professor
Director, Liggins Institute and National Research Centre for
   Growth and Development
University of Auckland
Private Bag 92019
Auckland, New Zealand

Professor Keith Godfrey, BM, PhD, FRCP
Reader in Epidemiology & Human Development
MRC Epidemiology Resource Centre
University of Southampton
Southampton General Hospital
Southampton S016 6YD, UK

Dr Carmen Guarino, MB
Department of General Pathology
II University of Naples
80131 Naples, Italy

Professor Mark Hanson, MA, DPhil, FRCOG
British Heart Foundation Professor of Cardiovascular Science
Director, Centre for Developmental Origins of Health and
   Disease
University of Southampton
Princess Anne Hospital
Southampton S016 5YA, UK

Professor Richard Harding, MSc, PhD, DSc
NH & MRC Senior Principal Research Fellow
Department of Physiology
Monash University
Clayton, VIC 3800, Australia

Dr Jerrold J. Heindel, PhD
Scientific Program Administrator
Division of Extramural Research and Training
National Institute of Environmental Health Sciences
Research Triangle Park
NC 27709, USA

Dr Paul Hofman, FRACP
Senior Lecturer in Paediatric Endocrinology
University of Auckland
Private Bag 92019
Auckland, New Zealand

Associate Professor Terrie Inder, MBChB, MD, FRACP
Neonatal Neurologist
Royal Children's Hospital
Murdoch Children's Research Institute, Parkville
VIC 3052, Australia

Dr Craig A. Jefferies, MBChB, FRACP
University Honorary Senior Lecturer
Paediatric Endocrinologist
Paediatrician
University of Auckland
Private Bag 92019
Auckland, New Zealand

Dr Luise Kalbe, PhD
Institute of Life Science
Université catholique de Louvain
B1348 Louvain-la-Neuve, Belgium

Professor Tom Kirkwood, PhD, FMedSci
Professor of Medicine; Co-Director
Institute for Ageing and Health
Henry Wellcome Laboratory for Biogerontology Research
University of Newcastle
Newcastle upon Tyne NE4 6BE, UK

Dr Jason Landon, BSc, MSc, PhD
Research Fellow
Liggins Institute
University of Auckland
Private Bag 92019
Auckland, New Zealand

Dr Catherine Law, MD, FRCPCH, FFPH
Reader in Children's Health
Institute of Child Health
University College London
30 Guilford Street, London WC1N 1EH, UK

Dr Cindy P. Lawler, PhD
Scientific Program Administrator
Division of Extramural Research and Training
National Institute of Environmental Health
   Sciences
Research Triangle Park
NC 27709, USA

Professor Gert S. Maritz, PhD, MBA
Department of Medical Biosciences
University of the Western Cape
7535 Bellville, South Africa

Dr Josie M. L. McConnell, BSc, PhD
Senior Research Fellow
Maternal and Fetal Research Unit
Division of Reproductive Health
Endocrinology & Development
King's College London
St Thomas' Hospital
London SE1 7EH, UK

Dr Karen Moritz, MSc, PhD
Research Fellow
Department of Anatomy and Cell Biology
Monash University
Clayton, VIC 3800, Australia

Dr Susan Morton, MBChB, PhD, FAFPHM
Senior Lecturer in Epidemiology
Liggins Institute and School of Population
   Health
University of Auckland
Private Bag 92019
Auckland, New Zealand

Dr Timothy J. M. Moss, PhD
Senior Research Fellow
School of Women's and Infants' Health
The University of Western Australia
M094, 35 Stirling Highway
Crawley, WA 6009, Australia

Professor Leslie Myatt, PhD
Professor of Obstetrics and Gynecology; Director
Physician Scientist Training Program; Director
Women's Reproductive Health Research Scholars
    Program
University of Cincinnati
College of Medicine, PO Box 670526
Cincinnati, OH 45267, USA

Professor Claudio Napoli, MD, PhD, MBE
Professor of Medicine and Clinical Pathology
Excellence Research Center on Cardiovascular Diseases and
    Department of General Pathology
II University of Naples
Naples 80131, Italy
and Adjunct Professor of Medicine
Whitaker Cardiovascular Institute
Boston University, MA 02118, USA

Professor John P. Newnham, MD, FRANZCOG
Professor of Obstetrics and Gynaecology (Maternal Fetal
    Medicine)
Head, School of Women's and Infants' Health
The University of Western Australia
King Edward Memorial Hospital
Bagot Road, Subiaco, WA 6008, Australia

Dr Ray Noble, BSc, PhD
Co-Director, Collaborative Centre for Reproductive Ethics
    and Rights
Institute for Women's Health
Department of Obstetrics and Gynaecology
University College London
London WC1E 6BT, UK

Professor Richard O. C. Oreffo, DPhil
Professor of Musculoskeletal Science
Bone and Joint Research Group
Developmental Origins of Health and
    Disease Division
University of Southampton
Southampton S016 6YD, UK

Dr Susan Ozanne, BSc, PhD
British Heart Foundation Lecturer
Department of Clinical Biochemistry
University of Cambridge
Addenbrookes's Hospital
Cambridge CB2 2QR, UK

Professor David I. W. Phillips, MA, PhD, FRCP
Professor of Metabolic and Endocrine Programming
MRC Epidemiology Resource Centre
University of Southampton
Southampton General Hospital
Southampton S016 6YD, UK

Dr Orlando Pignalosa, MD
Department of General Pathology
II University of Naples
80131 Naples, Italy

Professor Lucilla Poston, BSc, PhD, FRCOG
Director of Research
Maternal and Fetal Research Unit
Division of Reproductive Health
Endocrinology & Development
King's College London
St Thomas' Hospital
London SE1 7EH, UK

Associate Professor Sandra Rees, MSc, MPhil, PhD
Associate Professor and Reader
Department of Anatomy and Cell Biology
University of Melbourne
Parkville, VIC 3010, Australia

Professor Claude Remacle, PhD
University Full Professor
Institute of Life Science
Université catholique de Louvain
B1348 Louvain-la-Neuve, Belgium

Dr Brigitte Reusens, PhD
Senior Scientist
Institute of Life Science
Université catholique de Louvain
B1348 Louvain-la-Neuve, Belgium

Dr H. I. (Trudy) Roach, PhD
University Orthopaedics
Southampton General Hospital
Southampton SO16 6YD, UK

Dr Victoria Roberts, BSc, PhD
Postdoctoral Fellow
Department of Obstetrics and Gynecology
University of Cincinnati College of Medicine
231 Albert Sabin Way
Cincinnati, OH 45267, USA

Professor Michael G. Ross, MD, MPH
Professor of Obstetrics/Gynecology and Public Health
UCLA School of Medicine and Public Health
Chair, Department of Obstetrics and Gynecology
Harbor–UCLA Medical Center
1000 W. Carson Street, Torrance
CA 90502, USA

Dr Loredana Rossi, MB
Department of General Pathology
II University of Naples
80131 Naples, Italy

Professor H. P. S. Sachdev, MD, FIAP, FAMS
Professor and In-charge
Division of Clinical Epidemiology
Department of Pediatrics
Maulana Azad Medical College
New Delhi 110 002, India

Professor Vincenzo Sica, MD
Professor of Clinical Pathology
Department of General Pathology
II University of Naples
80131 Naples, Italy

Dr Deborah M. Sloboda, PhD
Forrest Fetal Research Scientist
Postdoctoral Research Fellow
School of Women's and Infants' Health
The University of Western Australia
King Edward Memorial Hospital
Bagot Road, Subiaco
WA 6008, Australia

Noel Smith, BSc
Department of Clinical Biochemistry
University of Cambridge
Addenbrookes's Hospital
Cambridge CB2 2QR, UK

Professor Michael E. Symonds, BSc, PhD
Professor of Developmental Physiology
Head of the Academic Division of Child Health
School of Human Development
Queen's Medical Centre
Nottingham NG7 2UH, UK

Professor Kent L. Thornburg, PhD
M. Lowell Edwards Chair for Research in Clinical Cardiology
Professor of Medicine (Cardiology)
Director, Heart Research Center
Oregon Health and Science University
3181 S.W. Sam Jackson Park Road
Portland, OR 97239, USA

Dr Christopher Torrens, BSc, PhD
Postdoctoral Research Fellow
Maternal, Fetal & Neonatal Physiology
Centre for Developmental Origins of Health & Disease
University of Southampton
Princess Anne Hospital
Southampton S016 5YA, UK

Dr Janelle Ward, PhD, BSc
Department of Physiology
University of Cambridge
Downing Street
Cambridge CB2 3EG, UK

Professor John O. Warner, MD, FRCP, FRCPCH
Professor of Child Health
Infection, Inflammation and Repair Division
School of Medicine
University of Southampton
Southampton General Hospital
Southampton S016 6YD, UK

Professor Emma Whitelaw, DPhil
School of Molecular and Microbial Biosciences
University of Sydney
NSW 2006, Australia
current address: Queensland Institute of Medical Research
Brisbane, QLD 4029, Australia

Professor E. Marelyn Wintour, PhD, DSc, FAA
Department of Physiology
Monash University
Clayton, VIC 3800, Australia

Preface

This book could not have been written ten years ago. In the first instance, the field it covers, that of developmental origins of health and disease (DOHaD) was at that stage embryonic and highly controversial. While there was compelling epidemiological data, there was a lack of experimental and mechanistic data on which to create consensus. But over the last decade the science of DOHaD has advanced rapidly. The epidemiological evidence for the DOHaD paradigm is now strongly supported by prospective clinical data, experimental observations and a growing understanding of the underlying molecular and developmental mechanisms. Further, the scope of physiological systems that may be involved has expanded. The relevance of the phenomenon to the ecology of human disease in different populations is now much clearer.

So there is now a pressing need for a book such as this. By the time of its publication, three world congresses on DOHaD will have occurred; an international learned society has been formed; and there are a substantial number of reviews on many aspects of the field and its implications. Yet to date there is no definitive textbook. Students, clinicians and researchers need a volume that brings current knowledge together, whether to introduce them to the subject as a whole or to help them broaden their knowledge of an expanding field.

Moreover, the implications of the DOHaD concept are now becoming clear. The scientific implications now extend not only into epidemiology, developmental biology and physiology, but also into evolutionary biology and anthropology. DOHaD has very important implications for public health policy, not only in developed but also in developing societies.

In this volume, we have assembled contributions from undisputed experts in the DOHaD field. Many are architects of the ideas that are reviewed throughout. We are enormously grateful to them for their timely and well constructed contributions to the volume. Our thanks must also go to Peter Silver, who commissioned the volume from Cambridge University Press, and to Deborah Peach, Cathy Pinal and Karen Goldstone who worked so hard on the preparation of the manuscripts for publication.

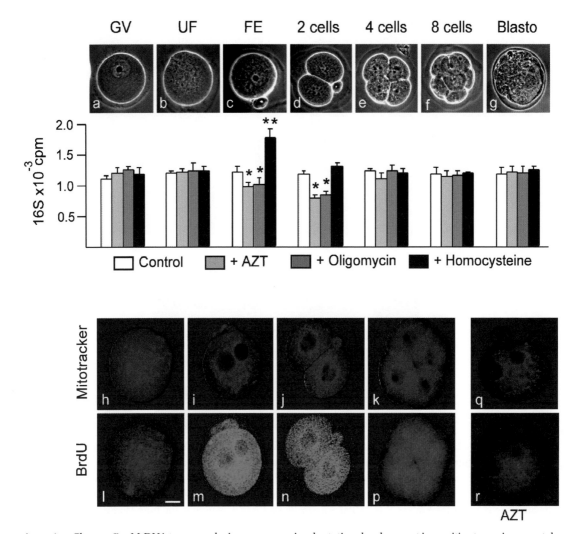

Plate 1 (*see Chapter 6*) MtDNA turnover during mouse preimplantation development is sensitive to environmental factors. Full-grown oocytes (GV) were isolated from ovaries, unfertilised eggs (UF) were collected 12 h after HCG injection, and fertilised eggs (FE), two-, four-, eight-cell and blastocyst-stage embryos were collected after successful mating at 24, 36, 48, 60 and 72 h post HCG (panels a–g). MtDNA copy number was measured in groups of embryos at each stage after being cultured alone, with AZT, with oligomycin or with homocysteine. The relative levels of mtDNA present in embryos at each stage after different culture conditions is represented by coded grouped histograms beneath a light-field image of the relevant stage. Unfertilised eggs (UF), fertilised eggs (FE), two-cell embryos and four-cell embryos were preincubated with aphidicolin to prevent nuclear replication and then cultured in aphidicolin plus BrdU 10 μg/ml for 4 h. All staged embryos were finally incubated in Mitotracker RedCM-H2Xros (Molecular Probes) 400 nm for 10 min prior to fixation to pinpoint mitochondria. All samples were subsequently processed so as to visualise BrdU incorporation. Red fluorescence (Mitotracker) panels h–q and green fluorescence (BrdU) panels l–r were monitored using confocal microscopy; all samples were measured at identical settings. Panels q and r show the effects of incubating fertilised eggs in aphidicolin, BrdU and AZT. Under these conditions all incorporation of BrdU into mtDNA is ablated.

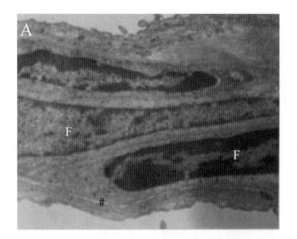

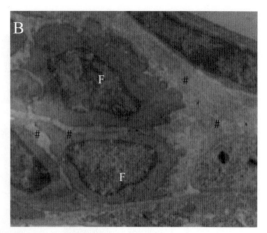

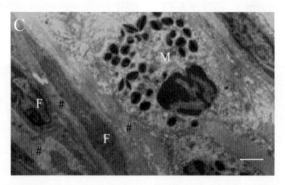

Plate 2 (*see Chapter 25*) Transmission electron micrographs of the alveolar walls of control (A) and IUGR (B and C) sheep at 2.3 years after birth. The basement membranes of adjacent interstitial cells in the alveolar walls of control lung are thin (#), resulting in the cells being in close contact. In the IUGR sheep the spaces between adjacent interstitial cells are prominent and filled with extracellular matrix (ECM) (#). The fibroblasts (F) and mast cells (M) are often separated by thick layers of ECM. Bar = 1 μm. Reproduced with permission from Maritz *et al.* (2003).

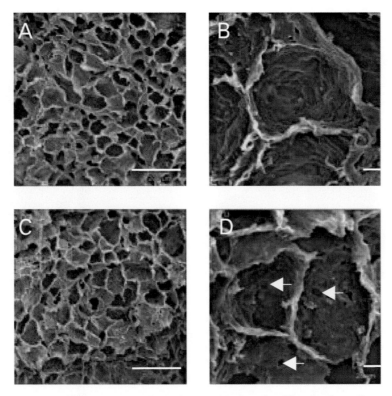

Plate 3 (*see Chapter 25*)   Scanning electron micrographs of the alveolar surface of lung tissue of 2-year-old control (A and B) and IUGR (C and D) sheep. The alveolar fenestrations (white arrows) in the lungs of the IUGR sheep are more numerous than in control sheep. A and C, bar = 20μm; B and D, bar = 200 μm. Reproduced with permission from Maritz *et al.* (2003).

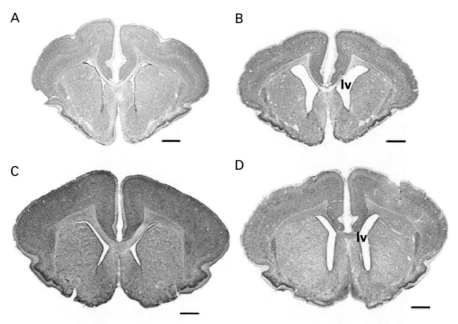

Plate 4 (*see Chapter 28*)   The effects of chronic placental insufficiency on brain development. Coronal thionin-stained sections of control term (A) and 8 weeks postnatal (C) and prenatally compromised term (B) and 8 weeks postnatal (D) guinea pig brains. The lateral ventricles (lv) are enlarged in the compromised brains compared to controls at both ages. Scale bars: 2.2 mm. Images: Dr Alexandra Rehn and Dr Carina Mallard.

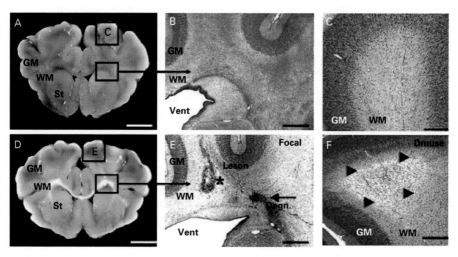

Plate 5 (*see Chapter 28*)   The effects of inflammatory agents on the fetal brain. Coronal thionin-stained sections of fetal sheep brain (B, C, E, F) and unstained slices (A, D) at 105 days of gestation (term ∼147 days). Compared to controls (A, B, C), LPS exposure (repeated injections from 95 to 100 days of gestation) resulted in diffuse subcortical damage (F, arrowheads) and cystic infarcts (E, *) and diffuse damage in the periventricular white matter (E). GM, grey matter; WM, white matter; Vent, lateral ventricle. Scale bars: A, D, 4.6 mm; B, E, 528 μm; C, F, 440 μm. Images: Dr Jhodie Duncan.

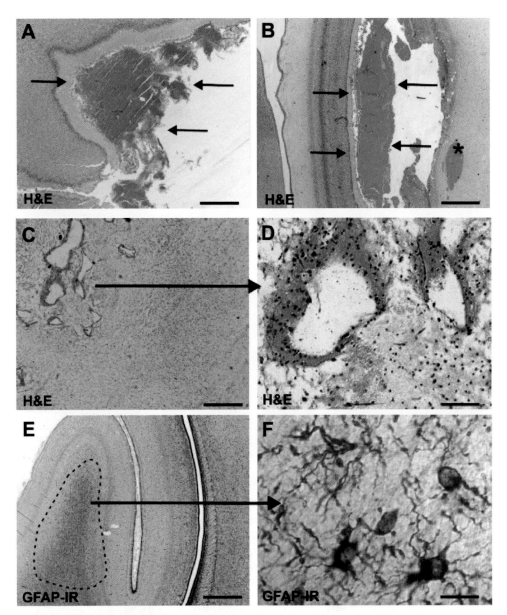

Plate 6 (*see Chapter 28*)   Injury in the brains of prematurely delivered baboons. (A–D) H&E stained sections: (A) subarachnoid haemorrhage (arrows); (B) intraventricular haemorrhage (not associated with the choroid plexus) in the lateral ventricle (arrows) and an intraparenchymal haemorrhage (asterisk); (C) coagulative necrosis and infarction in the periventricular white matter; (D) high-power view of coagulative necrosis from C. (E, F) GFAP-IR stained sections: (E) reactive astrocytes in the subcortical white matter; (F) high-power view of reactive astrocytes from E. GFAP, glial fibrillary acidic protein; H&E, hemotoxylin and eosin; IR, immunoreactive. Scale bars: A, B, E, 800 μm; C, 500 μm; D, 110 μm; F, 15 μm. Images: Drs Michelle Loeliger, Sandra Dieni and Emily Camm.

(A) Control diet

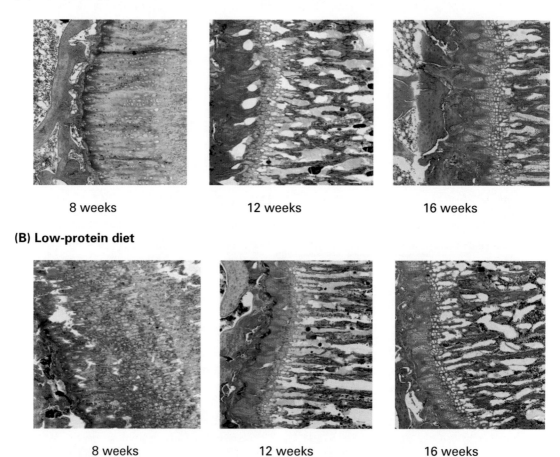

8 weeks   12 weeks   16 weeks

(B) Low-protein diet

8 weeks   12 weeks   16 weeks

Plate 7 (*see Chapter 30*)   Modulation of growth plate in offspring following maternal protein restriction during pregnancy. Histology of rat femurs from offspring of mothers on a (A) control diet (18% casein) or (B) maintained during pregnancy on a low-protein diet (9% casein) at 8, 12 and 16 weeks stained with Alcian Blue/Sirius Red. The growth plate can be seen as a distinct blue band separating the secondary ossification centre from the spongiosa of the diaphysis (original magnification × 50). In the low-protein group at 8 weeks the growth plates were wider; but by 12 and 16 weeks intrauterine diet appeared to have no significant effect on growth-plate height.

The developmental origins of health and disease: an overview

Peter D. Gluckman[1] and Mark A. Hanson[2]

[1]University of Auckland
[2]University of Southampton

The concept of developmental origins of health and disease (DOHaD) grew from the earlier concept of fetal origins of adult disease (FOAD) (reviewed in Barker 1995, 1998). There are two important reasons for the change. The first results from the large amount of research (much of it reviewed in this book) showing that the early life events which determine in part the risk of later disease occur not only in the fetal period specifically, but throughout the plastic phase of development. In this respect the use of the word 'development' is helpful because it implies not only effects operating during early stages of embryonic life (usually the preserve of developmental biology) but also those in infancy. Secondly, the DOHaD terminology emphasises that this area of science has implications not only for disease, and its prevention, but also for health promotion. The latter is of great importance in public health and education programmes in many parts of the world. But the accent on 'developmental origins' is more than just a flag of convenience under which several disciplines may sail: it represents a fundamental shift in thinking about the way in which early life processes affect later health and disease in humans.

Previously, proponents of FOAD championed the view that prenatal events were of utmost importance. Adopting this position was tactically necessary in the battle (now won) to gain widespread recognition that the aetiology of many chronic diseases, such as coronary heart disease (Barker and Osmond 1986), type 2 diabetes (Ravelli *et al.* 1998) or osteoporosis (Cooper *et al.* 2002), lay not only in genetic predisposition or in adult lifestyle, but also in the ways in which early life events could affect subsequent biology. As a result, both epidemiologists and experimentalists have expanded the period of interest to that around conception (Cnattingius *et al.* 1998, Kwong *et al.* 2000, Inskip *et al.* 2001, Bloomfield *et al.* 2003, Robinson *et al.* 2004, Crozier *et al.* in press). In parallel, other clinical and basic scientists were stressing the importance of the postnatal environment during suckling, infancy and childhood in setting an individual on the path to health or disease (Eriksson *et al.* 1999, 2003, Singhal *et al.* 2002, 2003). At times, these two schools of thought appeared to be at loggerheads, and the resulting conflict did little to promote understanding of the importance of the field that they shared. Development is a continuum extending on either side of birth – consider the wide variation in maturation at birth in different species. More recently, the recognition that the field of evolutionary developmental biology ('evo-devo') has enabled the development of a broader understanding of the phenomenon and, in turn, studies of the DOHaD phenomenon have led to new concepts in evo-devo biology. Both these advances in theoretical thinking and new experimental observations allow recognition that both pre- and postnatal environmental factors play vitally important roles, and that what matters most is the degree of match/mismatch between

Developmental Origins of Health and Disease, ed. Peter Gluckman and Mark Hanson. Published by Cambridge University Press.

them. This idea is more fully explained in Chapter 3. Suffice it to say here that the term 'development' helps to emphasise the importance of this continuity.

There are other ways in which the epidemiological work has continued to be controversial. The early concerns about confounding variables led to discussion on the relative importance of low birthweight versus other contributory factors. At times such discussions became rather sterile. Because the consensus in both animal and human research is now that phenotypes can be induced in offspring without necessarily being accompanied by low birthweight, it is clear that reduction of fetal growth per se does not lie on a causal pathway to later disease. Rather, low birthweight is a surrogate marker of the effects of the prenatal environment on the fetus, and one aspect of the fetal 'coping' responses to that environment. The problems in this area were compounded by an insufficient appreciation of the distinction between clinically manifest disease and other surrogate markers or risk factors for disease (Huxley *et al.* 2002). Examples included the use of elevated blood pressure as a marker for cardiovascular disease, or reduced insulin sensitivity as a marker of diabetes. With the wisdom of hindsight, it is not surprising that interpretation of the links between surrogates of fetal adaptation (birthweight) and later disease (blood pressure, insulin sensitivity) yielded different interpretations at the hands of different researchers. As the field has progressed, however, we have developed more sensitive markers of fetal adaptive responses and these can now directly relate to clinical disease. When this is done, the striking correlations that underpin the DOHaD hypothesis begin to emerge.

The work conducted by basic scientists, many of them using experimental animals, has not been without criticism either. Inevitably the use of a range of species to investigate the phenomenon, partly based on convenience, cost and suitability for experimental techniques, has produced a similarly sterile discussion about which provides the most suitable experimental model for the human (Symonds *et al.* 2000, Langley-Evans 2000, Bertram and Hanson 2001, Armitage *et al.* 2004). Ideas have become refined as

confirmation of similar aspects of the phenomenon across species has been made. Surprisingly, one of the features to emerge from the intense research activity in the area is how easy it is to manipulate the phenotype of offspring by changes in the early environment. This poses the problem of the relevance to humans of an observation made in animals. A key issue is to distinguish between factors that disrupt development and which are not regulated and those that are based on the processes of developmental plasticity and may have adaptive value – these ideas are expanded in Chapter 3. We have to accept that some environmental exposures, either clinical or experimental, simply disrupt the normal pattern of development. Such exposures do not necessarily lead to increased risk of disease (which cannot usually be ascertained in animals), nor have direct relevance to DOHaD in humans.

Notwithstanding these issues, studies in animals have revealed exciting insights into the mechanisms which underlie DOHaD. The first has been referred to above, and is the perception that changes in the developmental environment can induce phenotypic changes which are not necessarily accompanied by a reduction of birthweight or change in body proportions at birth (Hanson 2002). But perhaps the most exciting development relates to the area of gene–environment interactions, usually now referred to as epigenetics. As the reader will see (Chapter 5), it is now clear that graded changes in certain factors, such as histone acetylation and the degree of DNA methylation (Weaver *et al.* 2004), can produce subtle changes in the expression of genes. Coupled with our increasing knowledge about post-transcriptional and post-translational factors which influence gene expression, we are now beginning to see how developmental plasticity operates through environmental actions interceding between the genotype and the induction of the phenotype. Because such epigenetic processes depend on dietary availability of key nutrients and micronutrients, and because they can be affected by hormone levels (Waterland and Jirtle 2004), they are prime candidates for mechanisms underlying DOHaD, at least as regards the most commonly studied systems.

Moreover, whilst it was formerly thought that the methylation of DNA was established anew in the embryo at or before the blastocyst stage, it is now clear that levels of methylation can to a degree be transmitted from one generation to the next (Weaver *et al.* 2004). Research has revealed several ways in which transgenerational effects can be passed not only from the mother to her offspring but also to her grandchildren and possibly further down the lineage (Drake and Walker 2004).

In Chapter 3 we present a theoretical basis for the DOHaD phenomenon, in the context of previous theories that contribute substantially to it, such as metabolic teratogenesis, the thrifty genotype, thrifty phenotype and others. We believe that such an exercise is important for synthesising current ideas and allowing the incorporation of new experimental findings. It is surprising how easily current experimental findings fit into such a theory, but its real utility will probably be derived when a set of observations which do not fit is uncovered. In this sense using a theory makes the identification of such extraneous observations easier, and goes on to generate new experimental approaches, hypotheses and, ultimately, new theories. Even as it stands, however, the theory must ask questions about our tacit assumption that neo-Darwinian processes have contributed greatly to phenotypic diversity, including phenotypes susceptible to disease, in human populations. We think the implications of theoretical thinking regarding DOHaD for evolutionary biology will be substantial.

Most research in the field has been focused on metabolic disorders or on the cardiovascular system, reflecting the original epidemiological observations of Barker and his colleagues. Indeed, many of the chapters in this book reflect this emphasis. But now research in DOHaD is broadening to include other chronic diseases, such as osteoporosis (Cooper *et al.* 2002), cognitive decline (Richards *et al.* 2002, Gale *et al.* 2003), behavioural abnormalities (Thompson *et al.* 2001, Wahlbeck *et al.* 2001), obesity (Eriksson *et al.* 2001) and some forms of cancer (Dos Santos *et al.* 2004; see also Chapter 31). This does not mean that the phenomenon is so broad and all-

encompassing as to be meaningless. Rather it suggests that an entirely new way of viewing chronic disease will have to be developed in both developed and developing societies. The importance of this to public health policy makers is discussed in Chapter 34.

Many of the contributors to this volume make reference to the importance of the DOHaD concept to public health policy. Various estimates have been made of the impact of early-life factors in determining later risk of disease. A conservative estimate, based on the effects of low birthweight on later endothelial function in childhood, suggests that such early-life programming is equivalent in magnitude to the effect of smoking in later life (Leeson *et al.* 2001). More dramatic figures come from the retrospective studies of the Helsinki cohort (Chapters 3 and 15) which indicate that men who had a low ponderal index at birth and a high body mass index at age 12 had a five-fold greater risk of dying of coronary heart disease. In relation to the epidemic of obesity and associated diseases, data from India (Bhargava *et al.* 2004) suggest that the incidence of type 2 diabetes in adults who had an accelerated adiposity rebound as children will be about 25%. More work to define the magnitude of these effects is urgently needed.

Western societies are now characterised by increasing longevity, and this means that the number of those suffering from heart disease and related disorders will increase over the next few years, even though paradoxically those dying from such diseases will fall. There is no room for complacency in the latter statistic, as it may well be only temporary. Furthermore, there is increased interest in the effects of infection and inflammatory responses in early life in contributing to the increased longevity, but there are clearly many factors of equal importance. In earlier life the DOHaD concept is giving important insights into the epidemic of obesity developing in childhood and adolescence (see Chapter 18). The recognition that fat deposition (Vickers *et al.* 2000, Symonds *et al.* 2004), propensity to exercise (Vickers *et al.* 2003) and even dietary preference (Bellinger *et al.* 2003) may be programmed in early life now makes it essential to think how to intervene. It is possible that 'lifestyle' interventions may be effective in developed societies, in a way that may be less so in developing societies (see Chapter 3). However, even if this is the case it is likely that there will have to be a shift away from public health messages aimed at targeting the population as a whole towards more individually 'customised' dietary and exercise plans for those at risk. This will not be easy; the perception that the risk of later disease may be less in the infant who is fat and becomes obese as a young adolescent, in contrast to the small baby who later becomes fat, raises important issues of interpretation. These two children in their teens may in the end have identical body mass indices, but have arrived at that point by different paths and, hence, in later life have very different prospects for disease risk.

Many other factors contribute to the importance of DOHaD in the social policy arena. In particular, family size is decreasing in both industrialised/developed and developing nations. In industrialised societies, this may reflect the tendency for women to pursue careers and to start families later, and reflect social policy as in China with a 'one child' policy to limit population size. Moreover, well-meaning programmes to promote contraception accessibility in many developing countries will serve to limit family size further. Because of the maternal-constraint issues raised in Chapter 3, these initiatives may make the mismatch between the pre- and postnatal environments greater.

Our overall conclusion, therefore, is that environmental factors acting during the phase of developmental plasticity interact with genotypic variation to change the capacity of the organism to cope with its environment in later life. Because the postnatal environment can change dramatically, whereas the intrauterine environment is relatively constant over generations, it may well be that much of humankind is now living in an environment beyond that for which we evolved. The DOHaD phenomenon can explain how this manifests in the ecological patterns of human disease. It is no longer possible for adult medicine to ignore the developmental phase of life.

REFERENCES

Armitage, J. A., Khan, I. Y., Taylor, P. D., Nathanielsz, P. W. and Poston, L. (2004). Developmental programming of metabolic syndrome by maternal nutritional imbalance: how strong is the evidence from experimental models in mammals? *J. Physiol.*, **561**, 355–77.

Barker, D. J. P. (1995). Fetal origins of coronary heart disease. *BMJ*, **311**, 171–4.

(1998). *Mothers, Babies and Health in Later Life*, 2nd edn. Edinburgh: Churchill Livingstone.

Barker, D. J. P. and Osmond, C. (1986). Infant mortality, childhood nutrition, and ischaemic heart disease in England and Wales. *Lancet*, **1**, 1077–81.

Bellinger, L., Lilley, C. and Langley-Evans, S. C. (2003). Prenatal exposure to a low protein diet prgrammes a preference for high fat foods in the rat. *Pediatr. Res.*, **53**, 38A.

Bertram, C. E. and Hanson, M. A. (2001). Animal models and programming of the metabolic syndrome. *Br. Med. Bull.*, **60**, 103–21.

Bhargava, S. K., Sachdev, H. S., Fall, C. H. D. *et al.* (2004). Relation of serial changes in childhood body-mass index to impaired glucose tolerance in young adulthood. *N. Engl. J. Med.*, **350**, 865–75.

Bloomfield, F., Oliver, M., Hawkins, P. *et al.* (2003). A periconceptional nutritional origin for noninfectious preterm birth. *Science*, **300**, 606.

Cnattingius, S., Bergstrom, R., Lipworth, L. and Kramer, M. S. (1998). Prepregnancy weight and the risk of adverse pregnancy outcomes. *N. Engl. J. Med.*, **338**, 147–52.

Cooper, C., Javaid, M. K., Taylor, P., Walker-Bone, K., Dennison, E. and Arden, N. (2002). The fetal origins of osteoporotic fracture. *Calcif. Tissue. Int.*, **70**, 391–4.

Crozier, S., Borland, S., Robinson, S., Godrey, K. and Inskip, H. (in press). How effectively do young women prepare for pregnancy? *BJOG*.

Dos Santos, S. I., de Stavola, B. L., Hardy, R. J., Kuh, D. J., McCormack, V. A. and Wadsworth, M. E. (2004). Is the association of birth weight with premenopausal breast cancer risk mediated through childhood growth? *Br. J. Cancer*, **91**, 519–24.

Drake, A. J. and Walker, B. R. (2004). The intergenerational effects of fetal programming: non-genomic mechanisms for the inheritance of low birth weight and cardiovascular risk. *J. Endocrinol.*, **180**, 1–16.

Eriksson, J. G., Forsen, T., Tuomilehto, J., Winter, P. D., Osmond, C. and Barker, D. J. P. (1999). Catch-up growth in childhood and death from coronary heart disease: longitudinal study. *BMJ*, **318**, 427–31.

Eriksson, J., Forsen, T., Tuomilehto, J., Osmond, C. and Barker, D. (2001). Size at birth, childhood growth and obesity in adult life. *Int. J. Obes.*, **25**, 735–40.

Eriksson, J. G., Forsen, T. J., Osmond, C. and Barker, D. J. P. (2003). Pathways of infant and childhood growth that lead to type 2 diabetes. *Diabetes Care*, **26**, 3006–10.

Gale, C. R., Walton, S. and Martyn, C. N. (2003). Foetal and postnatal head growth and risk of cognitive decline in old age. *Brain*, **126**, 2273–8.

Hanson, M. (2002). Birth weight and the fetal origins of adult disease. *Pediatr. Res.*, **52**, 473–4.

Huxley, R., Neil, A. and Collins, R. (2002). Unravelling the fetal origins hypothesis: is there really an inverse association between birthweight and subsequent blood pressure? *Lancet*, **360**, 659–65.

Inskip, H., Hammond, J., Borland, S., Robinson, S. and Shore, S. (2001). Determinants of fruit and vegetable consumption in 5,630 women aged 20–34 years from the Southampton Women's Survey. *Pediatr. Res.*, **50**, 58A.

Kwong, W. Y., Wild, A. E., Roberts, P., Willis, A. C. and Fleming, T. P. (2000). Maternal undernutrition during the preimplantation period of rat development causes blastocyst abnormalities and programming of postnatal hypertension. *Development*, **127**, 4195–202.

Langley-Evans, S. C. (2000). Critical differences between two low protein diet protocols in the programming of hypertension in the rat. *Int. J. Food. Sci. Nutr.*, **51**, 11–17.

Leeson, C. P. M., Kattenhorn, M., Morley, R., Lucas, A. and Deanfield, J. E. (2001). Impact of low birth weight and cardiovascular risk factors on endothelial function in early adult life. *Circulation*, **103**, 1264–8.

Ravelli, A. C., van der Meulen, J. H., Michels, R. P. *et al.* (1998). Glucose tolerance in adults after prenatal exposure to famine. *Lancet*, **351**, 173–7.

Richards, M., Hardy, R., Kuh, D. and Wadsworth, M. E. J. (2002). Birthweight, postnatal growth and cognitive function in a national UK birth cohort. *Int. J. Epidemiol.*, **31**, 342–8.

Robinson, S. M., Crozier, S. R., Borland, S. E., Hammond, J., Barker, D. J. and Inskip, H. M. (2004). Impact of educational attainment on the quality of young women's diets. *Eur. J. Clin. Nutr.*, **58,** 1174–80.

Singhal, A., Farooqi, I. S., O'Rahilly, S., Cole, T. J., Fewtrell, M. and Lucas, A. (2002). Early nutrition and leptin concentrations in later life. *Am. J. Clin. Nutr.*, **75**, 993–9.

Singhal, A., Fewtrel, M., Cole, T. J. and Lucas, A. (2003). Low nutrient intake and early growth for later insulin resistance in adolescents born preterm. *Lancet*, **361**, 1089–97.

Symonds, M. E., Budge, H. and Stephenson, T. (2000). Limitations of models used to examine the influence of nutrition during pregnancy and adult disease. *Arch. Dis. Child.*, **83**, 215–19.

Symonds, M. E., Pearce, S., Bispham, J., Gardner, D. S. and Stephenson, T. (2004). Timing of nutrient restriction and programming of fetal adipose tissue development. *Proc. Nutr. Soc.*, **63**, 397–403.

Thompson, C., Syddall, H., Rodin, I., Osmond, C. and Barker, D. J. P. (2001). Birth weight and the risk of depressive disorder in late life. *Br. J. Psychiatry*, **179**, 450–5.

Vickers, M. H., Breier, B. H., Cutfield, W. S., Hofman, P. L. and Gluckman, P. D. (2000). Fetal origins of hyperphagia, obesity and hypertension and its postnatal amplification by hypercaloric nutrition. *Am. J. Physiol.*, **279**, E83–7.

Vickers, M., Breier, B. H., McCarthy, D. and Gluckman, P. (2003). Sedentary behaviour during postnatal life is determined by the prenatal environment and exacerbated by postnatal hypercaloric nutrition. *Am. J. Physiol.*, **285**, R271–3.

Wahlbeck, K., Forsen, T., Osmond, C., Barker, D. J. P. and Eriksson, J. G. (2001). Association of schizophrenia with low maternal body mass index, small size at birth and thinness during childhood. *Arch. Gen. Psychiatry*, **58**, 48–52.

Waterland, R. A. and Jirtle, R. L. (2004). Early nutrition, epigenetic changes at transposons and imprinted genes, and enhanced susceptibility to adult chronic diseases. *Nutrition*, **20**, 63–8.

Weaver, I. C. G., Cervoni, N., Champagne, F. A. *et al.* (2004). Epigenetic programming by maternal behavior. *Nat. Neurosci.*, **7**, 847–54.

2

The 'developmental origins' hypothesis: epidemiology

Keith Godfrey

University of Southampton

Introduction

Research worldwide has established that people who were small at birth and had poor growth in infancy have an increased risk of adult coronary heart disease and type 2 diabetes, particularly if this is followed by increased childhood weight gain. There is also evidence linking impaired early growth with other degenerative disorders in later life, including stroke, hypertension, obesity, osteoporosis, obstructive airways disease, reduced cognitive function and poor mental health. The relations between smaller infant size and an increased risk of ill health and adult disease extend across the normal range of infant size in a graded manner. Moreover, recent animal studies and epidemiological data have demonstrated that while maternal thinness and unbalanced diet during pregnancy may have modest effects on size at birth, they are nonetheless associated with raised blood pressure and altered glucose–insulin metabolism and stress responsiveness in the adult offspring. It is now clear that the associations do not simply reflect genetic influences; rather the findings indicate that interactions between the genetic influences and the early-life environment determine disease and susceptibility to adverse influences in the adult environment.

The observations have led to the hypothesis that cardiovascular disease, type 2 diabetes, osteoporosis and obstructive airways disease originate through developmental plastic responses made by the fetus and infant as part of a prediction of the subsequent environment to which it anticipates that it will be exposed. Critical periods in development result in irreversible changes; if the environment in childhood and adult life differs from that predicted during fetal life and infancy, the developmental responses may increase the risk of adult disease. This chapter provides an overview of some of the epidemiological evidence underpinning the developmental origins of degenerative disease. Evidence is also accumulating indicating important developmental influences on cancer, described in Chapter 31.

Fetal, infant and childhood growth in relation to health in later life

Ecological observations pointing to developmental influences on adult health

At the start of the twentieth century the incidence of coronary heart disease rose steeply in western countries so that it became the most common cause of death. In many of these countries the steep rise has been followed by a fall over recent decades that cannot be accounted for by changes in adult lifestyle. The incidence of coronary heart disease is now rising in other parts of the world to which western influences

Developmental Origins of Health and Disease, ed. Peter Gluckman and Mark Hanson. Published by Cambridge University Press.
© P. D. Gluckman and M. A. Hanson 2006.

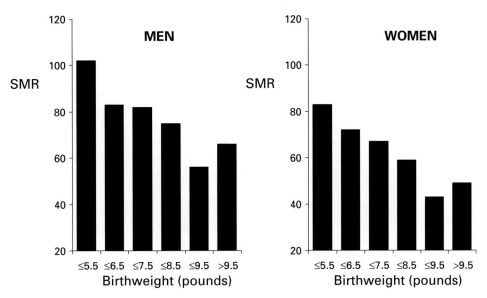

Figure 2.1 Coronary heart disease death rates, expressed as standardised mortality ratios (SMR), in 10 141 men and 5585 women born in Hertfordshire, UK, according to birthweight. Derived from Osmond *et al.* (1993).

are extending, including China, south Asia and eastern Europe.

A clue suggesting that coronary heart disease might originate during fetal development came from studies of death rates among babies in Britain during the early 1900s (Barker 1998). Perinatal mortality rates differed considerably between one part of the country and another, being highest in some of the northern industrial towns and the poorer rural areas in the north and west. This geographical pattern in death rates was shown to closely resemble today's large variations in death rates from coronary heart disease (Barker 1998). The usual certified cause of death in newborn babies during the early 1900s was low birthweight, and one possible conclusion suggested by the geographical association was that low rates of growth before birth are in some way linked to the development of coronary heart disease in adult life. Although it had previously been suggested that events in childhood influence the pathogenesis of coronary heart disease, the hypothesis that influences during fetal life and infancy play a critical role provided a new focus for research.

Coronary heart disease

Cohort studies of size at birth and coronary heart disease

The first direct evidence that an adverse intrauterine environment might have long-term consequences for the risk of coronary heart disease came from follow-up studies of men and women in middle and late life whose body measurements at birth had been recorded. A study of people born in Hertfordshire, UK, showed for the first time that those who had had low birthweights had increased death rates from coronary heart disease in adult life (Osmond *et al.* 1993, Barker 1998). Thus, among 15 726 people born during 1911 to 1930, death rates from coronary heart disease fell progressively with increasing birthweight in both men and women (Fig. 2.1). A small rise at the highest birthweights in men could relate to the macrosomic infants of women with gestational diabetes. Another study, of 1586 men born in Sheffield during 1907 to 1925, showed that it was particularly people who were small at birth as a result of growth restriction who were at increased risk of the disease (Barker *et al.* 1993a).

Replication of the UK findings has led to wide acceptance that low rates of fetal growth are associated with coronary heart disease in later life. For example, confirmation of a link between low birthweight and adult coronary heart disease has come from studies of 1200 men in Caerphilly, south Wales (Frankel *et al.* 1996) and of 70 297 nurses in the United States (Rich-Edwards *et al.* 1997). The latter study found a two-fold fall in the relative risk of non-fatal coronary heart disease across the range of birthweight. Similarly, among 517 men and women in Mysore, south India the prevalence of coronary heart disease in men and women aged 45 years or older fell from 15% in those who weighed 2.5 kg or less at birth, to 4% in those who weighed 3.2 kg or more (Stein *et al.* 1996).

Follow-up studies of populations with more detailed birth measurements suggest that altered birth proportions are more strongly associated with late outcomes than is birthweight per se (Forsen *et al.* 1997). The Hertfordshire records and the nurses and Caerphilly studies did not include measurements of body size at birth other than weight, but in populations where birth length was recorded, derivation of ponderal index (birthweight/length^3) allows a crude assessment of body composition and thinness at birth; ponderal index cannot, however, adequately distinguish variations in fat and lean mass. Where neonatal head circumference has also been recorded the baby whose body and trunk is small in relation to its head, as a result of 'brain sparing', can also be distinguished. Patterns of altered birth proportions and restricted fetal growth linked with later coronary heart disease may be summarised as a small head circumference, shortness or thinness (Barker *et al.* 1993a, Martyn *et al.* 1996a, Forsen *et al.* 1997, Barker 1998, Eriksson *et al.* 1999, 2001).

Although low placental weight (Forsen *et al.* 1997) and an altered ratio of placental weight to birthweight have also been linked with raised adult coronary heart disease death rates (Martyn *et al.* 1996a, Forsen *et al.* 1999), other studies have found no association with placental weight (Leon *et al.* 1998, Eriksson *et al.* 2001). Animal studies offer a possible explanation of this inconsistency. In sheep, the placenta enlarges in response to moderate undernutrition in mid pregnancy, presumably reflecting an adaptive response to extract more nutrients from the mother (Robinson *et al.* 1994); however, this effect is only seen in ewes that were well nourished before conception, and in ewes poorly nourished before conception undernutrition in mid pregnancy is associated with small placental size (Robinson *et al.* 1994).

Infant and childhood growth and coronary heart disease

Evidence suggesting both additive and interactive effects of poor prenatal and infant growth on the risk of subsequent coronary heart disease is now emerging from epidemiological studies. Follow-up of men born in Hertfordshire, UK, between 1911 and 1930 found that lower weight at age 1 year was strongly associated with higher hazard ratios for coronary heart disease (Osmond *et al.* 1993; Fig. 2.2), and subsequent analyses of this cohort have suggested additive effects of poor fetal and infant growth (Barker 1998).

Confirmation that smaller and thinner infants at age one year have increased rates of coronary heart disease in adulthood has come from people born in the 1930s and 1940s in Helsinki, Finland (Eriksson *et al.* 2001; Fig. 2.2). These findings, described in detail in Chapter 15, point to the possibility that interactions between the pre- and postnatal environments have an important influence of the risk of coronary heart disease. In the Helsinki study, hazard ratios for coronary heart disease fell with increasing birthweight and, more strongly, with increasing ponderal index at birth. These trends were found in babies born at term or prematurely and therefore reflect slow intrauterine growth. Consistent with the findings in Hertfordshire and with the known association between coronary heart disease and short adult stature (Marmot *et al.* 1984), men in Helsinki who developed the disease also tended to have poor

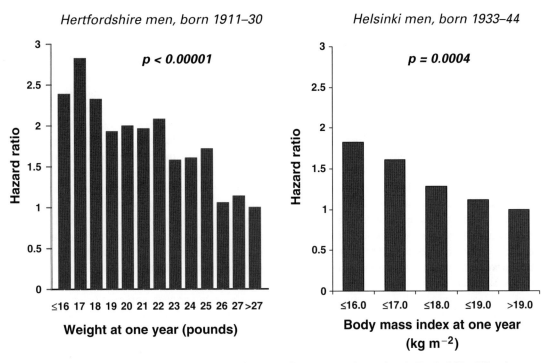

Figure 2.2 Hazard ratios for coronary heart disease according to weight at age 1 year in men born in Hertfordshire, UK, and according to body mass index at age 1 year in men born in Helsinki, Finland. Derived from Barker (1998) and Eriksson *et al.* (2001).

weight gain and low rates of height growth in infancy (Chapter 15). Although **infant** growth failure was deleterious in individuals that were both small and large at birth, **childhood** weight gain had very different effects in small and large neonates; in relation to the risk of adult coronary heart disease, there was a strong interaction between ponderal index at birth and body mass index in childhood. Among boys who were thin at birth with a below-average ponderal index, rapid weight gain and increasing body mass index during childhood was associated with higher rates of adult coronary heart disease; however, in boys who had an above-average ponderal index at birth, rapid childhood weight gain and increasing body mass index was unrelated to the risk of coronary heart disease (Eriksson *et al.* 2001). Findings among girls were similar, and again the risk of coronary heart disease was determined more by the tempo of weight gain than the body size attained (Forsen *et al.* 1999).

Size of effects and potential confounding influences

The findings described above suggest that influences linked to pre- and postnatal growth have an important effect on the risk of coronary heart disease. Assessment of the relative importance of early and later-life exposures is difficult as there is a paucity of well-characterised cohorts with both perinatal data and health outcomes documented well into later life. Some commentators have argued that the magnitude of developmental effects on adult cardiovascular risk is small (Hattersley and Tooke 1999, Huxley *et al.* 2002), although the only published estimate based upon the Helsinki cohort suggests that it is considerable when clinical disease is used as the outcome measure (Barker *et al.* 2002). Analysis of the magnitude of developmental effects on health 50 or more years later in life is challenging because concurrent risk factors can often be measured with greater precision and it is difficult to identify or attribute risk to distant, early-life factors. Moreover, the observed relationship between disease risk and birth size does not imply a causal role of being born small but reflects the sensitivity of fetal growth to adverse intrauterine influences. It is thought that it is the effect of environmental influences acting during early development that is the causal trigger. Indeed, much experimental and epidemiological evidence indicates that adverse developmental influences can affect disease risk without birth size being affected.

It has been argued that the associations between size at birth and later disease could primarily reflect genetic influences (Hattersley and Tooke 1999). Recent findings, however, indicate that it is interactions between the early-life environment and genetic influences that are likely to be the principal determinants of disease susceptibility (Eriksson *et al.* 2002; Chapter 15). Moreover, it is important to recognise that birth size has only a modest genetic component and primarily reflects the quality of the intrauterine environment (Morton 1955, Snow 1989, Brooks *et al.* 1995).

Other commentators have argued that people whose growth was impaired *in utero* may continue to be exposed to an adverse environment in childhood and adult life, and it is this later environment that produces the effects attributed to developmental influences. There is strong evidence that this argument cannot be sustained. In four of the studies which have replicated the association between birthweight and coronary heart disease, data on adult lifestyle factors including smoking, employment, diet, alcohol consumption and exercise were collected (Frankel *et al.* 1996, Rich-Edwards *et al.* 1997, Leon *et al.* 1997, Barker *et al.* 2001). Allowance for them had little effect on the association between birthweight and coronary heart disease. Influences in adult life, however, add to the effects of the intrauterine environment. For example, the prevalence of coronary heart disease is highest in people who had low birthweight but were obese as adults.

In studies exploring the mechanisms underlying the associations between early growth and later coronary heart disease, there are similar trends between birthweight and major risk factors for cardiovascular disease, including hypertension and type 2 diabetes (Hales *et al.* 1991, Huxley *et al.* 2000). Studies of cardiovascular risk factors have been extended to children, and suggest that developmental influences on cardiovascular risk are still acting in today's children and not simply of historical importance (Hofman *et al.* 1997, Leeson *et al.* 1997). These prospective clinical studies of children have again shown that the associations with smaller size at birth are independent of social class, cigarette smoking and alcohol consumption.

A further aspect, suggested by data from the Helsinki cohort, is that the early life and adult environments may not simply have **additive** effects, but may **interact** to influence the risk of coronary heart disease. Poverty and low household income have long been linked with coronary heart disease, but recent analyses suggest that this effect occurs in those who are thinner than average at birth, but not in those who are fatter than average (Barker *et al.* 2001). If interactions between the early-life and adult environments are confirmed, this will have important implications for our understanding of the evolutionary implications of developmental responses (see Chapter 3).

Stroke, hypertension and cardiovascular function

As compared with coronary heart disease, epidemiological studies of developmental influences on the risk of stroke have been hampered by the lower population prevalence of the disorder and the paucity of cohorts including both early-life data and information distinguishing occlusive and haemorrhagic stroke. The information that is available suggests that stroke is associated with low birthweight, but not with stunting or thinness (Martyn *et al.* 1996a). In the Helsinki cohort, the association between small size at birth and haemorrhagic stroke was only significant after adjustment for head circumference, and there was no association with occlusive stroke

(Eriksson *et al.* 2000a). Subsequent analyses in a larger Swedish cohort again found that impaired fetal growth was associated with haemorrhagic stroke, but not with occlusive stroke (Hypponen *et al.* 2001). In the Swedish cohort, the pronounced inverse association between birthweight and haemorrhagic stroke did not depend on adjustment for other birth dimensions, although adjustments for birth length and head circumference strengthened the association with birthweight. The strength of the association between impaired fetal growth and haemorrhagic stroke was appreciably greater than that found with coronary heart disease in the same cohort (Leon *et al.* 1998).

Hypertension is an important risk factor for both occlusive and haemorrhagic stroke, but there are established differences in the aetiological mechanisms underlying the two subtypes. One such mechanism is carotid atherosclerosis, which is associated with occlusive stroke. There is, however, some evidence linking low birthweight with carotid atherosclerosis. In a group of people aged 70 years, the prevalence and severity of carotid atherosclerosis was greatest in those with the lowest birthweights; when compared with people who weighed over 7.5 pounds (3.4 kg) at birth, the odds ratio of carotid stenosis was 5.3 in those who had weighed 6.5 pounds (2.9 kg) or less at birth (Martyn *et al.* 1998). Ultrasound measurement of intimal–medial thickness provides an indication of preclinical carotid atherosclerosis; among a group of men and women aged 27–30 years, intimal–medial thickness was increased in those who had experienced severe intrauterine growth restriction, particularly if they also had exaggerated postnatal growth (Oren *et al.* 2004).

Hypertension and blood pressure

Associations between low birthweight and raised blood pressure in childhood and adult life have been extensively demonstrated around the world. A systematic review of published papers described the associations between birthweight and blood pressure (Huxley *et al.* 2000) in 80 studies of people of all ages in many countries. These associations were not confounded by socioeconomic conditions at the time of birth or in adult life. The difference in systolic pressure associated with a 1-kg difference in birthweight was around 2.0 mm Hg. In clinical practice this would be a small difference but these are large differences between the mean values of populations and may correspond to a substantial proportion of total attributable mortality. Some observers have disputed the relevance of birthweight to blood pressure levels in later life (Huxley *et al.* 2002), but others have since cautioned about the dangers of extrapolating from a surrogate measure of disease risk, such as blood pressure, to clinical disorders (Gluckman and Hanson 2004). Where clinical disease has been used as the outcome measure, the effect of early environmental influences is clear. Among 22 846 men in the Health Professionals Follow-up Study there were strong relationships between birth size and the risk of developing clinically significant hypertension or diabetes mellitus, but no relationship with systolic blood pressure (Curhan *et al.* 1996). The findings demonstrate the importance of studying outcomes rather than surrogate measures of disease.

The association between low birthweight and raised blood pressure depends primarily on babies who were born small for dates, after reduced fetal growth, rather than on babies born preterm (Law *et al.* 1991, Barker *et al.* 1992, Moore *et al.* 1999, Eriksson *et al.* 2000b). In these studies alcohol consumption and higher body mass were also associated with raised blood pressure, but the associations between birthweight and blood pressure were independent of them. Nevertheless body mass remains an important influence on blood pressure and, in humans and animals, the highest pressures are found in those who were small at birth but become overweight as adults (Eriksson *et al.* 2000b). In some studies the blood pressures of the mothers during and after pregnancy have been recorded. They correlate with the offspring's blood pressure. However, the associations between body size and proportions at birth and later blood pressure are independent of the mothers' blood pressures (Law *et al.* 1991, Martyn *et al.* 1995a, Barker 1998).

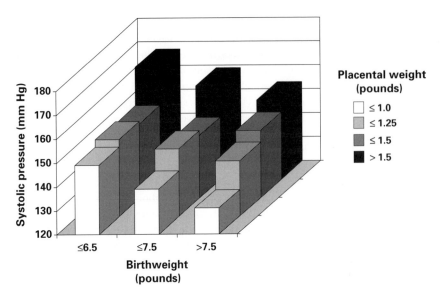

Figure 2.3 Mean systolic blood pressure (mm Hg) of men and women aged 50, born after 38 completed weeks of gestation, according to placental weight and birthweight. Derived from Barker *et al.* (1992).

As discussed previously, birthweight is a crude measure of fetal growth that does not distinguish thinness or short length, differences in head size, or variations in the balance of fetal and placental size. Analyses of babies born in Preston, UK, defined two groups who developed raised adult blood pressures (Barker *et al.* 1992). The first group had below-average placental weight and were thin with a low ponderal index and a below-average head circumference. The second had above-average placental weight and a short crown–heel length in relation to their head circumference; such short babies tend to be fat and may have above-average birthweight. In contrast to the associations between birth size and coronary heart disease, those between birthweight and blood pressure are generally as strong as those between thinness, shortness and blood pressure. Associations between blood pressure and thinness and shortness have been found in some studies but not in others (Barker 1998). In a longitudinal study of young people in Adelaide, Australia, associations between blood pressure and thinness and shortness were not apparent at age 8 years but emerged at age 20 (Moore *et al.* 1999).

Figure 2.3 shows the systolic pressure of a group of men and women who were born at term in Preston 50 years ago (Barker *et al.* 1992). Subjects are grouped according to their birthweights and placental weights. As in other studies, systolic pressure falls between subjects with low and high birthweight. In addition, however, there is an increase in blood pressure with increasing placental weight. Subjects with a mean systolic pressure of 150 mm Hg or more, a level sometimes used to define hypertension in clinical practice, comprise a group who as babies were relatively small in relation to the size of their placentas. There are similar trends with diastolic pressure.

A rise in blood pressure with increasing placental weight and a higher ratio of placental weight to birthweight was also found in 4-year-old children in Salisbury, UK, and among young adults in Adelaide, Australia (Law *et al.* 1991, Moore *et al.* 1999). In studies of children and adults the association between placental enlargement and raised blood pressure has, however, been inconsistent. As discussed in relation to coronary heart disease, variations in maternal nutritional status prior to conception may underlie some of the inconsistent relations with placental weight. For example, three studies that have reported an association between small placental size and raised blood pressure have been in populations in which the mother's nutritional status was poor or food intake was restricted (Campbell *et al.* 1996, Eriksson *et al.* 2000b, Thame *et al.* 2000).

Mechanisms underlying developmental effects on hypertension and raised blood pressure

There are a number of possible mechanisms by which restricted intrauterine growth could either initiate raised blood pressure or lead to accentuated amplification of blood pressure in later life. Studies in the USA, the UK and Holland have shown that blood pressure in childhood predicts the likelihood of developing hypertension in adult life. These predictions are strongest after adolescence. In children the rise of blood pressure with age is closely related to growth and is accelerated by the adolescent growth spurt. These observations led Lever and Harrap (1992) to propose that essential hypertension is a disorder of growth. The hypothesis that hypertension is a disorder of accelerated childhood growth can be reconciled with the association with low birthweight by postulating that rapid postnatal compensatory growth plays an important role in amplifying changes established in utero.

Much attention has focused on the possible role of impaired renal development in mediating early-life effects on later hypertension. If the materno-placental supply of nutrients does not match fetal requirements in the last trimester of pregnancy the fetus diverts blood and nutrients to maintain brain metabolism at the expense of the trunk and limbs. This adaptation reduces blood flow to the fetal kidneys and may underlie activation of the fetal renin–angiotensin system in intrauterine growth retardation. A follow-up study of men and women born in Sheffield found, however, that those who had been small at birth had *lower* plasma concentrations of inactive and active rennin (Martyn *et al.* 1996b). Causes of raised blood pressure that are not mediated by increased renin release tend to result in low concentrations of renin. These findings therefore suggest that the association between impaired fetal growth and raised blood pressure involves mechanisms other than the renin–angiotensin system. Low concentrations of renin in adult life do not, however, exclude the possibility of an earlier but lasting influence of the renin–angiotensin system, and the possible consequences of early activation of the system are discussed further in Chapter 23.

An alternative explanation for the low plasma renin concentrations of people who were small at birth is that they reflect a relative deficit of nephrons. Brenner suggested that retarded fetal growth leads to reduced numbers of nephrons, increasing pressure in the glomerular capillaries and glomerular sclerosis (Mackenzie and Brenner 1995). This sclerosis results in further loss of nephrons and a self-perpetuating cycle of hypertension and progressive glomerular injury. The numbers of nephrons is established during fetal life and varies widely in the normal population, with a normal range of around 300 000 to 1 100 000 or more (Mackenzie and Brenner 1995). Studies using fetal ultrasound have shown that babies that are small for gestational age have reduced renal growth during a critical period between 26 and 34 weeks of gestation. This reduces the antero-posterior size of the kidney but does not diminish kidney length (Konje *et al.* 1996). Direct support for the hypothesis that the number of nephrons plays an important role in primary hypertension has come from a case-control study of the number of glomeruli in 10 patients with primary hypertension and 10 matched normotensive subjects, all of whom had died in accidents. The median number of glomeruli per kidney was 702 379 in the hypertensive patients and 1 429 200 in the normotensive controls (Keller *et al.* 2003). Chapter 23 describes animal studies which provide substantial experimental evidence supporting the importance of impaired intrauterine renal development.

Animal studies also provide much evidence that re-setting of homeostatic neuroendocrine mechanisms controlling blood pressure is likely to be involved in mediating developmental effects on later blood pressure. A number of the maternal exposures that impair fetal growth are associated with alterations in the fetus's hypothalamic–pituitary–adrenal axis, and Chapter 13 describes evidence that this can alter the set-point of the biological response to stress. Altered sympathoadrenal and hypothalamic–pituitary–adrenal responses to stress are likely to be important mechanisms by which adverse influences during development affect the health of the offspring, and it is now known that people who had low birthweight have increased stress sensitivity, as indicated by cardiovascular responses, hypothalamic–pituitary–adrenal axis activity and sympathoadrenal responses. A review concluded that smaller birth size is associated with higher adult fasting plasma cortisol concentrations (Phillips *et al.* 2000); more detailed studies of the hypothalamic–pituitary–adrenal axis are required to define the underlying mechanism. People with high blood pressure tend to have features of increased sympathetic nervous system activity, including a high resting pulse rate, a high cardiac output and a hyperdynamic circulation. Among men and women in Preston, those who had low birthweight had a higher resting pulse rate (Phillips and Barker 1997). This is consistent with the hypothesis that retarded growth in utero establishes increased sympathetic nervous activity and contributes to raised blood pressure in later life.

Cardiovascular structure and function

Evidence that developmental influences can have long-term effects on cardiac structure came initially from a follow up study of 290 men born during 1920–30. Using echocardiography it was found that left ventricular mass increased with lower weight at age one-year, but was not related to birthweight (Vijayakumar *et al.* 1995). The relation with weight at 1 year was independent of adult body size, systolic blood pressure and age, leading to speculation that the left ventricular enlargement may be a long-term result of haemodynamic changes in utero or of persisting changes in growth factor concentrations. Subsequently, echocardiography of 210 children and young adults found a concentric increase in left ventricular mass, adjusted for sex and current body

size, with decreasing weight at 9 months or 2 years, even though there was no association between systolic pressure and weight at these ages (Zureik *et al.* 1996). Support for the hypothesis that left ventricular mass might be partly determined during fetal life and early infancy has come from experiments in pregnant guinea pigs and sheep; maternal food restriction in early pregnancy resulted in increased left ventricular mass in the postnatal offspring (Khan *et al.* 2005). Mechanisms underlying developmental effects on cardiac structure are discussed in Chapter 20.

The content and arrangement of elastin in the aorta and large conduit arteries plays an important part in minimising the rise of blood pressure in systole and maintaining blood pressure in diastole. Elastin is only synthesised in early life and the gradual loss or fracture of elastin fibres is thought to contribute to the rise in systolic and pulse pressure with ageing. These considerations have led to the hypothesis that impaired fetal development may be associated with a relative deficiency in elastin synthesis, resulting in stiffer arteries and raised blood pressure in postnatal life (Martyn and Greenwald 1997). This hypothesis is supported by a study of 50-year-old men and women showing that those who had a small abdominal circumference at birth tended to have a higher pulse wave velocity and decreased arterial elasticity in adult life (Martyn *et al.* 1995a).

Recent studies suggest that, in addition to its associations with compliance, low birthweight is also associated with persisting alterations in vascular structure and function. Hertfordshire men who had had low birthweight had narrow bifurcation angles in their retinal blood vessels (Chapman *et al.* 1997). People with hypertension have similar changes in retinal vascular geometry.

In the search for mechanisms which link reduced early growth with cardiovascular disease, evidence has emerged suggesting that functional abnormalities of the vasculature may be important. Vascular endothelial dysfunction is a key early event in atherosclerosis and is important in the development of the diseases associated with poor early growth. It is seen in subjects with coronary artery disease and type 2 diabetes and is closely associated with insulin resistance. Several studies have suggested that there is a relationship between birthweight and endothelial dysfunction that is present in children as early as the first decade of life. This was first reported in a study of 333 British children aged 9–11 years, which showed that the ability of the brachial artery to dilate in response to increased blood flow (induced by forearm cuff occlusion and release), an endothelium-dependent response, was reduced in children who had been small at birth (Leeson et al. 1997). It was confirmed in a study of 9-year-old children in Sweden (Martin et al. 2000). Other studies showed that this association persists into adult life, including a UK case–control study of 19 to 20-year-old subjects of low compared with normal birthweight (Goodfellow et al. 1998). The adult studies suggest that birthweight has a substantial effect similar in magnitude to the effect of smoking. Chapter 21 discusses the mechanisms underlying a developmental influence on endothelial function.

Serum cholesterol and blood clotting

Studies in Sheffield, UK, show that the neonate that has a short body and low birthweight in relation to the size of its head has persisting disturbances of cholesterol metabolism and blood coagulation (Barker 1998). Disproportion in body length relative to head size is associated with redistribution of blood flow away from the trunk to sustain the brain. This affects blood flow to the liver, two of whose functions, regulation of cholesterol and of blood clotting, seem to be permanently perturbed. Disturbance of cholesterol metabolism and blood clotting are both important features predisposing to cardiovascular disease.

The Sheffield records included abdominal circumference at birth, as well as length, and it was specifically reduction in this birth measurement that predicted raised serum concentrations of total and low-density-lipoprotein cholesterol and apolipoprotein B in men and women (Barker et al. 1993b). The differences in concentrations across the range

of abdominal circumference were large, statistically equivalent to 30 per cent differences in mortality from coronary heart disease. Findings for plasma fibrinogen concentrations, a measure of blood coagulability, were of similar size (Martyn et al. 1995b). Small abdominal circumference at birth also predicted death from coronary heart disease (Barker et al. 1995). Abdominal circumference in a neonate indicates liver size as well as the fatness of the abdominal wall, and one interpretation is that impaired liver growth is associated with persisting changes in liver metabolism. The Sheffield findings suggest that birthweight is a poor surrogate for developmental influences on liver metabolism and that caution should be exercised when making inferences from studies lacking more detailed information on prenatal growth and development (Huxley et al. 2004).

Animal experiments provide strong support for both pre- and postnatal influences on the 'setting' of lipid metabolism, as described in Chapter 11. The findings relating to postnatal influences on human lipid metabolism are less consistent. However, evidence from follow-up of men and women born in Hertfordshire, UK, suggests that poor infant growth, exclusive bottle-feeding and breast-feeding beyond 1 year may be associated with raised serum concentrations of total and low-density-lipoprotein cholesterol and apolipoprotein B (Fall et al. 1992).

Type 2 diabetes and the metabolic syndrome

Insulin has a central role in fetal growth, and disorders of glucose and insulin metabolism are therefore an obvious possible link between early growth and cardiovascular disease. Although obesity and a sedentary lifestyle are known to be important in the development of type 2 diabetes, they seem to lead to the disease only in predisposed individuals. Family and twin studies have suggested that the predisposition is familial, but the nature of this predisposition is unknown. The disease tends to be transmitted through the maternal rather than paternal side of the family.

Size at birth and type 2 diabetes

A number of studies have confirmed the association between birthweight and impaired glucose tolerance and type 2 diabetes first reported in Hertfordshire (Hales *et al.* 1991, McCance *et al.* 1994, Curhan *et al.* 1996, Lithell *et al.* 1996). In the Health Professionals Study, USA, the odds ratio for diabetes, after adjusting for current body mass, was 1.9 among men whose birthweights were less than 5.5 pounds (2.5 kg) compared with those who weighed 7.0 to 8.5 pounds (3.2–3.9 kg) (Curhan *et al.* 1996). Among the Pima Indians, USA, the odds ratio for diabetes was 3.8 in men and women who weighed less than 5.5 pounds (McCance *et al.* 1994). In Preston it was the thin babies who developed impaired glucose tolerance and diabetes (Phillips *et al.* 1994a). Lithell and colleagues (1996) confirmed the association with thinness in Uppsala, Sweden: the prevalence of diabetes was three times higher among men in the lowest fifth of ponderal index at birth. Among the Pima Indians diabetes in pregnancy is unusually common and the association between birthweight and type 2 diabetes is U-shaped, with an increased prevalence in young people with birthweights over 9.9 pounds (4.5 kg) (McCance *et al.* 1994). The increased risk of diabetes among those of high birthweight was associated with maternal diabetes in pregnancy.

Both deficiency in insulin production and insulin resistance are thought to be important in the pathogenesis of type 2 diabetes. There is evidence that both may be determined in fetal life. As discussed further in Chapter 16, infants who are small for dates have fewer pancreatic β cells and there is evidence that nutritional and other factors determining fetal and infant growth influence the size and function of the adult β cell complement (Hales and Barker 1992). Whether and when type 2 diabetes supervenes will be determined by the rate of attrition of β cells with ageing, and by the development of insulin resistance, of which obesity is an important determinant.

While some studies of adults have found no association between birthweight and insulin responses to infused glucose (Alvarsson *et al.* 1994), it is possible that insulin resistance in adult life changes insulin secretion and obscures associations with fetal growth. Studies of younger people may resolve this. A study of men aged 21 years showed that those with lower birthweight had reduced plasma insulin concentrations 30 minutes after a glucose challenge (Robinson *et al.*, 1992). Another study of men of similar age showed that a low insulin response to glucose was associated with high placental weight and a high ratio of placental weight to birthweight (Wills *et al.* 1996). In contrast, a study of young Pima Indians showed that those with low birthweight had evidence of insulin resistance but no defect in insulin secretion (Leger *et al.* 1997a).

In Mysore, south India, men and women with type 2 diabetes showed signs of both insulin resistance and deficiency (Fall *et al.* 1998). As in people from south India living in Britain, there was a high prevalence of insulin resistance and central adiposity in this population. Those in Mysore who had type 2 diabetes, however, also had a low insulin increment after a glucose challenge, indicating insulin deficiency as well as resistance. Whereas, however, insulin resistance was associated with low birthweight, type 2 diabetes was associated with shortness at birth in relation to birthweight, that is a high ponderal index, and with maternal adiposity (Fall *et al.* 1998). As set out in Chapter 35, these findings led to a novel hypothesis to account for the epidemic of type 2 diabetes in urban and migrant Indian populations (Fall *et al.*, 1998).

Insulin resistance and the metabolic syndrome

Men and women with low birthweight have a high prevalence of the 'insulin resistance syndrome' or 'metabolic syndrome' (Barker *et al.* 1993c), in which impaired glucose tolerance, hypertension and raised serum triglyceride concentrations occur in the same patient. Phillips *et al.* (1994b) carried out insulin tolerance tests on 103 men and women in Preston, UK. At each body mass, insulin resistance was greater in people who had a low ponderal index at birth. Conversely, at each ponderal index, resistance was greater in those with high body mass. The greatest insulin resistance was therefore in those with low ponderal index at birth but high current body mass.

A study in San Antonio, Texas, confirmed the association between low birthweight and the insulin resistance syndrome in 30-year-old Mexican-Americans and non-Hispanic white people (Valdez *et al.* 1994). Among men and women in the lowest third of the birthweight distribution and the highest third of current body mass 25% had the syndrome. By contrast, none of those in the highest third of birthweight and lowest third of current body mass had it. A study of young adults in France showed that those who had had intrauterine growth retardation had raised plasma insulin concentrations when fasting and after a glucose challenge (Leger *et al.* 1997b). They did not show any of the other abnormalities that occur in the insulin resistance syndrome. This suggests that insulin resistance may be a primary abnormality to which other changes are secondary. Follow-up of men and women who were in utero during the Dutch famine provides evidence that maternal undernutrition can programme insulin resistance and type 2 diabetes (Ravelli *et al.* 1998). Those exposed to famine in utero had higher two-hour plasma glucose and insulin concentrations than those born before or conceived after the famine.

Law *et al.* (1995) reported associations between thinness at birth and raised 30-minute plasma glucose concentrations in 7-year-old children in Salisbury, UK. In a group of older children, Whincup (1997) found that those who had lower birthweight had raised plasma insulin concentrations, both fasting and after oral glucose, suggesting insulin resistance. Among these children, however, those who had low birthweight had normal plasma glucose concentrations, which implies that despite being insulin resistant they were currently able to maintain glucose homeostasis. More recently, follow-up of children who were born prematurely has shown that they have an isolated reduction in insulin sensitivity as compared with controls (Hofman *et al.* 2004). These and other findings in children support an intrauterine origin for type 2 diabetes and suggest that the seeds of diabetes in the next generation have already been sown and are apparent in today's children (Chapter 14).

The processes that link thinness at birth with insulin resistance in adult life are not known, but experimental studies are now providing important clues (Chapter 17). Babies born at term with a low ponderal index have a reduced mid-arm circumference and low muscle bulk. It is possible that thinness at birth is associated with abnormalities in muscle structure and function that originate in mid gestation and have long term consequences that interfere with insulin's ability to promote glucose uptake in skeletal muscle. Magnetic resonance spectroscopy studies show that people who were thin at birth have lower rates of glycolysis and glycolytic ATP production during exercise (Taylor *et al.* 1995). More recently, magnetic resonance studies have investigated skeletal muscle metabolism in the healthy offspring of patients with type 2 diabetes; insulin resistance in the offspring was associated with dysregulation of intramyocellular fatty acid metabolism (Petersen *et al.* 2004). An inherited defect in mitochondrial oxidative phosphorylation is one explanation, but an intrauterine effect transmitted across generations is an alternative possibility. In response to undernutrition a fetus may reduce its metabolic dependence on glucose and increase oxidation of other substrates, including amino acids and lactate. This raises the possibility that a glucose-sparing metabolism persists into adult life, and that insulin resistance arises as a consequence of similar processes, possibly because of reduced rates of glucose oxidation in insulin-sensitive peripheral tissues.

When the availability of nutrients to the fetus is restricted, concentrations of anabolic hormones, including insulin and insulin-like growth factor 1, fall, while catabolic hormones, including glucocorticoids, rise. As discussed in Chapter 19, persisting hormonal changes could contribute to the development of the metabolic syndrome. Bjorntorp (1995) has postulated that glucocorticoids, growth hormone and sex steroids may play major roles in the evolution of the metabolic syndrome.

Table 2.1 Body mass index at 1 and 12 years and cumulative incidence of type 2 diabetes according to age at adiposity rebound. Data from Eriksson *et al.* (2003).

Age at adiposity rebound (yrs)	BMI at 1 year (kg m^{-2})	BMI at 12 years	Cumulative incidence of diabetes %
≤4	16.9	20.1	8.6
5	16.9	17.9	4.4
6	17.7	17.2	3.2
7	18.2	17.1	2.2
≥8	18.4	16.9	1.8
p for trend	< 0.001	< 0.001	< 0.001

Obesity and the adiposity rebound

The studies described earlier found that people who were small at birth and had low infant weight gain are at particular risk of adult coronary heart disease if they become overweight in childhood. After age 2 years the body mass index of normal young children falls to a minimum around 6 years before rising again, the so-called adiposity rebound (Rolland-Cachera *et al.* 1987). Early age at adiposity rebound has been related to obesity in childhood and adult life (Whitaker *et al.* 1997).

Data from Helsinki showed for the first time that early age at adiposity rebound is a strong predictor of type 2 diabetes (Eriksson *et al.* 2003); this observation has since been replicated in Delhi, India (Bhargava *et al.* 2004). Table 2.1 shows this trend is remarkably strong, even without taking adult obesity into account. Overall, the Helsinki observations showed that slow growth in utero, low weight gain in infancy and early age at adiposity rebound in later childhood are associated with large increases in the incidence of type 2 diabetes. The adiposity rebound may primarily reflect crossing of BMI centiles, but most cohort studies have lacked the detailed longitudinal pre- and postnatal anthropometric data to fully characterise the adiposity rebound and its causes; surprisingly, thinness at age 1 year was a strong predictor in the Helsinki data (Table 2.1). The importance of collecting detailed body-composition measurements in well-characterised children is emphasised by data

from the US National Collaborative Perinatal Project showing that greater weight gain from birth to age 4 months is also a major risk factor for later obesity (Stettler *et al.* 2003).

Musculoskeletal health

Osteoporosis is a common skeletal disorder in developed communities characterised by low bone mass and microarchitectural deterioration of bone tissue predisposing to fracture. The disorder has major health implications; among European people aged 50 years or older the lifetime risk of fracture at the hip, spine and wrist is 39% in women and 13% in men. Much recent evidence has shown that the risk of osteoporotic fracture is modified by environmental influences during intrauterine and early postnatal life (Harvey and Cooper 2004). Studies in the US, UK, Sweden and Australia have shown that low birthweight and weight at one year are associated with low bone mass in adult life, as assessed by dual energy X-ray absorptiometry (Cooper *et al.* 1997, Yarbrough *et al.* 2000, Javaid and Cooper 2002). The relationships are independent of known environmental risk factors for osteoporosis including smoking, alcohol consumption, lack of exercise and low calcium intakes. Longitudinal studies in Finland have shown that low birthweight and slow postnatal skeletal growth are associated with higher rates of hip fracture (Cooper *et al.* 2001).

Preliminary data suggest important interactions between birthweight and genes that predict adult bone mass, including the vitamin D receptor gene (Dennison *et al.* 2001). Follow-up of children to age 9 years has demonstrated that a low ionised calcium concentration in cord blood is associated with reduced childhood bone mass, and that both measurements correlate with reduced circulating maternal 25(OH) vitamin D levels (Javaid *et al.* 2003). Maternal vitamin D insufficiency may therefore lead to retarded intrauterine and postnatal skeletal development, with a consequent reduction in peak bone mass and elevated risk of fracture in late adulthood. Other maternal characteristics are now known to influence the bone mineral content of babies. Maternal smoking, low maternal fat stores and high maternal physical activity in late gestation are independently associated with reduced neonatal bone mineral content (Godfrey *et al.* 2001).

Developmental influences on skeletal muscle mass and function may contribute to the increased fracture risk in individuals whose early growth was restricted (Syddall *et al.* 2003, Sayer *et al.* 2004). Muscle strength also has a major impact on the age-related decline in physical performance, quality of life and mortality. Lower birthweight has been linked with lower adult muscle mass (Phillips 1995, Gale *et al.* 2001), altered muscle metabolism (Phillips *et al.* 1994c) and reduced muscle strength (Sayer *et al.* 1998). Follow-up of men and women aged 53 years in the Medical Research Council National Survey of Health and Development found that lower birthweight was associated with reduced adult grip strength, even after adjustment for height and weight in both childhood and adult life (Kuh *et al.* 2002). The mechanisms through which the early-life environment may influence musculoskeletal health in adult life are discussed further in Chapter 29.

Respiratory health and atopy

Chronic obstructive airways disease was one of the original disorders for which ecological studies suggested an important developmental influence (Barker 1998), but subsequent epidemiological studies have tended to neglect investigation of developmental influences on respiratory health and atopy. Several studies have suggested that maternal smoking before and after birth may be associated with impaired lung function of the offspring, but not all studies have found such as effect (Hanrahan *et al.* 1992, Murray *et al.* 2002, Stocks and Dezateux 2003). Independently of maternal smoking, children and adults who were small at birth tend to have reduced lung function (Barker *et al.* 1991, Rona *et al.* 1993, Stein *et al.* 1997, Nikolajev *et al.* 1998) and an increased risk of respiratory morbidity and

mortality (Barker *et al.* 1991, Svanes *et al.* 1998). The normal physiological growth and development patterns of the airways and parenchyma remain poorly understood, but epidemiological studies measuring premorbid lung function in infancy indicate the importance of genetic and environmental factors during fetal and early postnatal life (Clarke *et al.* 1995, Stick *et al.* 1996, Dezateux *et al.* 1999). In 131 normal infants aged 5–14 weeks, we recently found that smaller birth size and higher early-infancy weight gain were associated with lower forced expiratory volume at 0.4 s and lower forced expiratory flow at functional residual capacity (Lucas *et al.* 2004): these suggest impaired lung development and may predispose to obstructive airways disease, including asthma.

Although the mechanisms linking early lung development with lung function in later life are unknown, impaired airway and alveolar growth may be important. Airway branching is complete by 16 weeks gestation, and alveolar formation begins before birth. Between birth and 18 months of age there is a rapid increase in alveolar number and size, whilst airway diameter continues to grow. Environmental influences during both prenatal and early postnatal life therefore have the potential to affect lung development. These are discussed further in Chapter 25.

Fetal and postnatal growth have been associated with later atopy and asthma, and Chapter 26 describes evidence that early-life exposure to infections and pollutants may have long-term effects on immune function and atopy. Links between a large neonatal head circumference and a raised total serum IgE in childhood (Gregory *et al.* 1999, Leadbitter *et al.* 1999) and adulthood (Godfrey *et al.* 1994a) led to the hypothesis that factors influencing fetal growth may programme the developing immune system (Beasley *et al.* 1999). Birth length and weight have been associated with later asthma (Leadbitter *et al.* 1999), but this was not replicated in another study (Svanes *et al.* 1998). The conflicting results may reflect the age at which the relationship is examined, and whether persistent wheezing associated with atopy is considered separately from transient wheezing in children with small airways who are predisposed to wheeze with viral infections (Martinez *et al.* 1995).

Cognitive function and mental health

Brain growth and cognitive function in childhood and old age

There is evidence that elderly adults with larger head sizes not only tend to gain higher scores on tests of IQ and memory function, but are also less likely to show a decline in these scores over time (Gale *et al.* 2003) and less likely to develop Alzheimer's disease in later life (Schofield *et al.* 1997). Because head size is known to correlate closely with brain volume, these findings suggest that brain development in the first few years of life is important in determining how well cognitive abilities are preserved in old age. Developmental influences on ageing are discussed further in Chapter 32. Studies in children have shown the importance of brain growth in the early years after birth for the attainment of high levels of cognition. At 9 years, IQ scores were highest in those who had experienced a large increase in head circumference between birth and 9 months of age and a further large increase in head circumference between 9 months and 9 years of age (Gale *et al.* 2004). These associations persisted after controlling for maternal factors, including the mother's IQ, education and social class.

Schizophrenia and mood disorders

It has long been hypothesised that perinatal influences play an important role in the genesis of major brain disorders (Pasamanick *et al.* 1956). Advances in neuropathology and imaging have led to the conclusion that schizophrenia may indeed have a developmental basis (Pilowsky *et al.* 1993), perhaps originating through abnormal neuronal migration (Akbarian *et al.* 1996). This conclusion is supported by evidence that intrauterine exposures and obstetric complications are associated in later life with the brain dysfunction that characterises the disorder (Brixey *et al.* 1993, Cannon *et al.* 2002). Maternal influenza infection in mid trimester has been linked with an increased risk of schizophrenia in the offspring (Mednick *et al.* 1988), although other studies of maternal influenza have provided inconsistent findings (Weinberger 1995). Evidence for a role of maternal nutrition has come from follow-up studies of the offspring of women who were pregnant during the Dutch famine: famine exposure during the first trimester was found to double the risk of schizophrenia in adult life (Susser *et al.* 1996, Hoek *et al.* 1998).

Epidemiological studies of the Dutch famine suggest that intrauterine influences may also increase the risk of affective disorders and low mood in the offspring (Brown *et al.* 1995). Although adverse life events are often the proximal cause of depressive illness, these act selectively on vulnerable individuals, and it has been proposed that both genetic and intrauterine influences may determine this vulnerability (Thompson *et al.* 2001). Evidence for an effect of the intrauterine environment in determining the later risk of mental illness has come from observations in the 1958 British birth cohort study, in which Sacker *et al.* (1995) found lower birthweight in patients admitted with affective psychosis. Subsequent studies in Sweden (Mittendorfer-Rutz *et al.* 2004) and Hertfordshire, UK (Thompson *et al.* 2001) have found that low birthweight increases the risk of suicide and depression in adolescence and adult life. In the Swedish study of 713 370 young adults, restricted fetal growth and teenage motherhood were associated with both suicide completion and attempt in the offspring, influences that acted independently of the mother's parity and education (Mittendorfer-Rutz *et al.* 2004). The biological bases for these and other early-life effects on brain function are discussed further in Chapters 27 and 28.

Maternal influences on development and offspring health

The demonstration that normal variations in fetal size and proportions at birth have implications for health throughout life has prompted a re-evaluation of maternal influences on fetal growth and development. Much experimental and epidemiological

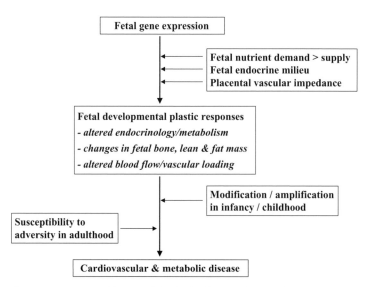

Figure 2.4 A conceptual framework for the developmental-origins hypothesis.

research now suggests that maternal diet, body composition and other influences can have important long-term effects on the health of the offspring, and that these long-term effects can operate without necessarily affecting usually measured pregnancy outcomes such as birthweight.

Research to date has linked specific maternal influences with the adult health of the offspring, notably: (1) the mother's own birthweight, (2) maternal body composition, including fat and lean mass, (3) maternal dietary intakes, including macro- and micronutrient balance, (4) maternal endocrine status. There is increasing evidence that fetal development can be affected by nutritional variation within the normal range of western diets, and many women eat unbalanced diets or constrain their weight by dieting (Godfrey 2000). Furthermore, studies of the Dutch famine indicate that the longer-term effects on offspring may depend on the duration and timing of famine exposure and can be independent of birth size (Roseboom *et al.* 2001a). Although nutrition has received the most focus (Langley and Jackson 1994, Vickers *et al.* 2000, Bertram and Hanson 2001), other early environmental factors such as infection, season of birth (Doblhammer and Vaupel 2001) and smoking (Power and Jefferis 2002) may also have long-term effects.

We have proposed that the mechanisms through which maternal influences lead to developmental plastic responses include (a) a mismatch between fetal nutrient demands, largely determined by the growth trajectory set in early pregnancy, and the maternoplacental capacity to meet this demand, (b) alterations in the fetal endocrine milieu, and (c) changes in placental vascular impedance, which impact on fetal cardiovascular loading. There is now evidence that the consequences of developmental plastic responses can be modified during infancy, and that their effects can be amplified by high childhood weight gain and perhaps by low levels of habitual physical activity, increasing vulnerability to adverse lifestyle influences during adulthood. This conceptual framework is illustrated in Fig. 2.4.

Periconceptional influences and the early trajectory of fetal growth

Size at birth is the product of the fetus's trajectory of growth, which is set at an early stage in development, and the maternoplacental capacity to supply sufficient nutrients to maintain that trajectory. In western communities, randomised controlled trials of maternal macronutrient supplementation have had relatively small effects on birthweight (Chapter 8 and Kramer 1993). This has led to the view that regulatory mechanisms in the maternal and placental systems act to ensure that human fetal growth and development is little influenced by normal variations in maternal nutrient intake, and that there is a simple relationship between a woman's body composition and the growth of her fetus. Subsequent experimental studies in animals and observational data in humans challenge these concepts. They suggest that a mother's dietary intakes and body composition around the time of conception and during pregnancy can exert major effects on the balance between the fetal demand for nutrients (Kwong et al. 2000) and the maternoplacental capacity to meet that demand (Duggleby and Jackson 2001).

A rapid trajectory of growth increases the fetus's demand for nutrients. Though fetal demand for nutrients is greatest late in pregnancy, the magnitude of this demand is thought to be primarily determined by genetic and environmental effects on the trajectory of fetal growth, which is set at an early stage in development. Experimental studies of pregnant ewes have shown that, although a fast growth trajectory is generally associated with larger fetal size and improved neonatal survival, it renders the fetus more vulnerable to a reduced maternoplacental supply of nutrients in late gestation. Thus, maternal undernutrition during the last trimester adversely affects the development of rapidly growing fetuses with high requirements, while having little effect on those growing more slowly (Harding et al. 1992). Rapidly growing fetal lambs were found to make a series of adaptations in order to survive, including fetal wasting and placental oxidation of fetal amino acids to maintain lactate output to the fetus (Barker et al. 1993d).

Experiments in animals have shown that alterations in maternal diet around the time of conception can change the fetal growth trajectory. In a recent study, rats were fed a 9% casein low-protein diet in the periconceptional period. This led to reduced stem cell populations being formed during embryonic development for later fetal and placental

lineage pathways, and to small size at birth, compensatory postnatal growth and raised blood pressure in the offspring during adult life (Kwong et al. 2000 and Chapter 4). Early embryos from sheep and cattle are also sensitive to environmental conditions leading to loss of fetal growth control known as 'large offspring syndrome' and increased postnatal disease (Walker et al. 2000). The sensitivity of the human embryo to its environment is being increasingly recognised with the development of assisted reproductive technology and the reported low birthweight of singleton IVF babies compared with those from natural conception (Walker et al. 2000, Winston and Hardy 2002). The trajectory of fetal growth is thought to increase with improvements in periconceptional nutrition, and is faster in male fetuses. The consequent greater vulnerability of male fetuses to undernutrition may contribute to the higher death rates from coronary heart disease among men. Characterisation of maternal influences on the early growth trajectory of the human fetus is now an important priority.

Transgenerational effects

The supply of nutrients to the human fetus depends on the long and vulnerable series of steps known as the fetal supply line; this includes the mother's body composition and size, her metabolism, and transport of nutrients to and across the placenta. Part of the fetal supply line is established during the mother's own intrauterine life. Strong evidence for major intergenerational effects in humans has come from studies showing that a woman's birthweight influences the birthweight of her offspring (Emanuel et al. 1992). A study in the UK showed that whereas low-birthweight mothers tended to have thin infants with a low ponderal index, the father's birthweight was unrelated to ponderal index at birth (Godfrey et al. 1997). The effect of maternal birthweight on thinness at birth is consistent with the hypothesis that in low-birthweight mothers the fetal supply line is compromised and unable to meet fetal nutrient demand. These and other observations have led to the conclusion that mothers constrain fetal growth and that the degree of constraint they exert is set when they are in utero. Potential mechanisms underlying this effect include alterations in the uterine or systemic vasculature, changes in maternal metabolism and impaired placentation.

A study in Preston, UK, showed that young men and women whose mothers had low birthweight have raised blood pressure even after allowing for their mothers' blood pressure; father's birthweight was not related to the offspring's blood pressure (Barker *et al.* 2000). This led to the conclusion that if the growth of a female fetus is constrained by lack of nutrients there are persisting changes in its physiology and metabolism which lead to reduced fetal nutrition and raised adult blood pressure in the next generation. Little is known about the effects of intergenerational transmission of retarded fetal growth on coronary heart disease, or other degenerative disorders, in the next generation, although it is known that women who had low-birthweight babies have increased rates of cardiovascular disease (Smith *et al.* 2000).

Experimental studies in animals have shown that undernutrition can have effects on reproductive performance, which may persist for several generations (Drake and Walker 2004). Among rats fed a protein-deficient diet over 12 generations there was a progressive fall in fetal growth rates. When restored to a normal diet it took three generations before growth and development were normalised (Stewart *et al.* 1980). The existence of strong intergenerational effects on fetal growth is important for public health today. Improvements in women's diets are likely to benefit more than one generation.

Maternal influences on placental size and transfer capabilities

Little is known about maternal influences on placental function, but there is more evidence in relation to placental growth and structure. This suggests effects of maternal metabolic and endocrine status, of maternal hypoxaemia and anaemia, and of maternal diet and nutritional status, particularly in the periconceptional period (Godfrey 2002).

Although the size of the placenta gives only an indirect measure of its capacity to transfer nutrients to the fetus, it is nonetheless strongly associated with fetal size at birth. Experiments in sheep have shown that maternal undernutrition in early pregnancy can exert major effects on the growth of the placenta, and thereby alter fetal development (Robinson *et al.* 1994). As previously referred to, the effects produced depend on the nutritional status of the ewe in the periconceptional period. In ewes poorly nourished around the time of conception, high nutrient intakes in early pregnancy increased the size of the placenta. Conversely, in ewes well nourished around conception, high intakes in early pregnancy resulted in smaller placental size (Robinson *et al.* 1994). Although this suppression of placental growth appears paradoxical, in sheep farming it is common practice for ewes to be put on rich pasture prior to mating and then on poor pasture for a period in early pregnancy. Support for important nutritional effects on placental growth and structure comes from studies in guinea pigs, in which food restriction before and during pregnancy reduced the exchange surface area and increased the arithmetic mean barrier thickness to diffusion (Roberts *et al.* 2001). In this model, maternal food restriction not only reduced placental weight, but also induced structural alterations that would result in functional impairment beyond that expected for the reduction in weight.

There is evidence that high dietary intakes in early pregnancy can suppress placental growth in humans (Godfrey *et al.* 1996). Among women who delivered at term in Southampton, UK, those with high dietary intakes in early pregnancy, especially intakes of carbohydrate, had smaller placentas, particularly if this was combined with low intakes of dairy protein in late pregnancy. These effects were independent of the mother's body size, social class and smoking, and resulted in alterations in the ratio of placental weight to birthweight and in a low ponderal index at birth (Godfrey *et al.* 1997). Further evidence that maternal diet can alter placental growth has come from the Dutch famine, in which famine exposure in early pregnancy increased placental weight (Lumey 1998).

The U-shaped relation between the placental ratio and later coronary heart disease found in men born earlier last century in Sheffield (Martyn *et al.* 1996a) suggests that effects on placental growth could be of long-term importance. Babies with a disproportionately small placenta may suffer as a consequence of an impaired placental supply capacity; those with a disproportionately large placenta may experience fetal catabolism and wasting to supply amino acids for placental consumption (Barker *et al.* 1993d). Consequent fetal adaptations may underlie the increased adult coronary heart death rates in those with both low and high placental ratios.

Maternal diet and body composition

Direct evidence supporting a long-term effect of levels of maternal nutrient intake during pregnancy has come from a follow-up study of children whose mothers took part in a randomised controlled trial of calcium supplementation in pregnancy in Argentina (Belizan *et al.* 1997). Supplementation was associated with lowering of the offspring's blood pressure in childhood. Follow-up studies of people exposed to the Dutch famine of 1944–5 showed that severe maternal caloric restriction at different stages of pregnancy was variously associated with obesity, dyslipidaemia and insulin resistance in the offspring, and there is preliminary evidence of an increased risk of coronary heart disease among people conceived during the famine (Ravelli *et al.* 1998, Roseboom *et al.* 2000a, 2000b).

In the Dutch studies, famine exposure per se was not associated with raised blood pressure in the offspring, but there was evidence for an effect of macronutrient balance. Maternal rations with a low protein density were associated with raised blood pressure in the adult offspring (Roseboom *et al.* 2001b). Similarly, among adolescent boys, systolic blood pressure was inversely related to the mothers' percentage of dietary energy from protein (Adair *et al.* 2001). This adds to the findings of studies in

Aberdeen, UK, which showed that maternal diets with either a low or a high ratio of animal protein to carbohydrate were associated with raised blood pressure in the offspring during adult life (Campbell *et al.* 1996). In the Aberdeen study maternal diets with a high protein density were associated not only with raised blood pressure in the offspring but also with insulin deficiency and impaired glucose tolerance (Shiell *et al.* 2000). While it may seem counterintuitive that a high-protein diet should have adverse effects, these findings are consistent with the results of controlled trials of protein supplementation in pregnancy, which show that high protein intakes are associated with reduced birthweight (Rush 1989).

The Aberdeen findings have recently been replicated in a follow-up study of men and women in Motherwell, UK, whose mothers were advised to eat a high-meat-protein, low-carbohydrate diet during pregnancy (Shiell *et al.* 2001). Those whose mothers had high intakes of meat and fish in late pregnancy, but low intakes of carbohydrate, had raised blood pressure – particularly if the mother also had a low intake of green vegetables. One possibility is that the effect on blood pressure may be a consequence of the metabolic stress imposed on the mother by an unbalanced diet in which high intakes of essential amino acids are not accompanied by the micronutrients required to utilise them. Evidence in support of this comes from analysis of the offspring's fasting plasma cortisol concentrations (Herrick *et al.* 2004). Men and women whose mothers had high intakes of meat and fish and low intakes of green vegetables had raised cortisol concentrations.

Fetal growth and development depends on maternal nutrient stores and the turnover of protein and fat in the mother's tissues at least as much as on the mother's diet: for the fetus to depend primarily on the mother's diet in pregnancy would be too dangerous a strategy (James 1997). Maternal size and body composition account for up to 20% of the variability in birthweight (Catalano *et al.*, 1998). Studies in Europe and India have shown that high maternal weight and adiposity are associated with insulin deficiency, type 2 diabetes and coronary heart disease in the offspring (Forsen *et al.* 1997, Fall *et al.* 1998, Shiell *et al.* 2001). In the data from Helsinki, increasing maternal body mass index had little effect on the offspring's death rates in tall women, but strong effects in short women (Forsen *et al.* 1997). One interpretation of these findings is that greater maternal body fatness may increase fetal growth and hence the fetal demand for nutrients; short women may not be able to meet this increased demand as a result of a constrained nutrient supply capacity determined during their own intrauterine development. These observations for high maternal weight and adiposity add to those linking gestational diabetes with adverse long-term outcomes in the offspring (Silverman *et al.* 1996).

Of considerable importance is an increasing body of consistent evidence showing strong links between low maternal weight and body mass index and insulin resistance in the adult offspring (Ravelli *et al.* 1998, Shiell *et al.* 2000, Mi *et al.* 2000). Although low maternal body mass index does not appear to be linked with raised blood pressure in the offspring, thin maternal skinfold thicknesses and low pregnancy weight gain have been consistently associated with raised offspring blood pressure (Margetts *et al.* 1991, Godfrey *et al.* 1994b, Clark *et al.* 1998, Adair *et al.* 2001). One of the metabolic links between maternal body composition and birth size is protein synthesis. Women with a greater lean body mass have higher rates of protein synthesis in pregnancy (Duggleby and Jackson 2001). Variation in rates of maternal protein synthesis explains around a quarter of the variability in birth length.

Prevention of adult degenerative disease

The experimental and epidemiological evidence indicates that prevention of a substantial proportion of degenerative disease, including cardiovascular disease, type 2 diabetes, cognitive decline and osteoporosis, together with obesity, may depend on interventions at a number of stages of development. Strategies that target infants and young children may give the most immediate benefit, but improving the intrauterine environment is an important long-term goal. In **mothers** we need to improve the macronutrient balance and micronutrient content of the diet before and during pregnancy. Animal studies now show how effective such measures can be in improving the development of the offspring (Brawley *et al.* 2004). We also need to improve women's body composition before pregnancy, with avoidance of excessive thinness or overweight. In **infants** we need to protect growth in weight, length and head circumference during the first year after birth by good infant feeding practices, avoidance of recurrent infections, and cognitive stimulation. We need to prevent rapid weight gain among **children** especially those who were small or thin at birth or at one year. **Adults** who were small at birth are more vulnerable to obesity and psychosocial stress in adult life: we need to understand this more deeply in order to prevent it.

The complexities of fetal growth and development are such that currently available data form only a limited basis for changing dietary recommendations to young women. Future work will need to identify the factors that set the trajectory of fetal growth, and the influences that limit the maternoplacental delivery of nutrients and oxygen to the fetus. We also need to define how the fetus adapts to a limited nutrient supply, how these adaptations change the structure and physiology of the body, and by what molecular mechanisms nutrients and hormones alter gene expression. A strategy of interdependent clinical, animal and epidemiological research is required to identify specific recommendations both for whole populations and for vulnerable groups such as teenage pregnancies and single parents. Research is also required to identify the barriers to healthy eating among young women, whose diets are important both for their own health and for the health of the next generation. Such an approach may allow us to reduce the prevalence of major chronic diseases and diminish social inequalities in health.

If, as we believe, a woman's own fetal growth, and her diet and body composition before and during pregnancy, play a major role in programming the future health of her children, mothers will want to know what they can do to optimise the intrauterine environment they provide for their babies. A recent technical consultation organised by the United States Department of Agriculture, the World Bank and UNICEF concluded that a key area of focus to reduce the burden of low birthweight and its associated morbidities is to improve the nutritional status of adolescent girls and of pregnant women. Similarly, one of the two main recommendations of an Independent Inquiry into Inequalities in Health (1998) in the United Kingdom was that 'a high priority is given to policies aimed at improving health and reducing inequalities in women of childbearing age, expectant mothers and young children.'

Conclusion

Degenerative diseases, including cardiovascular disease, type 2 diabetes, osteoporosis and obstructive airways disease, have higher rates among poorer people and cause much disability in both developed and developing communities. The evidence that links the combination of poor maternal nutrition, impaired fetal/infant development and increased weight gain in early childhood to later cardiovascular disease is now strong. Many women have diets with a suboptimal balance of nutrients, and wide variations between women in the amounts of lean and fat tissue alter the partitioning of food between mothers and babies. However, little is known about how maternal nutrition influences early growth and development, or about interactions with genetic influences and with nutrition and physical activity after birth. In order to improve the health of future generations we need to identify the factors that now affect fetal, infant and childhood growth and development.

REFERENCES

Adair, L. S., Kuzawa, C. W. and Borja, J. (2001). Maternal energy stores and diet composition during pregnancy program adolescent blood pressure. *Circulation*, **104**, 1034–9.

Akbarian, S., Kim, J. J., Potkin, S. G., Hetrick, W. P., Bunney, W. E. Jr. and Jones, E. G. (1996). Maldistribution of interstitial neurons in prefrontal white matter of the brains of schizophrenic patients. *Arch. Gen. Psychiatry*, **53**, 425–36.

Alvarsson, M., Efendic, S. and Grill, V. E. (1994). Insulin responses to glucose in healthy males are associated with adult height but not with birth weight. *J. Intern. Med.*, **236**, 275–9.

Barker, D. J. P. (1998). *Mothers, Babies and Health in Later Life*, 2nd edn. Edinburgh: Churchill Livingstone.

Barker, D. J. P., Bull, A. R., Osmond, C. and Simmonds, S. J. (1990). Fetal and placental size and risk of hypertension in adult life. *BMJ*, **301**, 259–62.

Barker, D. J. P., Godfrey, K. M., Fall, C., Osmond, C., Winter, P. D. and Shaheen, S. O. (1991). Relation of birth weight and childhood respiratory infection to adult lung function and death from chronic obstructive airways disease. *BMJ*, **303**, 671–5.

Barker, D. J. P., Godfrey, K. M., Osmond, C. and Bull, A. (1992). The relation of fetal length, ponderal index and head circumference to blood pressure and the risk of hypertension in adult life. *Paediatr. Perinat. Epidemiol.*, **6**, 35–44.

Barker, D. J. P., Osmond, C., Simmonds, S. J. and Wield, G. A. (1993a). The relation of small head circumference and thinness at birth to death from cardiovascular disease in adult life. *BMJ*, **306**, 422–6.

Barker, D. J. P., Martyn, C. N., Osmond, C., Hales, C. N. and Fall, C. H. (1993b). Growth in utero and serum cholesterol concentrations in adult life. *BMJ*, **307**, 1524–7.

Barker, D. J. P., Hales, C. N., Fall, C. H. D., Osmond, C., Phipps, K. and Clark, P. M. S. (1993c). Type 2 (non-insulin-dependent) diabetes mellitus, hypertension and hyperlipidaemia (syndrome X): relation to reduced fetal growth. *Diabetologia*, **36**, 62–7.

Barker, D. J. P., Gluckman, P. D., Godfrey, K. M., Harding, J. E., Owens, J. A. and Robinson, J. S. (1993d). Fetal nutrition and cardiovascular disease in adult life. *Lancet*, **341**, 938–41.

Barker, D. J. P., Martyn, C. N., Osmond, C. and Wield, G. A. (1995). Abnormal liver growth in utero and death from coronary heart disease. *BMJ*, **310**, 703–4.

Barker, D. J. P., Shiell, A. W., Barker, M. E. and Law, C. M. (2000). Growth in utero and blood pressure levels in the next generation. *J. Hypertens.*, **18**, 843–6.

Barker, D. J. P., Forsen, T., Uutela, A., Osmond, C. and Eriksson. J. G. (2001). Size at birth and resilience to the effects of poor living conditions in adult life: longitudinal study. *BMJ*, **323**, 1273–6.

Barker, D. J. P., Eriksson, J. G., Forsen, T. and Osmond, C. (2002). Fetal origins of adult disease: strength of effects and biological basis. *Int. J. Epidemiol.*, **31**, 1235.

Beasley, R., Leadbitter, P., Pearce, N. and Crane, J. (1999). Is enhanced fetal growth a risk factor for the development of atopy or asthma? *Int. Arch. Allergy Immunol.*, **118**, 408–10.

Belizan, J. M., Villar, J., Bergel, E. *et al.* (1997). Long term effect of calcium supplementation during pregnancy on the blood pressure of offspring: follow up of a randomised controlled trial. *BMJ*, **315**, 281–5.

Bertram, C. E. and Hanson, M. A. (2001). Animal models and programming of the metabolic syndrome. *Br. Med. Bull.*, **60**, 103–21.

Bhargava, S. K., Sachdev, H. S., Fall, C. H. D. *et al.* (2004). Relation of serial changes in childhood body-mass index to impaired glucose tolerance in young adulthood. *N. Engl. J. Med.*, **350**, 865–75.

Bjorntorp, P. (1995). Insulin resistance: the consequence of a neuroendocrine disturbance? *Int. J. Obes.*, **19** (suppl 1), S6–10.

Brawley, L., Torrens, C., Anthony, F. W. *et al.* (2004). Glycine rectifies vascular dysfunction induced by dietary protein imbalance during pregnancy. *J. Physiol.*, **554**, 497–504.

Brixey, S. N., Gallagher, B. J., McFalls, J. A. Jr. and Parmelee, L. F. (1993). Gestational and neonatal factors in the etiology of schizophrenia. *J. Clin. Psychol.*, **49**, 447–56.

Brooks, A. A., Johnson, M. R., Steer, P. J., Pawson, M. E. and Abdalla, H. I. (1995). Birth weight: nature or nurture? *Early Hum. Dev.*, **42**, 29–35.

Brown, A. S., Susser, E. S., Lin, S. P., Neugebauer, R. and Gorman, J. M. (1995). Increased risk of affective disorders in males after second trimester prenatal exposure to the Dutch hunger winter of 1944–45. *Br. J. Psychiatry*, **166**, 601–6.

Campbell, D. M., Hall, M. H., Barker, D. J. P., Cross, J., Shiell, A. W. and Godfrey, K. M. (1996). Diet in pregnancy and the offspring's blood pressure 40 years later. *Br. J. Obstet. Gynaecol.*, **103**, 273–80.

Cannon, M., Jones, P. B. and Murray, R. M. (2002). Obstetric complications and schizophrenia: historical and meta-analytic review. *Am. J. Psychiatry*, **159**, 1080–92.

Catalano, P. M., Thomas, A. J., Huston, L. P. and Fung, C. M. (1998). Effect of maternal metabolism on fetal growth and body composition. *Diabetes Care*, **21**, B85–90.

Chapman, N., Mohamudally, A., Cerutti, A. *et al.* (1997). Retinal vascular network architecture in low-birth-weight men. *J. Hypertens.*, **15**, 1449–53.

Clark, P. M., Atton, C., Law, C. M., Shiell, A., Godfrey, K. and Barker, D. J. P. (1998). Weight gain in pregnancy, triceps skinfold thickness and blood pressure in the offspring. *Obstet. Gynaecol.*, **91**, 103–7.

Clarke, J. R., Salmon, B. and Silverman, M. (1995). Bronchial responsiveness in the neonatal period as a risk factor for wheezing in infancy. *Am. J. Respir. Crit. Care Med.*, **151**, 1434–40.

Cooper, C., Fall, C., Egger, P., Hobbs, R., Eastell, R. and Barker, D. (1997). Growth in infancy and bone mass in later life. *Ann. Rheum. Dis.*, **56**, 17–21.

Cooper, C., Eriksson, J. G., Forsen, T., Osmond, C., Tuomilehto, J. and Barker, D. J. P. (2001). Maternal height, childhood growth and risk of hip fracture in later life: a longitudinal study. *Osteoporos. Int.*, **12**, 623–9.

Curhan, G. C., Willett, W. C. and Rimm, E. B. *et al.* (1996). Birth weight and adult hypertension and diabetes mellitus in US men. *Am. J. Hypertens.*, **9**, 11A.

Dennison, E. M., Arden, N. K., Keen, R. W. *et al.* (2001). Birthweight, vitamin D receptor genotype and the programming of osteoporosis. *Paediatr. Perinat. Epidemiol.*, **15**, 211–19.

Dezateux, C., Stocks, J., Dundas, I. and Fletcher, M. E. (1999). Impaired airway function and wheezing in infancy: the influence of maternal smoking and a genetic predisposition to asthma. *Am. J. Respir. Crit. Care Med.*, **159**, 403–10.

Doblhammer, G. and Vaupel, J. W. (2001). Lifespan depends on month of birth. *Proc. Natl. Acad. Sci. USA*, **98**, 2934–9.

Drake, A. J. and Walker, B. R. (2004). The intergenerational effects of fetal programming: non-genomic mechanisms for the inheritance of low birth weight and cardiovascular risk. *J. Endocrinol.*, **180**, 1–16.

Duggleby, S. L. and Jackson, A. A. (2001). Relationship of maternal protein turnover and lean body mass during pregnancy and birth length. *Clin. Sci.*, **101**, 65–72.

Emanuel, I., Filakti, H., Alberman, E. and Evans, S. J. W. (1992). Intergenerational studies of human birthweight from the 1958 birth cohort. I. Evidence for a multigenerational effect. *Br. J. Obstet. Gynaecol.*, **99**, 67–74.

Eriksson, J. G., Forsen, T., Tuomilehto, J., Winter, P. D., Osmond, C. and Barker, D. J. P. (1999). Catch-up growth in childhood and death from coronary heart disease: longitudinal study. *BMJ*, **318**, 427–31.

Eriksson, J. G., Forsen, T., Tuomilehto, J., Osmond, C. and Barker, D. J. P. (2000a). Early growth, adult income, and risk of stroke. *Stroke*, **31**, 869–74.

(2000b). Fetal and childhood growth and hypertension in adult life. *Hypertension*, **36**, 790–4.

(2001). Early growth and coronary heart disease in later life: longitudinal study. *BMJ*, **322**, 949–53.

Eriksson, J. G., Lindi, V., Uusitupa, M. *et al.* (2002). The effects of the Pro12Ala polymorphism of the peroxisome proliferator-activated receptor-gamma2 gene on insulin sensitivity and insulin metabolism interact with size at birth. *Diabetes*, **51**, 2321–4.

Eriksson, J. G., Forsen, T., Tuomilehto, J., Osmond, C. and Barker, D. J. P. (2003). Early adiposity rebound in childhood and risk of type 2 diabetes in adult life. *Diabetologia*, **46**, 190–4.

Fall, C. H., Barker, D. J. P., Osmond, C., Winter, P. D., Clark, P. M. and Hales, C. N. (1992). Relation of infant feeding to adult serum cholesterol concentration and death from ischaemic heart disease. *BMJ*, **304**, 801–5.

Fall, C. H. D., Stein, C. E., Kumaran, K. *et al.* (1998). Size at birth, maternal weight, and type 2 diabetes in South India. *Diabet. Med.*, **15**, 220–7.

Forsen, T., Eriksson, J. G., Tuomilehto, J., Teramo, K., Osmond, C. and Barker, D. J. P. (1997). Mother's weight in pregnancy and coronary heart disease in a cohort of Finnish men: follow up study. *BMJ*, **315**, 837–40.

Forsen, T., Eriksson, J. G., Tuomilehto, J., Osmond, C. and Barker, D. J. P. (1999). Growth in utero and during childhood among women who develop coronary heart disease: longitudinal study. *BMJ*, **319**, 1403–7.

Frankel, S., Elwood, P., Sweetnam, P., Yarnell, J. and Davey Smith, G. (1996). Birthweight, body-mass index in middle age, and incident coronary heart disease. *Lancet*, **348**, 1478–80.

Gale, C. R., Martyn, C. N., Kellingray, S. *et al.* (2001). Intrauterine programming of adult body composition. *J. Clin. Endocrinol. Metab.*, **86**, 267–72.

Gale, C. R., Walton, S. and Martyn, C. N. (2003). Foetal and postnatal head growth and risk of cognitive decline in old age. *Brain*, **126**, 2273–8.

Gale, C. R., O'Callaghan, F. J., Godfrey, K. M., Law, C. M. and Martyn, C. N. (2004). Critical periods of brain growth and cognitive function in children. *Brain*, **127**, 321–9.

Gluckman, P. D. and Hanson, M. A. (2004). Living with the past: evolution, development, and patterns of disease. *Science*, **305**, 1733–6.

Godfrey, K. M. (2000). Maternal nutrition and fetal development: implications for fetal programming. In *Fetal Origins of Cardiovascular and Lung Disease* In (ed. D. J. P. Barker. New York: National Institutes of Health, pp. 249–71.

Godfrey, K. M. (2002). The role of the placenta in fetal programming: a review. *Placenta*, **23** (Suppl. A, Trophoblast Res), S20–27.

Godfrey, K. M., Barker, D. J. P. and Osmond, C. (1994a). Disproportionate fetal growth and raised IgE concentration in adult life. *Clin. Exp. Allergy*, **24**, 641–8.

Godfrey, K. M., Forrester, T., Barker, D. J. P. *et al.*, (1994b). Maternal nutritional status in pregnancy and blood pressure in childhood. *Br. J. Obstet. Gynaecol.*, **101**, 398–403.

Godfrey, K., Robinson, S., Barker, D. J. P., Osmond, C. and Cox, V. (1996). Maternal nutrition in early and late pregnancy in relation to placental and fetal growth. *BMJ*, **312**, 410–4.

Godfrey, K. M., Barker, D. J. P., Robinson, S. and Osmond, C. (1997). Maternal birthweight and diet in pregnancy in relation to the infant's thinness at birth. *Br. J. Obstet Gynaecol.*, **104**, 663–667.

Godfrey, K. M., Walker-Bone, K., Robinson, S. *et al.* (2001). Neonatal bone mass: influence of parental birthweight and maternal smoking, body composition and activity during pregnancy. *J. Bone Mineral Res.*, **16**, 1694–703.

Goodfellow, J., Bellamy, M. F. and Gorman, S. T. *et al.* (1998). Endothelial function is impaired in fit young adults of low birth weight. *Cardiovasc. Res.*, **40**, 600–6.

Gregory, A., Doull, I., Pearce, N. *et al.* (1999). The relationship between anthropometric measurements at birth: asthma and atopy in childhood. *Clin. Exp. Allergy*, **29**, 330–3.

Hales, C. N. and Barker, D. J. P. (1992). Type 2 (non-insulin-dependent) diabetes mellitus: the thrifty phenotype hypothesis. *Diabetologia*, **35**, 595–601.

Hales, C. N., Barker, D. J. P., Clark, P. M. S. *et al.* (1991). Fetal and infant growth and impaired glucose tolerance at age 64. *BMJ*, **303**, 1019–22.

Hanrahan, J. P., Tager, I. B., Segal, M. R. *et al.* (1992). The effect of maternal smoking during pregnancy on early infant lung function. *Am. Rev. Respir. Dis.*, **145**, 1129–35.

Harding, J. E., Liu, L., Evans, P., Oliver, M. and Gluckman, P. (1992). Intrauterine feeding of the growth-retarded fetus: can we help? *Early Hum. Dev.*, **29**, 193–7.

Harvey, N. and Cooper, C. (2004). The developmental origins of osteoporotic fracture. *J. Br. Menopause Soc.*, **10**, 14–29.

Hattersley, A. T. and Tooke, J. E. (1999). The fetal insulin hypothesis: an alternative explanation of the association of low birthweight with diabetes and vascular disease. *Lancet*, **353**, 1789–92.

Herrick, K., Phillips, D. I. W., Haselden, S., Shiell, A. W., Campbell-Brown, M. and Godfrey. K. M. (2004). Maternal consumption of a high-meat, low-carbohydrate diet in late pregnancy: relation to adult cortisol concentrations in the offspring. *J. Clin. Endocrin. Metab.*, **88**, 3554–60.

Hoek, H. W., Brown, A. S. and Susser, E. (1998). The Dutch famine and schizophrenia spectrum disorders. *Soc. Psychiatry Psychiatr. Epidemiol.*, **33**, 373–9.

Hofman, P. L., Cutfield, W. S., Robinson, E. M. *et al.* (1997). Insulin resistance in short children with intrauterine growth retardation. *J. Clin. Endocrinol. Metab.*, **82**, 402.

Hofman, P. L., Regan, F., Jackson, W. E. *et al.* (2004). Premature birth and later insulin resistance. *N. Engl. J. Med.*, **351**, 2179–86.

Huxley, R. R., Shiell, A. W. and Law, C. M. (2000). The role of size at birth and postnatal catch-up growth in determining systolic blood pressure: a systematic review of the literature. *J. Hypertens.*, **18**, 815–31.

Huxley, R., Neil, A. and Collins, R. (2002). Unravelling the fetal origins hypothesis: is there really an inverse association between birthweight and subsequent blood pressure? *Lancet*, **360**, 659–65.

Huxley, R., Owen, C. G., Whincup, P. H., Cook, D. G., Colman, S. and Collins, R. (2004). Birth weight and subsequent cholesterol levels: exploration of the 'fetal origins' hypothesis. *JAMA*, **292**, 2755–64.

Hypponen, E., Leon, D. A., Kenward, M. G. and Lithell, H. (2001). Prenatal growth and risk of occlusive and haemorrhagic stroke in Swedish men and women born 1915–29: historical cohort study. *BMJ*, **323**, 1033–4.

Independent Inquiry into Inequalities in Health (1998). *Report of the Independent Inquiry into Inequalities in Health.* London: The Stationery Office.

James, W. P. T. (1997). Long-term fetal programming of body composition and longevity. *Nutr. Rev.*, **55**, S41–3.

Javaid, M. K. and Cooper, C. (2002). Prenatal and childhood influences on osteoporosis. *Best Pract. Res. Clin. Endocrinol. Metab.*, **16**, 349–67.

Javaid, M. K., Shore, S. R., Taylor, P. *et al.* (2003). Maternal vitamin D status during late pregnancy and accrual of childhood bone mineral. *J. Bone Mineral Res.*, **18** suppl. 2, S13.

Keller, G., Zimmer, G., Mall, G., Ritz, E. and Amann, K. (2003). Nephron number in patients with primary hypertension. *N. Engl. J. Med.*, **348**, 101–8.

Khan, I. Y., Dekou, V., Douglas, G. *et al.* (2005). A high-fat diet during rat pregnancy or suckling induces cardiovascular dysfunction in adult offspring. *Am. J. Physiol. Regul. Integr. Comp. Physiol.*, **288**, R127–33.

Konje, J. C., Bell, S. C., Morton, J. J., de Chazal, R. and Taylor, D. J. (1996). Human fetal kidney morphometry during gestation and the relationship between weight, kidney morphometry and plasma active renin concentration at birth. *Clin. Sci.*, **91**, 169–75.

Kramer, M. S. (1993). Effects of energy and protein intakes on pregnancy outcome: an overview of the research evidence from controlled clinical trials. *Am. J. Clin. Nutr.*, **58**, 627–35.

Kuh, D., Bassey, J., Hardy, R., Sayer, A. A., Wadsworth, M. and Cooper, C. (2002). Birth weight, childhood size, and muscle strength in adult life: evidence from a birth cohort study. *Am. J. Epidemiol.*, **156**, 627–33.

Kwong, W. Y., Wild, A., Roberts, P., Willis, A. C. and Fleming, T. P. (2000). Maternal undernutrition during the pre-implantation period of rat development causes blastocyst abnormalities and programming of postnatal hypertension. *Development*, **127**, 4195–202.

Langley, S. C. and Jackson, A. A. (1994). Increased systolic blood pressure in adult rats induced by fetal exposure to maternal low protein diets. *Clin. Sci. (Lond.)*, **86**, 217–22.

Law, C. M., Barker, D. J. P., Bull, A. R. and Osmond, C. (1991). Maternal and fetal influences on blood pressure. *Arch. Dis. Child.*, **66**, 1291–5.

Law, C. M., Gordon, G. S., Shiell, A. W., Barker, D. J. P. and Hales, C. N. (1995). Thinness at birth and glucose tolerance in seven year old children. *Diabet. Med.*, **12**, 24–9.

Leadbitter, P., Pearce, N., Cheng, S. *et al.* (1999). Relationship between fetal growth and the development of asthma and atopy in childhood. *Thorax*, **54**, 905–10.

Leeson, C. P. M., Whincup, P. H., Cook, D. G. *et al.* (1997). Flow-mediated dilation in 9- to 11-year old children. The influence of intrauterine and childhood factors. *Circulation*, **96**, 2233–8.

Leger, J., Levy-Marchal, C., Bloch, J. *et al.*, (1997a). Evidence for insulin-resistance developing in young adults with intra-uterine growth retardation. *Diabetologia*, **40**, A53.

(1997b). Reduced final height and indications for insulin resistance in 20 year olds born small for gestational age: regional cohort study. *BMJ*, **315**, 341–7.

Leon, D. A., Lithell, H., Vagero, D. *et al.* (1997). Biological and social influences on mortality in a cohort of 15,000 Swedes followed from birth to old age. *J. Epidemiol. Community Health*, **51**, 594.

(1998). Reduced fetal growth rate and increased risk of death from ischaemic heart disease: cohort study of 15 000 Swedish men and women born 1915–29. *BMJ*, **317**, 241–5.

Lever, A. F. and Harrap, S. B. (1992). Essential hypertension: a disorder of growth with origins in childhood? *J. Hypertens.*, **10**, 101–20.

Lithell, H. O., McKeigue, P. M., Berglund, L., Mohsen, R., Lithell, U. B. and Leon, D. A. (1996). Relation of size at birth to non-insulin dependent diabetes and insulin concentrations in men aged 50–60 years. *BMJ*, **312**, 406–10.

Lucas, J. S., Inskip, H., Godfrey, K. M. *et al.* (2004). Small size at birth and greater postnatal weight gain: relations to diminished infant lung function. *Am. J. Resp. Critical Care Med.*, **170**, 534–40.

Lumey, L. H. (1998). Compensatory placental growth after restricted maternal nutrition in early pregnancy. *Placenta*, **19**, 105–11.

Mackenzie, H. S. and Brenner, B. M. (1995). Fewer nephrons at birth: a missing link in the etiology of essential hypertension? *Am. J. Kidney Dis.*, **26**, 91–8.

Margetts, B. M., Rowland, M. G. M., Foord, F. A., Cruddas, A. M., Cole, T. J. and Barker, D. J. P. (1991). The relation of maternal weight to the blood pressures of Gambian children. *Int. J. Epidemiol.*, **20**, 938–43.

Marmot, M. G., Shipley, M. J. and Rose, G. (1984). Inequalities in death: specific explanations of a general pattern? *Lancet*, **I**, 1003–6.

Martin, H., Hu, J., Gennser, G. and Norman, M. (2000). Impaired endothelial function and increased carotid stiffness in 9-year-old children with low birthweight. *Circulation*, **102**, 2739–44.

Martinez, F. D., Wright, A. L., Taussig, L. M., Holberg, C. J., Halonen, M. and Morgan, W. J. (1995). Asthma and wheezing in the first six years of life. The Group Health Medical Associates. *N. Engl. J. Med.*, **332**, 133–8.

Martyn, C. N. and Greenwald, S. E. (1997). Impaired synthesis of elastin in walls of aorta and large conduit arteries during early development as an initiating event in pathogenesis of systemic hypertension. *Lancet*, **350**, 953–5.

Martyn, C. N., Barker, D. J. P., Jespersen, S., Greenwald, S., Osmond, C. and Berry, C. (1995a). Growth in utero, adult blood pressure, and arterial compliance. *Br. Heart J.*, **73**, 116–21.

Martyn, C. N., Meade, T. W., Stirling, Y. and Barker, D. J. P. (1995b). Plasma concentrations of fibrinogen and factor VII in adult life and their relation to intra-uterine growth. *Br. J. Haematol.*, **89**, 142–6.

Martyn, C. N., Barker, D. J. P. and Osmond, C. (1996a). Mothers' pelvic size, fetal growth, and death from stroke and coronary heart disease in men in the UK. *Lancet*, **348**, 1264–8.

Martyn, C. N., Lever, A. F. and Morton, J. J. (1996b). Plasma concentrations of inactive renin in adult life are related to indicators of foetal growth. *J. Hypertens.*, **14**, 881–6.

Martyn, C. N., Gale, C. R., Jespersen, S. and Sherriff, S. B. (1998). Impaired fetal growth and atherosclerosis of carotid and peripheral arteries. *Lancet*, **352**, 173–8.

McCance, D. R., Pettitt, D. J., Hanson, R. L., Jacobsson, L. T. H., Knowler, W. C. and Bennett, P. H. (1994). Birth weight and non-insulin dependent diabetes: thrifty genotype, thrifty phenotype, or surviving small baby genotype? *BMJ*, **308**, 942–5.

Mednick, S. A., Machon, R. A., Huttunen, M. O. and Bonett, D. (1988). Adult schizophrenia following prenatal exposure to an influenza epidemic. *Arch. Gen. Psychiatry*, **45**, 189–92.

Mi, J., Law, C., Zhang, K.-L., Osmond, C., Stein, C. and Barker, D. J. P. (2000). Effects of infant birthweight and maternal body mass index in pregnancy on components of the insulin resistance syndrome in China. *Ann. Intern. Med.*, **132**, 253–60.

Mittendorfer-Rutz, E., Rasmussen, F. and Wasserman, D. (2004). Restricted fetal growth and adverse maternal psychosocial and socioeconomic conditions as risk factors for suicidal behaviour of offspring: a cohort study. *Lancet*, **364**, 1135–40.

Moore, V. M., Cockington, R. A., Ryan, P. and Robinson, J. S. (1999). The relationship between birth weight and blood pressure amplifies from childhood to adulthood. *J. Hypertens.*, **17**, 883–8.

Morton, N. E. (1955). The inheritance of human birth weight. *Ann. Hum. Genet.*, **20**, 123–34.

Murray, C. S., Pipis, S. D., McArdle, E. C., Lowe, L. A., Custovic, A. and Woodcock, A. (2002). Lung function at one month of age as a risk factor for infant respiratory symptoms in a high risk population. *Thorax*, **57**, 388–92.

Nikolajev, K., Heinonen, K., Hakulinen, A. and Lansimies, E. (1998). Effects of intrauterine growth retardation and prematurity on spirometric flow values and lung volumes at school age in twin pairs. *Pediatr. Pulmonol.*, **25**, 367–70.

Oren, A., Vos, L. E., Uiterwaal, C. S., Gorissen, W. H., Grobbee, D. E. and Bots, M. L. (2004). Birth weight and carotid intima-media thickness: new perspectives from the atherosclerosis risk in young adults (ARYA) study. *Ann. Epidemiol.*, **14**, 8–16.

Osmond, C., Barker, D. J. P., Winter, P. D., Fall, C. H. D. and Simmonds, S. J. (1993). Early growth and death from cardiovascular disease in women. *BMJ*, **307**, 1519–24.

Pasamanick, B., Rogers, M. E. and Lilienfeld, A. M. (1956). Pregnancy experience and the development of behavior disorders in children. *Am. J. Psychiatry*, **112**, 613–18.

Petersen, K. F., Dufour, S., Befroy, D., Garcia, R. and Shulman, G. I. (2004). Impaired mitochondrial activity in the insulin-resistant offspring of patients with type 2 diabetes. *N. Engl. J. Med.*, **350**, 664–71.

Phillips, D. I. W. (1995). Relation of fetal growth to adult muscle mass and glucose tolerance. *Diabet Med.* **12**, 686–90.

Phillips, D. I. W. and Barker, D. J. P. (1997). Association between low birthweight and high resting pulse in adult life: is the sympathetic nervous system involved in programming the insulin resistance syndrome? *Diabet. Med.*, **14**, 673–7.

Phillips, D. I. W., Barker, D. J. P., Hales, C. N., Hirst, S. and Osmond, C. (1994a). Thinness at birth and insulin resistance in adult life. *Diabetologia*, **37**, 150–4.

Phillips, D. I. W., Hirst, S., Clark, P. M. S., Hales, C. N. and Osmond, C. (1994b). Fetal growth and insulin secretion in adult life. *Diabetologia*, **37**, 592–6.

Phillips, D. I. W., Taylor, D. J. and Kemp, G. J. *et al.* (1994c). Programming of muscle metabolism in adults who experienced growth retardation in utero. *Diabetologia*, **37**, A57.

Phillips, D. I. W., Walker, B. R., Reynolds, R. M. *et al.* (2000). Low birth weight predicts elevated plasma cortisol concentrations in adults from 3 populations. *Hypertension*, **35**, 1301–6.

Pilowsky, L. S., Kerwin, R. W. and Murray, R. M. (1993). Schizophrenia: a neurodevelopmental perspective. *Neuropsychopharmacology*, **9**, 83–91.

Power, C. and Jefferis, B. J. (2002). Fetal environment and subsequent obesity: a study of maternal smoking. *Int. J. Epidemiol.*, **31**, 413–19.

Ravelli, A. C. J., van der Meulen, J. H. P. and Michels, R. P. J. *et al.* (1998). Glucose tolerance in adults after prenatal exposure to famine. *Lancet*, **351**, 173–7.

Rich-Edwards, J. W., Stampfer, M. J., Manson, J. E. *et al.* (1997). Birth weight and risk of cardiovascular disease in a cohort of women followed up since 1976. *BMJ*, **315**, 396–400.

Roberts, C. T., Sohlstrom, A., Kind, K. L. *et al.* (2001). Maternal food restriction reduces the exchange surface area and increases the barrier thickness of the placenta in the guinea-pig. *Placenta*, **22**, 177–85.

Robinson, J. S., Owens, J. A., de Barro, T., *et al.* (1994). Maternal nutrition and fetal growth. In *Early Fetal Growth and Development* (ed. R. H. T. Ward, S. K. Smith and D. Donnai). London: Royal College of Obstetricians and Gynaecologists, pp. 317–34.

Robinson, S., Walton, R. J., Clark, P. M., Barker, D. J. P., Hales, C. N. and Osmond, C. (1992). The relation of fetal growth to plasma glucose in young men. *Diabetologia*, **35**, 444–6.

Rolland-Cachera, M. F., Deheeger, M., Guilloud-Bataille, M., Avons, P., Patois, E. and Sempe, M. (1987). Tracking the development of adiposity from one month of age to adulthood. *Ann. Hum. Biol.*, **14**, 219–29.

Rona, R. J., Gulliford, M. C. and Chinn, S. (1993). Effects of prematurity and intrauterine growth on respiratory health and lung function in childhood. *BMJ*, **306**, 817–20.

Roseboom, T. J., van der Meulen, J. H., Osmond, C., Barker, D. J. P., Ravelli, A. C. and Bleker, O. P. (2000a). Plasma lipid profiles in adults after prenatal exposure to the Dutch famine. *Am. J. Clin. Nutr.*, **72**, 1101–6.

Roseboom, T. J., van der Meulen, J. H. and Osmond, C. *et al.*, (2000b). Coronary heart disease after prenatal exposure to the Dutch famine, 1944–45. *Heart*, **84**, 595–8.

Roseboom, T. J., van der Meulen, J. H., Ravelli, A. C., Osmond, C., Barker, D. J. P. and Bleker, O. P. (2001a). Effects of prenatal exposure to the Dutch famine on adult disease in later life: an overview. *Mol. Cell. Endocrinol.*, **185**, 93–8.

Roseboom, T. J., van der Meulen, J. H., van Montfrans, G. A. *et al.* (2001b). Maternal nutrition during gestation and blood pressure in later life. *J. Hypertens.*, **19**, 29–34.

Rush, D. (1989). Effects of changes in maternal energy and protein intake during pregnancy, with special reference to fetal growth. In *Fetal Growth* (ed. F. Sharp, R. B. Fraser and R. D. G., Milner). London: Royal College of Obstetricians and Gynaecologists, pp. 203–33.

Sacker, A., Done, D. J., Crow, T. J. and Golding, J. (1995). Antecedents of schizophrenia and affective illness: obstetric complications. *Br. J. Psychiatry*, **166**, 734–41.

Sayer, A. A., Cooper, C. and Evans, J. R. *et al.* (1998). Are rates of ageing determined in utero? *Age Ageing*, **27**, 579–83.

Sayer, A. A., Syddall, H. E., Gilbody, H. J., Dennison, E. M. and Cooper, C. (2004). Does sarcopenia originate in early life? Findings from the Hertfordshire cohort study. *J. Gerontol. A Biol. Sci. Med. Sci.*, **59**, M930–4.

Schofield, P. W., Logroscino, G., Andrews, H. F., Albert, S. and Stern, Y. (1997). An association between head circumference and Alzheimer's disease in a population-based study of aging and dementia. *Neurology*, **49**, 30–37.

Shiell, A. W., Campbell, D. M., Hall, M. H. and Barker, D. J. P. (2000). Diet in late pregnancy and glucose-insulin metabolism of the offspring 40 years later. *Br. J. Obstet. Gynaecol.*, **107**, 890–5.

Shiell, A. W., Campbell-Brown, M., Haselden, S., Robinson, S., Godfrey, K. M. and Barker, D. J. P. (2001). A high meat, low carbohydrate diet in pregnancy: relation to adult blood pressure in the offspring. *Hypertension*, **38**, 1282–8.

Silverman, B. L., Purdy, L. P. and Metzger, B. E. (1996). The intrauterine environment: implications for the offspring of diabetic mothers. *Diabetes Rev.*, **4**, 21–35.

Smith, G. D., Whitley, E., Gissler, M. and Hemminki, E. (2000). Birth dimensions of offspring, premature birth, and the mortality of mothers. *Lancet*, **356**, 2066–7.

Snow, M. H. L. (1989). Effects of genome on fetal size at birth. In *Fetal Growth*. (ed. F. Sharp, R. B. Fraser and R. D. G. Milner). London: Royal College of Obstetricians and Gynaecologists, pp. 1–11.

Stein, C. E., Fall, C. H. D., Kumaran, K., Osmond. C., Cox, V. and Barker, D. J. P. (1996). Fetal growth and coronary heart disease in south India. *Lancet*, **348**, 1269–73.

Stein, C. E., Kumaran, K., Fall, C. H., Shaheen, S. O., Osmond, C. and Barker, D. J. P. (1997). Relation of fetal growth to adult lung function in south India. *Thorax*, **52**, 895–9.

Stettler, N., Kumanyika, S. K., Katz, S. H., Zemel, B. S. and Stallings, V. A. (2003). Rapid weight gain during infancy and obesity in young adulthood in a cohort of African Americans. *Am. J. Clin. Nutr.*, **77**, 1374–8.

Stewart, R. J. C., Sheppard, H., Preece, R. and Waterlow, J. C. (1980). The effect of rehabilitation at different stages of development of rats marginally malnourished for ten to twelve generations. *Br. J. Nutr.*, **43**, 403–12.

Stick, S. M., Burton, P. R., Gurrin, L., Sly, P. D. and LeSouef, P. N. (1996). Effects of maternal smoking during pregnancy and a family history of asthma on respiratory function in newborn infants. *Lancet*, **348**, 1060–4.

Stocks, J. and Dezateux, C. (2003). The effect of parental smoking on lung function and development during infancy. *Respirology*, **8**, 266–85.

Susser, E., Neugebauer, R., Hoek, H. W. *et al.* (1996). Schizophrenia after prenatal famine: further evidence. *Arch. Gen. Psychiatry*, **53**, 25–31.

Svanes, C., Omenaas, E., Heuch, J. M., Irgens, L. M. and Gulsvik, A. (1998). Birth characteristics and asthma symptoms in young adults: results from a population-based cohort study in Norway. *Eur. Respir. J.*, **12**, 1366–70.

Syddall, H., Cooper, C., Martin, F., Briggs, R. and Sayer A. A. (2003). Is grip strength a useful single marker of frailty? *Age Ageing*, **32**, 650–6.

Taylor, D. J., Thompson, C. H., Kemp, G. J. *et al.* (1995). A relationship between impaired fetal growth and reduced muscle glycolysis revealed by ^{31}P magnetic resonance spectroscopy. *Diabetologia*, **38**, 1205–12.

Thame, M., Osmond, C., Wilks, R. J., Bennett, F. I., McFarlane-Anderson, N. and Forrester, T. E. (2000). Blood pressure is related to placental volume and birth weight. *Hypertension*, **35**, 662–7.

Thompson, C., Syddall, H., Rodin, I., Osmond, C. and Barker, D. J. P. (2001). Birth weight and the risk of depressive disorder in late life. *Br. J. Psychiatry*, **179**, 450–5.

Valdez, R., Athens, M. A., Thompson, G. H., Bradshaw, B. S. and Stern, M. P. (1994). Birthweight and adult health outcomes in a biethnic population in the USA. *Diabetologia*, **37**, 624–31.

Vickers, M. H., Breier, B. H., Cutfield, W. S., Hofman, P. L. and Gluckman, P. D. (2000). Fetal origins of hyperphagia, obesity, and hypertension and postnatal amplification by hypercaloric nutrition. *Am. J. Physiol. Endocrinol. Metab.*, **279**, E83–7.

Vijayakumar, M., Fall, C. H., Osmond, C. and Barker, D. J. P. (1995). Birth weight, weight at one year, and left ventricular mass in adult life. *Br. Heart. J.*, **73**, 363–7.

Walker, S. K., Hartwick, K. M. and Robinson, J. S. (2000). Long-term effects on offspring of exposure of oocytes and embryos to chemical and physical agents. *Hum. Reprod. Update*, **6**, 564–7.

Weinberger, D. R. (1995). From neuropathology to neurodevelopment. *Lancet*, **346**, 552–7.

Whincup, P. H., Cook, D. G., Adshead, F. *et al.* (1997). Childhood size is more strongly related than size at birth to glucose and insulin levels in 10–11-year-old children. *Diabetologia*, **40**, 319–26.

Whitaker, R. C., Wright, J. A., Pepe, M. S., Seidel, K. D. and Dietz, W. H. (1997). Predicting obesity in young adulthood from childhood and parental obesity. *N. Engl. J. Med.*, **337**, 869–73.

Wills, J., Watson, J. M., Hales, C. N. and Phillips, D. I. W. (1996). The relation of fetal growth to insulin secretion in young men. *Diabet. Med.*, **13**, 773–4.

Winston, R. M. L. and Hardy, K. (2002). Are we ignoring potential dangers of in vitro fertilization and related treatments? *Nat. Cell Biol.*, **2**, S14–18.

Yarbrough, D. E., Barrett-Connor, E. and Morton, D. J. (2000). Birth weight as a predictor of adult bone mass in postmenopausal women: the Rancho Bernardo study. *Osteoporos. Int.*, **11**, 626–30.

Zureik, M., Bonithon-Kopp, C., Lecomte, E., Siest, G. and Ducimetiere, P. (1996). Weights at birth and in early infancy, systolic pressure, and left ventricular structure in subjects aged 8 to 24 years. *Hypertension*, **27**, 339–45.

3

The conceptual basis for the developmental origins of health and disease

Peter D. Gluckman[1] and Mark A. Hanson[2]

[1]University of Auckland
[2]University of Southampton

Introduction

The fundamental assumption underlying the DOHaD model is that environmental factors acting in early life have consequences which become manifest as an altered disease risk in later life. The concept that multiple phenotypes can arise during development from a single genotype ('developmental plasticity') is not new: these different phenotypes are based on the nature of the gene–environment interactions, a feature well recognised in developmental biology and the range of phenotypes that can be induced is termed the reaction norm (Gilbert 2001). Given the universality of developmental plasticity, particular sets of phenotypic outcomes may be manifest as variable disease risk (Bateson et al. 2004). As a result, one part of the reaction norm may be associated with better survival in one type of environment, while another is better suited to a different environment. One example comes from the desert locust Schistocerca gregaria, where factors acting in the larval stage induce a phenotype appropriate for migratory or non-migratory situations (Applebaum and Heifetz 1999, Simpson et al., 2002). Having a wing shape appropriate for a non-migratory lifestyle will compromise the locust in a situation of overcrowding and nutritional compromise.

While in comparative biology the concept of environmentally influenced developmental trajectories has been accepted, its influence on our understanding of human disease has taken time to be accepted. This delay has impacted on how the developmental-origins field has developed since the early epidemiological observations in humans relating birth size to later disease risk (Forsdahl 1977, Barker and Osmond 1986).

It is now generally accepted that the original observations relating birth size to later disease risk were not due to a causal pathway whereby being small directly caused disease. Rather, the statistical relationship existed because altered birth size is one measure of a disturbed fetal environment. As reviewed in Chapter 1, it is now apparent that the period of early life in which external factors can influence biology extends at least from conception to the neonatal period (Kwong et al. 2000, Singhal et al. 2003, 2004, Bloomfield et al. 2004). Moreover, through the course of human evolution one generally did not live long past the post-reproductive years; hence, there would have been little selection pressure against any processes that had deleterious effects in later life, provided that they conferred fitness earlier in life. Thus, comparative biology and human evolutionary history provide examples of the phenomenon that early-life environmental factors can have lifelong effects and can manifest as disease in modern society. Contemporary human observations must be reinterpreted in view of this understanding.

Developmental Origins of Health and Disease, ed. Peter Gluckman and Mark Hanson. Published by Cambridge University Press.
© P. D. Gluckman and M. A. Hanson 2006.

While the focus of this chapter must be on the mammal and how influences on pregnancy have consequences for the progeny, there is ample evidence of comparable transgenerational influences even in non-mammalian species. These are generally called **maternal effects**, and can be demonstrated in organisms ranging from plants to mammals (Agrawal *et al.* 1999). If such observations are relevant to DOHaD, and we would propose that they are, then they imply a broader evolutionary importance to the phenomenon.

Developmental disruption and developmental plasticity

Developmental plasticity can act early in life to change the course of development, leading to irreversible trajectories that manifest as different phenotypes. These may be very distinct, as in the axolotl, which chooses to be either aquatic or amphibious depending on the availability and size of freshwater ponds during early development (Wolpert 2002). Alternatively, the range of phenotypes may be continuous, as in the case of the timing of metamorphosis in toads, which is determined by population density in the pond (Denver 1997). The greater the population density, the earlier the spade toad will metamorphose from a tadpole to a toad and end its aquatic existence. In the tiger snake, jaw size is matched to prey size a feature determined not by genetics but by exposure during the neonatal phase to prey of different sizes. This matches prey resources to the capacity to eat the prey and demonstrates the adaptive value of phenotypic plasticity (Aubret *et al.* 2004).

Developmental plasticity is the term that encompasses these physiologically and environmentally determined patterns of development (West-Eberhard 2003, Bateson *et al.* 2004). Three characteristics are important in understanding developmental plasticity. First, the nature of the response will in part be dependent on the nature of the environmental cue. Second, there are critical windows for plasticity in different systems (i.e.,

when a system may be most vulnerable to change) that relate, in turn, to the necessary order of development. For instance, an environmental influence may have a lifelong impact if the cue acts during the critical developmental window, but will not have analogous effect if acting outside this window. The neonatal rat brain provides a well-known example of a critical window in development in that exposure to testosterone determines lifelong sexual behaviours (Christensen and Gorski 1978, Jacobson *et al.* 1981). Third, the duration of developmental plasticity is time-limited: once organogenesis is complete structurally and functionally, plasticity is no longer possible. The timing will be different for different systems and it would appear that the span over which developmental plasticity operates is longer for processes associated with growth and metabolism, as in, for example, the brain versus organs such as the heart. Presumably indefinite plasticity is not realistic because of the energetics required to support it in all tissues and structures.

However, not all environmental factors act during early development through these plastic processes (Gluckman *et al.* 2005a). Some environmental influences are clearly pathological and lead to disruption of development rather than channelling development. Teratogenesis is the most obvious manifestation of pathology, whereby an environmental toxin may grossly disrupt development with anatomic malformation as the consequence. The organism either dies or is left to cope with the consequences.

Teratogenesis or developmental disruption may also occur at a less overt level. The change may not be in gross structure, leading to a malformation, but in the substructure or function of the organ. This change in structure or function has no adaptive value at any stage in the organism's life – evident, for example, in the functional consequences of intrauterine iodine deficiency leading to hearing impairment (Valeix *et al.* 1994). The key point here is that some environmental factor induces a developmental change that has no adaptive advantage for the organism. Another example is the reduced neuronal number found in the hippocampus of animals born with fetal growth retardation (Mallard *et al.* 2000). It is difficult to conceive of a situation where a reduced number of neurons could be advantageous, yet the growth-retarded animal must cope with the consequences.

This discussion has important implications. One limitation of animal experiments is that when an environmental stress imposed during development is extreme (e.g., following very severe nutritional challenges or very high-dose glucocorticoid exposure), it may be inducing a teratogenic effect. The relevance of such disruptive consequences to the DOHaD phenomenon seems remote. Similarly, the extrapolation from observations made on severely growth-retarded children or prematurely delivered children to the biology of programming must be done with caution. The possibility that an abnormal phenotype represents some form of developmental disruption must be considered. The seminal observations on programming were made on children with birth phenotypes within the normal range, not with extreme abnormal phenotypes. We would argue that phenomena acting across the broad range of the normal population are unlikely to be underpinned by non-regulated disruptive processes.

Adaptive responses during development

The developing organism can respond to its environment with transient, homeostatic responses; these do not change its developmental trajectory and are generally only of immediate consequence. This is clearly evident in the developing fetus who in the process of brief periods of asphyxial insult experiences a transient cessation of breathing movements. This type of response has immediate adaptive value in that it allows the fetus to conserve oxygen by stopping an activity that has no survival consequences. However, if the environmental stimulus is chronic or repeated, then transient homeostatic responses may not be sufficient and the trajectory of development may have to change. This process was termed

homeorhesis by Waddington (1957). If the trajectory chosen has immediate adaptive advantage but is followed by long-term cost, then a **trade-off** has been created.

The concept of biological trade-offs is the basis of life-history theory. Trade-offs are common, particularly between growth, reproduction and longevity. For example, under conditions of nutritional stress many invertebrate and vertebrate species will grow more slowly, but enter puberty/reproductive competence earlier (Ibáñez *et al.* 2000a, Metcalfe and Monaghan 2003). A biological trade-off is a way to survive an environmental challenge with immediate adaptive advantage but long-term disadvantage – but it is only a successful strategy if the species lives long enough to reproduce. Lifelong stunting after a period of intrauterine growth retardation due to maternal undernutrition is such a trade-off. It has clear advantage to the fetus in that it can survive to birth on lesser nutritional support and still reach reproductive competence. The disadvantage is a lesser chance of reproductive success and a greater chance of earlier death, as it has been observed that smaller members of a species may have lesser survival and lower social status in pecking orders that influence reproductive opportunities (Albon *et al.* 1987, Metcalfe and Monaghan 2003), with strikingly similar observations in humans (Phillips *et al.* 2001). Premature delivery in response to maternal undernutrition can be demonstrated in many species, including humans (Bloomfield *et al.* 2003, King 2003, Kramer 2003). This is a form of trade-off by which exit from a potentially dangerous situation of maternal food deprivation allows the organism to be more likely to able to obtain food postnatally. The trade-off is the compromise to health that arises from prematurity.

The 'thrifty phenotype' hypothesis, one of the first models developed to explain the DOHaD phenomenon, is based on trade-off theory (Hales and Barker 1992). In brief, it describes how the fetus grows more slowly in response to a deprived intrauterine environment, the consequence of which is an altered biology that the organism must then cope with postnatally. This trade-off contributes to increased disease risk in later life. This model, which was a valuable step in the development of our current understanding, will be discussed later in this chapter.

More recently we have pointed out that there is a further class of environmental response that is unique to the phase of developmental plasticity, whereby the adaptive advantage is not immediate, but occurs later in life. This type of response is termed a **predictive adaptive response** (PAR) (Gluckman and Hanson 2004a, 2005). In the desert locust, the choice of wing and metabolic phenotype is determined in the larval phase in response to a pheromonic signal from the mother at egg-laying about population density. The wing shape and metabolism will be set for a migratory form if the population density is high and for the solitary non-migratory form if the density is low (Applebaum and Heifetz 1999, Simpson *et al.* 2002). Clearly, the choice of wing shape has no advantage to the larva, but is a response for future advantage to an environmental cue about population density. Mammals experience PARs as well, as evident in the meadow vole. The vole pup is born with a coat thickness that is thick if winter is approaching and thin if summer is approaching (Lee and Zucker 1988). Yet the fetal thermal environment and nest temperatures are similar. It has been shown that coat thickness is determined in response to the maternal melatonin cycle (Lee *et al.* 1989). There can be no advantage to the fetal or infant vole in either trajectory of hair density, but by making a choice in expectation of the future environment the developing vole has an adaptive advantage: it is more likely to survive the oncoming winter or summer, depending on its coat thickness, and successfully reproduce.

PARs have a number of characteristics (see Box 3.1). Using the processes of developmental plasticity, the organism establishes a mature phenotype it expects will be advantageous in the adult environment it predicts to be exposed to (Bateson 2001, Gluckman and Hanson 2004a). The developmental path chosen need not have any immediate adaptive value, as the consequences to the organism depend on the accuracy of the prediction. If the meadow vole was transported to an environment for which the

coat thickness was inappropriate, then the vole's fitness would be compromised.

Box 3.1 The characteristics of predictive adaptive responses

- Predictive adaptive responses are induced by environmental factors acting in early life, most often in pre-embryonic, embryonic or fetal life, not as an immediate physiological adaptation, but as a predictive response in expectation of some future environment.
- Predictive adapted responses are manifest in permanent change in the physiology of the organism and are likely underpinned by epigenetic processes.
- There are multiple pathways to the induction of these responses involving different environmental cues acting at different times in development.
- Predictive adaptive responses are not restricted in direction and occur across the full range of fetal environments.
- The induction of predictive adaptive responses will confer a survival advantage in the predicted reproductive environment (that is, appropriate prediction) and this will be manifest as increased fitness.
- The predictive adaptive response thus defines an environmental range in which the organism can optimally thrive until and through the reproductive phase of its postnatal life.
- Predictive adaptive responses may well lead to disease or disadvantage when the predicted reproductive or post-reproductive environmental boundaries are exceeded (that is, inappropriate prediction).
- These responses are neo-Darwinian adaptations permitting a species to survive short-term environmental challenges whilst preserving maximum genotypic variation for later environmental challenges and evolutionary fitness.
- It is to be anticipated that PARs may operate across several generations, depending for example on the duration of gestation in relation to an environmental change, the time to sexual maturity of offspring, etc.

Modified from Gluckman and Hanson (2005).

There is latitude for some adaptive responses to have both short- and long-term advantage. For example, the choice to have an activated hypothalamic–pituitary–adrenal axis (HPAA) in response to maternal stress may have advantage in those species where parturition is dependent on the fetal HPAA (e.g., sheep), as this allows the fetus to advance parturition and exit from a stressed fetal environment (Hawkins *et al.* 2001, Bloomfield *et al.* 2004). On the other hand, resetting the postnatal HPAA to be hyper-responsive may also have adaptive value in a stressful mature environment (Bolt *et al.* 2002). It is also obvious that there is not a clear boundary between disruptive, homeorhetic, and adaptive processes (Gluckman *et al.* 2005a) (Fig. 3.1).

The central issue is the accuracy of the prediction (Bateson 2001, Gluckman and Hanson 2004a). For the mammal, there is much potential for the prediction made early in life to be mismatched to the actual environment the mature organism will grow into. Such inaccurate prediction can arise because of imprecise transmission of environmental information from mother to egg/embryo/fetus either due to maternal or placental disease or because the postnatal environment changes. As we will discuss later, a key issue for human evolution is that while the extrauterine environment can rapidly change, the intrauterine environment is relatively constant over generations. Modelling demonstrates that provided the prediction is correct and confers fitness more than 50% of the time, it is advantageous to a species (Jablonka *et al.* 1995).

The PARs concept suggests that the relationship between the predicted and actual mature environment is not linear (Fig. 3.2). During development, the embryo/fetus/infant predicts its future environment based on maternal information and sets its mature physiology accordingly by choosing a developmental channel or trajectory. (See the classical work of Waddington (1957) for more discussion on the concepts of developmental channels.) This will establish a range of physiology associated with maximal fitness during its reproductive stage of life. But because fetal growth is constrained by maternal factors (see below), optimal fetal growth reflects less than its genetic capacity. The maximal fetal growth attainable thus establishes an adult environmental range for optimal fitness, and this will have an upper limit. Irrespective of the actual maternal environment, the

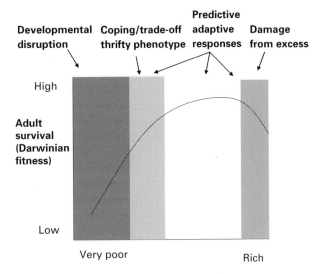

Figure 3.1 Developmental disruption and plasticity and their consequences. Extreme developmental environments lead to developmental disruption, while less extreme environments may lead to immediate adaptive responses, including induction of a 'thrifty phenotype'. Both may lead to long-term consequences with which the organism must cope. Within the normal range of variation, an individual's developmental environment maximal fitness is conferred by the action of predictive adaptive responses. Modified from Gluckman *et al.* (2005a).

limiting nature of maternal and placental influences on fetal growth constrains the intrauterine environment experienced, and this has long-term consequences for the individual's physiology. We define appropriate PARs as those which destine the organism to have physiology associated with maximal fitness in adulthood, and inappropriate PARs as those that are associated with physiological settings leading to reduced fitness – in humans, becoming manifest as greater disease risk (Gluckman and Hanson 2004b).

Explanations of the developmental origins of adult disease

The initial epidemiological associations between disease risk and measures of birth size led to a variety

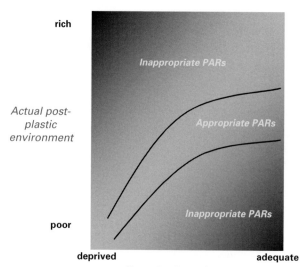

rich

Actual post-plastic environment

Inappropriate PARs

Appropriate PARs

poor

Inappropriate PARs

deprived   adequate

*Post-plastic environment
predicted from environment
during the plastic phase*

Figure 3.2 The nature of PARs is determined by the actual mature (post-plastic) environment relative to that predicted during the plastic phase. In general, one can think of the plastic phase as equivalent to the fetal and neonatal life and the post-plastic phase as equivalent to childhood and beyond. Modified from Gluckman and Hanson (2004b).

of conceptual models. Initial criticism focused on the issues of epidemiological confounders such as socioeconomic status, but once that matter had been addressed, attention turned to the linkage between fetal growth and later disease risk. (See Osmond and Barker (2000) for a discussion of these confounders and subsequent data; Huxley (2002) for additional commentary.) Initial explanations considered a causal role for fetal growth in the pathway, in other words, that being born small conferred disease risk. It is now generally agreed that being born small is only a surrogate measure for a less-than-optimal fetal environment. This was reinforced for example by observations made of the Dutch winter famine where early-pregnancy famine had long-term consequences for the offspring without effects on birth size (Kannisto *et al.* 1997, Roseboom *et al.* 2001). A plethora of observations in experimental animals reinforces this point, and more recent data

show that prematurity can also have long-term consequences independent of birth size (Cutfield *et al.* 2004).

The 'thrifty genotype' hypothesis

Pure genotypic explanations were proposed many years ago to explain regional differences in the incidence of disease. Neel developed the concept of the **thrifty genotype**, whereby populations developed a propensity for insulin resistance, either through selection or through genetic drift (Neel 1962). This would have been advantageous for such populations in uncertain nutritional environments. A modification of the 'thrifty genotype' concept was subsequently suggested as the basis of the apparent birth weight/disease risk relationship. As insulin is a regulator of birth size, via regulating fetal IGF1 release and promoting somatic growth, as well as through its direct adipogenic actions, it has been suggested that any genes conferring a degree of insulin resistance would reduce birth size and also have long-term consequences manifest as an increased risk of diabetes (Hales and Barker 1992). Several candidate genes were proposed, including glucokinase, there being some evidence for relatively common mutations in this gene affecting birth size, as well as being associated with some forms of diabetes (e.g. MODI) (Hattersley *et al.* 1998, Hattersley and Tooke 1999).

While there can be no doubt that genetic polymorphisms play a role in determining the strength of developmental gene–environment interactions, it has been difficult to reconcile a purely genetic explanation with the observations from the Dutch famine (Lumey 1992, Roseboom *et al.* 2001), or with (a) the widespread evidence of such relationships between early environment and long-term outcomes in different populations – e.g. European (Forsen *et al.* 2000), Asian, Indian subcontinent (Yajnik 2004); (b) evidence relating to different outcomes – e.g. dyslipidaemia (Jaquet *et al.* 2003), diabetes (Curhan *et al.* 1996, Ravelli *et al.* 1998), heart disease (Barker and Osmond 1986), osteoporosis (Cooper *et al.* 2002), mood disorders (Wahlbeck *et al.* 2001); (c) the rapid increase in the scale of the phenomenon in populations in transition (Popkin 2004, Yajnik 2004). Further, the ease with which 'programming' can be induced experimentally in a variety of organ systems and across species suggests that the basic underlying mechanisms are non-genetic (Bertram and Hanson 2001).

The 'thrifty phenotype' hypothesis

Barker and Hales, playing off the 'thrifty' terminology, suggested an alternative **thrifty phenotype** model, which was essentially a description of a developmental trade-off. They proposed that under conditions of intrauterine deprivation the fetus would grow more slowly and thus become committed to a developmental path associated with insulin resistance and other changes appropriate for a deprived environment (Hales and Barker 1992). This has immediate adaptive value in that by reducing somatic growth to preserve available energy for the heart and brain, it promotes survival in an otherwise deprived intrauterine environment. The cost of the trade-off would be that the individual is set for life with a physiology more appropriate for a deprived environment. The implication of the model is that the intrauterine environment need be sufficiently impaired to reduce fetal growth. This might occur if the external environment to which the mother was exposed was very harsh, as in time of famine, in which case the adaptive strategy might prove to be effective. However, reduced fetal growth is also frequently associated with maternal or placental disease, which does not reflect an impaired external environment. Here, the fetal adaptive responses will produce a phenotype not suited to the future environment.

Thus, the 'thrifty phenotype' model originally gave centrality to the degree of growth retardation occurring in utero. The model is most easily envisaged under conditions when a poor environment exceeds a threshold beyond which the immediate compensatory mechanisms of the fetus are inadequate; it is less easy to envisage as operating in a graded manner across the normal birthweight range, which

is what the epidemiological data show. While the model could explain the long-term consequences of extreme intrauterine growth retardation, it could not, for example, readily explain how a reduction in birth size from the 80th centile to the 60th could be associated with increased disease risk. It could not explain how transient fetal insults (evident from clinical data, and more so from experimental data) could lead to long-term consequences. Lastly, whilst the explanation fitted the induction of metabolic phenotypes, it did not sit easily with programming of systems, such as fluid balance (Ross *et al.* 2005) or thermogenesis (Gate *et al.* 1999), where the mechanisms of fluid and thermal homeostasis in utero conferred no immediate adaptive value. We (Gluckman and Hanson 2004a) and Bateson (2001) alternatively proposed that the fetal responses were in part made in prediction of the future environment.

Gene–environment interactions and the explanation of the DOHaD paradigm

The thrifty-phenotype model was also criticised, perhaps unfairly, as excluding a genetic component. Indeed, epidemiological studies demonstrated that there were links between genotype and disease risk but that these links were modified by developmental and presumed environmental factors. Studies of polymorphisms of $PPAR\gamma$ illustrate the nature of these interactions. A common polymorphism of $PPAR\gamma$ is associated with insulin resistance in adulthood, but the association is dependent on low birthweight. Not all of those with the polymorphism develop insulin resistance or have low birthweight; but only those with low birthweight and the polymorphism develop insulin resistance, so that the correlation between birthweight and disease risk is restricted to those with this polymorphism (Eriksson *et al.* 2002). Whether this interaction is restricted to the population studied is not known. However, other examples of comparable interactions are now being reported: for instance, a polymorphism in the vitamin D receptor determines the strength of the relationship between birth size and the risk of later osteoporosis (Dennison *et al.* 2001).

Such interactions are, of course, not incompatible with an environmental explanation. Essentially all interactions between an organism and its environment depend on gene–environment interactions, and both the nature of the stressor and the precise genotype determine the outcome of the interaction. Indeed, such observations, as made in the case of the effect of the *PPARγ* haplotype, give strength to the arguments for the environmental component. Many candidate genes are likely to be identified in which polymorphisms affect the gene–environment interaction in a given physiological system. On the one hand this adds considerable complexity to the field, but on the other it may assist in identifying those at particular risk.

A further question, which is as yet unanswerable, is whether different polymorphisms lead to different capacities for epigenetic modification. If indeed epigenetic change is fundamental to how the environment impacts on developmental plasticity (as opposed to disruption), then this will create a further layer of complexity in unravelling gene–environment interactions during development.

The role of catch-up growth

Another important feature, which emerged first from epidemiological studies followed later by experimental observations, is the role of catch-up growth. Barker's group found that people of lower birth size (weight or ponderal index) who as children showed rapid growth or weight gain, or who had higher ponderal indices in adolescence or adulthood, were at particular risk of disease (Eriksson *et al.* 1999, 2003). Rats born to dams undernourished in pregnancy developed insulin resistance and hypertension postnatally, but the magnitude of the hypertension, insulin resistance, visceral obesity and other features was far greater if the animals were placed on a high-fat 'cafeteria' diet (Vickers *et al.* 2000). This suggested an interaction between the environmental exposure in utero and the environmental exposure that occurred postnatally. Subsequent studies were able to show in rat pups that postnatal high-

fat diets alone could induce programming of insulin resistance and obesity in later life (Khan *et al.* 2005).

More recently, clinical studies have suggested that high caloric intakes in infancy in premature infants have long-term consequences (Singhal *et al.* 2003), while other studies suggest that rapid childhood growth alone might have consequences (Eriksson *et al.* 2001). It is not known whether these postnatal effects involve different processes from those underlying 'fetal origins' or whether they are all part of a spectrum of biological responses during development. One unresolved issue is the extent to which these two components of growth are independent of each other. Is it that the trajectories chosen in utero induce changes in postnatal growth regulation such that earlier and more rapid growth is more likely, or are they independent mechanisms? If the latter, it may still be that there is effective linkage between the two because the natural response to being born small or thin is to induce maternal and societal responses that promote growth. This research highlights the importance of considering both the offspring and their environment, including the environment created by the mother.

Constraint of fetal growth

Mammalian fetuses do not grow to their maximum genetic potential but are constrained by non-genetic, maternal-uterine factors, such as maternal size, possibly age, nutritional status, and whether or not it is a primiparous pregnancy (Ounsted and Ounsted 1973, Gluckman and Liggins 1984). These effects are generally grouped under the term **maternal constraint**. The presence of maternal constraint is critical to our current conceptual understandings of the programming phenomenon, as all fetal development is influenced by maternal constraint to some degree, mediated in part by metabolic and endocrine signals (Gluckman and Liggins 1984, Gluckman *et al.* 1992, Gluckman and Hanson 2004a). It also implies that in some pregnancies, factors will act in the extreme to induce even greater constraint on the fetus, with pathological consequences, as evident in maternal–placental disease. At birth these constraints are lifted and the consequences are then manifest.

Maternal constraint is particularly important in the bipedal hominid, as the development of a narrow pelvis required that fetal growth was constrained to match maternal size. Maternal constraint is accordingly greater in smaller women – manifested as reduced birth size in women with short stature (or those of low birthweight). It is also the basis of the original observations of maternal constraint made by Walton and Hammond in crossing horses from breeds of very different size (Walton and Hammond 1938). So significant is the impact of maternal constraint, that it has been possible to show that the effect of primiparous pregnancy on birthweight is not that dissimilar from the effects of maternal smoking (Ong *et al.* 2002). Maternal constraint is also greater in adolescent pregnancies, where nutrients are preferentially allocated towards the young mother's ongoing somatic growth instead of to her fetus (Wallace *et al.* 2001), and in multiple pregnancies, where it is associated with reduced birth size because limitations on nutrients across the uteroplacenta restrict nutrient availability to each fetus (Gluckman *et al.* 1992). Maternal age at first pregnancy also significantly impacts on birthweight and is associated with increased pregnancy complications that may lead to preterm delivery (Naeye 1983, Aldous and Edmonson 1993).

Match–mismatch, PARs and DOHaD: towards a conceptual synthesis

Our unifying model recognises that there are common features to the induction of programming by fetal/neonatal manipulation, and to induction by rapid childhood growth. Both represent situations where there is a degree of mismatch between the fetal/neonatal environment and the later environment. In the first case, it is caused by restraining environmental factors impacting on fetal/infant development followed by a relatively normal postnatal environment. In the second, it is due to a relatively

normal but constrained fetal environment followed by an abundant postnatal environment. Both are situations where there is an anticipated mismatch between the fetal/neonatal environment, in what we may term a plastic phase of development, and that in a post-plastic phase.

These concepts, together with the recognition of predictive adaptive responses, have allowed for the development of an integrated explanation of the programming paradigm at the systems level. The recognition that epigenetic modification of the genome could be influenced by environmental factors, such as maternal nutrition or behaviour, provides a mechanistic basis (Waterland and Jirtle 2004, Weaver *et al.* 2004).

The PARs model suggests that the developing organism constantly senses its environment during its plastic phase. In the case of mammals this depends on maternal transmission of environmental information through to the embryo, fetus or neonate, including potentially independent effects on placental function and lactation. The plastic organism uses this information to predict aspects of its adult environment and, using the mechanisms of PARs, sets its physiology accordingly.

As the nutritional environment is the most critical for species survival, it is not surprising that the systems most likely to be programmed are those associated with metabolism, growth, reproduction and coping with stress. Provided that across a species the prediction is more often right than wrong, the genetic infrastructure of PARs (e.g. epigenetic processes) will be positively selected during evolution. The presence of PARs confers enormous survival advantage to a species. PARs allow a genotype to survive *transient* environmental change, where the duration of the change spans a generation or more, unlike homeostasis, which allows an individual to survive very transient environmental change, or Darwinian selection, which generally operates over a long time base and assumes a constant direction of change in the environment. Instead, the PARs model allows a broader range of genotypes in a population to be preserved, and this in itself creates a long-term Darwinian advantage (Fig. 3.3). This modelling

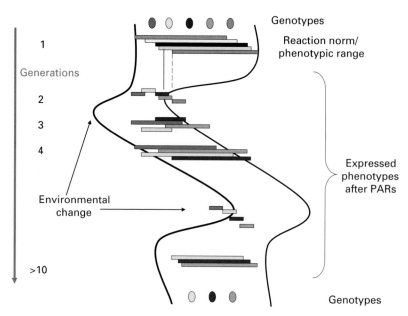

Figure 3.3 The advantage of PARs in preserving genotypic variation in a population during rapid environmental changes occurring over 1–3 generations. Consider a range of genotypes (shown by the patterned dots) within a population. They convey adult phenotypic types shown by the horizontal bars of the same pattern. Each bar represents many individuals each sharing a phenotypic characteristic. The individuals will be able to survive as long as the capabilities of the phenotype are not exceeded by an environmental challenge. The range of environment that the individual phenotypes can tolerate is indicated by the length of the horizontal bars and will generally equal the reaction norm for the genotype. Therefore, the reaction norm for the whole population for any generation is the maximum extent of these different ranges. When the population is in a stable state with respect to its environmental niche, the extent of the range bounded by the lines and the varying environmental conditions, e.g. with seasons, coincide. If the environment changes drastically so that its boundaries shift between one generation and the next (here, indicated by the curvature of the boundaries), the population is no longer in a stable state. By tracing the vertical broken line we can see by way of example that all of the offspring from the phenotype on the right (generation 2) now lie outside this range, and may perish; so will the majority of the other phenotypes. Their corresponding genotypes will also be lost from the gene pool. The species is in trouble: its offspring will be poorly equipped to deal with the environment they will face and they are unlikely to survive to reproduce. Worse still, if the environment shifts back again to beyond its original range we can see that any phenotypes which had survived the first shift will find themselves outside the range after the second. The species may become extinct in a few generations.

But this effect is obviated by the action of PARs. If the environmental change had occurred during the pregnancy of the first generation, then there will have been the chance for PARs to shift the development of generation 2 towards the traits that convey survival. The horizontal bars are now shifted, but also shortened. More individuals will be bunched up with phenotypic traits that convey a fitness advantage. The process is not perfect: even with the operation of PARs, the phenotype on the right will not have been able to shift far enough, and they may all die, as will a proportion of the next two phenotypes. But the attrition rate will be far less than without this strategy. When the environment shifts back in the opposite direction, phenotypes (and hence genotypes) on the left will be lost, but we can see that by the time the environment stabilises again at least three of the original five genotypes have been preserved. Modified from Gluckman and Hanson (2005).

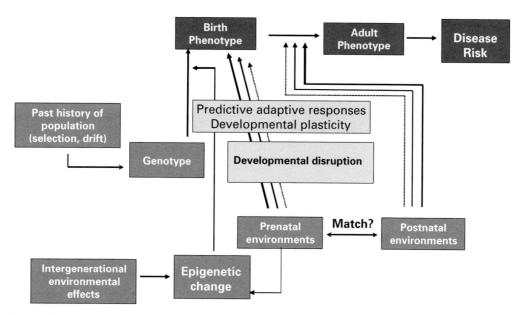

Figure 3.4 A general model of how genomic, epigenetic and environmental factors interact during development to affect developmental plasticity and alter disease risk in adulthood. If the prenatal and postnatal environments match, then the risk of disease is reduced because PARs will have left the developing organism well prepared for its postnatal environment. Conversely, a mismatch between the prenatal and postnatal environments may be pathogenic. Modified from Gluckman and Hanson (2004a).

is supported by earlier estimates of the value of phenotypic memory (Jablonka *et al.* 1995).

A further consideration is that of intergenerational effects. In the Dutch winter famine, the effects of undernutrition in the first trimester were reflected in reduced birthweight of the grandchildren (Lumey 1992), and there is considerable experimental evidence for multigenerational impacts of transient environmental influences. In rodents, it takes at least three generations before the effects of undernutrition on growth disappear (Stewart *et al.* 1980). Maternal diet has effects on endothelial function extending to the F2 generation that are transmitted both by male and by female progeny (Torrens *et al.* 2002). The male-mediated transmission excludes mitochondrial mechanisms as an explanation. In humans, there is a report of transmission of type 2 diabetes to men as a consequence of poor nutrition in their grandfathers during the prepuberty period (Kaati *et al.* 2002). The recent recognition that not all epigenetic modification of the genome is lost

at meiosis (see Chapter 5), and that there can be intergenerational transmission of non-genomic epigenetic effects, provides a probable explanation of these intergenerational effects (Jablonka and Lamb 1989). Other possible explanations include effects on the development of the reproductive tract during fetal life as a result of maternal undernutrition (Ibáñez *et al.* 2000b) and the effects of programming on the progeny's metabolic adaptations to pregnancy.

Thus, a general model can be developed (Fig. 3.4). The genomic and epigenetic state of the conceptus is established by long-term population characteristics (genetic drift, selection), the parental genomes and intergenerational epigenetic influences reflecting recent environmental exposures experienced by the parents and grandparents. On this genetic and epigenetic background, the conceptus senses its future environment by means of metabolic and hormonal signals from the mother and selects its developmental strategy accordingly (Bateson 2001,

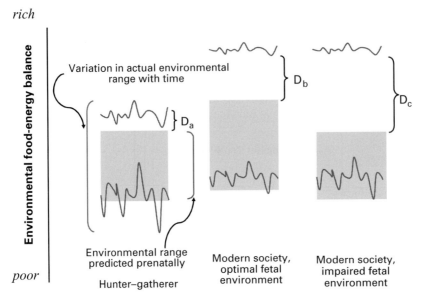

Figure 3.5 The predictive adaptive (*PARs*) model is illustrated with respect to the nutritional environment for humans at different evolutionary times and environmental space. The ordinate is an arbitrary measure of the nutritional quality of the postnatal environment. For each of three scenarios, the relationship is shown between the postnatal environmental range, as predicted by the fetus based on information available to it during fetal development (shaded region), and the actual environmental range (the range between the two curves). The PARs model suggests that the fetus sets its postnatal physiology for the predicted, rather than actual, range. (a) Hunter–gatherer (left). The upper limit of the predicted range may be below the upper limit of the actual range due to maternal constraint – this range (D_a) creates a region where there is a risk of mismatch between the prenatal and postnatal environments. (b) Optimal fetal development in a modern society (middle). The upper limit of the actual nutritional range has shifted upward from that of the hunter–gatherer. Maternal constraint continues to restrict the upper limit of predicted environmental range, creating a wider gulf between the predicted and actual postnatal environments (D_b), which increases the probability of disease risk. (c) Modern situation complicated by pathology or extreme maternal constraint (right). PARs reduce the upper limit of the predicted postnatal environment even further, widening D_c and increasing the risk of mismatch and disease. Additionally, irreversible plastic changes with immediate adaptive value in utero have further restricted the range of postnatal environments the fetus can adapt to.

Gluckman and Hanson 2004a). If the environmental challenge is extreme it may induce developmental disruption, and the individual must cope with the consequences. If the environmental challenge is somewhat less severe it may induce a homeorhetic change, conferring immediate advantage but possible long-term disadvantage (i.e. a trade-off). However, under most circumstances the developing conceptus chooses its developmental trajectory in a continuous manner based on its prediction of its adult environment. To do so the organism uses PARs, the underlying mechanisms of which have

been selected for because they confer survival advantage to the species. We stress that PARs confer no immediate advantage to the conceptus but, depending on the fidelity of the prediction, they may confer increased fitness in adult life.

The fidelity of the prediction is influenced by physiological factors, such as maternal constraint, and by pathophysiological factors, such as maternal or placental disease or changes in maternal nutrition, which are recognised by the fetus. Recent clinical observations show that fetal growth patterns can be affected by maternal nutritional balance within

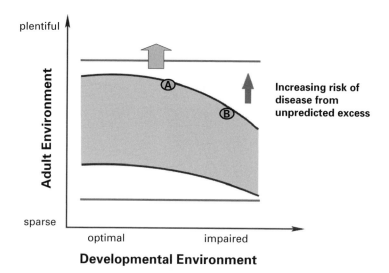

Figure 3.6 The relationship between the developmental and adult environment is shown with respect to nutritional signals. The horizontal lines show the environmental limits an individual might be exposed to. The upper line is shifting upwards as a result of availability of food and sedentary behaviour in many societies. The shaded area represents the zone of appropriate *PARs*, associated with reduced disease risk. It is apparent that the risk of disease due to nutritional excess increases as the developmental environment is more compromised. An individual at point A, exposed to a better intrauterine environment, can tolerate a greater postnatal nutritional load without disease than an individual at point B. Modified from Gluckman and Hanson (2004a).

the normal absolute-intake range (Godfrey *et al.* 1996). There is also much evidence that micronutrient intakes can affect both fetal structural development and physiology (Rao *et al.* 2001, Brawley *et al.* 2003, 2004). If the PARs prediction is correct, then the risk of disease is low. If the prediction is faulty, then the risk of disease will be greater. This disease is most likely to manifest itself in middle age or beyond. There is little or no selection pressure against such risk of disease, so such detrimental aspects of inappropriate PARs have not been selected out by evolution. The risk of disease thus reflects the degree of match or mismatch between the environments during the plastic phase of life and that actually experienced in mature life.

Consideration of hominid evolution provides a further perspective (Fig. 3.5). Humans evolved as hunter–gatherers with low carbohydrate intakes. Maternal constraint ensured successful pelvic delivery. As hominids adopted an upright posture this became more important, reflected somewhat by

the relative neoteny of the human skull at birth (Penin *et al.* 2002) and the relatively immature neurological state compared to other primates, including *Homo erectus*. Because of maternal constraint, the hominid fetus had PARs which predicted a relatively constrained postnatal nutritional environment. This probably conferred an advantage in the uncertain nutritional environment of the hunter–gatherer, resulting in a reasonably good match between fetal and postnatal environments (excluding the impact of disease). As agriculture developed, the postnatal environment had the capacity to change, but the intrauterine environment less so, primarily because of the considerations of pelvic size, maternal constraint, and so on, which increased the risk of mismatch. This mismatch was probably of little significance when life span was short, as the disease manifestations of inappropriate PARs would not be exhibited. Furthermore, because PARs determine the range for mature physiological homeostasis rather than an absolute operating point, the range of environments the adult could cope with was probably adequate until the post-industrial era. But the very rapid shifts in nutrition due to advances in agriculture, food manufacture and population migration, have meant that there is increasing risk of mismatch between the environment sensed in utero in the presence of limiting factors, and that experienced in the post-plastic period of life. We have proposed elsewhere that this is responsible for the changing patterns of disease (Gluckman and Hanson 2004a, 2004b, Gluckman *et al.* 2005b). In addition, because of the absolute limitation on the fetal environment, excessive postnatal environments alone can create a mismatch between the plastic and post-plastic phases, creating the consequences of inappropriate PARs.

The PARs model provides the basis for a continuous relationship between the induced fetal phenotype (as reflected in surrogates such as birth size) and long-term health consequences. It also provides a pathway by which the transition from an optimal or highly nourished fetal environment to a poor postnatal environment might produce greater disease risk from inappropriate PARs. The evidence for this latter path is less clear, but there are human data (see Chapter 15) supporting its existence. In reports from African famines it appears to be the children of largest birth size who are more likely to develop clinical evidence of vitamin D deficiency (Chali *et al.* 1998).

A point central to the PARs model is shown with respect to nutritional stimulus in Fig. 3.6. Theoretically, as the fetal environment becomes more compromised, the maximum postnatal environmental level that the individual may adapt to without disease risk is reduced. In other words, an individual exposed in utero to a poor environment will tolerate a lower nutritional range without developing disease than one born following an optimal intrauterine environment. Thus, the nutritional range associated with optimal health in adulthood is determined by the individual's experience during the plastic phase.

In developed countries the degree of mismatch with respect to nutrition and energy is enhanced by increasing nutritional excess and a sedentary

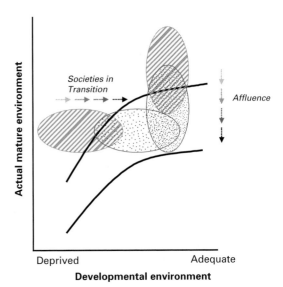

Figure 3.7 The *PARs* model has implications for interventional strategies in different societies. The physiology of the mature organism is influenced by *PARs* operative during the plastic phase; these establish a mature environmental range for which the organism's physiology is adapted. This range is shown between the two curved lines. If the actual postnatal environment is within this range, the disease risk is lower. If it is beyond this range (outside these lines) then the disease risk in adult life will be higher. The nutritional status of two hypothetical societies is shown – one that is typical of 'affluent' nations with access to plentiful food resources; the other more typical of 'societies in transition,' where food may be limited, maternal health likely to be compromised, and fetal growth retardation common. It can be seen that in a society of affluence, a focus on postnatal environmental factors (diet and exercise) is likely to have a major influence on disease risk, whereas in the society in transition, it may be that greater health gains can be achieved by a focus on improving maternal, fetal and infant health. Reprinted from Gluckman *et al.* (2005b).

lifestyle. Prenatal factors which accentuate the mismatch are primiparity, adolescent pregnancy, possibly advanced maternal age, poor maternal nutrition, and diseases of pregnancy and the placenta. In developing countries the same factors operate, but are further compounded by the problems of short maternal stature, chronic maternal disease, infections (e.g. HIV, malaria), and chronically poor female nutritional status from social and cultural factors. There are compelling data that the nutritional status of women prior to conception has major effects on pregnancy outcome, and these effects are likely to be mediated in part by the mechanisms we have discussed (Inskip *et al.* 2001, Robinson *et al.* 2004, Crozier *et al.* in press). Elsewhere we have pointed out that the strategy for intervention to promote adult health in a population depends on the shape of the PARs relationship (Gluckman *et al.* 2005b). As shown in Fig. 3.7, it may well be that for a developing country prenatal interventions are more likely to be effective, whereas postnatal lifestyle intervention will remain the most important component of managing the epidemics of obesity and related diseases in westernised societies.

ACKNOWLEDGMENTS

MAH is supported by the British Heart Foundation.

REFERENCES

Agrawal, A. A., Laforsch, C. and Tollrian, R. (1999). Transgenerational induction of defences in animals and plants. *Nature*, **401**, 60–3.

Albon, S. D., Clutton-Brock, T. H. and Guinness, F. E. (1987). Early development and population dynamics in red deer. II. Density-independent effects and cohort variation. *J. Anim. Ecol.*, **56**, 69–81.

Aldous, M. B. and Edmonson, M. B. (1993). Maternal age at first childbirth and risk of low birth weight and preterm delivery in Washington State. *JAMA*, **270**, 2574–7.

Applebaum, S. W. and Heifetz, Y. (1999). Density-dependent physiological phase in insects. *Ann. Rev. Entomol.*, **44**, 317–41.

Aubret, F., Shine, R. and Bonnet, X. (2004). Evolutionary biology: adaptive developmental plasticity in snakes. *Nature*, **431**, 261–2.

Barker, D. J. and Osmond, C. (1986). Infant mortality, childhood nutrition, and ischaemic heart disease in England and Wales. *Lancet*, **1**, 1077–81.

Bateson, P. (2001). Fetal experience and good adult design. *Int. J. Epidemiol.*, **30**, 928–34.

Bateson, P., Barker, D., Clutton-Brock, T. *et al.* (2004). Developmental plasticity and human health. *Nature*, **430**, 419–21.

Bertram, C. E. and Hanson, M. A. (2001). Animal models and programming of the metabolic syndrome. *Br. Med. Bull.*, **60**, 103–21.

Bloomfield, F., Oliver, M., Hawkins, P. *et al.* (2003). A periconceptional nutritional origin for noninfectious preterm birth. *Science*, **300**, 606.

(2004). Periconceptional undernutrition in sheep accelerates maturation of the fetal hypothalamic–pituitary–adrenal axis in late gestation. *Endocrinology*, **145**, 4278–85.

Bolt, R. J., van Weissenbruch, M. M., Lafeber, H. N. and Delemarre-Van De Waal, H. A. (2002). Development of the hypothalamic–pituitary–adrenal axis in the fetus and preterm infant. *J. Pediatr. Endocrinol. Metab.*, **15**, 759–69.

Brawley, L., Dance, C. S., Dunn, R. L. *et al.* (2003). Dietary folate supplementation prevents the attenuated relaxation to vascular endothelial growth factor (VEGF) in the uterine artery of protein-restricted pregnant rats. *Pediatr. Res.*, **53**, 37A.

Brawley, L., Torrens, C., Anthony, F. W. *et al.* (2004). Glycine rectifies vascular dysfunction induced by dietary protein imbalance during pregnancy. *J. Physiol.*, **554**, 497–504.

Chali, D., Enquselassie, F. and Gesese, M. (1998). A case–control study on determinants of rickets. *Ethiop. Med. J.*, **36**, 227–34.

Christensen, L. W. and Gorski, R. A. (1978). Independent masculinization of neuroendocrine systems by intracerebral implants of testosterone or estradiol in the neonatal rat. *Brain Res.*, **146**, 325–40.

Cooper, C., Javaid, M. K., Taylor, P., Walker-Bone, K., Dennison, E. and Arden, N. (2002). The fetal origins of osteoporotic fracture. *Calc. Tissue Int.*, **70**, 391–4.

Crozier, S., Borland, S., Robinson, S., Godrey, K. and Inskip, H. (in press). How effectively do young women prepare for pregnancy? *BJOG*.

Curhan, G. C., Willett, W. C., Rimm, E. B., Spiegelman, D., Ascherio, A. L. and Stampfer, M. J. (1996). Birth weight and adult hypertension, diabetes mellitus, and obesity in US men. *Circulation*, **94**, 3246–50.

Cutfield, W. S., Regan, F. A., Jackson, W. E. *et al.* (2004). The endocrine consequences for very low birth weight premature infants. *Growth Horm. IGF. Res.*, **14**, S130–5.

Dennison, E. M., Arden, N. K., Keen, R. W. *et al.* (2001). Birthweight, vitamin D receptor genotype and the programming of osteoporosis. *Paediatr. Perinat. Epidemiol.*, **15**, 211–19.

Denver, R. J. (1997). Environmental stress as a developmental cue: corticotropin-releasing hormone is a proximate mediator of adaptive phenotypic plasticity in amphibian metamorphosis. *Horm. Behav.*, **31**, 169–79.

Eriksson, J. G., Forsen, T., Tuomilehto, J., Winter, P. D., Osmond, C. and Barker, D. J. (1999). Catch-up growth in childhood and death from coronary heart disease: longitudinal study. *BMJ*, **318**, 427–31.

Eriksson, J. G., Forsen, T., Tuomilehto, J., Osmond, C. and Barker, D. J. (2001). Early growth and coronary heart disease in later life: longitudinal study. *BMJ*, **322**, 949–53.

Eriksson, J. G., Lindi, V., Uusitupa, M. *et al.* (2002). The effects of the Pro12Ala polymorphism of the peroxisome proliferator-activated receptor-gamma2 gene on insulin sensitivity and insulin metabolism interact with size at birth. *Diabetes*, **51**, 2321–4.

Eriksson, J. G., Forsen, T., Tuomilehto, J., Osmond, C. and Barker, D. J. (2003). Early adiposity rebound in childhood and risk of type 2 diabetes in adult life. *Diabetologia*, **46**, 190–4.

Forsdahl, A. (1977). Are poor living conditions in childhood and adolescence an important risk factor for arteriosclerotic heart disease? *Br. J. Prevent. Soc. Med.*, **31**, 91–5.

Forsen, T., Eriksson, J., Tuomilehto, J., Reunanen, A., Osmond, C. and Barker, D. (2000). The fetal and childhood growth of persons who develop type 2 diabetes. *Ann. Intern. Med.*, **133**, 176–82.

Gate, J. J., Clarke, L., Lomax, M. A. and Symonds, M. E. (1999). Chronic cold exposure has no effect on brown adipose tissue in newborn lambs born to well-fed ewes. *Reprod. Fertil. Dev.*, **11**, 415–18.

Gilbert, S. F. (2001). Ecological developmental biology: developmental biology meets the real world. *Dev. Biol.*, **233**, 1–12.

Gluckman, P. D. and Hanson, M. A. (2004a). Living with the past: evolution, development and patterns of disease. *Science*, **305**, 1773–6.

(2004b). The developmental origins of the metabolic syndrome. *Trends Endocrinol. Metab.*, **15**, 183–7.

(2004c). Maternal constraint of fetal growth and its consequences. *Semin. Fetal Neonatal Med.*, **9**, 419–25.

(2005). *The Fetal Matrix: Evolution, Development, and Disease*. Cambridge: Cambridge University Press.

Gluckman, P. D. and Liggins, G. C. (1984). The regulation of fetal growth. In *Fetal Physiology and Medicine* (ed. R. W. Beard and P. W. Nathanielsz). New York: Dekker, pp. 511–58.

Gluckman, P. D., Morel, P. C. H., Ambler, G. R., Breier, B. H., Blair, H. T. and McCutcheon, S. N. (1992). Elevating maternal insulin-like growth factor-I in mice and rats alters the pattern of fetal growth by removing maternal constraint. *J. Endocrinol.*, **134**, R1–3.

Gluckman, P. D., Hanson, M. A., Spencer, H. G. and Bateson, P. (2005a). Environmental influences during development and their later consequences for health and disease: impli-cations for the interpretation of empirical studies. *Proc. Biol. Soc.*, **272**, 671–7.

Gluckman, P. D., Hanson, M. A., Morton, S. M. and Pinal, C. S. (2005b). life-long echoes: a critical analysis of the developmental origins of adult disease model. *Biol. Neonate*, **87**, 127–39.

Godfrey, K., Robinson, S., Barker, D. J., Osmond, C. and Cox, V. (1996). Maternal nutrition in early and late pregnancy in relation to placental and fetal growth. *BMJ*, **312**, 410–14.

Hales, C. N. and Barker, D. J. (1992). Type 2 (non-insulin-dependent) diabetes mellitus: the thrifty phenotype hypothesis. *Diabetologia*, **35**, 595–601.

Hattersley, A. T. and Tooke, J. E. (1999). The fetal insulin hypothesis: an alternative explanation of the association of low birthweight with diabetes and vascular disease. *Lancet*, **353**, 1789–92.

Hattersley, A. T., Beards, F., Ballantyne, E., Appleton, M., Harvey, R. and Ellard, S. (1998). Mutations in the glucokinase gene of the fetus result in reduced birth weight. *Nat. Genet.*, **19**, 209–10.

Hawkins, P., Hanson, M. A. and Matthews, S. G. (2001). Maternal undernutrition in early gestation alters molecular regulation of the hypothalamic–pituitary–adrenal axis in the ovine fetus. *J. Neuroendocrinol.*, **13**, 855–61.

Huxley, R., Neil, A. and Collins, R. (2002). Unravelling the fetal origins hypothesis: is there really an inverse association between birthweight and subsequent blood pressure? *Lancet*, **360**, 659–65.

Ibáñez, L., Ferrer, A., Marcos, M. V., Hierro, F. R. and de Zegher, F. (2000a). Early puberty: rapid progression and reduced final height in girls with low birth weight. *Pediatrics*, **106**, 72–4.

Ibáñez, L., Potau, N., Enriquez, G. and de Zegher, F. (2000b). Reduced uterine and ovarian size in adolescent girls born small for gestational age. *Pediatr. Res.*, **47**, 575–7.

Inskip, H., Hammond, J., Borland, S., Robinson, S. and Shore, S. (2001). Determinants of fruit and vegetable consumption in 5,630 women aged 20–34 years from the Southampton Women's Survey. *Pediatr. Res.*, **50**, 58A.

Jablonka, E. and Lamb, M. J. (1989). The inheritance of acquired epigenetic variations. *J. Theor. Biol.*, **139**, 69–83.

Jablonka, E., Oborny, B., Molnar, I., Kisdi, E., Hofbauer, J. and Czaran, T. (1995). The adaptive advantage of phenotypic memory in changing environments. *Phil. Trans. R. Soc. Lond. B.*, **350**, 133–41.

Jacobson, C. D., Csernus, V. J., Shryne, J. E. and Gorski, R. A. (1981). The influence of gonadectomy, androgen exposure, or a gonadal graft in the neonatal rat on the volume of the sexually dimorphic nucleus of the preoptic area. *J. Neurosci.*, **1**, 1142–7.

Jaquet, D., Léger, J., Lévy-Marchal, C. and Czernichow, P. (2003). Low birth weight: effect on insulin sensitivity and lipid metabolism. *Horm. Res.*, **59**, 1–6.

Kaati, G., Bygren, L. O. and Edvinsson, S. (2002). Cardiovascular and diabetes mortality determined by nutrition during parents' and grandparents' slow growth period. *Eur. J. Hum. Genet.*, **10**, 682–8.

Kannisto, V., Christensen, K. and Vaupel, J. W. (1997). No increased mortality in later life for cohorts born during famine. *Am. J. Epidemiol.*, **145**, 987–94.

Khan, I. Y., Dekou, V., Douglas, G. *et al.* (2005). A high-fat diet during rat pregnancy or suckling induces cardiovascular dysfunction in adult offspring. *Am. J. Physiol. Regul. Integr. Comp. Physiol.*, **288**, R127–33.

King, J. C. (2003). The risk of maternal nutritional depletion and poor outcomes increases in early or closely spaced pregnancies. *J. Nutr.*, **133**, 1732–6S.

Kramer, S. (2003). The epidemiology of adverse pregnancy outcomes: an overview. *J. Nutr.*, **133**, 1592–6S.

Kwong, W. Y., Wild, A. E., Roberts, P., Willis, A. C. and Fleming, T. P. (2000). Maternal undernutrition during the preimplantation period of rat development causes blastocyst abnormalities and programming of postnatal hypertension. *Development*, **127**, 4195–202.

Lee, T. M. and Zucker, I. (1988). Vole infant development is influenced perinatally by maternal photoperiodic history. *Am. J. Physiol.*, **255**, R831–8.

Lee, T. M., Spears, N., Tuthill, C. R. and Zucker, I. (1989). Maternal melatonin treatment influences rates of neonatal development of meadow vole pups. *Biol. Reprod.*, **40**, 495–502.

Lumey, L. H. (1992). Decreased birthweights in infants after maternal *in utero* exposure to the Dutch famine of 1944–1945. *Paediatr. Perinat. Epidemiol.*, **6**, 240–53.

Mallard, C., Loeliger, M., Copolov, D. and Rees, S. (2000). Reduced number of neurons in the hippocampus and the cerebellum in the postnatal guinea-pig following intrauterine growth-restrictionG. *Neuroscience*, **100**, 327–33.

Metcalfe, N. B. and Monaghan, P. (2003). Growth versus lifespan: perspectives from evolutionary ecology. *Exp. Gerontol.*, **38**, 935–40.

Naeye, R. L. (1983). Maternal age, obstetric complications, and the outcome of pregnancy. *Obstet. Gynecol.*, **61**, 210–16.

Neel, J. V. (1962). Diabetes mellitus: a 'thrifty' genotype rendered detrimental by 'progress'? *Am. J. Hum. Genet.*, **14**, 353–62.

Ong, K. K., Preece, M., Emmett, P. M., Ahmed, M. L. and Dunger, D. B. (2002). Size at birth and early chidhood growth in relation to maternal smoking, parity and infant breast-feeding: Longitudinal birth cohort study and analysis. *Pediatr. Res.*, **52**, 863–7.

Osmond, C. and Barker, D. J. P. (2000). Fetal, infant, and childhood growth are predictors of coronary heart disease, diabetes, and hypertension in adult men and women. *Environ. Health Perspect.*, **108**, 545–53.

Ounsted, M. and Ounsted, C. (1973). *On Fetal Growth Rate: Its Variations and Their Consequences*. London: Heinemann.

Penin, X., Berge, C. and Baylac, M. (2002). Ontogenetic study of the skull in modern humans and the common chimpanzees: neotenic hypothesis reconsidered with a tridimensional procrustes analysis. *Am. J. Phys. Anthropol.*, **118**, 50–62.

Phillips, D. I. W., Handelsman, D. J., Eriksson, J. G., Forsen, T., Osmond, C. and Barker, D. J. P. (2001). Prenatal growth and subsequent marital status: longitudinal study. *BMJ*, **322**, 771.

Popkin, B. M. (2004). The nutrition transition: an overview of world patterns of change. *Nutr. Rev.*, **62**, S140–3.

Rao, S., Yajnik, C. S., Kanade, A. *et al.* (2001). Intake of micronutrient-rich foods in rural Indian mothers is associated with the size of their babies at birth: Pune maternal nutrition study. *J. Nutr.*, **131**, 1217–24.

Ravelli, A. C., van der Meulen, J. H., Michels, R. P. *et al.* (1998). Glucose tolerance in adults after prenatal exposure to famine. *Lancet*, **351**, 173–7.

Robinson, S. M., Crozier, S. R., Borland, S. E., Hammond, J., Barker, D. J. and Inskip, H. M. (2004). Impact of educational attainment on the quality of young women's diets. *Eur. J. Clin. Nutr.*, **58**, 1174–80.

Roseboom, T. J., van der Meulen, J. H., Ravelli, A. C., Osmond, C., Barker, D. J. P. and Bleker, O. P. (2001). Effects of prenatal exposure to the Dutch famine on adult disease in later life: an overview. *Mol. Cell. Endocrinol.*, **185**, 93–8.

Ross, M. G., Desai, M., Guerra, C. and Wang, S. (2005). Prenatal programming of hypernatremia and hypertension in neonatal lambs. *Am. J. Physiol. Regul. Integr. Comp. Physiol.*, **288**, R97–103.

Simpson, S. J., Raubenheimer, D., Behmer, S. T., Whitworth, A. and Wright, G. A. (2002). A comparison of nutritional regulation in solitarious- and gregarious-phase nymphs of the desert locust *Schistocerca gregaria*. *J. Exp. Biol.*, **205**, 121–9.

Singhal, A., Fewtrel, M., Cole, T. J. and Lucas, A. (2003). Low nutrient intake and early growth for later insulin resistance in adolescents born preterm. *Lancet*, **361**, 1089–97.

Singhal, A., Cole, T. J., Fewtrell, M. and Lucas, A. (2004). Breastmilk feeding and lipoprotein profile in adolescents born preterm: follow-up of a prospective randomised study. *Lancet*, **363**, 1571–8.

Stewart, R. J. C., Sheppard, H., Preece, R. and Waterlow, J. C. (1980). The effect of rehabilitation at different stages of development of rats marginally malnourished for ten to twelve generations. *Br. J. Nutr.*, **43**, 403–12.

Torrens, C., Brawley, L., Dance, C. S., Itoh, S., Poston, L. and Hanson, M. A. (2002). First evidence for transgenerational vascular programming in the rat protein restriction model. *J. Physiol.*, **543**, 41–2P.

Valeix, P., Preziosi, P., Rossignol, C., Farnier, M. A. and Hercberg, S. (1994). Relationship between urinary iodine concentration and hearing capacity in children. *Eur. J. Clin. Nutr.*, **48**, 54–9.

Vickers, M. H., Breier, B. H., Cutfield, W. S., Hofman, P. L. and Gluckman, P. D. (2000). Fetal origins of hyperphagia, obesity, and hypertension and postnatal amplification by hypercaloric nutrition. *Am. J. Physiol. Endocrinol. Metab.*, **279**, E83–7.

Waddington, C. H. (1957). *The Strategy of Genes: a Discussion of Some Aspects of Theoretical Biology*. London: George Allen & Unwin.

Wahlbeck, K., Forsen, T., Osmond, C., Barker, D. J. P. and Eriksson, J. G. (2001). Association of schizophrenia with low maternal body mass index, small size at birth, and thinness during childhood. *Arch. Gen. Psychiatry.*, **58**, 48–52.

Wallace, J., Bourke, D., Da Silva, P. and Aitken, R. (2001). Nutrient partitioning during adolescent pregnancy. *Reproduction*, **122**, 347–57.

Walton, A. and Hammond, J. (1938). The maternal effects on growth and conformation in shire horse–Shetland pony crosses. *Proc. Royal. Soc. Lond. B.*, **125**, 311–35.

Waterland, R. A. and Jirtle, R. L. (2004). Early nutrition, epigenetic changes at transposons and imprinted genes, and enhanced susceptibility to adult chronic diseases. *Nutrition*, **20**, 63–8.

Weaver, I. C. G., Cervoni, N., Champagne, F. A. *et al.* (2004). Epigenetic programming by maternal behavior. *Nat. Neurosci.*, **7**, 847–54.

West-Eberhard, M. J. (ed.) (2003). *Developmental Plasticity and Evolution*. New York: Oxford University Press.

Wolpert, L. (2002). Evolution and development. In *Principles of Development*, (ed. L. Wolpert, R. Beddington, T. Jessell, P. Lawrence, E. Meyerowitz and J. Smith). Oxford: Oxford University Press, pp. 493–519.

Yajnik, C. S. (2004). Early life origins of insulin resistance and type 2 diabetes in India and other Asian countries. *J. Nutr.*, **134**, 205–10.

4

The periconceptional and embryonic period

Tom P. Fleming

University of Southampton

Introduction

The periconceptional period of mammalian development has long been recognised as an early 'developmental window' during which environmental conditions may influence the pattern of future growth and physiology. For example, in early studies, it was found that in-vitro culture of mouse preimplantation embryos prior to transfer to recipient females lead to reduced fetal growth compared to in-vivo-derived fetuses (Bowman and McLaren 1970). The culture of ruminant embryos prior to transfer has also been linked with abnormal future growth and the so-called 'large offspring syndrome' (LOS), where fetal organomegaly is associated with perinatal mortality (reviewed in Sinclair *et al.* 2000). The concern from animal studies that preimplantation environment may alter embryo developmental potential has led to retrospective analysis of possible effects resulting from human in vitro fertilisation and assisted reproduction treatment (ART). Indeed, a number of 'outcome' studies in different parts of the world have identified a small increase in preterm delivery, low birthweight and perinatal mortality in singleton pregnancies following ART compared with that following natural conception (Hansen *et al.* 2002, Schieve *et al.* 2002).

The concept that embryo environment in vitro may modulate future development has been further expanded by a growing literature demonstrat-ing that similar phenomena may occur in vivo, in response to maternal diet and physiological status. Thus, in rats, maternal low-protein diet administered exclusively during the preimplantation period caused abnormal postnatal growth and organ size and onset of high blood pressure in a gender-specific manner (Kwong *et al.* 2000). High-protein diets fed to sheep during the periconceptional period associate with reduced developmental viability and increased fetal and birth weight, similar to the LOS phenotype (McEvoy *et al.* 1997). Periconceptional undernutrition in sheep also disturbs later fetal development and physiology (Edwards and McMillen 2002a, 2002b), and similar effects have been proposed for poor fetal growth and low birthweight in the human (Wynn and Wynn 1988). In addition, the link between periconceptional micronutrient intake, particularly folic acid and B12 vitamin, and suppression of neural tube defects later in development has been established (Ashworth and Antipatis 2001).

The sensitivity of the early embryo from diverse species to environmental conditions both in vitro and in vivo and the consequences for later development has clear implications and relevance for the developmental origins of health and disease (DOHaD) hypothesis. Changes in postnatal phenotype that can be traced back to embryo environment are broad and not restricted directly to growth, metabolic and/or cardiovascular status. For example, a recent study involving mouse in vitro culture

Developmental Origins of Health and Disease, ed. Peter Gluckman and Mark Hanson. Published by Cambridge University Press.
© P. D. Gluckman and M. A. Hanson 2006.

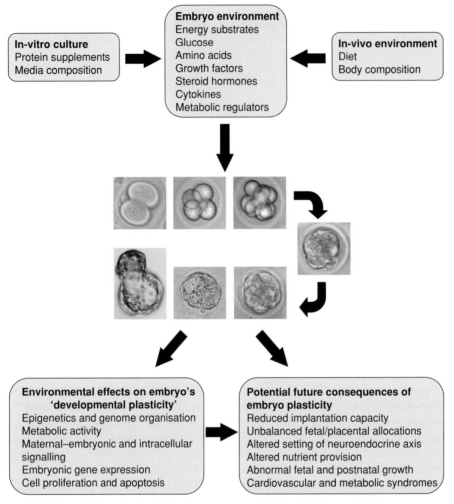

Figure 4.1 Schematic representing the interactions between the environment of the embryo and potential consequences. Potential key components of the embryo environment, modulated either in vitro or in vivo, are depicted. The embryo may elicit immediate responses demonstrating developmental plasticity which may result in future consequences. Different stages of preimplantation mouse embryo development are shown through early cleavage, compaction, cavitation and hatching.

has shown that culture conditions can associate with changed postnatal behaviour and memory characteristics (Ecker *et al.* 2004). From an evolutionary perspective, these diverse long-term alterations in phenotype accredited to early embryonic environment suggest a pivotal role for maternal–embryonic interactions and cues in the setting of fetal growth and development. We can perhaps consider a critical role for the early embryo in the 'perception' of mater-

nal nutrient supply and therefore what it is likely to be during later gestation, and in converting this information into a mechanistic process controlling its own development. Thus, developmental plasticity can be viewed as a pathway leading from maternal physiology through the embryo to a 'selected' and appropriate phenotype for fetal development and physiology. In this chapter, the mechanisms linking embryo environment to fetal and postnatal phenotype are considered (Fig. 4.1). Five critical aspects of embryo biology appear central to this discussion, namely epigenesis, metabolism, developmental signalling, gene expression and proliferation. The integration of these parameters, coupled with continued maternal interactions with the conceptus after implantation, are likely mediators of the developmental programme that may link periconceptional environment with postnatal health and physiology.

Embryos and epigenesis

Imprinted genes show parental allele-specific expression in response to heritable epigenetic modification at regulatory CpG domains, mediated by the pattern of DNA methylation (differentially methylated regions, DMRs) (Lucifero *et al.* 2004). Chromatin modelling is further dynamically organised by histone methylation and acetylation events (Reik *et al.* 2003) which collectively may coordinate imprinted gene expression. Imprinted genes are involved particularly in control of fetal growth (e.g., *Igf2*, *Igf2-r*) and placental growth and nutrient supply (e.g., *Igf2*, *Mash2*, *Ip1*, *Peg3*), and hence their activity in response to embryo environmental conditions are critical to understand (Constancia *et al.* 2002, Reik *et al.* 2003, Lucifero *et al.* 2004). Significantly, gametogenesis and preimplantation development are periods during which genomic imprints and structural organisation are subject to modification, such that susceptibility to environmental conditions may be heightened. Thus, demethylation of non-imprinted genes occurs consecutively on paternal and maternal alleles during mouse cleavage but the methylation status of imprinted genes needs to be maintained for control of allele-specific expression (Reik *et al.* 2003, Lucifero *et al.* 2004). A specific 'oocyte' DNA methyl transferase 1 (DNMT1o) appears responsible for this critical activity (Howell *et al.* 2001, Santos *et al.* 2002).

Mouse embryo culture conditions have been shown to alter the methylation pattern of specific imprinted genes. Thus, embryos cultured in Whitten's medium exhibit loss of allele-specific

methylation of *H19*, the regulator of *Igf2*, whilst embryos cultured in KSOM plus amino acids maintain normal *H19* methylation status (Doherty *et al.* 2000). Mouse embryos cultured in medium containing serum have been shown, after transfer, to give rise to fetuses that are smaller and exhibit reduced *H19* and *Igf2* expression and hypermethylated *H19* DMR compared to fetuses from embryos cultured in the absence of serum (Khosla *et al.* 2001), indicating that epigenetic alterations in the embryo appear heritable during development. Mouse extra-embryonic tissues also show disturbed *H19* methylation following embryo culture (Sasaki *et al.* 1995). In fetal sheep exhibiting LOS following embryo culture in medium containing serum, *Igf2-r* expression is retarded, thereby increasing the bioavailability of Igf2, a likely mediator of the enhanced growth associated with this syndrome (Young *et al.* 2001). Bovine fetuses derived from in vitro cultured embryos show elevated Igf2 in liver compared with in vivo controls (Blondin *et al.* 2000). Epigenetically derived changes in imprinted gene expression have recently also been identified in vivo; in response to maternal undernutrition, male rat blastocysts show reduced *H19* expression in the trophectoderm lineage compared to blastocysts from mothers fed normal diet (Kwong *et al.* 2003).

Embryo metabolism in response to environmental conditions

Adverse environmental conditions may influence embryo metabolism, inducing a stress response, which may lead to altered long-term growth and development. This phenomenon is perhaps best illustrated with respect to hyperglycaemic conditions and amino acid availability. The preferred substrate for embryo energy metabolism during cleavage in different species switches from pyruvate during early cycles to glucose during morula and blastocyst stages (Hardy *et al.* 1989, Leese 2003), and this change appears to be reflected in the nutrient composition of the female tract (Gardner *et al.* 1996). Thus, glucose consumption increases in late cleavage, and this capacity has been shown to correlate positively with fetal developmental potential after transfer (Gardner and Leese 1987). However, in hyperglycaemic conditions evident in rodent diabetic models, glucose levels are substantially increased and act negatively on embryo developmental potential, since this condition induces a reduction in glucose transporter expression at both mRNA and protein levels (Chi *et al.* 2000). As a consequence, glucose starvation may result, leading to a stress response including increased apoptosis and chromatin degradation, and reduced cellular proliferation within the blastocyst (Lea *et al.* 1996, Hinck *et al.* 2003). Embryos derived from a diabetic environment, after transfer, show increased pregnancy loss and fetal growth retardation (Lea *et al.* 1996, Moley 2001).

The mechanism of embryo-derived hyperglycaemic reduction in future developmental potential may in part reside in disturbed cellular interactions around the time of implantation. Thus, the blastocyst inner cell mass (ICM) lineage, the progenitor of the entire fetus, expresses *Fgf4*, which acts as a proliferative signal on the outer trophectoderm lineage, the progenitor of the chorioallantoic placenta. In diabetic models, this signal cascade is perturbed and may underlie a dysregulation of differentiative pathways associated with nutrient support (Leunda-Casi *et al.* 2001). The embryo responsiveness to the glucose/insulin balance associated with hyperglycaemia is substantiated by the capacity of insulin both to stimulate mouse ICM proliferation (Kaye 1997) and, after embryo transfer, to induce an increase in fetal growth rate (Kaye and Gardner 1999). Hyperglycaemia is also implicated as a contributor to embryo sensitivity to maternal low-protein diet in the rat. Thus, this dietary treatment has been shown to induce elevated glucose and reduced insulin levels in mothers during blastocyst development, coinciding with reduced blastocyst cellular proliferation and leading to postnatal growth alteration and hypertension (Kwong *et al.* 2000). Maternal low-protein diet in rats has also been associated with an increase in glycolysis in conceptuses during organogenesis after implantation (Leese and Isherwood-Peel 1999).

Amino acid availability is a second potential mediator of altered embryo metabolism in response to environmental conditions with long-term consequences. Amino acids have multiple roles in the embryo evident in different species; apart from protein synthesis, they stimulate blastocyst formation and contribute to energy production, osmoregulation, pH control and signal transduction pathways coordinating the developmental programme (Van Winkle 2001). Sodium-dependent and -independent amino acid transport systems are expressed in embryos to accommodate amino acid uptake and turnover (Van Winkle 2001). A key link between amino acid turnover, measured non-invasively in the human embryo during early cleavage, and potential to form a blastocyst has been demonstrated (Houghton *et al.* 2002). Interestingly, this association takes the form of a reduced turnover pattern coinciding with an increased developmental potential, suggesting that amino acid flux, like glycolytic rate, is an indicator of stress (Leese 2002). Culture of mouse and sheep embryos in media containing amino acids stimulates early development, and has been shown to significantly improve fetal development after transfer (Thompson *et al.* 1995, Lane and Gardner 1997). Whilst the relative amino acid composition in the embryo environment is clearly critical with respect to developmental potential, it has also been identified that breakdown of amino acids in culture to produce ammonium ions can cause a reduction in blastocyst cellular proliferation, increased apoptosis, abnormal imprinted gene *H19* expression and, after transfer, lead to impaired fetal development (Lane and Gardner 1994, 2003).

Maternal low-protein diet in rats during the periconceptional period also leads to depletion in serum essential amino acids, associated with postnatal changes in growth and physiology (Kwong *et al.* 2000). Diet-induced reductions in amino acid levels directly impact on embryo environment in vivo since analysis of uterine fluid in mice shows similar reductions to those identified in maternal serum (Porter *et al.* 2003). The importance of amino acids to embryo potential in this respect is considered further below in terms of signal transduction pathways.

For consideration of the importance of mitochondrial metabolism in embryo potential, see Chapter 6.

Signal transduction and embryo developmental potential

At the time of fertilisation, the sperm induces a signal transduction cascade within the egg which collectively blocks further sperm fusion, induces cortical granule exocytosis, activates the egg to resume the cell cycle, and initiates expression from the embryonic genome, most significantly of the programme controlling early development of the embryo (Carroll 2001). This cascade is mediated by sperm-released phospholipase C, which activates the oocyte phosphatidylinositol second-messenger pathway, causing intracellular calcium release and regular oscillations and activation of conventional protein kinase C (cPKC). The amplitude, frequency and duration of calcium oscillations during the first few hours following fertilisation, together with cPKC activation, mediate the diverse downstream effectors required to initiate the developmental programme (Ducibella *et al.* 2002, Halet *et al.* 2004). When the number and pattern of calcium oscillations are modified experimentally, later developmental processes are affected, including the number of cells within blastocyst ICM and trophectoderm lineages, the rate of apoptosis and the extent of fetal development in parthenogenetic embryos (Bos-Mikich *et al.* 1997, Gordo *et al.* 2000, Ozil *et al.* 2001). These intriguing findings require further study to elucidate mechanisms, but it is clear that signal transduction events associated with fertilisation have a profound influence on future development and may be subject to environmental sensitivity.

Amino acid signalling via the mammalian target of rapamycin (mTOR) may also be susceptible to environmental conditions. mTOR is a serine–threonine kinase pathway with broad roles in activating, through phosphorylation, regulatory proteins involved in protein translation and biosynthesis (Meijer *et al.* 2004, Tokunaga *et al.* 2004), and it has been implicated in several roles in growth,

patterning and differentiation during development (e.g., Hentges *et al.* 2001). During early development, mTOR signalling is required to induce an invasive and migratory phenotype within blastocyst trophectoderm cells necessary for implantation and continued proliferative activity (Martin and Sutherland 2001, Martin *et al.* 2003). mTOR signalling is controlled by leucine bioavailability, and this essential amino acid has been shown to be significantly and consistently depleted both in rodent serum and in uterine fluid during the time of blastocyst development, in response to maternal low-protein diet (Kwong *et al.* 2000, Porter *et al.* 2003). It will be of interest to establish how important this signalling pathway may be in the maternal–embryonic interactions that set developmental plasticity.

A further signalling pathway of particular relevance in embryo environmental sensitivity is that involving ghrelin, the ligand for the growth hormone secretogogue receptor (GHSR) which is implicated in modulating feeding behaviour and embryo metabolism. Ghrelin is detectable within mouse blastocysts as well as in uterine fluid and endometrium, and GHSR is expressed within the embryo (Kawamura *et al.* 2003). Uterine levels of ghrelin increase during fasting and this hormone can suppress the rate of embryo development in vitro, indicating that this pathway may provide a mechanism to coordinate embryo metabolic demands and proliferative potential with maternal nutrient availability (Kawamura *et al.* 2003).

Gene expression changes in embryos in response to environment

Clearly, changes in metabolic and signalling activity in response to in vivo or in vitro environment will be accompanied by phenotypic changes within embryos associated with gene expression and homeostasis. Changes in stress gene expression including *hsp70.1* and *CHOP10* occur in bovine and rodent embryos in response to various conditions (Christians *et al.* 1995, Fontanier-Razzaq *et al.* 2001). Growth regulators such as *IGf1* and *IGf2* are expressed at lower levels in mouse embryos in vitro compared to in vivo (Stojanov *et al.* 1999, Stojanov and O'Neill 2001), while culture medium containing amino acids causes increased expression of these factors and their receptors, compared with medium lacking amino acids (Ho *et al.* 1995). The types of genes found to be susceptible to environmental conditions in embryos include those genes known to be critical for incipient differentiation (Niemann and Wrenzycki 2000). For example, genes important in trophectoderm epithelial maturation and adhesion are significantly down-regulated in bovine embryos cultured in vitro compared with in vivo embryos (Miller *et al.* 2003). Whilst it is difficult to evaluate the human embryo in this way, it has been shown that wide variation in the level of expression of genes involved in differentiation and apoptosis do occur in human embryos in vitro, alongside a similar variation in their developmental potential (Hardy 1997, Spanos *et al.* 2002, Ghassemifar *et al.* 2003).

Embryo environment and cellular proliferation

One consistent feature of embryo development across species in response to adverse culture or in-vivo environment is a reduction in the proliferation of the blastocyst stem cell lineages for fetal and placental development, the ICM and trophectoderm, respectively. Thus, cell numbers for these lineages are reduced in cultured human embryos in the absence of sufficient growth factors, amino acids and metabolites (Hardy *et al.* 2002). Similarly, the in-vivo environment with respect to maternal age (Jurisicova *et al.* 1998), dietary protein level (Kwong *et al.* 2000) and zinc composition (Peters *et al.* 1993) all may alter the normal pattern of cellular proliferation occurring within the rodent blastocyst.

The consequences of depleted proliferation within the embryo for subsequent fetal development have been examined mainly in the mouse. Different methods used to reduce these stem cell populations, such as cell ablation and embryo bisection in early cleavage, have demonstrated the resilient nature of embryos after transfer, such that compensatory proliferative activity can occur during post-implantation development up to mid gestation with good rates of fetal survival. However, where blastocyst ICM cell numbers have been artificially depleted, the proportion of ICM derivatives during later gestation remains decreased, the rate of development including primitive endoderm formation and gastrulation can be slowed down, and pregnancy loss can increase (Tsunoda and McLaren 1983, Rands 1986, Tam 1988, Power and Tam 1993, Papaioannou and Ebert 1995, Hishinuma *et al.* 1996). It is not surprising, therefore, that the mouse preimplantation embryo is equipped with cell biological mechanisms associated with cell–cell interactions, spindle orientation and cell shape that collectively maintain the number and ratio of cells within ICM and trophectoderm lineages within a relatively narrow range (Fleming 1987, Pickering *et al.* 1988).

Changes in blastocyst cell numbers brought about by varied environmental conditions have also been shown to correlate with changes in fetal or postnatal development. For example, this has been demonstrated in response to rodent maternal diet (Kwong *et al.* 2000), mouse in vitro embryo culture in relation to amino acid availability (Lane and Gardner 1997), and bovine embryo culture compared with in vivo embryos (Van Soom *et al.* 1997). Similar evidence is available for the human embryo in that quantitative measurements of the ICM size is positively correlated with implantation rate (Richter *et al.* 2001).

From embryo plasticity to fetal physiology

We have seen that preimplantation embryos may interact with their environment either in vitro or in vivo in diverse ways which may alter their phenotype with respect to epigenetic status of the genome, metabolic activity and energy production, signalling pathways, gene and protein expression profile, and cellular proliferation. All of these examples of embryo developmental plasticity have been associated with long-term changes in potential, affecting either fetal or postnatal growth, metabolism and physiology. We need now to consider how these early markers of environmental sensitivity may lead on to changes in fetal growth and physiology.

Maternal–fetal neuroendocrinal signalling is believed to play a pivotal role in coordinating the intrauterine growth trajectory following sustained dietary undernutrition throughout pregnancy. Thus, maternal undernutrition during gestation increases the level of expression of the maternal glucocorticoids (GC, cortisol, corticosterone) which can affect the physiological status of the developing fetus (Lesage et al. 2001). Whilst the conceptus would normally be protected against rising maternal GC by placental 11β-hydroxysteroid dehydrogenase type 2 (11β-HSD2), which converts GC into an inactive state (Brown et al. 1996), placental levels of 11β-HSD2 become depleted under conditions of maternal undernutrition, causing enhanced fetal exposure to maternal GC (Langley-Evans et al. 1996, Bertram et al. 2001). Consequently the setting of the fetal hypothalamus–pituitary–adrenal (HPA) axis may alter, leading to elevation of fetal GC levels, which, through GC receptors, can change several gene expression pathways underlying growth and metabolism, including cardiovascular and renal physiology (O'Regan et al. 2001, Bertram and Hanson 2002).

Neuroendocrinal signalling has been shown to be similarly affected in animal models following maternal undernutrition during the periconceptional period where embryo plasticity has been altered. Thus, maternal dietary restriction in sheep before mating and up to seven days of development, before return to normal diet for the remainder of gestation, leads to higher levels of fetal plasma pituitary adrenocorticotropic hormone (ACTH), a greater GC response to corticotropin-releasing hormone, and an increase in fetal blood pressure in twin pregnancies (Edwards and McMillen 2002a, 2002b). This change in fetal physiology may derive from reduced trophectoderm development, from which placental hormones such as prostaglandin E$_2$ derive, and which influence ACTH secretion later in gestation (Hollingsworth et al. 1995, Edwards and McMillen 2002a). In the rat, maternal low-protein diet during the preimplantation period causes reduced trophectoderm proliferation and altered postnatal growth and hypertension (Kwong et al. 2000). This also results in fetal liver elevation of 11β-HSD type 1 gene expression which converts GC to an active state (Kwong et al. in preparation). This in turn indicates a link between early embryonic environment and maternal–fetal neuroendocrine signalling.

Further mechanisms which may associate early embryonic environment with altered postnatal physiology are likely to derive from effects upon the balance of placental–fetal growth and function, which may derive from effects on embryo lineage allocation and epigenetics. Sensitivity of imprinted gene expression within embryos (discussed above) may include those contributing to placental growth and nutrient exchange. Thus, the Igf2 gene includes a placental-specific isoform, Igf2P0, which is expressed exclusively in the labyrinthine trophoblast; deletion of Igf2P0 causes reduced placental growth and transport activity and subsequently reduced fetal growth (Constancia et al. 2002). Similarly, there is evidence that the LOS phenotype in ruminants may derive from abnormal allantoic development and defective placentation (Thompson and Peterson 2000, Bertolini and Anderson 2002).

Conclusions

The concept that the early embryo is merely the conduit by which cellularisation of the new zygotic genome occurs for the purposes of shaping morphogenesis and segregation of fetal and extraembryonic lineages is now obsolete. The evidence is now overwhelming, pointing to a dynamic relationship between the embryo and its environment. This relationship is multifactorial, operating at epigenetic, metabolic, cellular and signalling levels, and results not only in the plasticity evident within the embryonic phenotype but also in a legacy that persists throughout gestation and beyond. Whilst our understanding of these complex associations, both between environment and embryo and between embryo and future developmental potential, is still very sketchy and descriptive, it is now a major focus internationally to decipher mechanisms which can ultimately be translated into health care and protection against adverse consequences.

ACKNOWLEDGMENTS

I am grateful for financial support within my laboratory from the Medical Research Council, UK, and National Institutes of Health, USA, for research into mechanisms of embryo environmental sensitivity.

REFERENCES

Ashworth, C. J. and Antipatis, C. (2001). Micronutrient programming of development throughout gestation. *Reproduction*, **122**, 527–35.

Bertolini, M. and Anderson, G. B. (2002). The placenta as a contributor to production of large calves. *Theriogenology*, **57**, 181–7.

Bertram, C. E. and Hanson, M. A. (2002). Prenatal programming of postnatal endocrine responses by glucocorticoids. *Reproduction*, **124**, 459–67.

Bertram. C., Trowern, A. R., Copin, N., Jackson, A. A. and Whorwood, C. B. (2001). The maternal diet during pregnancy programs altered expression of the glucocorticoid receptor and type 2 11beta-hydroxysteroid dehydrogenase: potential molecular mechanisms underlying the programming of hypertension in utero. *Endocrinology*, **142**, 2841–53.

Blondin, P., Farin, P. W., Crosier, A. E., Alexander, J. E. and Farin, C. E. (2000). In vitro production of embryos alters levels of insulin-like growth factor-II messenger ribonucleic acid in bovine fetuses 63 days after transfer. *Biol. Reprod.*, **62**, 384–9.

Bos-Mikich, A., Whittingham, D. G. and Jones, K. T. (1997). Meiotic and mitotic Ca^{2+} oscillations affect cell composition in resulting blastocysts. *Dev. Biol.*, **182**, 172–9.

Bowman, P. and McLaren, A. (1970). Viability and growth of mouse embryos after in vitro culture and fusion. *J. Embryol. Exp. Morphol.*, **23**, 693–704.

Brown, R. W., Diaz, R., Robson, A. C. *et al.* (1996). The ontogeny of 11 beta-hydroxysteroid dehydrogenase type 2 and mineralocorticoid receptor gene expression reveal intricate control of glucocorticoid action in development. *Endocrinology*, **137**, 794–7.

Carroll, J. (2001). The initiation and regulation of Ca^{2+} signalling at fertilization in mammals. *Semin. Cell Dev. Biol.*, **12**, 37–43.

Chi, M. M., Pingsterhaus, J., Carayannopoulos, M. and Moley, K. H. (2000). Decreased glucose transporter expression triggers BAX-dependent apoptosis in the murine blastocyst. *J. Biol. Chem.*, **275**, 40252–7.

Christians, E., Campion, E., Thompson, E. M. and Renard, J. P. (1995). Expression of the HSP 70.1 gene, a landmark of early zygotic activity in the mouse embryo, is restricted to the first burst of transcription. *Development*, **121**, 113–22.

Constancia, M., Hemberger, M., Hughes, J. *et al.* (2002). Placental-specific IGF-II is a major modulator of placental and fetal growth. *Nature*, **417**, 945–8.

Doherty, A. S., Mann, M. R., Tremblay, K. D., Bartolomei, M. S. and Schultz, R. M. (2000). Differential effects of culture on imprinted H19 expression in the preimplantation mouse embryo. *Biol. Reprod.*, **62**, 1526–35.

Ducibella. T., Huneau, D., Angelichio, E. *et al.* (2002). Egg-to-embryo transition is driven by differential responses to Ca(2+) oscillation number. *Dev. Biol.*, **250**, 280–91.

Ecker, D. J., Stein, P., Xu, Z. *et al.* (2004). Long-term effects of culture of preimplantation mouse embryos on behavior. *Proc. Natl. Acad. Sci. USA*, **101**, 1595–1600.

Edwards, L. J. and McMillen, I. C. (2002a). Impact of maternal undernutrition during the periconceptional period, fetal number, and fetal sex on the development of the hypothalamo-pituitary adrenal axis in sheep during late gestation. *Biol. Reprod.*, **66**, 1562–9.

(2002b). Periconceptional nutrition programs development of the cardiovascular system in the fetal sheep. *Am. J. Physiol. Regul. Integr. Comp. Physiol.*, **283**, R669–79.

Fleming, T. P. (1987). A quantitative analysis of cell allocation to trophectoderm and inner cell mass in the mouse blastocyst. *Dev. Biol.*, **119**, 520–31.

Fontanier-Razzaq, N., McEvoy, T. G., Robinson, J. J. and Rees, W. D. (2001). DNA damaging agents increase gadd153 (CHOP-10) messenger RNA levels in bovine preimplantation embryos cultured in vitro. *Biol. Reprod.*, **64**, 1386–91.

Gardner, D. K. and Leese, H. J. (1987). Assessment of embryo viability prior to transfer by the noninvasive measurement of glucose uptake. *J. Exp. Zool.*, **242**, 103–5.

Gardner, D. K., Lane, M., Calderon, I. and Leeton, J. (1996). Environment of the preimplantation human embryo in vivo: metabolite analysis of oviduct and uterine fluids and metabolism of cumulus cells. *Fertil. Steril.*, **65**, 349–53.

Ghassemifar, M. R., Eckert, J. J., Houghton, F. D., Picton, H. M., Leese, H. J. and Fleming, T. P. (2003). Gene expression regulating epithelial intercellular junction biogenesis during human blastocyst development in vitro. *Mol. Hum. Reprod.*, **9**, 245–52.

Gordo, A. C., Wu, H., He, C. L. and Fissore, R. A. (2000). Injection of sperm cytosolic factor into mouse metaphase II oocytes induces different developmental fates according to the frequency of [Ca(2+)](i) oscillations and oocyte age. *Biol. Reprod.*, **62**, 1370–9.

Halet, G., Tunwell, R., Parkinson, S. J. and Carroll, J. (2004). Conventional PKCs regulate the temporal pattern of Ca^{2+} oscillations at fertilization in mouse eggs. *J. Cell. Biol.*, **164**, 1033–44.

Hansen, M., Kurinczuk, J. J., Bower, C. and Webb, S. (2002). The risk of major birth defects after intracytoplasmic sperm injection and in vitro fertilization. *N. Engl. J. Med.*, **346**, 725–30.

Hardy, K. (1997). Cell death in the mammalian blastocyst. *Mol. Hum. Reprod.*, **3**, 919–25.

Hardy, K. and Spanos, S. (2002). Growth factor expression and function in the human and mouse preimplantation embryo. *J. Endocrinol.*, **172**, 221–36.

Hardy, K., Hooper, M. A. K., Handyside, A. H., Rutherford, A. J., Winston, R. M. L. and Leese, H. J. (1989). Non-invasive measurement of glucose and pyruvate uptake by individual human oocytes and preimplantation embryos. *Hum. Reprod.*, **4**, 188–91.

Hentges, K. E., Sirry, B., Gingeras, A. C. *et al.* (2001). FRAP/mTOR is required for proliferation and patterning during embryonic development in the mouse. *Proc. Natl. Acad. Sci. USA*, **98**, 13796–801.

Hinck, L., Thissen, J. P. and De Hertogh, R. (2003). Identification of caspase-6 in rat blastocysts and its implication in the induction of apoptosis by high glucose. *Biol. Reprod.*, **68**, 1808–12.

Hishinuma, M., Takahashi, Y. and Kanagawa, H. (1996). Post-implantation development of demi-embryos and induction of decidual cell reaction in mice. *Theriogenology*, **45**, 1187–1200.

Ho, Y., Wigglesworth, K., Eppig, J. J. and Schultz, R. M. (1995). Preimplantation development of mouse embryos in KSOM: augmentation by amino acids and analysis of gene expression. *Mol. Reprod. Dev.*, **41**, 232–8.

Hollingsworth, S. A., Deayton, J. M., Young, I. R. and Thorburn, G. D. (1995). Prostaglandin E_2 administered to fetal sheep increases the plasma concentration of adreno-corticotropin (ACTH) and the proportion of ACTH in low molecular weight forms. *Endocrinology*, **136**, 1233–40.

Houghton, F. D., Hawkhead, J. A., Humpherson, P. G. *et al.* (2002). Non-invasive amino acid turnover predicts human embryo developmental capacity. *Hum. Reprod.*, **17**, 999–1005.

Howell, C. Y., Bestor, T. H., Ding, F. *et al.* (2001). Genomic imprinting disrupted by a maternal effect mutation in the Dnmt1 gene. *Cell*, **104**, 829–38.

Jurisicova, A., Rogers, I., Fasciani, A., Casper, R. F. and Varmuza, S. (1998). Effect of maternal age and conditions of fertilization on programmed cell death during murine preimplantation embryo development. *Mol. Hum. Reprod.*, **4**, 139–45.

Kawamura, K., Sato, N., Fukuda, J. *et al.* (2003). Ghrelin inhibits the development of mouse preimplantation embryos in vitro. *Endocrinology*, **144**, 2623–33.

Kaye, P. L. (1997). Preimplantation growth factor physiology. *Rev. Reprod.*, **2**, 121–7.

Kaye, P. L. and Gardner, H. G. (1999). Preimplantation access to maternal insulin and albumin increases fetal growth rate in mice. *Hum. Reprod.*, **14**, 3052–9.

Khosla, S., Dean, W., Brown, D., Reik, W. and Feil, R. (2001). Culture of preimplantation mouse embryos affects fetal development and the expression of imprinted genes. *Biol. Reprod.*, **64**, 918–26.

Kwong, W. Y., Wild, A. E., Roberts, P., Willis, A. C. and Fleming, T. P. (2000). Maternal undernutrition during the preimplantation period of rat development causes blastocyst abnormalities and programming of postnatal hypertension. *Development*, **127**, 4195–202.

Kwong, W. Y., Miller, D. J., Wild, A. E., Osmond, C. and Fleming, T. P. (2003). Effect of maternal low protein diet on imprinted gene expression in the rat preimplantation embryo. *Pediatr. Res.*, **53**, 46A.

Lane, M. and Gardner, D. K. (1994). Increase in postimplantation development of cultured mouse embryos by amino acids and induction of fetal retardation and exencephaly by ammonium ions. *J. Reprod. Fertil.*, **102**, 305–12.

(1997). Differential regulation of mouse embryo development and viability by amino acids. *J. Reprod. Fertil.*, **109**, 153–64.

(2003). Ammonium induces aberrant blastocyst differentiation, metabolism, pH regulation, gene expression and subsequently alters fetal development in the mouse. *Biol. Reprod.*, **69**, 1109–17.

Langley-Evans, S. C., Phillips, G. J., Benediktsson, R. *et al.* (1996). Protein intake in pregnancy, placental glucocorticoid metabolism and the programming of hypertension in the rat. *Placenta*, **17**, 169–72.

Lea, R. G., McCracken, J. E., McIntyre, S. S., Smith, W. and Baird, J. (1996). Disturbed development of preimplantation embryo in the insulin-dependent diabetic BB/E rat. *Diabetes*, **45**, 1463–70.

Leese, H. J. (2002). Quiet please, do not disturb: a hypothesis of embryo metabolism and viability. *Bioessays*, **24**, 845–9.

(2003). What does an embryo need? *Hum. Fertil. (Camb.)*, **6**, 180–5.

Leese, H. J. and Isherwood-Peel, G. (1999). Early embryo nutrition and disorders in later life. In *Fetal Programming:*

Influences on Development and Disease in Later Life (ed. P. M. S. O'Brien, T. Wheeler and D. J. P. Barker). London: RCOG Press, pp. 104–16.

Lesage, J., Blondeau, B., Grino, M., Breant, B. and Dupouy, J. P. (2001). Maternal undernutrition during late gestation induces fetal overexposure to glucocorticoids and intrauterine growth retardation, and disturbs the hypothalamo-pituitary adrenal axis in the newborn rat. *Endocrinology*, **142**, 1692–1702.

Leunda-Casi, A., De Hertogh, R. and Pampfer, S. (2001). Decreased expression of fibroblast growth factor-4 and associated dysregulation of trophoblast differentiation in mouse blastocysts exposed to high D-glucose in vitro. *Diabetologia*, **44**, 1318–25.

Lucifero, D., Chaillet, J. R. and Trasler, J. M. (2004). Potential significance of genomic imprinting defects for reproduction and assisted reproductive technology. *Hum. Reprod. Update*, **10**, 3–18.

Martin, P. M. and Sutherland, A. E. (2001). Exogenous amino acids regulate trophectoderm differentiation in the mouse blastocyst through an mTOR-dependent pathway. *Dev. Biol.*, **240**, 182–93.

Martin, P. M., Sutherland, A. E. and Van Winkle, L. J. (2003). Amino acid transport regulates blastocyst implantation. *Biol. Reprod.*, **69**, 1101–8.

McEvoy, T. G., Robinson, J. J., Aitken, R. P., Findlay, P. A. and Robertson, I. S. (1997). Dietary excesses of urea influence the viability and metabolism of preimplantation sheep embryos and may affect fetal growth among survivors. *Anim. Reprod. Sci.*, **47**, 71–90.

Meijer, A. J. and Dubbelhuis, P. F. (2004). Amino acid signalling and the integration of metabolism. *Biochem. Biophys. Res. Commun.*, **313**, 397–403.

Miller, D. J., Eckert, J. J., Lazzari, G. *et al.* (2003). Tight junction mRNA expression levels in bovine embryos are dependent upon the ability to compact and in vitro culture methods. *Biol. Reprod.*, **68**, 1394–1402.

Moley, K. H. (2001). Hyperglycemia and apoptosis: mechanisms for congenital malformations and pregnancy loss in diabetic women. *Trends Endocrinol. Metab.*, **12**, 78–82.

Niemann, H. and Wrenzycki, C. (2000). Alterations of expression of developmentally important genes in preimplantation bovine embryos by in vitro culture conditions: implications for subsequent development. *Theriogenology*, **53**, 21–34.

O'Regan, D., Welberg, L. L., Holmes, M. C. and Seckl, J. R. (2001). Glucocorticoid programming of pituitary–adrenal function: mechanisms and physiological consequences. *Semin. Neonatol.*, **6**, 319–29.

Ozil, J. P. and Huneau, D. (2001). Activation of rabbit oocytes: the impact of the Ca^{2+} signal regime on development. *Development*, **128**, 917–28.

Papaioannou, V. E. and Ebert, K. M. (1995). Mouse half embryos: viability and allocation of cells in the blastocyst. *Dev. Dyn.*, **203**, 393–8.

Peters, J. M., Wiley, L. M., Zidenberg-Cherr, S. and Keen, C. L. (1993). Influence of periconceptional zinc deficiency on embryonic plasma membrane function in mice. *Teratog. Carcinog. Mutagen.*, **13**, 15–21.

Pickering, S. J., Maro, B., Johnson, M. H. and Skepper, J. N. (1988). The influence of cell contact on the division of mouse 8-cell blastomeres. *Development*, **103**, 353–63.

Porter, R., Humpherson, P., Fussing, P., Cameron, I., Osmond, C. and Fleming, T. P. (2003). Metabolic programming of the blastocyst within the uterine environment. *Pediatr. Res.*, **53**, 46A.

Power, M. A. and Tam, P. P. L. (1993). Onset of gastrulation, morphogenesis and somitogenesis in mouse embryos displaying compensatory growth. *Anat. Embryol.*, **187**, 493–504.

Rands, G. F. (1986). Size regulation in the mouse embryo. II. The development of half embryos. *J. Embryol. Exp. Morphol.*, **98**, 209–17.

Reik, W., Santos, F. and Dean, W. (2003). Mammalian epigenomics: reprogramming the genome for development and therapy. *Theriogenology*, **59**, 21–32.

Richter, K. S., Harris, D. C., Daneshmand, S. T. and Shapiro, B. S. (2001). Quantitative grading of a human blastocyst: optimal inner cell mass size and shape. *Fertil. Steril.*, **76**, 1157–67.

Santos, F., Hendrich, B., Reik, W. and Dean, W. (2002). Dynamic reprogramming of DNA methylation in the early mouse embryo. *Dev. Biol.*, **241**, 172–82.

Sasaki, H., Ferguson-Smith, A. C., Shum, A. S., Barton, S. C. and Surani, M. A. (1995). Temporal and spatial regulation of H19 imprinting in normal and uniparental mouse embryos. *Development*, **121**, 4195–202.

Schieve, L. A., Meikle, S. F., Ferre, C., Peterson, H. B., Jeng, G. and Wilcox, L. S. (2002). Low and very low birth weight in infants conceived with use of assisted reproductive technology. *N. Engl. J. Med.*, **346**, 731–7.

Sinclair, K. D., Young, L. E., Wilmut, I. and McEvoy, T. G. (2000). In-utero overgrowth in ruminants following embryo culture: lessons from mice and a warning to men. *Hum. Reprod. Suppl.*, **5**, 68–86.

Spanos, S., Rice, S., Karagiannis, P. *et al.* (2002). Caspase activity and expression of cell death genes during development of human preimplantation embryos. *Reproduction*, **124**, 353–63.

Stojanov, T. and O'Neill, C. (2001). In vitro fertilization causes epigenetic modifications to the onset of gene expression from the zygotic genome in mice. *Biol. Reprod.*, **64**, 696–705.

Stojanov, T., Alechna, S. and O'Neill, C. (1999). In vitro fertilization and culture of mouse embryos in vitro significantly retards the onset of insulin-like growth factor-II expression from the zygotic genome. *Mol. Hum. Reprod.*, **5**, 116–124.

Tam, P. P. (1988). Postimplantation development of mitomycin C-treated mouse blastocysts. *Teratology*, **37**, 205–12.

Thompson, J. G. and Peterson, A. J. (2000). Bovine embryo culture in vitro: new developments and post-transfer consequences. *Hum. Reprod.*, **15**, (Suppl. 5), 59–67.

Thompson, J. G., Gardner, D. K., Pugh, P. A., McMillan, W. H. and Tervit, H. R. (1995). Lamb birth weight is affected by culture system utilized during in vitro pre-elongation development of ovine embryos. *Biol. Reprod.*, **53**, 1385–91.

Tokunaga, C., Yoshino, K. and Yonezawa, K. (2004). mTOR integrates amino acid- and energy-sensing pathways. *Biochem. Biophys. Res. Commun.*, **313**, 443–6.

Tsunoda, Y. and McLaren, A. (1983). Effect of various procedures on the viability of mouse embryos containing half the normal number of blastomeres. *J. Reprod. Fertil.*, **69**, 315–22.

Van Soom, A., Boerjan, M. L., Bols, P. E. *et al.* (1997). Timing of compaction and inner cell allocation in bovine embryos produced in vivo after superovulation. *Biol. Reprod.*, **57**, 1041–9.

Van Winkle, L. J. (2001). Amino acid transport regulation and early embryo development. *Biol. Reprod.*, **64**, 1–12.

Wynn, M. and Wynn, A. (1988). Nutrition around conception and the prevention of low birthweight. *Nutr. Health*, **6**, 37–52.

Young, L. E., Fernandes, K., McEvoy, T. G. *et al.* (2001). Epigenetic change in IGF2R is associated with fetal overgrowth after sheep embryo culture. *Nat. Genet.*, **27**, 153–4.

5

Epigenetic mechanisms

Emma Whitelaw[1] and David Garrick[2]

[1]University of Sydney
[2]Oxford University

Introduction

There is a growing awareness that whether or not a gene is actively expressed within a particular cell is determined not only by the primary nucleotide sequence of the gene and its regulatory elements, but also by changes in the way the DNA is modified and packaged within the nucleus. This non-sequence-based information is termed epigenetic. Epigenetic changes include methylation of the DNA itself, and modifications of the histone proteins that package the DNA within chromosomes. The pattern of epigenetic information varies from cell type to cell type and is reflected by the cell-specific profile of gene expression. Once established in a differentiated cell type, these epigenetic signals are stably inherited through mitosis, and are essential to maintain the correct gene expression profile within cells of that type for the life of the organism. The acquisition and maintenance of the correct epigenetic profile is therefore essential for normal development. The past decade has witnessed an explosion in our understanding of so-called 'epigenetic diseases', where the disruption of an epigenetic signal results in the inappropriate expression or silencing of one or more genes, giving rise to the disease phenotype. The aims of this chapter are to introduce the chemical nature of the major epigenetic signals, to discuss epigenetic processes which take place during normal development, and to briefly review some

of the important examples of human diseases arising due to breakdowns in epigenetic processes.

The nature of epigenetic information

DNA methylation

DNA methylation, the best-characterised epigenetic modification, refers to the enzymatic attachment of methyl moieties at the C^5 position of cytosine residues in genomic DNA. DNA methylation is not universal but has been conserved among higher eukaryotes with complex genomes. In mammals, the majority of methylated cytosines are situated within the symmetrical dinucleotide 5'-CpG-3', and in human somatic cells some 70–90% of all CpG dinucleotides exist in the methylated form. Those CpGs that escape methylation are tightly clustered within the genome, forming so-called CpG islands. These short stretches of unmethylated CpG-rich DNA are usually located close to the promoter regions of genes, including all housekeeping genes and many tissue-restricted genes.

The genomic methylation pattern observed in adult somatic tissues is established by the DNA methyltransferase enzymes (DNMTs). Three active DNMTs have been identified in mammals. DNMT1 is responsible for the maintenance methyltransferase activity, as it preferentially methylates the nascent

Developmental Origins of Health and Disease, ed. Peter Gluckman and Mark Hanson. Published by Cambridge University Press.

strand within hemi-methylated CpG dinucleotides that arise after DNA replication, thereby restoring the methylation pattern to both DNA strands (Pradhan *et al.* 1999). DNMT1 is ubiquitously expressed and its function is essential to maintain the DNA methylation pattern through multiple cell divisions in proliferating cells. In contrast, DNMT3A and DNMT3B are active at CpGs that are completely unmethylated, and together these enzymes constitute the *de novo* methyltransferase activity. These enzymes are highly expressed in embryonic stem (ES) cells and early embryos and are responsible for establishing new DNA methylation patterns during development. The patterns thus established are then stably propagated in differentiated tissues by the maintenance activity of DNMT1. Mice which lack either Dnmt1 or one or both of the *de novo* Dnmts fail to develop normally (Li *et al.* 1992, Okano *et al.* 1999), confirming that the establishment and maintenance of a proper genomic DNA methylation pattern is critical for normal mammalian development.

It has long been recognised that the fundamental role of DNA methylation is as a mechanism for regulating gene expression. A clear correlation has been established between the transcriptional repression of a gene and the methylation of associated CpG dinucleotides. DNA methylation can bring about transcriptional silencing by several distinct mechanisms. In some rare cases, methylation can directly interfere with the binding of transcription factors to their recognition sites within gene promoters and regulatory elements. More commonly, silencing of methylated genes is achieved by the recruitment of cofactors that specifically recognise the methyl–CpG moieties. A family of six methyl-CpG-binding proteins (MECP2, MBD1–4 and Kaiso) have been identified in mammals. These proteins themselves recruit large corepressor complexes to sites of DNA methylation. These complexes include histone-modifying enzymes and chromatin-remodelling factors that bring about transcriptional silencing by inducing the formation of a repressive chromatin structure (Ballestar and Wolffe 2001).

Methylation-mediated transcriptional silencing is essential in several developmentally important processes, including allele-specific gene expression (parental imprinting) and X-chromosome inactivation (see below). Further, DNA methylation is involved in silencing the expression of parasitic DNA elements (transposons and retroviruses), and thereby limiting their spread throughout the host genome (Yoder *et al.* 1997). Apart from these specific instances, it has long been suggested that gene repression by DNA methylation is also more generally critical for the establishment and maintenance of the correct tissue-specific gene expression profile (Holliday and Pugh 1975), based on the observation that for many tissue-restricted genes there is a correlation between transcriptional activation and a loss of DNA methylation. However, there is little direct evidence that methylation plays a direct causative role in silencing the expression of tissue-restricted genes (Walsh and Bestor 1999), and the general role of DNA methylation in establishing gene expression profiles during development remains speculative.

Epigenetic information of chromatin

Within the eukaryotic nucleus, DNA is packaged into a condensed state referred to as chromatin. The basic unit of chromatin is the nucleosome, in which the DNA double helix is wrapped twice around an octamer of histone proteins (comprised of two molecules each of histones H2A, H2B, H3 and H4). This initial fibre of core particles undergoes many further stages of folding and compaction to establish the native chromatin, although the nature of these higher-order packaging events is not entirely understood. The chromatin fibre established is not uniform with respect to its degree of compaction, and chromatin can be broadly classified into two cytologically distinguishable states. Euchromatin is cytologically lightly staining, reflecting its loosely compacted, decondensed state, and is generally rich in transcriptionally active genes. In contrast, heterochromatin is tightly compacted and so darkly staining, rich in repetitive DNA and contains few actively transcribed genes. It is now very clear that the precise chromatin structure has important functional ramifications for gene transcription and other

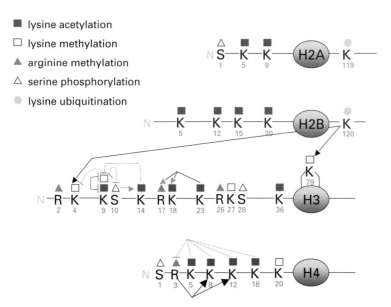

Figure 5.1 Covalent modifications of histone tails. The globular histone-fold domains (grey discs) and the protruding N- and C-terminal tails are shown for each of the four core histones. The sites of known covalent modifications (a compilation of observations from different organisms) are shown by symbols, according to the key. Histone H4 can also be modified by sumoylation, but the lysine residues targeted have not yet been determined (Shiio and Eisenman 2003). Mono-, di- or tri-methylated residues are not distinguished. Regulatory interactions between different modifications are illustrated. Arrows represent a stimulatory influence (exerted in the direction of the arrowhead). Repressive interactions are indicated by dotted lines (with the direction of the repressive influence indicated by a crossed line).

DNA-templated processes. It is therefore not surprising that mechanisms that modify chromatin structure are fundamentally involved in regulating gene transcription.

Chromatin remodelling

The obvious effect of the formation of chromatin on gene expression is that nucleosomes and higher-order structures act simply as physical barriers, to prevent the binding of factors to DNA and the assembly of the transcription machinery. Gene expression can therefore be regulated by repositioning or 'remodelling' the nucleosome core particles so as to expose (to activate expression) or obscure (to repress expression) core regulatory DNA elements. This repositioning is carried out by a number of well-conserved multi-subunit complexes, termed 'chromatin remodelling complexes'. Remodelling of nucleosomes is an energy-dependent process and

all remodelling complexes appear to be based on an ATPase core subunit. The major remodelling complexes characterised to date have been extensively described in recent reviews (Narlikar *et al.* 2002, Lusser and Kadonaga 2003) and mutations in several of these chromatin remodelling factors are responsible for a number of human epigenetic diseases (see *Defects in histone modifications*, below).

Covalent histone modifications

As well as compacting the DNA, it is now well established that the histones themselves also carry epigenetic information. The exposed N-terminal tails of the histones are subject to a variety of different enzyme-catalysed covalent modifications, including acetylation, methylation, phosphorylation, ubiquitination and ATP-ribosylation (summarised in Fig. 5.1). Since multiple modifications can occur on a single histone tail, and since all four histone tails can be modified, there is an enormous number of possible combinations of the different modifications which can mark the surface of a single nucleosome. It has been suggested that these different combinations constitute an epigenetic language or 'histone code' which exerts effects on chromatin-associated functions, including DNA replication and gene expression (Strahl and Allis 2000). These modifications either act directly by altering the physical properties of the chromatin (for example, histone acetylation weakens the interaction between DNA and the nucleosome, thereby decondensing and opening up the fibre (Hong *et al.* 1993)), or act indirectly by recruiting other mediatory factors that implement the downstream event.

The biological consequences of the different modifications are gradually being unravelled. For example, histone hyperacetylation is associated with transcriptional activation and conversely, hypoacetylated histones are found at inactive genes and within heterochromatic regions. The level of histone acetylation at a chromosomal locus is determined by the opposing activities of histone acetyltransferases (HATs) and histone deacetylases (HDACs), which are often recruited to promoters as part of multicomponent coactivator or corepressor complexes respectively. Histone methylation can bring about either activation or repression of a gene, depending on which residues within the histone tail are methylated, and the number of methyl moieties attached (Lachner and Jenuwein 2002). Methylation at lysine 9 within the N terminus of histone H3 (H3–K9) is associated with transcriptional inactivity. This modification is observed not only at silenced promoters, but also marks large inactive (heterochromatic) chromosomal regions at centromeres and telomeres, and the inactive X chromosome. Similarly, trimethylation of histone H3 at lysine 27 (3meH3–K27) is a repressive modification observed at the inactive X chromosome (Plath *et al.* 2003), and has recently been observed also at silenced promoters on autosomes (Kirmizis *et al.* 2004). In contrast to these repressive signals, methylation at lysine 4 of histone H3 is specifically associated with the promoters of active genes (Santos-Rosa *et al.* 2002). Among other histone modifications,

methylation of arginine residues is generally associated with transcriptional activation, while serine phosphorylation is observed at active genes during interphase, but is also associated with chromosome condensation and gene silencing during mitosis (Nowak and Corces 2004). Sumoylation of histone H4 has recently been implicated in the initiation of transcriptional silencing and gene repression (Shiio and Eisenman 2003) while histone lysine ubiquitination has been reported to exert both positive and negative effects on transcription (Zhang 2003). As well as understanding the biological consequences of individual modifications, there is an increasing awareness of the extent to which the different covalent modifications can affect each other. The major known cases of regulatory crosstalk between individual modifications are also summarised in Fig. 5.1.

Epigenetics and development

Clearing and establishing epigenetic marks during development

It is clear that epigenetic signals are critical for normal mammalian development. Part of this requirement derives from the involvement of epigenetic information in the specific processes of genomic imprinting and X-chromosome inactivation (see below). Apart from these specific instances, normal development also requires a complex process whereby the epigenetic pattern of DNA methylation inherited from the parents is erased early during development, so that a new epigenetic programme can be established in the embryo. The methylation pattern is removed first from the paternally derived chromosomes by an active enzymatic process (Oswald *et al.* 2000) (although the DNA demethylase responsible has not yet been identified), while the maternally inherited chromosomes become demethylated more slowly. As a result of these active and passive processes, most of the epigenetic information inherited from the gametes has been erased in the embryo by the blastocyst stage of development (Monk *et al.* 1987). The cells of the blastocyst are thus rendered pluripotent, and now have the potential to generate the multiple different cell types and tissues which will constitute the embryo. Following this general clearing, the new embryonic patterns of DNA methylation begin to be re-established. A wave of *de novo* methylation begins in the inner cell mass of the blastocyst and continues beyond implantation in the primitive ectodermal layer, which gives rise to the tissues of the embryo itself (Santos *et al.* 2002). The proper establishment of methylation patterns in the post-implantation embryo requires both *de novo* and maintenance methyltransferase activities. It is not yet entirely clear exactly why this programme of clearing and re-establishing DNA methylation patterns is required for normal mammalian development. The preferred model is that the single inherited pattern must be erased, to clear the way for the establishment of multiple new tissue-specific patterns, which are in turn integral to the ultimate determination of different cell types. While the dynamics of DNA methylation have been well documented, it is quite likely that dynamic changes in other epigenetic signals are also involved in genomic reprogramming during early mammalian development.

It should be noted that despite the general erasure of epigenetic signals prior to the blastocyst stage, at some alleles the inherited patterns are preserved. These include the epigenetic marks which are required to ensure allele-specific gene expression at imprinted loci. Relatively recently it has also become clear that there is a failure to clear inherited epigenetic marks from a number of unusual mouse alleles, now referred to as metastable epialleles (Rakyan *et al.* 2002). Because the epigenetic state (usually DNA methylation) determines transcriptional activity of these alleles, these metastable epialleles represent an important case in which the ultimate phenotype of the animal is determined by inherited epigenetic as well as genetic information (Morgan *et al.* 1999). The epigenetic modification and expression of these alleles may also be subject to external environmental influence (see below). It is not yet clear whether such alleles exist in humans.

Parental imprinting

Parental or genomic imprinting refers to the process whereby a gene is expressed from only one allele (either the maternally or paternally inherited allele). In the mouse, some 60–100 genes have been shown to exhibit monoallelic expression in at least some tissues, and most of those that have been investigated have also been found to be imprinted in humans (Morison and Reeve 1998). Some imprinted genes are expressed exclusively from the paternal allele, while others are expressed only from the maternal allele. Many of the genes that are imprinted are associated with embryonic and fetal growth. While it is not clear exactly why imprinting has evolved, it is clear that it is essential for normal development. Mouse embryos bearing either two maternally inherited (gynogenetic) or two paternally inherited (androgenetic) chromosome complements (from which monoallelic expression of imprinted genes is not achieved) fail to develop beyond implantation (McGrath and Solter 1984).

At imprinted genes, the paternally and maternally inherited alleles are functionally non-equivalent because they bear different epigenetic modifications. Imprinted genes tend to be clustered at a small number of chromosomal locations, and most of these locations are associated with a so-called differentially methylated region (DMR), a small segment which shows a different pattern of DNA methylation between the paternal and maternal alleles. For a number of clusters, it has been demonstrated that deletion of the DMR results in a failure of imprinting (Thorvaldsen *et al.* 1998), confirming the importance of methylation as the distinguishing mark. It has recently been demonstrated using gene knockouts that the *de novo* methyltransferase Dnmt3a is essential for achieving monoallelic expression of imprinted genes (Kaneda *et al.* 2004), as is a related but enzymatically inactive member of the Dnmt3 family (Dnmt3L) (Hata *et al.* 2002). The mechanisms by which the allele-specific marking of the DMR results in differential expression of the imprinted genes are various and often complex, as demonstrated at the well-characterised *Igf2/H19* locus

(Hark *et al.* 2000). The different methylation patterns are actually established in the gametes of the parents, when the alleles are still physically separated, prior to coming together in a single nucleus at fertilisation. As mentioned above, unlike most genomic methylation, these allele-specific methylation marks are not erased during the general wave of demethylation which occurs prior to the blastocyst stage of development, and so are maintained in the adult somatic tissues. It is not yet clear how methylation at imprinted loci is specifically protected during this demethylation process. The methylation imprints are only erased in the primordial germ cells (Hajkova *et al.* 2002) so that the new mark can be established in the gametes according to the sex of the new embryo. While DNA methylation is clearly integral to the imprinting process, it is likely that other epigenetic signals such as histone modifications are also involved (Grandjean *et al.* 2001), although whether these signals are upstream or downstream of DNA methylation remains unknown.

X-chromosome inactivation

The process of X-chromosome inactivation refers to a highly regulated programme in female mammals in which one of the two X chromosomes is converted from the transcriptionally active form observed in the pluripotent cell types of the implanting embryo, to a highly condensed, transcriptionally silent form in differentiated tissues. The silencing of one X chromosome in females is required to compensate for the dosage difference with the XY male. Within the cells of embryonic tissues there is a random choice whether to inactivate the paternally or maternally inherited X chromsome (X_p and X_m respectively), while in extra-embryonic tissues X inactivation is a non-random process, with the X_p being preferentially silenced.

As with genomic imprinting, X inactivation establishes a functional distinction between two alleles that are present within the same nucleus, and it is clear that this functional difference is the result of differential epigenetic modification. Unlike imprinting, the epigenetic differences between the active

and inactive X chromosomes are initially established while they are physically together within the same nucleus. The first step in silencing occurs when expression of the *XIST* gene, which produces a large, non-coding transcript, is upregulated specifically on the future inactive X chromosome (X_i). These transcripts accumulate and coat the arms of the chromosome from which they are expressed. This initial coating of X_i by the *XIST* transcript triggers a programme of epigenetic changes that render the chromosome stably repressed. The earliest epigenetic modification detected to date is the specific enrichment at X_i of histone H3 which is trimethylated at Lys 27 (3meH3–K27) (Plath *et al.* 2003). This modification is catalysed by a member of the Polycomb (PcG) protein family, ENX1/EZH2, which appears to be recruited to X_i by the accumulated *Xist* transcript (Silva *et al.* 2003). This initial signal is followed by other covalent modifications to histones on X_i; as well as a global histone deacetylation (Belyaev *et al.* 1996), X_i is also generally depleted (relative to the active X) of histone H3 which is methylated at Lys 4 (meH3–K4) (Boggs *et al.* 2002). DNA methylation has also been implicated in the process of X inactivation, although it is believed to play a role in maintaining the inactive state once established, rather than in the initial transcriptional silencing itself (Sado *et al.* 2000). While the transcriptional silencing of X_i is initially dependent on the presence of the *XIST* transcript, the progressive accumulation of these epigenetic changes transforms the chromosome into a stably repressed, *Xist*-independent state. It should be noted that the order of events described above has been largely obtained from studies of differentiating mouse ES cells, and there is evidence that at least some of the specific features of the inactivation process differ between mouse and humans (Vasques *et al.* 2002).

Epigenetics and nuclear cloning

Somatic cell nuclear cloning (SCNC) refers to a burgeoning technology in which the nucleus from an adult somatic cell is transferred into a previously enucleated oocyte, which is then activated to undergo embryonic development. The resulting embryo will be genetically identical or a 'clone' of the adult from whom the somatic cell was taken. In cases of reproductive cloning, the cloned embryo is carried to term by a surrogate mother, to give rise to a cloned adult animal. Cloned animals have already been successfully produced in several mammalian species (Rhind *et al.* 2003), although no cloned human has yet been conclusively reported and reproductive cloning of humans is currently banned under law in Europe, North America and Australia. However, it is the vast medical potential presented by non-reproductive or therapeutic cloning which is responsible for the enormous interest in this area. In therapeutic cloning, the cloned embryo is not carried to term, but develops only to the blastocyst stage of development. The blastocyst can be used as a source of pluripotent ES cells, which are genetically identical to the adult from whom the somatic nucleus was taken (in this case the patient). In theory, these cloned ES cells could potentially be used to replace any damaged or diseased tissue in the patient (with whom they will be immunologically compatible). Moreover, the potential exists to genetically manipulate cloned ES cells to correct an underlying genetic defect prior to returning them to the patient. At present, many of these processes remain beyond our current technologies, but the potential offered by therapeutic cloning strategies has generated an enormous interest in understanding the cloning process.

Initial experiments have established that epigenetic factors are going to have important implications for cloning technology. As described above, in a fertilised zygote derived from a normal mating, most inherited epigenetic information is erased prior to implantation to clear the way for the appropriate new tissue-specific patterns to be imposed in the differentiating cells of the developing embryo. In the case of nuclear cloning, the genome transferred into the oocyte will bear the epigenetic profile of the somatic cell type from which it was acquired. These somatic epigenetic markers must be erased to regain a pluripotent state. The successful production of cloned animals indicates that in some

cases it has been possible for the adult nucleus to be 'de-differentiated' and undergo almost normal epigenetic reprogramming. However, it appears that this process is highly inefficient, as the vast majority of cloned embryos derived from late somatic nuclei die in utero, and those that are carried to term often have developmental abnormalities and shortened lifespan (Ogonuki *et al.* 2002, Tamashiro *et al.* 2002). That these developmental defects are due to epigenetic rather than genetic abnormalities (such as chromosomal aberrations arising during the process of nuclear transfer) is proven by the fact that the abnormalities are not transmitted to the progeny derived from natural matings between affected cloned parents (Tamashiro *et al.* 2002). A number of epigenetic abnormalities have now been detected in cloned animals, indicating a failure to achieve full epigenetic reprogramming of the donor-cell DNA. These include abnormalities of histone modifications (Santos *et al.* 2003) and highly aberrant patterns of DNA methylation (resembling that observed in the donor nucleus) (Kang *et al.* 2001). As a result of this abnormal reprogramming, defects in processes regulated by epigenetic signals, including parental imprinting (Mann *et al.* 2003) and X inactivation (Wrenzycki *et al.* 2002), have been observed in cloned embryos. There is evidence that donor nuclei from different somatic cell types vary in the extent to which they can be epigenetically reprogrammed during cloning (Santos *et al.* 2003). A more complete understanding of the factors affecting the efficiency of nuclear reprogramming will be essential if the enormous medical potential of therapeutic cloning is to be fully realised.

Epigenetic modifications are influenced by the environment

A number of recent studies have raised the interesting possibility that epigenetic marks can be influenced by external environmental factors. Due to the labile nature of DNA methylation, there has been considerable debate about whether dietary manipulation in utero could influence the extent of cytosine methylation. *S*-adenosylmethionine (SAM) serves as the methyl donor for cytosine methylation. Dietary sources including choline, betaine, methionine and folic acid contribute to the production of SAM in humans.

Wolff *et al.* (1998) demonstrated that the phenotype of offspring could be modulated by micronutrient supplementation of maternal diet using a murine locus, *agouti viable yellow*, A^{vy}. The A^{vy} allele results from the insertion of an intracisternal A particle (IAP) retrotransposon upstream of the *agouti* gene. A cryptic promoter in the retrotransposon can drive constitutive expression of the downstream *agouti* gene, which is involved in coat colour. The expression state of the cryptic promoter correlates with DNA methylation; an active promoter is hypomethylated, while a silenced promoter is hypermethylated. An inbred population of mice (all members of which are genetically identical) carrying this epiallele display variable expressivity, with some mice having completely yellow coats and others a brown (agouti) coat. Some mice in the inbred strain have various degrees of mottling, a trait that stems from variegation of agouti expression from clonally derived patches. Supplementation of maternal diets with methyl donors and cofactors involved in SAM production demonstrated that the proportion of coat-colour phenotypes found in the offspring could be shifted from those on a control diet. With maternal micronutrient supplementation, an increased proportion of offspring were found to carry more heavily mottled coats. These effects were found to be influenced by the strain background, suggesting that the differences in the sensitivity to dietary supplements were due to genetic differences in methyl metabolism between the strains (Wolff *et al.* 1998).

This finding suggests that methyl supplementation, by providing more substrate, created hypermethylated A^{vy} alleles in the offspring, which in turn resulted in more coat-colour mottling. This interpretation was subsequently supported by Waterland and Jirtle (2003), who used bisulphite sequencing to show that increased methylation of the A^{vy} retrotransposon correlated with the shift in coat colours that resulted when dams were fed methyl-group enriched diets. This work not only demonstrates a link between maternal diet and offspring coat-colour phenotype, but has implications for the long-term health of the offspring. Overexpression of agouti, which is a paracrine signalling molecule, results in deleterious health effects in adult mice including obesity, hyperinsulinaemia, diabetes, increased susceptibility to cancer and a shorter life span (Cooney *et al.* 2002, Waterland and Jirtle, 2003). So, at least in the case of the A^{vy} allele, micronutrient maternal supplementation impacts on the long-term health of an individual through epigenetic mechanisms. However, it is worth pointing out that alleles like A^{vy}, which are particularly sensitive to epigenetic state, are not common in the mouse genome, and none has yet been identified in humans. These alleles are now termed metastable epialleles, and to date only a handful have been identified in the mouse (Rakyan *et al.* 2002). There is now intense interest in the identification of similar alleles in humans, but this is a challenging task due to the outbred nature of our population.

Even more exciting is the possibility that these marks are a read-out of external environmental events in the past history of that organism. A recent study carried out in rats describes the role of epigenetic modifications at the glucocorticoid receptor (*GR*) gene in establishing the level of stress felt by adult animals. The 'stressability' of rats is known to be affected by whether their mothers lick them in the first week of life (Meaney 2001). Weaver *et al.* (2004) have recently shown that the promoter of the *GR* gene becomes methylated in response to licking, and that this is maintained for the life of the rat and permanently affects its phenotype.

These two pieces of work, on the effect of maternal diet on expression of a coat-colour gene in the mouse, and on the role of DNA methylation in the maternal effect on stress response in rats, raise the interesting possibility that by studying the epigenotype of an individual we may learn something about its environmental history and be better able to predict disease risk.

Epigenetics and disease

A number of important human diseases are now known to occur either due to mutations in factors which implement epigenetic signals, or as a direct result of a failure of normal epigenetic processes (such as imprinting). Because the disruption of epigenetic pathways is likely to perturb expression of multiple downstream genes, diseases involving epigenetic abnormalities tend to be complex syndromal disorders affecting many systems.

Defects in DNA methylation as a cause of disease

Pathological conditions can arise as a result of either abnormal DNA hypermethylation or hypomethylation, leading to inappropriate gene repression or activation, respectively. Abnormal DNA methylation profiles are frequently associated with tumorigenesis and neoplastic transformation (see below). A disease phenotype can also arise if abnormalities of DNA methylation occur in DMRs associated with imprinted loci, resulting in deregulated expression of normally imprinted genes. For example, Beckwith–Wiedemann syndrome, a developmental disease of organ overgrowth, is associated with abnormal methylation within one or more DMRs near chromosome 11p15.5, and the inappropriate biallelic expression (*IGF2*) or silencing (*CDKN1C*) of associated genes (Engel *et al.* 2000). Two other diseases of imprinting, the Angelman and Prader–Willi syndromes, are associated with oppositely imprinted genes within a cluster on chromosome 15, and can involve either loss or mutation of the normally expressed (non-imprinted) allele or a failure of the imprinting process (Nicholls *et al.* 1998). Other human diseases involving DNA methylation include the ICF (immunodeficiency, centromere instability and facial anomalies) and Rett syndromes. ICF is a rare recessive disorder caused by mutations in the gene encoding the DNMT3B *de novo* methyltransferase, and is associated with hypomethylation of specific heterochromatic repeat sequences leading to centromere instability and chromosomal

rearrangements (Xu *et al.* 1999). Rett syndrome is an X-linked dominant disease causing intellectual disability in affected females. This disease is caused by mutations in the gene encoding MeCP2 (Amir *et al.* 1999), one of the methyl–CpG binding proteins involved in implementing transcriptional silencing at methylated genes. Thus Rett syndrome does not result from a defect in DNA methylation per se, but from the downstream silencing events normally following from methylation.

Defects in histone modifications and nucleosome remodelling as a cause of disease

There are now several human diseases whose aetiology is known to involve disruption of the normal pattern of histone modifications. For example, mutations which affect the histone acetyltransferase activity of the CREB binding protein (CBP) give rise to the Rubinstein–Taybi syndrome, an autosomal dominant mental retardation and congenital malformation disorder (Murata *et al.* 2001). Another complex mental retardation disorder, the Coffin–Lowry syndrome, is caused by mutations in Rsk-2, a protein kinase involved in mitogen-stimulated phosphorylation of histone H3, suggesting that the phenotype may reflect failed chromatin modification and transcriptional activation of mitogen-responsive promoters (Sassone-Corsi *et al.* 1999). As well as disruptions to covalent histone modifications, disease can arise due to mutations affecting the cellular nucleosome remodelling machinery (Huang *et al.* 2003). One of the best-characterised disorders of chromatin remodelling is the α-thalassaemia / mental retardation syndrome, X-linked (ATR-X), a pleiotropic developmental disorder involving many systems (Gibbons and Higgs 2000). The gene mutated in this syndrome (*ATRX*) encodes a member of the SWI/SNF protein family, which displays ATPase and nucleosome remodelling activities in vitro (Xue *et al.* 2003) and associates with heterochromatic domains within the nucleus (McDowell *et al.* 1999). Apart from the α-globin genes, which are down-regulated in ATRX patients, other developmentally important genes whose expression is dependent on ATRX are yet to be identified. Mutations in chromatin remodelling factors and factors involved in covalent histone modifications have also been implicated in the aetiology of numerous human tumours.

Epigenetics and cancer

One of the most significant impacts of epigenetics on human disease derives from the involvement of abnormal epigenetic signalling pathways in cancer. The frequency with which epigenetic abnormalities are associated with both rare and common human tumours has led to the acceptance that an epigenetic event, either inherited or somatically acquired, can constitute one of the two 'hits' required for tumorigenesis, according to Knudson's model (Knudson 1971). The first epigenetic abnormality observed in cancer was a general loss of DNA methylation in malignant cells relative to matched normal tissues (Gama-Sosa et al. 1983), and hypomethylation has now been detected in a wide variety of human tumours. It is believed that this demethylation may result in the aberrant derepression of one or more genes important for cancer growth, and indeed overexpression associated with loss of promoter methylation has now been demonstrated for a number of oncogenes. DNA hypomethylation may also contribute more generally to chromosome instability, either directly (since hypomethylated satellite sequences predispose centromeric regions to chromosome breakage (Qu et al. 1999)), or indirectly (through the activation and spreading of retroviral elements, promoting illegitimate recombination events). The molecular basis for the general loss of methylation observed in cancer is not yet understood.

As well as general DNA hypomethylation in malignant tissues, aberrant hypermethylation of specific sequences has also been associated with a number of human tumours. The oncogenic mechanism in this case involves specific promoter methylation and associated transcriptional silencing of one or more tumour-suppressor genes. Methylation-dependent silencing was first demonstrated for the *RB* gene in retinoblastomas (Greger *et al.* 1989), and has now been observed for other key tumour-suppressor proteins. It is not always clear whether abnormal hypermethylation is the primary silencing event, and for some tumour suppressors it appears that the role of methylation may be to 'lock in' and maintain an inactive state arising from other epigenetic change (Bachman *et al.* 2003). More recently research has extended beyond methylation to links between cancer and chromatin. Many tumour suppressors are themselves involved in some aspect of chromatin structure, and so mutations are likely to exert their oncogenic effect by deregulating the expression of one or more important downstream targets. Mutations or chromosomal translocations affecting HATs, HDACs, histone methyltransferases, components of SWI/SNF-related chromatin remodelling complexes, and factors which recruit these to genomic targets, have been identified in a wide range of human malignancies (reviewed in Hake *et al.* 2004, Roberts and Orkin 2004).

Because tumour-suppressor genes silenced by epigenetic mechanisms remain structurally intact, the potential exists for so called 'epigenetic chemotherapy', targeting drugs to modify the epigenetic profile and revert the gene to its active state. Inhibitors of DNA methylation have been shown to reactivate a number of genes silenced in cancer, and have shown moderate success against haematological malignancies in clinical trials (Issa *et al.* 2004). Since epigenetic mechanisms of gene silencing frequently involve histone deacetylation, HDAC inhibitors have also been investigated as potential anti-cancer drugs. At least one, suberoylanilide hydroxamic acid (SAHA) has shown anti-tumour effect associated with an accumulation of acetylated histones and is well tolerated in clinical trials (Kelly *et al.* 2003). Further trial regimes combining the use of methylation inhibitors and HDAC inhibitors are planned (Shaker *et al.* 2003). However, due to their non-targeted nature, the clinical use of these epigenetic modifiers raises a number of concerns. These include the potential activation of non-specific genes and retroviral elements, as well as genome instability resulting from general DNA hypomethylation. These concerns will have to be closely monitored.

Concluding remarks

In the past decade there has been a huge increase in our understanding of the impact of epigenetic signals on nuclear processes, and in particular on the regulation of gene expression. Epigenetic signals are fundamental to normal mammalian development, and epigenetic abnormalities are now known to underlie several important human diseases. Elucidating and understanding the entire spectrum of epigenetic mechanisms during normal and abnormal development should improve the rational design of therapeutic agents, and will be fundamental in developing somatic stem cell therapy.

REFERENCES

Amir, R. E., Van den Veyver, I. B., Wan, M., Tran, C. Q., Francke, U. and Zoghbi, H. Y. (1999). Rett syndrome is caused by mutations in X-linked MECP2, encoding methyl-CpG-binding protein 2. *Nat. Genet.*, **23**, 185–8.

Bachman, K. E., Park, B. H., Rhee, I. *et al.* (2003). Histone modifications and silencing prior to DNA methylation of a tumor suppressor gene. *Cancer Cell*, **3**, 89–95.

Ballestar, E. and Wolffe, A. P. (2001). Methyl-CpG-binding proteins: targeting specific gene repression. *Eur. J. Biochem.*, **268**, 1–6.

Belyaev, N., Keohane, A. M. and Turner, B. M. (1996). Differential underacetylation of histones H2A, H3 and H4 on the inactive X chromosome in human female cells. *Hum. Genet.*, **97**, 573–8.

Boggs, B. A., Cheung, P., Heard, E., Spector, D. L., Chinault, A. C. and Allis, C. D. (2002). Differentially methylated forms of histone H3 show unique association patterns with inactive human X chromosomes. *Nat. Genet.*, **30**, 73–6.

Cooney, C. A., Dave, A. A. and Wolff, G. L. (2002). Maternal methyl supplements in mice affect epigenetic variation and DNA methylation of offspring. *J. Nutr.*, **132**, 2393S–400S.

Engel, J. R., Smallwood, A., Harper, A. *et al.* (2000). Epigenotype–phenotype correlations in Beckwith–Wiedemann syndrome. *J. Med. Genet.*, **37**, 921–6.

Gama-Sosa, M. A., Slagel, V. A., Trewyn, R. W. *et al.* (1983). The 5-methylcytosine content of DNA from human tumors. *Nucleic Acids Res.*, **11**, 6883–94.

Gibbons, R. J. and Higgs, D. R. (2000). Molecular-clinical spectrum of the ATR-X syndrome. *Am. J. Med. Genet.*, **97**, 204–12.

Grandjean, V., O'Neill, L., Sado, T., Turner, B. and Ferguson-Smith, A. (2001). Relationship between DNA methylation, histone H4 acetylation and gene expression in the mouse imprinted Igf2–H19 domain. *FEBS Lett.*, **488**, 165–9.

Greger, V., Passarge, E., Hopping, W., Messmer, E. and Horsthemke, B. (1989). Epigenetic changes may contribute to the formation and spontaneous regression of retinoblastoma. *Hum. Genet.*, **83**, 155–8.

Hajkova, P., Erhardt, S., Lane, N. *et al.* (2002). Epigenetic reprogramming in mouse primordial germ cells. *Mech. Dev.*, **117**, 15–23.

Hake, S. B., Xiao, A. and Allis, C. D. (2004). Linking the epigenetic 'language' of covalent histone modifications to cancer. *Br. J. Cancer*, **90**, 761–9.

Hark, A. T., Schoenherr, C. J., Katz, D. J., Ingram, R. S., Levorse, J. M. and Tilghman, S. M. (2000). CTCF mediates methylation-sensitive enhancer-blocking activity at the H19/Igf2 locus. *Nature*, **405**, 486–9.

Hata, K., Okano, M., Lei, H. and Li, E. (2002). Dnmt3L cooperates with the Dnmt3 family of de novo DNA methyltransferases to establish maternal imprints in mice. *Development*, **129**, 1983–93.

Holliday, R. and Pugh, J. E. (1975). DNA modification mechanisms and gene activity during development. *Science*, **187**, 226–32.

Hong, L., Schroth, G. P., Matthews, H. R., Yau, P. and Bradbury, E. M. (1993). Studies of the DNA binding properties of histone H4 amino terminus: thermal denaturation studies reveal that acetylation markedly reduces the binding constant of the H4 'tail' to DNA. *J. Biol. Chem.*, **268**, 305–14.

Huang, C., Sloan, E. A. and Boerkoel, C. F. (2003). Chromatin remodeling and human disease. *Curr. Opin. Genet. Dev.*, **13**, 246–52.

Issa, J. P., Garcia-Manero, G., Giles, F. J. *et al.* (2004). Phase 1 study of low-dose prolonged exposure schedules of the hypomethylating agent 5-aza-2'-deoxycytidine (decitabine) in hematopoietic malignancies. *Blood*, **103**, 1635–40.

Kaneda, M., Okano, M., Hata, K. *et al.* (2004). Essential role for de novo DNA methyltransferase Dnmt3a in paternal and maternal imprinting. *Nature*, **429**, 900–3.

Kang, Y. K., Koo, D. B., Park, J. S. *et al.* (2001). Aberrant methylation of donor genome in cloned bovine embryos. *Nat. Genet.*, **28**, 173–7.

Kelly, W. K., Richon, V. M., O'Connor, O. *et al.* (2003). Phase I clinical trial of histone deacetylase inhibitor: suberoylanilide hydroxamic acid administered intravenously. *Clin. Cancer. Res.*, **9**, 3578–88.

Kirmizis, A., Bartley, S. M., Kuzmichev, A. *et al.* (2004). Silencing of human polycomb target genes is associated with methylation of histone H3 Lys 27. *Genes Dev.*, **18**, 1592–1605.

Knudson, A. G., Jr. (1971). Mutation and cancer: statistical study of retinoblastoma. *Proc. Natl. Acad. Sci. USA*, **68**, 820–3.

Lachner, M. and Jenuwein, T. (2002). The many faces of histone lysine methylation. *Curr. Opin. Cell. Biol.*, **14**, 286–98.

Li, E., Bestor, T. H. and Jaenisch, R. (1992). Targeted mutation of the DNA methyltransferase gene results in embryonic lethality. *Cell*, **69**, 915–26.

Lusser, A. and Kadonaga, J. T. (2003). Chromatin remodeling by ATP-dependent molecular machines. *Bioessays*, **25**, 1192–1200.

Mann, M. R., Chung, Y. G., Nolen, L. D., Verona, R. I., Latham, K. E. and Bartolomei, M. S. (2003). Disruption of imprinted gene methylation and expression in cloned preimplantation stage mouse embryos. *Biol. Reprod.*, **69**, 902–14.

McDowell, T. L., Gibbons, R. J., Sutherland, H. *et al.* (1999). Localization of a putative transcriptional regulator (ATRX) at pericentromeric heterochromatin and the short arms of acrocentric chromosomes. *Proc. Natl. Acad. Sci. USA*, **96**, 13983–8.

McGrath, J. and Solter, D. (1984). Completion of mouse embryogenesis requires both the maternal and paternal genomes. *Cell*, **37**, 179–83.

Meaney, M. J. (2001). Maternal care, gene expression, and the transmission of individual differences in stress reactivity across generations. *Annu. Rev. Neurosci.*, **24**, 1161–92.

Monk, M., Boubelik, M. and Lehnert, S. (1987). Temporal and regional changes in DNA methylation in the embryonic, extraembryonic and germ cell lineages during mouse embryo development. *Development*, **99**, 371–82.

Morgan, H. D., Sutherland, H. G., Martin, D. I. and Whitelaw, E. (1999). Epigenetic inheritance at the agouti locus in the mouse. *Nat. Genet.*, **23**, 314–18.

Morison, I. M. and Reeve, A. E. (1998). A catalogue of imprinted genes and parent-of-origin effects in humans and animals. *Hum. Mol. Genet.*, **7**, 1599–1609.

Murata, T., Kurokawa, R., Krones, A. *et al.* (2001). Defect of histone acetyltransferase activity of the nuclear transcriptional coactivator CBP in Rubinstein–Taybi syndrome. *Hum. Mol. Genet.*, **10**, 1071–6.

Narlikar, G. J., Fan, H. Y. and Kingston, R. E. (2002). Cooperation between complexes that regulate chromatin structure and transcription. *Cell*, **108**, 475–87.

Nicholls, R. D., Saitoh, S. and Horsthemke, B. (1998). Imprinting in Prader–Willi and Angelman syndromes. *Trends Genet.*, **14**, 194–200.

Nowak, S. J. and Corces, V. G. (2004). Phosphorylation of histone H3: a balancing act between chromosome condensation and transcriptional activation. *Trends Genet.*, **20**, 214–20.

Ogonuki, N., Inoue, K., Yamamoto, Y. *et al.* (2002). Early death of mice cloned from somatic cells. *Nat. Genet.*, **30**, 253–4.

Okano, M., Bell, D. W., Haber, D. A. and Li, E. (1999). DNA methyltransferases Dnmt3a and Dnmt3b are essential for de novo methylation and mammalian development. *Cell*, **99**, 247–57.

Oswald, J., Engemann, S., Lane, N. *et al.* (2000). Active demethylation of the paternal genome in the mouse zygote. *Curr. Biol.*, **10**, 475–8.

Plath, K., Fang, J., Mlynarczyk-Evans, S. K. *et al.* (2003). Role of histone H3 lysine 27 methylation in X inactivation. *Science*, **300**, 131–5.

Pradhan, S., Bacolla, A., Wells, R. D. and Roberts, R. J. (1999). Recombinant human DNA (cytosine-5) methyltransferase. I. Expression, purification, and comparison of de novo and maintenance methylation. *J. Biol. Chem.*, **274**, 33002–10.

Qu, G. Z., Grundy, P. E., Narayan, A. and Ehrlich, M. (1999). Frequent hypomethylation in Wilms tumors of pericentromeric DNA in chromosomes 1 and 16. *Cancer Genet. Cytogenet.*, **109**, 34–9.

Rakyan, V. K., Blewitt, M. E., Druker, R., Preis, J. I. and Whitelaw, E. (2002). Metastable epialleles in mammals. *Trends Genet.*, **18**, 348–51.

Rhind, S. M., Taylor, J. E., De Sousa, P. A., King, T. J., McGarry, M. and Wilmut, I. (2003). Human cloning: can it be made safe? *Nat. Rev. Genet.*, **4**, 855–64.

Roberts, C. W. and Orkin, S. H. (2004). The SWI/SNF complex: chromatin and cancer. *Nat. Rev. Cancer*, **4**, 133–42.

Sado, T., Fenner, M. H., Tan, S. S., Tam, P., Shioda, T. and Li, E. (2000). X inactivation in the mouse embryo deficient for Dnmt1: distinct effect of hypomethylation on imprinted and random X inactivation. *Dev. Biol.*, **225**, 294–303.

Santos, F., Hendrich, B., Reik, W. and Dean, W. (2002). Dynamic reprogramming of DNA methylation in the early mouse embryo. *Dev. Biol.*, **241**, 172–82.

Santos, F., Zakhartchenko, V., Stojkovic, M. *et al.* (2003). Epigenetic marking correlates with developmental potential in cloned bovine preimplantation embryos. *Curr. Biol.*, **13**, 1116–21.

Santos-Rosa, H., Schneider, R., Bannister, A. J. *et al.* (2002). Active genes are tri-methylated at K4 of histone H3. *Nature*, **419**, 407–11.

Sassone-Corsi, P., Mizzen, C. A., Cheung, P. *et al.* (1999). Requirement of Rsk-2 for epidermal growth factor- activated phosphorylation of histone H3. *Science*, **285**, 886–91.

Shaker, S., Bernstein, M., Momparler, L. F. and Momparler, R. L. (2003). Preclinical evaluation of antineoplastic activity of inhibitors of DNA methylation (5-aza-2'-deoxycytidine) and histone deacetylation (trichostatin A, depsipeptide) in combination against myeloid leukemic cells. *Leuk. Res.*, **27**, 437–44.

Shiio, Y. and Eisenman, R. N. (2003). Histone sumoylation is associated with transcriptional repression. *Proc. Natl. Acad. Sci. USA*, **100**, 13225–30.

Silva, J., Mak, W., Zvetkova, I. *et al.* (2003). Establishment of histone h3 methylation on the inactive X chromosome requires transient recruitment of Eed–Enx1 polycomb group complexes. *Dev. Cell*, **4**, 481–95.

Strahl, B. D. and Allis, C. D. (2000). The language of covalent histone modifications. *Nature*, **403**, 41–5.

Tamashiro, K. L., Wakayama, T., Akutsu, H. *et al.* (2002). Cloned mice have an obese phenotype not transmitted to their offspring. *Nat. Med.*, **8**, 262–7.

Thorvaldsen, J. L., Duran, K. L. and Bartolomei, M. S. (1998). Deletion of the H19 differentially methylated domain results in loss of imprinted expression of H19 and Igf2. *Genes Dev.*, **12**, 3693–702.

Vasques, L. R., Klockner, M. N. and Pereira, L. V. (2002). X chromosome inactivation: how human are mice? *Cytogenet. Genome Res.*, **99**, 30–5.

Walsh, C. P. and Bestor, T. H. (1999). Cytosine methylation and mammalian development. *Genes Dev.*, **13**, 26–34.

Waterland, R. A. and Jirtle, R. L. (2003). Transposable elements: targets for early nutritional effects on epigenetic gene regulation. *Mol. Cell. Biol.*, **23**, 5293–5300.

Weaver, I. C., Cervoni, N., Champagne, F. A. *et al.* (2004). Epigenetic programming by maternal behavior. *Nat. Neurosci.*, **7**, 847–54.

Wolff, G. L., Kodell, R. L., Moore, S. R. and Cooney, C. A. (1998). Maternal epigenetics and methyl supplements affect agouti gene expression in Avy/a mice. *Faseb. J.*, **12**, 949–57.

Wrenzycki, C., Lucas-Hahn, A., Herrmann, D., Lemme, E., Korsawe, K. and Niemann, H. (2002). In vitro production and nuclear transfer affect dosage compensation of the X-linked gene transcripts G6PD, PGK, and Xist in preimplantation bovine embryos. *Biol. Reprod.*, **66**, 127–34.

Xu, G. L., Bestor, T. H., Bourc'his, D. *et al.* (1999). Chromosome instability and immunodeficiency syndrome caused by mutations in a DNA methyltransferase gene. *Nature*, **402**, 187–91.

Xue, Y., Gibbons, R., Yan, Z. *et al.* (2003). The ATRX syndrome protein forms a chromatin-remodeling complex with Daxx and localizes in promyelocytic leukemia nuclear bodies. *Proc. Natl. Acad. Sci. USA*, **100**, 10635–40.

Yoder, J. A., Walsh, C. P. and Bestor, T. H. (1997). Cytosine methylation and the ecology of intragenomic parasites. *Trends Genet.*, **13**, 335–40.

Zhang, Y. (2003). Transcriptional regulation by histone ubiquitination and deubiquitination. *Genes Dev.*, **17**, 2733–40.

6

A mitochondrial component of developmental programming

Josie M. L. McConnell

King's College London

Introduction

Evidence both from epidemiological studies and from experimental animal models supports the concept of developmental programming (Osmond and Barker 2000, Sorensen *et al.* 2000, Barker 2002, Eriksson and Forsen 2002, Ozanne and Hales 2002). In studies of genetically homogeneous animals there are now unequivocal data demonstrating that environmental stress during the period from peri-implantation development through to the end of suckling can impact on the health status of the adult offspring, and can also have behavioural consequences (Langley-Evans and Jackson 1996, Ozanne *et al.* 1998, Khan *et al.* 2003, Vickers *et al.* 2003, Weaver *et al.* 2004). Amongst the disorders that have been reported after suboptimal maternal nutrition, the most common are hypertension, insulin resistance, dyslipidaemia, obesity and endothelial dysfunction. In one particularly well-characterised animal model adult offspring display all these symptoms, which in humans are collectively known as syndrome X (Khan *et al.* 2003, 2005). This constellation of disorders is predicted to be increasing at an alarming rate and is currently affecting large numbers of adults in the western world. A molecular understanding of developmental programming is not only a challenging academic problem, but also one that may enable us to devise preventative strategies, which will benefit human health and reduce medical care costs in the future.

Addressing the molecular mechanisms of developmental programming is difficult because the cellular disorders that lead to disease susceptibility in the adult occur long after the initial causative stress has been removed. Any effective strategy aimed at defining contributory molecular mechanisms must be multidisciplinary. Most importantly, the experimental system must allow precise and measurable manipulations of molecular parameters during early development, and provide a means of monitoring such changes throughout development and into adulthood, and careful and detailed definitions of physiological endpoints must be made so as to establish a direct causal link between molecular changes in early development and altered adult physiology. Without such an experimental paradigm, studies may show tantalising correlations but will not be able to provide proof of the molecular mechanisms underpinning developmental programming (Rees *et al.* 2000, Young *et al.* 2001).

A plausible molecular hypothesis of developmental programming is that the heritable material, namely the DNA, within each cell of the early embryo is altered by environmental stress. These environmentally induced changes remain dormant during early life and only contribute to adult disease by causing cellular dysfunction in adult tissue (Waterland

Developmental Origins of Health and Disease, ed. Peter Gluckman and Mark Hanson. Published by Cambridge University Press.
© P. D. Gluckman and M. A. Hanson 2006.

and Garza 1999). Each one of our cells contains a large nuclear genome containing 10^8 base pairs (bps) of nuclear DNA (nDNA), and epigenetic changes to this nDNA, which may be associated with developmental programming (Young *et al.* 1998, Rees *et al.* 2000), are discussed elsewhere in this volume. There is, however, an alternative genome in almost all our cells, and that is contained within each mitochondrion. Different cell types may contain different amounts of mitochondria with varying numbers of copies of mtDNA. Mitochondrial DNA (mtDNA) is very much smaller than nDNA; it is a small circular genome of only 16 000 bps (Attardi and Schatz 1988). Until recently mitochondria and mtDNA were thought to play a relatively minor role in cellular function. However, over the past ten years it has become clear that this small organelle containing its own genome can have far-reaching and pervasive effects on many different aspects of cellular function (Wallace 1999). It is the involvement of mitochondria in developmental programming that will be the focus of this chapter. The unusual developmental characteristics of mitochondria that make them a good transmission vector of early developmental stress will be reviewed, highlighting their association with disorders related to developmental programming. Finally, future experimental manipulations that may prove a direct link between environmentally induced changes in mitochondria and the consequences of developmental programming will be explored. The repercussions that these findings may have on apparently unrelated fields such as assisted-conception programmes in humans and evolution studies will be considered.

Mitochondrial dysfunction in disease and in tissues of 'programmed' animals

If stress-induced changes in mitochondria contribute to the constellation of disorders known as syndrome X it would be expected that abnormal mitochondrial dysfunction be associated with all of the disorders associated with this syndrome, namely hypertension, insulin resistance, dyslipidaemia,

obesity and endothelial dysfunction. Clinical studies show that this is indeed the case (Ballinger *et al.* 2002, Lamson and Plaza 2002, Wilson *et al.* 2004). Additionally, several learning disorders and behavioural abnormalities are associated with dysfunctional mitochondria (Swerdlow and Kish 2002, Aliev *et al.* 2003, Cardoso *et al.* 2004). This may of course be merely a consequence of cellular dysfunction in general, but, there are recent clinical and experimental reports showing that mtDNA mutations are linked to and precede the development of diabetes and hypertension in humans, implying a causal link (Song *et al.* 2001, Ballinger *et al.* 2002). Furthermore, experimental manipulations of mtDNA in mice, either in vitro in pancreatic cell lines (Soejima *et al.* 1996) or in vivo using conditional tissue-specific gene ablation studies, show a direct link with altered mtDNA and altered pancreatic and cardiac function (Larsson *et al.* 1998, Silva *et al.* 2000). Furthermore, recent elegant studies employing a mouse model with a defective mtDNA-specific DNA polymerise displayed chronic cellular dysfunction and more rapid rates of ageing (Trifunovic *et al.* 2004).

There is also evidence from models of developmental programming that both mitochondrial function and mtDNA are altered in the tissue of such animals (Rasschaert *et al.* 1995, McConnell *et al.* 2003, Park *et al.* 2003, Taylor *et al.* 2005). It is surprising that such very different maternal diets should all produce changes in mtDNA. These unexpectedly similar outcomes from such diverse stressors might suggest that mitochondria are a common vector through which different stressors permanently reset the mitochondrial inheritance of cells. Recent studies of the mtDNA content of the cells of adult tissue of developmentally programmed animals bear out the predictions based on a recently proposed hypothesis of developmental programming by Gluckman and Hanson (2004a, 2004b, 2004c). They proposed that maternal nutritional status sets up a predictive adaptive response such that offspring monitor the nutrient status of the mother and consider it 'normal'. If subsequently the dietary intake of the offspring markedly differs from that of the mother during pregnancy then the programmed adaptive response may be inappropriate, and an adverse health outcome may ensue. This hypothesis has been verified experimentally: animals exposed to a poor diet in utero and then reared on a rich diet have a reduced life span and cellular abnormalities (Ozanne and Hales 2004). Recent reports using a similar recuperative protocol recorded that mtDNA content within cells from different adult tissue was more severely reduced when animals were exposed to rich diets after birth to a mother fed a poor diet (Park et al. 2004).

Developmental programming by suboptimal maternal nutrition can be reversed by folate or taurine supplementation (Joshi et al. 2003, Franconi et al. 2004). Both these metabolites contribute to multiple pathways within cells, but it is notable that both can act as antioxidants, possibly ameliorating the damaging extrinsic and intrinsic consequences of the generation of additional radical oxygen species by mitochondria and their lasting effects on mtDNA.

Unique qualities of mitochondria

The findings discussed in the previous section are consistent with the involvement of mitochondria in developmental programming, but these molecular 'snapshots', mainly in adult tissue, do not address the central question of developmental programming, namely, how are early stresses perpetuated through development, and how do they eventually cause cellular dysfunction? In this respect the unusual properties of mitochondria and mtDNA in general, and their developmental characteristics in particular, may equip these small organelles with the ideal properties to act as molecular transmitters of early developmental stresses and the eventual cause of cellular dysfunction in adult offspring tissue.

Mitochondria are exclusively female in origin. They are small endosymbiotic organelles that exist in almost all cell types and require nuclear transcripts for activity (Attardi and Schatz 1988). Each mitochondrion contains many copies of its own circular genome, which is continuously turned over, being synthesised by a mitochondrial-specific DNA polymerase γ (Lestienne 1987). Levels of mtDNA are very sensitive to environmental stress, and a suboptimal environment can cause a reduction in both the efficiency and the fidelity of mtDNA synthesis, with an associated reduction in the quantity of mtDNA and an increase in random mutations within it (Graziewicz et al. 2002). MtDNA mutations can be induced as a result of both extrinsic and intrinsic stress and tolerated for many years before reaching a damaging threshold level (Chinnery et al. 2002). This latent nature of mtDNA mutations allows this genome to act as an ideal undetected transmitter of early developmental stress. During oocyte maturation, whilst the nuclear genome does not replicate its DNA and is therefore not susceptible to environmental changes, mtDNA on the other hand accumulates to high levels, being expanded from 10^1 copies per primordial germ cell to 10^5 copies in each mature oocyte (Cummins 2002). Although there are constant levels of mtDNA during preimplantation development (Piko and Taylor 1987), it has recently been shown that there is a short window of mtDNA synthesis between the one- and two-cell stages that is particularly susceptible to environmental stress (McConnell and Petrie 2004) (Plate 1). During preimplantation development a constant amount of mtDNA is divided between increasing numbers of cells, and each founder cell of the developing embryo at embryonic day 6 will consequently contain very few copies of mtDNA. This restriction, and any environmental factors which change mtDNA prior to this stage, will be pivotal in determining the mtDNA template for all cells of the developing fetus (Cummins 2002), including the primordial germ cells, which will in turn contribute to the next generation.

Given the unique characteristics of mitochondria, stress-induced changes in mtDNA could be induced soon after fertilisation. These abnormalities would persist during embryonic development and then be transmitted to all cells of the developing fetus, but because of the threshold effect they could remain dormant through fetal and early life. Cellular function may appear perfectly normal until additional cellular stresses in specific adult tissue tipped the cell over a damaging level of mtDNA mutation. Only at this point would mitochondria behave abnormally and contribute to adult disease. It is notable that the organs most affected in models of developmental programming are those with the highest energy needs, such as kidney, heart and pancreas. Energy-demanding cell types may be particularly prone to suffer from mitochondrial dysfunction if they carry aberrant mtDNA for two reasons: first, energy-demanding cells tend to display mitochondrial dysfunction at a lower threshold level, and second, high-energy-producing cells will inevitably have higher rates of oxidative phosphorylation, and this may produce more damaging free radicals which will further damage mtDNA (Larsson *et al.* 1998, Esposito *et al.* 1999). Thus early changes in mtDNA may establish a predisposition for cellular dysfunction, but this may first become apparent in energy-demanding cells.

There are additional data to support the proposition that the very earliest stages of development immediately after fertilisation may be particularly prone to insults which will alter adult phenotype. Stress arising from suboptimal nutrition or culture conditions during the preimplantation phases of mammalian development can lead to altered physiology in adult offspring (Kwong *et al.* 2000, Tamashiro *et al.* 2002, Ecker *et al.* 2004, Fernandez-Gonzalez *et al.* 2004). Further evidence implicating early environmental stress to mitochondria in the permanent resetting of adult phenotype comes from detailed experimental manipulations in a simple animal model system, the nematode *Caenorhabditis elegans* (Dillin *et al.* 2002). Additionally, we have shown that preimplantation embryos isolated from dams fed a low-protein diet contained reduced amounts of mtDNA when compared to controls, and that these alterations persist at the very least into fetal life (McConnell and Petrie 2003).

Proof of involvement of mtDNA in developmental programming

The great advantage of the proposal that early changes in mtDNA are involved in developmental programming is that there are clear predictions which can be immediately tested using current technology. There are two very obvious predictions. If early changes in mtDNA contribute to the disorders associated with developmental programming, then specific and measurable alteration of the mitochondrial genome during this phase alone will cause abnormalities in adult offspring. Secondly, since mitochondrial inheritance is exclusively female we would expect to see transmission into the second generation but only through the female line. Experiments involving in vitro embryo treatments followed by embryo replacement and transgenerational studies that directly address these two predictions are ongoing in the laboratory.

Studies on developmental programming and mtDNA replication in the very early embryo have already provided interesting insights into the basic biology of early mammalian development and altered a belief which had been accepted for the past 30 years (McConnell and Petrie 2004). There may also be important clinical implications of our observations. Even though there may be minor interspecies differences from humans, mouse models have been invaluable in discovering the molecular basis of mammalian development in general. In-vitro culture of human preimplantation embryos is required for assisted-conception programmes, for pre-genetic diagnosis, and for the powerful emerging technologies associated with customised human embryonic stem cell production and regenerative cell therapy (Pickering and Braude 2003, Pickering *et al.* 2003). We have recently observed a similar but extended period of mtDNA replication during human preimplantation development (Pickering and McConnell, unpublished). If deleterious changes were irreversibly programmed into the mitochondrial genome of human preimplantation embryos by suboptimal culture, then these progressive new technologies may inadvertently be contributing to disease in future human populations, at least in advanced western societies where these therapies are becoming common.

The possibility that environmental factors such as stress may accelerate the rates of acquired mutation in mtDNA also has implications for the field of evolutionary science. The Eve theory of evolution (Lewin 1987) assumes that we originated from Africa, based on the observation that there is a great number of mtDNA mutations in African populations. Since it has been assumed that numbers of different mutations accumulate with time it has been proposed that humans have lived in Africa for longer than elsewhere (Ayala 1995, Watson *et al.* 1997). However, if stress, such as particularly rapid and unexpected changes in food supply, may increase the rate of mutation, then levels of mutation in mtDNA may reflect not only time but also environmental stress.

In this chapter I have concentrated exclusively on the earliest changes to mtDNA because they are most likely to feed into the genetic bottleneck which occurs in mammals shortly after implantation as a result of the dilution of mtDNA by cell division in the absence of mtDNA replication. However, it is clear that this kind of developmental programming, which acts through alterations in mtDNA, could occur at stages other than immediately after fertilisation – but it may be likely to affect some tissues more than others, and the effects are likely to be less all-pervasive since they will have occurred after the earlier developmental bottleneck. The molecular mechanisms involved in developmental programming are likely to be complex, involving both nuclear and mitochondrial components. Experimental methods are currently available to define exactly the contribution of early changes in mtDNA in the enigmatic problem of developmental programming. Once it is defined, it will be interesting to identify interplay between nDNA and mtDNA; since mitochondria rely on nDNA encoded transcripts to function it is inevitable that alterations in nuclear gene expression will affect mitochondrial function and mitochondrial DNA replication. For instance, it is also known that mtDNA is stabilised by a binding factor, TFAm, the expression of which has recently been shown to be modulated by DNA methylation of the promoter region of another nuclear encoded gene, NRF1 (Choi *et al.* 2004). If the amount of TFAm within a cell type is reduced there is a corresponding decline in the content of mtDNA (Larsson *et al.* 1998). Thus epigenetic changes to nDNA may influence mitochondrial inheritance. With the growing interest in

the field of developmental programming, exciting new insights are inevitable during the next few years. It is ironic that a new and some would say imprecise and applied field, which is necessarily long-term and whole-animal-based, is already beginning to challenge assumptions in some more sophisticated fields of science, such as genetic inheritance, mitochondria replication and evolutionary biology

ACKNOWLEDGMENTS

I would like to thank Lesley Clayton for critical reading of the manuscript.

REFERENCES

Aliev, G., Seyidova, D., Lamb, B. T. *et al.* (2003). Mitochondria and vascular lesions as a central target for the development of Alzheimer's disease and Alzheimer disease-like pathology in transgenic mice. *Neurol. Res.*, **25**, 665–74.

Attardi, G. and Schatz, G. (1988). Biogenesis of mitochondria. *Annu. Rev. Cell Biol.*, **4**, 289–333.

Ayala, F. J. (1995). The myth of Eve: molecular biology and human origins. *Science*, **270**, 1930–6.

Ballinger, S. W., Patterson, C., Knight-Lozano, C. A. *et al.* (2002). Mitochondrial integrity and function in atherogenesis. *Circulation*, **106**, 544–9.

Barker, D. J. P. (2002). Fetal programming of coronary heart disease. *Trends Endocrinol. Metab.*, **13**, 364–8.

Cardoso, S. M., Santana, I., Swerdlow, R. H. and Oliveira, C. R. (2004). Mitochondria dysfunction of Alzheimer's disease cybrids enhances Abeta toxicity. *J. Neurochem.*, **89**, 1417–26.

Chinnery, P. F., Samuels, D. C., Elson, J. and Turnbull, D. M. (2002). Accumulation of mitochondrial DNA mutations in ageing, cancer, and mitochondrial disease: is there a common mechanism? *Lancet*, **360**, 1323–5.

Choi, Y. S., Kim, S., Kyu Lee, H., Lee, K. U. and Pak, Y. K. (2004). In vitro methylation of nuclear respiratory factor-1 binding site suppresses the promoter activity of mitochondrial transcription factor A. *Biochem. Biophys. Res. Commun.*, **314**, 118–22.

Cummins, J. M. (2002). The role of maternal mitochondria during oogenesis, fertilization and embryogenesis. *Reprod. Biomed. Online*, **4**, 176–82.

Dillin, A., Hsu, A. L., Arantes-Oliveira, N. *et al.* (2002). Rates of behavior and aging specified by mitochondrial function during development. *Science*, **298**, 2398–401.

Ecker, D. J., Stein, P., Xu, Z. *et al.* (2004). Long-term effects of culture of preimplantation mouse embryos on behavior. *Proc. Natl. Acad. Sci. USA*, **101**, 1595–600.

Eriksson, J. G. and Forsen, T. J. (2002). Childhood growth and coronary heart disease in later life. *Ann. Med.*, **34**, 157–61.

Esposito, L. A., Melov, S., Panov, A., Cottrell, B. A. and Wallace, D. C. (1999). Mitochondrial disease in mouse results in increased oxidative stress. *Proc. Natl. Acad. Sci. USA*, **96**, 4820–5.

Fernandez-Gonzalez, R., Moreira, P., Bilbao, A. *et al.* (2004). Long-term effect of in vitro culture of mouse embryos with serum on mRNA expression of imprinting genes, development, and behavior. *Proc. Natl. Acad. Sci. USA*, **101**, 5880–5.

Franconi, F., Di Leo, M. A., Bennardini, F. and Ghirlanda, G. (2004). Is taurine beneficial in reducing risk factors for diabetes mellitus? *Neurochem. Res.*, **29**, 143–50.

Gluckman, P. D. and Hanson, M. A. (2004a). Developmental origins of disease paradigm: a mechanistic and evolutionary perspective. *Pediatr. Res.*, **56**, 311–17.

(2004b). The developmental origins of the metabolic syndrome. *Trends Endocrinol. Metab.*, **15**, 183–7.

(2004c). Living with the past: evolution, development, and patterns of disease. *Science*, **305**, 1733–6.

Graziewicz, M. A., Day, B. J. and Copeland, W. C. (2002). The mitochondrial DNA polymerase as a target of oxidative damage. *Nucleic Acids Res.*, **30**, 2817–24.

Joshi, S., Rao, S., Golwilkar, A., Patwardhan, M. and Bhonde, R. (2003). Fish oil supplementation of rats during pregnancy reduces adult disease risks in their offspring. *J. Nutr.*, **133**, 3170–4.

Khan, I. Y., Taylor, P. D., Dekou, V. *et al.* (2003). Gender-linked hypertension in offspring of lard-fed pregnant rats. *Hypertension*, **41**, 168–75.

Khan, I. Y., Dekou, V., Douglas, G. *et al.* (2005). A high-fat diet during rat pregnancy or suckling induces cardiovascular dysfunction in adult offspring. *Am. J. Physiol. Regul. Integr. Comp. Physiol.*, **288**, R127–33.

Kwong, W., Wild, A., Roberts, P., Willis, A. and Fleming, T. (2000). Maternal undernutrition during the preimplantation period of rat development causes blastocyst abnormalities and programming of postnatal hypertension. *Development*, **127**, 195–202.

Lamson, D. W. and Plaza, S. M. (2002). Mitochondrial factors in the pathogenesis of diabetes: a hypothesis for treatment. *Altern. Med. Rev.*, **7**, 94–111.

Langley-Evans, S. and Jackson, A. (1996). Intrauterine programming of hypertension: nutrient–hormone interactions. *Nutr. Rev.*, **54**, 163–9.

Larsson, N. G., Wang, J., Wilhelmsson, H. *et al.* (1998). Mitochondrial transcription factor A is necessary for mtDNA maintenance and embryogenesis in mice. *Nat. Genet.*, **18**, 231–6.

Lestienne, P. (1987). Evidence for a direct role of the DNA polymerase gamma in the replication of the human mitochondrial DNA in vitro. *Biochem. Biophys. Res. Commun.*, **146**, 1146–53.

Lewin, R. (1987). The unmasking of mitochondrial Eve. *Science*, **238**, 24–6.

McConnell, J. M. L. and Petrie, L. (2003). Analyses of the effects of maternal protein restriction and elevated homocysteine on mitochondrial respiratory activity and mtDNA copy number in preimplantation embryos. *Pediatr. Res.*, **53**, 816.

(2004). Mitochondrial DNA turnover occurs during preimplantation development and can be modulated by environmental factors. *Reprod. Biomed. Online*, **9**, 418–24.

McConnell, J. M. L., Petrie, L., Taylor, P. and Poston, L. (2003). A high fat diet during pregnancy results in reduced mitochondrial copy number in offspring. *J. Soc. Gynecol. Investig.*, **10**, 732.

Osmond, C. and Barker, D. J. P. (2000). Fetal, infant, and childhood growth are predictors of coronary heart disease, diabetes, and hypertension in adult men and women. *Environ. Health Perspect.*, **108** (Suppl 3), 545–53.

Ozanne, S. E. and Hales, C. N. (2002). Early programming of glucose-insulin metabolism. *Trends Endocrinol. Metab.*, **13**, 368–73.

(2004). Lifespan: catch-up growth and obesity in male mice. *Nature*, **427**, 411–12.

Ozanne, S. E., Martensz, N. D., Petry, C. J., Loizou, C. L. and Hales, C. N. (1998). Maternal low protein diet in rats programmes fatty acid desaturase activities in the offspring. *Diabetologia*, **41**, 1337–42.

Park, K. S., Kim, S. K., Kim, M. S. *et al.* (2003). Fetal and early postnatal protein malnutrition cause long-term changes in rat liver and muscle mitochondria. *J. Nutr.*, **133**, 3085–90.

Park, H. K., Jin, C. J., Cho, Y. M. *et al.* (2004). Changes of mitochondrial DNA content in the male offspring of protein-malnourished rats. *Ann. NY Acad. Sci.*, **1011**, 205–16.

Pickering, S. and Braude, P. (2003). Further advances and uses of assisted conception technology. *BMJ*, **327**, 1156–8.

Pickering, S. J., Braude, P. R., Patel, M. *et al.* (2003). Preimplantation genetic diagnosis as a novel source of embryos for stem cell research. *Reprod. Biomed. Online*, **7**, 353–64.

Piko, L. and Taylor, K. D. (1987). Amounts of mitochondrial DNA and abundance of some mitochondrial gene transcripts in early mouse embryos. *Dev. Biol.*, **123**, 364–74.

Rasschaert, J., Reusens, B., Dahri, S. *et al.* (1995). Impaired activity of rat pancreatic islet mitochondrial glycerophosphate dehydrogenase in protein malnutrition. *Endocrinology*, **136**, 2631–4.

Rees, W. D., Hay, S. M., Brown, D. S., Antipatis, C. and Palmer, R. M. (2000). Maternal protein deficiency causes hypermethylation of DNA in the livers of rat fetuses. *J. Nutr.*, **130**, 1821–6.

Silva, J. P., Kohler, M., Graff, C. *et al.* (2000). Impaired insulin secretion and beta-cell loss in tissue-specific knockout mice with mitochondrial diabetes. *Nat. Genet.*, **26**, 336–40.

Soejima, A., Inoue, K., Takai, D. *et al.* (1996). Mitochondrial DNA is required for regulation of glucose-stimulated insulin secretion in a mouse pancreatic beta cell line, MIN6. *J. Biol. Chem.*, **271**, 26194–9.

Song, J., Oh, J. Y., Sung, Y. A., Pak, Y. K., Park, K. S. and Lee, H. K. (2001). Peripheral blood mitochondrial DNA content is related to insulin sensitivity in offspring of type 2 diabetic patients. *Diabetes Care*, **24**, 865–9.

Sorensen, H. T., Thulstrup, A. M., Norgdard, B. *et al.* (2000). Fetal growth and blood pressure in a Danish population aged 31–51 years. *Scand. Cardiovasc. J.*, **34**, 390–5.

Swerdlow, R. H. and Kish, S. J. (2002). Mitochondria in Alzheimer's disease. *Int. Rev. Neurobiol.*, **53**, 341–85.

Tamashiro, K., Wakayama, T., Akutsu, H. *et al.* (2002). Cloned mice have an obese phenotype not transmitted to their offspring. *Nat. Med.*, **8**, 262–7.

Taylor, P. D., McConnell, J. M. L., Khan, I. Y. *et al.* (2005). Impaired glucose homeostasis and mitochondrial abnormalities in offspring of rats fed a fat-rich diet in pregnancy. *Am. J. Physiol. Regul. Integr. Comp. Physiol.*, **288**, R134–9.

Trifunovic, A., Wredenberg, A., Falkenberg, M. *et al.* (2004). Premature ageing in mice expressing defective mitochondrial DNA polymerase. *Nature*, **429**, 417–23.

Vickers, M. H., Breier, B. H., McCarthy, D. and Gluckman, P. D. (2003). Sedentary behavior during postnatal life is determined by the prenatal environment and exacerbated by postnatal hypercaloric nutrition. *Am. J. Physiol. Regul. Integr. Comp. Physiol.*, **285**, R271–3.

Wallace, D. C. (1999). Mitochondrial diseases in man and mouse. *Science* **283**, 1482–8.

Waterland, R. A. and Garza, C. (1999). Potential mechanisms of metabolic imprinting that lead to chronic disease. *Am. J. Clin. Nutr.*, **69**, 179–97.

Watson, E., Forster, P., Richards, M. and Bandelt, H. J. (1997). Mitochondrial footprints of human expansions in Africa. *Am. J. Hum. Genet.*, **61**, 691–704.

Weaver, I. C., Cervoni, N., Champagne, F. A. *et al.* (2004). Epigenetic programming by maternal behavior. *Nat. Neurosci.*, **7**, 847–54.

Wilson, F. H., Hariri, A. *et al.* (2004). A cluster of metabolic defects caused by mutation in a mitochondrial tRNA. *Science*, **306**, 1190–4.

Young, L. E., Sinclair, K. D. and Wilmut, I. (1998). Large offspring syndrome in cattle and sheep. *Rev. Reprod.*, **3**, 155–163.

Young, L. E., Fernandes, K., McEvoy, T. G. *et al.* (2001). Epigenetic change in IGF2R is associated with fetal overgrowth after sheep embryo culture. *Nat. Genet.*, **27**, 153–4.

7

Role of exposure to environmental chemicals in developmental origins of health and disease

Jerrold J. Heindel and Cindy Lawler

National Institute of Environmental Health Sciences

Introduction

Between two and five per cent of all live-born infants have a major developmental defect. Up to 40 per cent of these defects have been estimated to result from maternal exposure(s) to harmful environmental agents that directly or indirectly create an unfavourable intrauterine environment. A spectrum of adverse effects can occur, including death, structural malformation, and/or functional alteration of the fetus/embryo. The traditional focus of the science of developmental toxicology has been on the role of agents (environmental or drugs) that cause either premature death of the fetus or birth defects. In recent years, attention has turned to examining the effects of in-utero or neonatal exposure to environmental agents on functional changes in tissues, e.g. permanent changes in tissue function that are not the result of overtly or grossly teratogenic effects but that result in increased susceptibility to disease/dysfunction later in life.

The epidemiology data that support the concept of the fetal basis of adult disease, together with the preliminary data showing alterations in gene expression and tissue imprinting due to in-utero exposures to some environmental agents, provide an attractive framework for understanding delayed functional effects of toxicant exposures. We propose that exposure to certain environmental chemicals, alone or in combination with altered nutrition, leads to aberrant developmental programming that permanently alters gland, organ or system potential. These states of altered potential or compromised function are hypothesised to result from epigenetic changes, e.g. altered gene expression due to toxicant-induced effects on imprinting, and the underlying methylation-related protein-DNA relationships associated with chromatin remodelling. The end result is an animal that is sensitised such that it will be more susceptible to diseases later in life.

The following key points serve to elaborate our general hypothesis:
- Time-specific (vulnerable window) and tissue-specific effects may occur.
- The initiating in-utero environmental insult may act alone or in concert with in-utero nutrition and/or with later exposures. That is, there could be an in-utero exposure that would lead by itself to pathophysiology later in life, or there could be in-utero exposure combined with a neonatal exposure (same or different compounds) or adult exposure that would trigger or exacerbate the pathophysiology.
- The pathophysiology may manifest as (a) the occurrence of a disease that otherwise would not have happened, (b) an increase in risk for a disease that would normally be of lower prevalence, or (c) either an earlier onset of a disease that would normally have occurred or an exacerbation of the disease.

- The pathophysiology may have a variable latent period from onset in the neonatal period, to early childhood, puberty, early or late adulthood depending on the toxicant, time of exposure and tissue/organ affected. Importantly, the effects may be transmitted to future generations through the germ line.
- The effects of in-utero exposure to toxic environmental chemicals may occur in the absence of reduced birthweight. This makes them more difficult to assess than effects due to severe nutritional deficits during development.

This review is selective in focus and is intended to highlight data that show proof of principle for the hypothesis that in-utero exposures to environmental agents alone or in combination with altered nutrition can provide the developmental basis for a number of later-occurring diseases. This is a unique perspective that focuses on an emerging component of the developmental basis of disease continuum. Although this topic appears relatively new it was proposed over 20 years ago (reviewed in Bern 1992, McLachlan *et al.* 2001) but received little attention until recently, when increased knowledge of the action of environmental chemicals during development provided a plausible basis for these concepts.

The main focus of this review is on animal studies. Research in this area is relatively new, however, and many of the animal studies cited will not fulfil all of the tenets of the fetal-origins hypothesis proposed above. Studies are organised by class of disease/dysfunction, and include examples from the areas of reproductive toxicity, neurodegeneration, obesity and immune/autoimmune disease. These studies are presented to show the state of the science in this area and to highlight data gaps and needs. Only a few human studies will be described, as the fetal-origins hypothesis is particularly difficult to assess in humans, because in-utero exposures must be linked to gene expression or other tissue-potential changes at birth and then to an adult disease. Nonetheless, humans are exposed to a variety of environmental chemicals in-utero, and many are the same chemicals that have been shown to cause increased incidence of disease/dysfunction later in

life in animal studies (Needham *et al.* 2000, Mori *et al.* 2002, Younglai *et al.* 2002) and at similar concentrations to those used in the animal studies. Thus the potential exists for extrapolation of the animal data to human health.

Reproductive toxicity/diseases and developmental exposures to environmental agents

Female effects

Neonatal xenoestrogen exposure during critical developmental windows can alter hormonal programming so that tissues respond abnormally to hormones later in life. This can lead to a number of adverse effects, including increased incidence of tumors in several endocrine-sensitive tissues.

The example of DES

In the reproductive tract, the classic example of this phenomenon is diethylstilboestrol (DES). In humans, in-utero exposure to DES (presumed to reduce miscarriage and early labour) resulted in an increased incidence of vaginal adenocarcinomas at puberty (Herbst *et al.* 1971) and increased breast cancer (Palmer *et al.* 2002). In CD-1 mice, neonatal low-dose DES ($0.1\ \mu g\ kg^{-1}$) resulted in animals without gross alterations in uterine morphology but that showed an altered response to oestrogen at puberty and altered uterine gene expression that was irreversible. These mice developed an increased incidence of uterine adenocarcinomas in adulthood. Importantly, the effect was transgenerational, with the F2 mice also showing an increased incidence of uterine cancers (McLachlan *et al.* 1980, Newbold *et al.* 1990). This finding is of special significance, as the ability to induce a transgenerational effect suggests an epigenetic change occurred and was transmitted through the germ line. Consistent with this hypothesis, the increased uterine adenocarcinomas observed in mice were accompanied by altered methylation of specific oestrogen-responsive genes in the uterus (Shuanfang *et al.* 2003). Neonatal DES treatment has also been shown to result in increased and persistent phosphorylation of EGFR, erbB2 and ERα along with an elevation of c-fos expression, effects capable of activating the receptor-mediated pathways in a ligand-independent manner, providing a possible mechanism for the effects of neonatal DES exposure (Li *et al.* 2003, Miyagawa *et al.* 2004). It is not clear if these effects are also related to epigenetic changes. Neonatal exposure of rats to DES also induces morphological and functional abnormalities in the adult ovary, including altered gene expression of steroidogenic enzymes (Nagai *et al.* 2003).

Additional xenobiotic endocrine disruptors

While there is unequivocal evidence for in-utero exposure to DES in the causation of cancers in humans and animals, as noted above, there are also data on developmental exposures to other oestrogenic endocrine disrupting chemicals in human and animal studies and increased cancer risk later in life. Birnbaum and Fenton's (2003) recent review concluded that there is good evidence for increased tumour formation induced by pre- or neonatal exposure to a variety of environmental chemicals, direct-acting carcinogens and drugs. Indeed, animal studies have shown that in-utero exposures to bisphenol A (a component of polycarbonate plastic and resins that line food and beverage containers, and that has been shown to leach out under harsh conditions (Hunt *et al.* 2003)), atrazine (a heavily used chlorotriazine herbicide) or dioxin can alter development and organisation of the mammary gland in mice and rats, effects that increase susceptibility to cancer later in life. For example, Markey *et al.* (2001) reported that the CD-1 mouse mammary gland responds to in-utero exposure to bisphenol A with altered DNA synthesis in the epithelium and stroma, resulting in atypical histoarchitecture (increase in terminal ducts and end buds) that became significant at 6 months of age. These changes have been associated with enhanced susceptibility to tumour formation in both rodents and humans (Birnbaum and Fenton 2003). Prenatal treat-

ment with dioxin also alters mammary gland development, resulting in fewer primary ducts, stunted epithelial progression into the fat pad, fewer terminal buds, decreased lateral branching, delayed lobule formation and absence of full maturation of the gland, effects that were correlated with increased tumour development later in life (Brown *et al.* 1998, Fenton *et al.* 2002). This effect of in-utero dioxin exposure on mammary gland development and tumour formation in rats was transgenerational, with disrupted mammary gland development observed in second-generation pups. Thus in-utero exposure to DES in mice and dioxin in rats can both lead to transgenerational effects. Similarly, prenatal exposure to atrazine inhibits mammary gland development (Fenton *et al.* 2002).

The mechanism by which delays in mammary gland development increase cancer risk is unclear at present. One possibility is that the delays in mammary gland development by dioxin or atrazine exposures in-utero confer an extended window of sensitivity to potential carcinogens after sexual maturity (Birnbaum and Fenton 2003). These studies suggest that animal and human studies of breast cancer that focus on adult exposures to environmental chemicals may be trying to correlate exposure and effect at the wrong time, and suggest the focus should be on in-utero exposures that increase susceptibility to tumour formation later in life. Indeed, Palmer *et al.* (2002) reported an overall 40 per cent increased risk of breast cancer in women exposed in-utero to DES, an effect that may increase as these women are just now reaching the age at which the incidence of breast cancer increases.

The effects observed with fetal exposure to DES have been shown to occur with other oestrogenic environmental chemicals, including the chlorinated hydrocarbon pesticide methoxychlor (Alworth *et al.* 2002) and the phytoestrogen genestein (Jefferson *et al.* in press). For example, Hughes *et al.* (2003) reported that developmental exposure of rat pups to soy milk or genestein at levels comparable to the ranges of human exposures permanently modified the expression of the oestrogen-regulated progesterone receptor in the uterus (Hughes *et al.* 2003).

In-utero exposure to low doses of genestein also caused earlier puberty and abnormal oestrous cycles in Wistar rats, effects probably related to masculinisation of the female brain (Kouki *et al.* 2003). An increased incidence of uterine adenocarcinomas (Newbold *et al.* 2001), multioocyte follicles in the maturing ovary (Jefferson *et al.* 2002) and carcinogen-induced mammary gland tumours in adulthood (Hilakivi-Clarke *et al.* 1999) in mice have been noted in other studies examining in-utero effects of genestein.

Prenatal exposure of the female rhesus monkey to androgen produces a syndrome of effects that provide a nonhuman primate model for the aetiology and mechanism of polycystic ovary syndrome (PCOS). This monkey model develops delayed menarche accompanied by increased body mass and ovarian dysfunction that by adulthood is accompanied by LH hypersecretion and impaired insulin resistance, hyperandrogenism, anovulation and infertility (Abbott *et al.* 1997, Eisner *et al.* 2002). These results have been verified in a sheep model (Padmanabhan *et al.* 1998). It appears that the prenatal androgen exposure reprogrammes multiple fetal organs, resulting in the hyperandrogenism that leads to increased LH and encourages preferential abdominal adiposity, which predisposes to insulin resistance (Abbott *et al.* 2002). While it is not likely that humans are exposed to environmental androgens, it is possible that they are exposed to environmental oestrogens that could be converted to androgens via aromatase or that could indirectly alter androgen programming; or increased androgen exposure might arise from altered ovarian or adrenal function in-utero. There is also increasing evidence suggesting a prenatal aetiology of PCOS-like syndromes in humans, indicating that the monkey model may be useful in understanding both aetiology and mechanism of PCOS induction.

Male effects

As for the female, the male is also sensitive to in-utero exposures to oestrogenic compounds. There is also significant data on in-utero exposures to antiandrogens and dioxin and their effects on disease/dysfunction later in life. In some instances (see below) the actual link from in-utero exposures to adult disease has not been developed and this is thus an area where future research is needed.

Dioxin and environmental oestrogens and the prostate

In-utero and lactational exposure to low doses of dioxin, e.g. doses close to background body levels in humans (Lin *et al.* 2003), alters prostate development (lobe-specific, with the ventral prostate the most sensitive, then the anterior, then the dorsolateral lobes) related to decreased formation of prostatic buds and agenesis of ventral buds. Dioxin essentially prevents the ventral prostate from developing. This effect is related to activation of the Ah receptor and is susceptible to regulation by oestrogen levels in the developing fetus (Timms *et al.* 2002). The in-utero exposure to dioxin in this experimental paradigm thus causes visible changes in tissue morphology. However, the changes would not be considered teratogenic as the prostate is present and appears to function normally; thus these data fit the fetal-origins paradigm. A major goal of this work is to determine if the in-utero exposure could be related to prostate cancer-like effects later in life, effects that could be extrapolated to human prostate hyperplasia and cancers. To this end, mice born to dams given dioxin or vehicle were examined at 100 and 510 days of age. Half were castrated ten days prior to necropsy to assess androgen dependence. Responses to castration were similar in vehicle- and dioxin-exposed mice at 100 days of age. However, dioxin-exposed mice were substantially more responsive to castration, by most measured indices, than vehicle-exposed mice at 510 days of age. Thus the decline in androgen-dependent prostate growth that occurs normally with age is prevented by in-utero and lactational dioxin exposure. This suggests that gene expression is altered by in-utero exposure to dioxin and that the alterations are permanent. The mechanisms for these permanent changes in gene expression may be altered tissue imprinting, and this aspect is under examination.

Histological examination of the dorsolateral prostates from 510-day-old mice exposed to dioxin perinatally showed that while 2–3% of ducts in the controls had cribriform structures, this was increased to 16% in the dioxin-exposed group (R. Peterson, personal communication). While mice do not develop prostate cancer, cribriform lesions are often considered a precancerous lesion in humans. Because the AhR signalling pathway is expressed in human fetal prostate, in benign prostate hyperplasia and in prostate cancer, the transcriptional machinery is present in the prostate of men to respond to dioxin exposures throughout life. This raises the important question of whether dioxin exposure during human fetal development could increase susceptibility to prostate cancer later in life.

The developing prostate is also sensitive to oestrogen levels. In-utero exposure to the environmental oestrogens bisphenol A, methoxychlor (an oestrogenic pesticide) or DES at low levels produced an increase in number and size of dorsolateral prostate ducts and an overall increase in prostate volume due to increased proliferation of basal epithelial cells, resulting in increased prostate weight in adulthood (Welshons *et al.* 1999, Ramos *et al.* 2001, B. G. Timms, unpublished). There is a permanent increase in prostatic androgen receptors in adult male mice due to the fetal exposure to low doses of DES, bisphenol A, oestradiol or ethynyloestradiol (vom Saal *et al.* 1997). These studies have not been extended to determine if the increased prostate weight and number of androgen receptors will result in hyperplastic or hyperplasic prostate later in life. However, it is interesting that in 1936 Zuckerman (noted in vom Saal *et al.* 1997) speculated that exposure to elevated oestrogens during development could predispose men to have an enlarged prostate in old age. It should be noted that higher doses of these chemicals or natural oestradiol above the physiological range led to the opposite effect, a reduction in adult prostate weight. Indeed, Woodham *et al.* (2003) showed that neonatal exposure to high doses of oestradiol benzoate down-regulates the prostate androgen receptor, an effect that persists into adulthood, indicat-

ing a permanent imprinting of the receptor levels in mice. Similarly, high doses of phytoestrogens during development result in reduced prostate androgen receptor levels that persist into adulthood and result in reduced prostate weight when the high phytoestrogen diet is maintained throughout life (Lund *et al.* 2004).

Environmental oestrogens and testis function and fertility

Neonatal DES (0.01 and 1 μg/animal) exposure in hamsters results in males that appear normal at birth with no evidence of cryptorchidism, testicular tumours or other testicular abnormalities, and with qualitatively normal and complete spermatogenesis up to 40 days of age. By 60 days of age, spermatogenesis declined and spermatids and secondary spermatocytes were absent in many seminiferous tubules, with some containing only Sertoli cells and spermatogonia. These effects were not reversed by testosterone treatment but are proposed to be due to reduced androgen receptor gene expression due to altered neonatal programming (Karri *et al.* 2004). These data highlight an in-utero exposure that does not appear to cause any toxicity at birth but leads to an increased disease which does not appear until adulthood. At present, however, there are no data showing an effect on gene expression or other parameters of reproductive function at birth that could be responsible for the altered disease state in adulthood.

Exposure of pregnant rats to vinclozolin, a systemic dicarboximide fungicide used on fruits and vegetables, at doses over 100 mg/kg, show teratogenic effects on sexual differentiation, apparently due to its antiandrogenic actions (Kelce *et al.* 1997, Gray *et al.* 1999). At doses of 100 mg/kg (significantly above potential human exposures) vinclozolin appears not to have any significant effects on external genitalia or other physiological parameters such as testis weight or serum testosterone. Nonetheless, this in-utero exposure to vinclozolin causes a delayed stage-specific germ cell apoptosis noticeable by day 20 and continuing onto adulthood at day

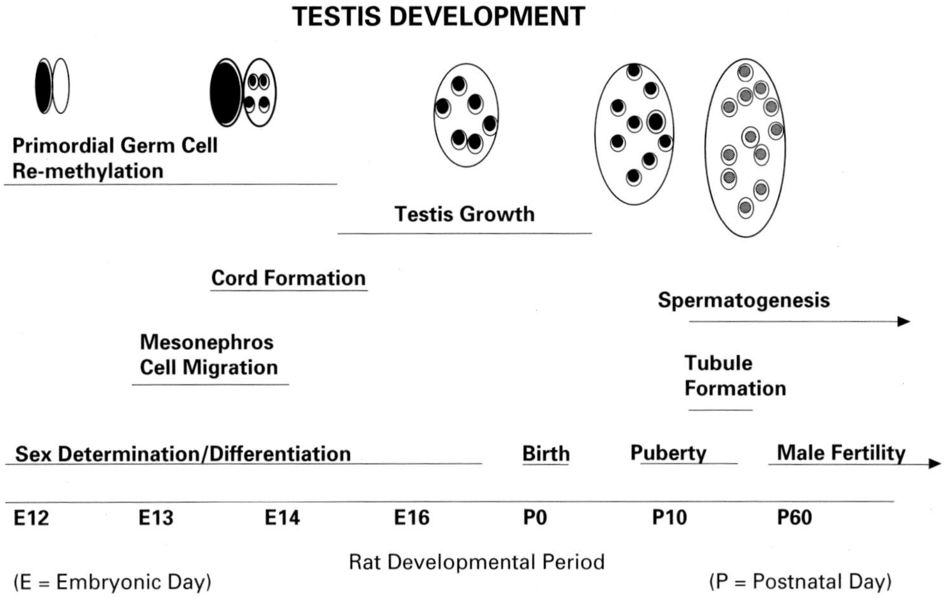

TESTIS DEVELOPMENT

Primordial Germ Cell
Re-methylation

Testis Growth

Cord Formation

Spermatogenesis

Mesonephros
Cell Migration

Tubule
Formation

Sex Determination/Differentiation   **Birth**   **Puberty**   **Male Fertility**

E12	E13	E14	E16	P0	P10	P60

Rat Developmental Period

(E = Embryonic Day)   (P = Postnatal Day)

Figure 7.1 Overview of testis development and windows of susceptibility to methoxychlor. As described in the text, exposure to methoxychlor at days E12–13 resulted in fertility problems later in life after age 60 days, an effect that was transmitted via the germ line for at least four generations. If the exposure in utero occurred later during the period of cord formation the effects on fertility were evident at 60 days of age but the effect was not transgenerational

60 (Uzumcu *et al.* 2004). While fertility was normal in these adult animals at 60 days of age, treated males started to develop infertility after 100 days of age (M. Skinner, personal communication) that correlated with altered testis histology. Thus the in-utero exposure clearly had adverse effects that became evident as spermatogenesis was initiated and progressed with age.

Perhaps the most compelling data on the role of exposures to environmental agents in the developmental basis of adult disease comes from the work on methoxychlor in male mice. In-utero exposure to methoxychlor not only resulted in effects in the adult due to in-utero exposure (e.g. increased testicular apoptosis leading to infertility starting at 100 days of age in up to 20% of the animals) but showed that the effects could be transmitted through the male germ line over at least four generations (Anway *et al.* 2005). The transgenerational effects were only noted when the in-utero exposure correlated with critical devel-

opmental processes such as cord formation and sex determination and the time of germ-cell remethylation. If dosing occurred later during testis development the transgenerational effects were absent, while other adverse effects still could be shown in the adult. Figure 7.1 outlines the dosing protocol and the timing of subsequent events. While other researchers have found significant adult male reproductive effects due to in-utero exposures to various environmental chemicals, they either did not look for transgenerational effects or did not find them; perhaps this was due to dosing too late during development, at the time of tissue development rather than during the time of epigenetic remodelling of germ-cell DNA. This transgenerational effect, along with that of dioxin on mammary gland function and DES on uterine tumours, when repeated and extended to other agents, has the potential to have a major impact on public health and evolutionary biology.

Obesity and developmental exposures to environmental agents

Obesity is a disease for which the prevalence has risen dramatically in developed countries over the past two to three decades, reaching epidemic proportions in the United States. It is considered to be caused by prolonged positive energy balance due to a combination of overeating and lack of physical activity on a background of genetic predisposition. The alarming rate of increase in obesity over only two to three decades indicates that the primary cause must lie in environmental and behavioural changes rather than in genetics. The environmental influence of interest to obesity has been in-utero, postnatal and adult nutrition. A large number of epidemiological studies have demonstrated a direct relationship between birthweight and body mass index attained later in life. These data support the seeming paradox of increased adult adiposity associated with both ends of the birthweight spectrum: higher body mass index with higher birthweight and increased central adiposity with lower birthweight (Oken and Gillman 2003, Rogers *et al.* 2003).

Recent data support the hypothesis that nutrition is not the only developmental environmental influence that may have an effect on obesity (Heindel 2003). The obesity epidemic is recent in origin, and Baillie-Hamilton (2002) notes a correlation with increasing exposure to manmade chemicals in occupational and environmental settings. The increase in obesity also correlates with living in the inner city, an area more highly exposed to environmental contaminants. Although such data are only correlational, it is tempting to speculate that there may be a role for increased exposures to environmental chemicals in the recent epidemic of obesity. It is well established that many substances including organophosphate pesticides, carbamates, antithyroid drugs, anabolic steroids and DES have been used to promote fattening and growth of animals (reviewed in Baillie-Hamilton 2002). In addition, as will be shown below, there is increasing evidence in animal models that in-utero exposure to environmental chemicals at environmentally relevant concentrations may alter developmental programming of adipose tissue and/or gastrointestinal–hypothalamic centres. The subsequent obesity observed in these models has been linked to irreversible alterations in tissue-specific function as a result of altered gene expression.

Environmental oestrogens and obesity

The most likely candidates for altering in-utero tissue function in ways that may result in obesity later in life include environmental oestrogens such as DES or bisphenol A as well as dioxin and nicotine. Newbold *et al.* (2004) have shown that low doses of DES ($1 \, \mu g/kg/day$), either pre- or neonatally, caused an increase in body weight of CD-1 mice that was not evident at birth but reached significance by 6 weeks of age. At 16 weeks of age the DES-exposed animals had a body fat of 27.6%, compared to controls with 20.9%. Neonatal exposure to other oestrogens, 2OH oestradiol, 4OH oestradiol, and the naturally occurring phytoestrogen genestein at approximately equal oestrogenic doses to DES also caused a significantly increased body weight at 4 months of age, suggesting that DES is not unique and that in-utero exposures to low doses of agents with oestrogenic activity can alter the set-point of body-weight control (Fig. 7.2). Genestein has effects that differ with dose and timing of exposure. This effect of genestein is opposite to that seen in the adult mouse, where high-dose genestein exposure decreases adipose tissue deposition (Naaz *et al.* 2003), and in adult humans, where soy has beneficial effects on obesity, indicating that the dose and timing of exposure to phytoestrogens will be critical in determining their effect (Bhathena and Velasquez 2002).

In-utero exposure to environmentally relevant doses of bisphenol A, which has been found in human fetal blood and amniotic fluid at low doses (Mori *et al.* 2002), also results in increased body weight of mice (Howdeshell *et al.* 1999, Rubin *et al.* 2001, Akingbemi *et al.* 2004). Bisphenol A exposure even during just the preimplantation period resulted in rats with increased weight at postnatal day 21

Developmental Exposure to Environmental Estrogens is Associated with Obesity Later in Life

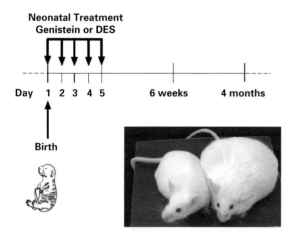

Figure 7.2 Timeline of exposure of mice to genestein or DES and subsequent obesity at 4 months of age.

(Takai *et al.* 2001). The site and mechanism of action of these agents is unstudied. However, it is known that mouse and human adipose stromal cells have aromatase that can produce oestrogens, and adipose cells contain oestrogen receptor subtypes that vary with adipose tissue location (Joyner *et al.* 2001, Anwar *et al.* 2001, Catalano *et al.* 2003), suggesting oestrogen may affect adipose tissue function directly. In addition, bisphenol A has been shown in vitro to increase glucose transport in preadipocytes (Sakurai *et al.* 2004) and in combination with insulin to increase conversion of mouse 3T3-L1 fibroblasts into adipocytes while also increasing lipoprotein lipase activity and triacylglycerol accumulation (Masuno *et al.* 2002).

Nicotine and obesity

In addition to possible direct effects on adipose cells that result in increased weight gain, weight gain can be caused by alterations in sympathetic innervation of adipose tissue. Chronic administration of a low dose of nicotine during gestation of rats resulted in normal birthweight but a significant increase in weight gain after birth (Levin 2005) and a significant increase in body fat (Williams and Kanagasabai 1984). Recent epidemiological evidence provides support for the relationship between prenatal nicotine exposure and subsequent obesity, as maternal smoking in pregnancy is associated with childhood and adult obesity in the offspring (Toschke *et al.* 2002, Wideroe *et al.* 2003). Further, since hypothalamic control of appetite is likely set during the fetal or neonatal period, exposure to environmental agents that affect hypothalamic development may alter appetite set-points and contribute to programming of adult obesity. This is an underdeveloped area that needs attention.

Nervous system disease/dysfunction and developmental exposures to environmental agents

Neurodegenerative disease

Some forms of neurodegenerative disease, including Parkinson's disease (PD), may have their origins in exposures in utero. PD is a neurodegenerative disorder that is caused by death of dopamine neurons in the substantia nigra, leading to a range of motor symptoms. While genetics and age are important risk factors for this disease, there are data suggesting that exposure to neurotoxicants may interact with age to increase the incidence of the disease. Thiruchelvam *et al.* (2003) have developed a model of PD that incorporates not only the fetal-origins paradigm but also includes exposures to multiple environmental agents; multiple exposures are typical in the case of humans. In this mouse model, in-utero or postnatal exposures on days 5–19 of age to paraquat, a herbicide/dessicant, and maneb, a fungicide, produced a permanent nigrostriatal dopamine neuron toxicity that was progressive over time, dose-related and brain-region-specific, thus mimicking the PD phenotype. Importantly, mice exposed developmentally showed enhanced vulnerability to the effects of the paraquat/maneb mixture

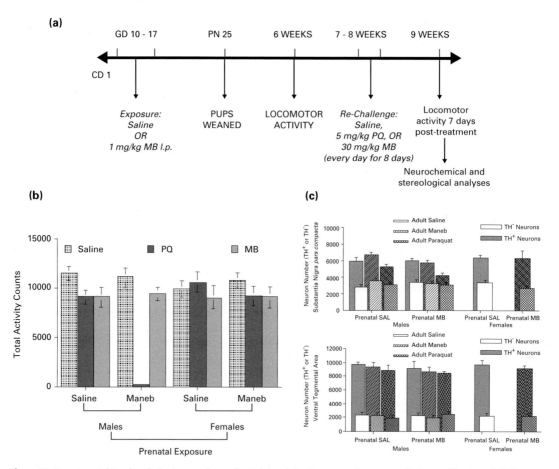

Figure 7.3 Experimental timeline, behaviour, and stereological data following prenatal exposure of mice to either maneb (MB) or paraquat (PQ). (a) shows the experimental timeline for exposure and outcome measures. (b) shows the locomotor activity data seven days after adult re-exposure. (c) shows the stereological cell counts one week after adult re-exposure.

administered later in life. In-utero or postnatal exposures to the paraquat/maneb mixture was more toxic than either agent alone. Even when the developmental exposures appeared to produce minimal toxicity, subsequent pesticide exposures later in life were significantly more toxic when preceded by developmental exposures, suggesting that the developmental exposure sensitised the brain to subsequent exposures. Adult mice were less sensitive to the neurotoxicity of these pesticides when exposed as adults compared to developmental exposures, adding additional evidence for the developmental

basis of PD. Figure 7.3 shows a schematic of the relation between exposures, dopamine neurons and Parkinson's-like disease in this model.

Exposure to the bacteriotoxin lipopolysaccharide (LPS) at embryonic day 10.5 in rats also results in animals born with fewer than normal dopamine neurons (Ling *et al.* 2004) as assessed at days 10 and 21 after birth; this effect was still evident at 120 days of age. There was some indication that normal age-related dopamine neuron loss was accelerated by this exposure. A role for inflammation was indicated by the fact that these animals had an accompanying inflammatory response, as measured by an increase in the proinflamatory cytokine tumour necrosis factor in the striatum. Tumour necrosis factor is increased in the brains of patients with PD, indicating that the LPS model may be relevant to humans.

While there are no conclusive human data supporting a role for in-utero exposures to either pesticides or LPS in the aetiology of PD there are data that human exposures to these agents do occur. Exposures to neurotoxic pesticides can be occupational and/or environmental, and several epidemiological studies have linked an individual's pesticide exposure to risk of PD. No human data are yet available, however, to determine whether maternal pesticide exposure poses a special risk of later PD to the offspring. Bacterial vaginosis is a common complication of pregnancy (14% of women) and has been shown to increase levels of LPS and proinflamatory cytokines in the fetal environment in utero. Thus, according to Ling *et al.* (2004), it is likely that a significant proportion of the adult population would have been exposed to either LPS, pesticides or both in utero and thus have brains that may be sensitised to develop PD on exposures to neurotoxic agents later in life, risk depending on the exposure, timing and background genetics.

Behavioural and cognitive dysfunction

Organophosphate insecticides are also of major concern because of their known developmental neurotoxicity. Indeed, Aldridge *et al.* (2004) have shown that chlorpyrifos (CPF), an organophosphate insecticide with worldwide usage, elicits immediate alterations in the ontogenesis of serotonin projections characterised by adverse effects on the 5HT presynaptic transporter, 5HT receptor binding sites and cell signalling mediated by 5HT receptors. Importantly, these effects can be detected at exposures below those that show maternal, fetal or neonatal overt toxicity. It has been proposed that developmental exposures to CPF may lead to increased susceptibility to diseases later in life including obesity and altered behaviour, e.g. depression. This work has

recently been expanded to show that developmental exposure to CPF led to distinct regional and sex-specific effects depending on the exposure regime (Aldridge *et al.* 2004). Indeed, sex differences in the effects of in-utero CPF were present only when exposure occurred in late gestation or neonatally and not with exposures during the neurulation stage of brain development. In addition, it is clear that deficits in brain cell numbers and synaptic communications emerge in adolescence and continue into adulthood, indicating that programming of synaptic development has clearly been altered by in-utero exposure to CPF (Qiao *et al.* 2003).

In-utero exposure to polycyclic biphenols (PCBs) leads to altered thyroid function and subsequent learning disabilities later in life in humans (Jacobson and Jacobson 2004). Data are needed, however, to ascertain whether the in-utero exposures lead to altered programming at the molecular level and whether the disease/dysfunction is a direct result, albeit temporally discordant in its onset and/or progression, of that altered programming. These data on PCBs and CPF are examples of the fetal-origins paradigm with behaviour as the endpoint, an area of significant interest but currently with minimal data available. However, there are conflicting data from some human studies, in that a study which examined in-utero exposure to a combination of low levels of PCBs and methylmercury in children found cognitive deficits attributable to the mixture (Stewart *et al.* 2003) at 38 months of age but not at 54 months. Thus some in-utero effects may not be permanent.

In-utero exposure to heavy metals alone has been implicated in developmental deficits relating to cognitive and behavioural function. A longitudinal developmental study conducted in the Faeroe Islands (Grandjean *et al.* 1997) reported that maternal methylmercury exposure in the range of 4–44 ppm, as measured in hair, was correlated with mild learning disabilities that seemed to persist into adolescence. The population under study was exposed to methylmercury primarily from ingestion of whale meat and fish. Another large study reported that maternal exposures to methylmercury in the same range, but solely from fish sources, did not produce adverse cognitive effects (Davidson *et al.* 1998). Well-controlled animal studies are needed to clarify these apparently disparate results.

Both in-utero and postnatal lead exposure at levels in the range of 10–20 µg/dl, for which there are extensive data, have been shown to have effects on cognition and behaviour that emerge and/or persist well after childhood. Studies have reported that adolescent delinquency is correlated with early and cumulative lead absorption (Needleman *et al.* 2002, Ris *et al.* 2004). Several excellent animal studies have corroborated the range of deficits seen in humans. Delville (1999) has reported that early exposure to lead increases aggressive behaviour in adult hamsters, while Cory-Slechta *et al.* (2004), in her extensive research on the effect of early lead exposure on rodents, has found that in-utero lead exposure and maternal stress produced multiplicative effects in the offspring. Rice (1996) confirmed the effects of in-utero lead in the nonhuman primate, and documented behaviours akin to attention deficit hyperactivity disorder in children.

While there are many targets for lead's neurotoxic effects, one of the important sites for cognitive effects may be hippocampal NMDA glutamate receptors. Marchioro *et al.* (1996) have shown that lead preferentially disrupts the developmental form of the NMDA receptor in the hippocampus, but does not have a similar effect on the adult form. These data support the idea that lead is much more neurotoxic to the developing brain and that in-utero exposures can lead to learning and memory problems throughout life.

Immune/autoimmune effects of developmental exposures to environmental agents

The potential impact of environmental prenatal exposures on immune-system programming, and consequent altered immune-system function and increased susceptibility to autoimmune diseases, represents another promising area of investigation. The development of the immune system, including the repertoire of reactive lymphocytes that will exist in postnatal life, begins prenatally. Alterations of the fetal immune environment might pre-programme the highly sensitive fetal immune system for aberrant immune regulation, leading to a loss of tolerance to self-antigens and resulting in an increased risk for autoimmune disease. These changes might then become manifest in adult life, although perhaps only after a second exposure to related environmental chemicals.

A growing body of data supports the notion that immune dysfunction induced prenatally can have consequences throughout the life span. Mice exposed prenatally to environmental agents such as DES, chlordane, DDT, dioxin, mycotoxins, cadmium, mercury and benzopyrene, as well as some therapeutic agents, showed altered immune-system development and sustained postnatal immunosupression (reviewed in Holladay 1999). As one example, gestational exposure to low-dose dioxin has been shown to result in suppressed delayed-type hypersensitivity at 4–5 months of age in F344 rats. This effect persisted through at least 19 months of age and was more pronounced in males than in females (Gehrs *et al.* 1997, Gehrs and Smialowicz 1999). Similarly, in-utero exposure to chlordane in mice led to a significant depression of cell-mediated immunity, delayed type 1 hypersensitivity and lymphocyte reactivity as adults (reviewed in Holladay 1999). There is evidence in both humans and experimental animals that prenatal exposure to immunosuppressant therapeutic drugs can lead to immune alterations at maturity, including development of autoantibodies and a higher risk of autoimmune disease in susceptible individuals. Holladay *et al.* (1993) reported that in-utero exposure of mice to DES resulted in significant thymic hypoplasia and reduced thymocyte maturation. When this study was repeated in SNF1 mice, a strain susceptible to autoimmune nephritis, male offspring developed the autoimmune disease significantly earlier than control mice (Holladay *et al.* 1993, Silverstone *et al.* 1998). Finally, there are preliminary data suggesting that humans exposed to DES in-utero may display hyperactive immune responses, including increased incidence of autoimmune diseases as well as of asthma and arthritis (Turiel and Wingard 1988). Continued monitoring of this population is needed to develop more definitive data. Taken together, these data show that exposure to environmental agents in utero can lead to altered immune responses, which could predispose to adult disease and dysfunction including autoimmune disease.

Mechanism responsible for altered programming due to in-utero exposure to environmental agents

Throughout this chapter, mention has been made of altered programming as the mechanism for the adult effects which result from in-utero exposures. But what is meant by altered programming? What is obvious is that in-utero exposure to the environmental agents described in this chapter results in altered expression of genes in a tissue- and time-dependent manner: genes may be turned on at inappropriate times or, perhaps more importantly, they may remain active when they should be turned off. The altered gene expression can lead to alterations at the intracellular, cellular and tissue level. This can result in tissues which may appear normal but may contain altered numbers or ratios of cell types and/or altered intracellular pathways due to the consequences of specific genes being expressed at the wrong time. It is easy to understand how an environmental chemical with oestrogenic activity, for example, can stimulate oestrogen-sensitive gene expression at the wrong time if the cells are exposed to the agent when oestrogen levels are usually low and oestrogen-sensitive genes should not be active. What is not so clear is how some of these activated genes remain so long after the oestrogenic stimulus is removed. The mechanism responsible for this phenomenon is termed epigenetic regulation of gene activity (Nakao 2001). Epigenetics literally means 'on top of genetics' and deals with chemical modification of DNA and chromatin that affects genome function (transcription, replication, recombination etc. – see Chapter 5). At the DNA level, DNA can be methylated at CpG islands

(areas of concentrated CpG repeats) due to DNA methyltransferases. Methyl-binding proteins then bind to these sites and attract other proteins with the result that there is a change in chromatin structure, leading to a silencing of the methylated gene. Hypomethylation of genes can generate increased and inappropriate gene expression (Novik et al. 2002). At the chromatin level, nucleosomal proteins, histones, can be covalently modified via acetylation, phosphorylation, methylation, ubiquination or ADP ribosylation or combinations of these processes: these modifications are termed the histone code, and they control gene expression by altering DNA availability (Jones and Baylin 2002, van Driel et al. 2003). Hyperacetylation of DNA leads to open DNA and transcriptional activation. DNA methylation can lead either to compaction and gene silencing or to activation, depending on the site, and it is unclear how ADP ribosylation, phosphorylation or ubiquination of histones affects DNA availability. These epigenetic marking systems work together to remodel chromatin. DNA methylation, histone deacetylation and histone methylation all lead to gene silencing.

There are two roles for imprinting (Reik et al. 2003). Imprinting in the germ line via gene methylation leads to activation of only one maternal or paternal copy of a gene and this methylation pattern is heritable, resulting in transgenerational effects (Murphy and Jirtle 2003). Only about 1% of genes are imprinted in this manner. There is still discussion of the importance and role of parent-of-origin imprinting (Kaneko-Ishino et al. 2003). Imprinting of somatic cells controls gene expression in a time- and tissue-specific manner.

Exactly how exposure in-utero or neonatally to environmental chemicals alters the patterns of epigenetic marking is not clear. However, there are already data showing that in-utero exposure to DES results in altered methylation of specific genes (Shuanfang et al. 2003). This suggests that the fetal basis of adult diseases induced by exposure to environmental chemicals, as discussed in this chapter, is the result of epigenetic changes which lead to altered gene expression and hence to altered tissue function. This produces increased susceptibility to disease and dysfunction later in life. It will take many years to determine the details of these interactions. Perhaps this review will stimulate research in this direction.

REFERENCES

Abbott, D. H., Dumesic, D. A., Eisner, J. W., Kemnitz, R. J. and Goy, R. W. (1997). The prenatally androgenized female rhesus monkey as a model for polycystic ovarian syndrome. In *Androgen Excess Disorders in Women*, (ed. R. Assiz, J. E. Nestler and D. Dewailly). Philadelphia, PA: Lippincott-Raven, pp. 369–82.

Abbott, D. H., Dumesic, D. A. and Franks, S. (2002). Developmental origins of polycystic ovary syndrome: a hypothesis. *J. Endocrinol.*, **174**, 1–5.

Akingbemi, B. T., Sottas, C. M., Koulova, A. I., Klindfelter, G. R. and Hardy, M. P. (2004). Inhibition of testicular steroidogenesis by the xenoestrogen bisphenol A is associated with reduced pituitary luteinizing hormone secretion and decreased steroidogenic enzyme gene expression in rat Leydig cells. *Endocrinology*, **145**, 592–603.

Aldridge, J. E., Seidler, F. J. and Slotkin, T. A. (2004). Developmental exposure to chlorpyrifos elicits sex-selective alterations of serotonergic synaptic function in adulthood: critical periods and regional selectivity for effects on the serotonin transporter, receptor subtypes, and cell signaling. *Environ. Health Perspect.*, **112**, 148–55.

Alworth, L. C., Howdeshell, K. L., Ruhlen, R. L. *et al.* (2002). Uterine responsiveness to estradiol and DNA methylation are altered by fetal exposure to diethylstilbestrol and methoxychlor in CD-1 mice: effects of low versus high doses. *Toxicol. Appl. Pharmacol.*, **183**, 10–22.

Anwar, A., McTernan, P. G., Anderson, L. A. *et al.* (2001). Site-specific regulation of oestrogen receptor a and b by estradiol in human adipose tissue. *Diabetes Obes. Metab.*, **3**, 338–49.

Anway, M. D., Cupp, A. S., Uzumcu, M. and Skinner. M. K. (2005). Epigenetic transgenerational actions of endocrine disruptors on male fertility. *Science*, **308**, 1466–9.

Baillie-Hamilton, P. F. (2002). Chemical toxins: a hypothesis to explain the global obesity epidemic. *J. Altern. Complement. Med.*, **8**, 185–92.

Bern, H. (1992). The fragile fetus. In *Chemically Induced Alterations in Sexual and Functional development: the Wildlife/Human Connection* (ed. T. Colborn and C. Clement). Princeton: Princeton Scientific Publishing, pp. 9–15.

Bhathena, S. J. and Velasquez, M. T. (2002). Beneficial role of dietary phytoestrogens in obesity and diabetes. *Am. J. Clin. Nutr.*, **76**, 1191–201.

Birnbaum, L. S. and Fenton, S. E. (2003). Cancer and developmental exposures to endocrine disruptors. *Environ. Health Perspect.*, **111**, 389–94.

Brown, N. M., Manzolillo, P. A., Ahang, J. X., Wang, J. and Lamartiniere, C. A. (1998). Prenatal TCDD and predisposition to mammary cancer in the rat. *Carcinogenesis*, **19**, 1623–9.

Catalano, S., Marsico, S., Giodano, C. *et al.* (2003). Leptin enhances, via AP-1, expression of aromatase in the MCF-7 cell line. *J. Biol. Chem.*, **278**, 28668–76.

Cory-Slechta, D. A., Virgolini, M. D., Thiruchelvam, M., Weston, D. D. and Bauter, M. R. (2004). Maternal stress modulates the effects of developmental lead exposure. *Environ. Health Perspect.*, **112**, 717–30.

Davidson, P. W., Myers, G. J., Cox, C. *et al.* (1998). Effects of prenatal and postnatal methylmercury exposures from fish consumption on neurodevelopment: outcomes at 66 months of age in the Seychelles Child Development Study. *JAMA*, **280**, 701–7.

Delville, Y. (1999). Exposure to lead during development alters aggressive behavior in golden hamsters. *Neurotoxicol. Teratol.*, **21**, 445–9.

Eisner, J. R., Barnett, M. A., Dumesic, D. A. and Abbott, D. H. (2002). Ovarian hyperandrogenism in adult female rhesus monkeys exposed to prenatal androgen excess. *Fertil. Steril.*, **77**, 167–72.

Fenton, S. E., Hamm, J. T., Birnbaum, L. S. and Youngblood, G. l. (2002). Persistant abnormalities in the rat mammary gland following gestational and lactational exposure to 2,3,7,8-tetrachlorodibenzo-p-dioxin (TCDD). *Toxicol. Sci.*, **67**, 63–74.

Gehrs, B. C. and Smialowicz, R. J. (1999). Persistent suppression of delayed-type hypersensitivity in adult F344 rats after exposure to 2,3,7,8-tetrachlorodibenzo-p-dioxin. *Toxicology*, **134**, 79–88.

Gehrs, B. C., Riddle, M. M., Williams, W. C. and Smialowicz, R. J. (1997). Alterations in the developing immune system of the F344 rat after prenatal exposure to 2,3,7,8-tetrachlorodibenzo-p-dioxin II: effects on the pup and the adult. *Toxicology*, **122**, 229–40.

Grandjean, P., Weihe, P., White, R. F. *et al.* (1997). Cognitive deficits in 7-year old children with prenatal exposures to methylmercury. *Neurotoxicol. Teratol.*, **19**, 417–28.

Gray, L. E., Ostby, J., Monosson, E. and Kelce, W. R. (1999). Environmental antiandrogens: low doses of the fungicide vinclozolin alter sex differentiation of the male rat. *Toxicol. Ind. Health*, **15**, 48–64.

Heindel, J. J. (2003). Endocrine disruptors and the obesity epidemic. *Toxicol. Sci.*, **76**, 247–9.

Herbst, A. L., Ulfelder, H., Poskanzer, D. C. and Longo, L. D. (1971). Adenocarcinoma of the vagina: association of maternal stilbestrol therapy with tumour appearance in young women. *N. Engl. J. Med.*, **284**, 878–81.

Hilakivi-Clarke, L., Cho, E., Onojafe, I., Raygada, M. and Clarke, R. (1999). Maternal exposure to genistein during pregnancy increases carcinogen-induced mammary tumourigenesis in female rat offspring. *Oncol. Rep.*, **6**, 1089–95.

Holladay, S. D. (1999). Prenatal immunotoxicant exposure and postnatal autoimmune disease. *Environ. Health Perspect.*, **107** (suppl. 5), 687–91.

Holladay, S. D., Blaylock B. L., Comment, C. E., Heindel, J. J., Fox, W. M. and Luster, M. I. (1993). Selective prothymocyte targeting by prenatal diethylstilbestrol exposure. *Cell. Immunol.*, **152**, 131–42.

Howdeshell, K. L., Hotchkiss, A. K., Thayer, K. A., Vandenbergh, J. G. and vom Saal, F. S. (1999). Exposure to bisphenol A advances puberty. *Nature*, **401**, 763–4.

Hughes, C. L., Liu, G., Beall, S., Foster, W. G. and Davis, V. (2004). Effects of genistein or soy milk during late gestation and lactation on adult uterine organisation in the rat. *Exp. Biol. Med.*, **229**, 108–17.

Hunt, P. A., Koehler, K. E., Susiarjo, M. *et al.* (2003). Bisphenol A exposure causes meiotic aneuploidy in the female mouse. *Curr. Biol.*, **13**, 546–53.

Jacobson, J. L. and Jacobson, S. W. (2004). Prenatal exposure to polychlorinated biphenols and attention at school age. *Obstet. Gynecol. Surv.*, **59**, 412–13.

Jefferson, W. N., Couse, J. F., Padilla-Banks, E., Korach, K. S. and Newbold, R. (2002). Neonatal exposure to genistein induces oestrogen receptor (ERa) expression and multioocyte follicles in the maturing mouse ovary: evidence for ERb-mediated and nonestrogenic actions. *Biol. Reprod.*, **67**, 1285–96.

Jefferson, W. N., Padilla-Banks, E., Couse, J. F., Korach, K. S. and Newbold, R. R. (in press). Neonatal genistein exposure induces oestrogen receptor mediated alterations in gene expression in the developing mouse uterus: differential effects of low versus high doses. *Mol. Endocrinol.*

Jones, P. A. and Baylin, S. B. (2002). The fundamental role of epigenetic events in cancer. *Nat. Rev. Genet.*, **3**, 415–28.

Joyner, J. K., Hutley, L. J. and Cameron, D. P. (2001). Estrogen receptors in human preadipocytes. *Endocrine*, **15**, 225–30.

Kaneko-Ishino, T., Kohda, T. and Ishino, F. (2003). The regulation and biological significance of genomic imprinting. *J. Biochem.*, **133**, 699–711.

Karri, S., Johnson, H., Hendry, W. J., Williams, S. C. and Kahn, S. A. (2004). Neonatal exposure to diethylstilbestrol leads to impaired action of androgens in adult male hamsters. *Reprod. Toxicol.*, **19**, 53–63.

Kelce, W. R., Gray, L. E. and Wilson, E. M. (1998). Antiandrogens as environmental endocrine disruptors. *Reprod. Fertil. Dev.*, **10**, 105–11.

Kouki, T., Kishitake, M., Okamoto, M., Talebe, M. and Yamanouchiu I. (2003). Effects of neonatal treatment with phytoestrogens, genestein and daidzein on sex difference in female rat brain function: estrous cycle and lordosis. *Horm. Behav.*, **44**, 140–5.

Levin, E. D. (2005). Fetal nicotinic overload, blunted sympathetic responsivity and weight gain. *Birth Defects Res. A Clin. Mol. Teratol.*, epub. June 2005.

Li, S., Hansman, R., Newbold, R., Davis, B. and McLachlan, J. (2003). Neonatal diethylstilbestrol exposure induces persistent elevation of c-fos expression and hypomethylation of its exon-4 in mouse uterus. *Mol. Carcinog.*, **38**, 78–84.

Lin, T. M., Rasmussen, N. T., Moore, R. W., Albrecht, R. M. and Peterson, R. E. (2003). Region-specific inhibition of prostatic epithelial bud formation in the urogenital sinus of C57BL/6 mice exposed in-utero to 2,3,7,8-tetrachlorodibenzo-p-dioxin. *Toxicol. Sci.*, **76**, 171–81.

Ling, Z. D., Chang, Q., Lipiton, J. W., Tong, C. W., Landers, T. M. and Carvey, P. M. (2004). Combined toxicity of prenatal bacterial endotoxin exposure and postnatal 6-hydroxydopamine in the adult rat midbrain. *Neuroscience*, **124**, 619–28.

Lund, T. D., Munson, D. J., Adlercreutz, H., Handa, R. J. and Lephart, E. D. (2004). Androgen receptor expression in the rat prostate is down regulated by dietary phytoestrogens. *Reprod. Biol. Endocrinol.*, **16**, 5–11.

Marchioro, M., Swanson, K. L., Aracava, Y. and Albuquerque, E. X. (1996). Glycine and calcium-dependent effects of lead on N-methyl-D-aspartate receptor function in rat hippocampal neurons. *J. Pharmacol. Exp. Ther.*, **279**, 143–53.

Markey, C. M., Luque, E. H., Munoz de Toro, M., Sonnenschein, C. and Soto S. M. (2001). In utero exposure to bisphenol A alters the development and tissue organisation of the mouse mammary gland. *Biol. Reprod.*, **65**, 1215–23.

Masuno, H., Kidani, T., Sekiya, *et al.* (2002). Bisphenol A in combination with insulin can accelerate the conversion of 3T3-L1 fibroblasts to adipocytes. *J. Lipid Res.*, **43**, 676–84.

McLachlan, J. A., Newbold, R. R. and Bullock, B. C. (1980). Long term effects on the female mouse genital tract associated with prenatal exposure to diethylstilbestrol. *Cancer Res.*, **40**, 3988–99.

McLachlan, J. A., Newbold, R. R., Burrow, M. E. and Li, S. F. (2001). From malformations to molecular mechanisms in the male: three decades of research on endocrine disruptors. *APMIS*, **109**, 263–72.

Miyagawa, S., Katsu, Y., Watanabe, H. and Iguchi, T. (2004). Estrogen-independent activation of erbBs signaling and estrogen receptor α in the mouse vagina exposed neonatally to diethylstilbestrol. *Oncogene*, **23**, 340–9.

Mori, C., Komiyama, M., Adachi, T. *et al.* (2002). Application of toxicogenomic analysis to risk assessment of delayed long-term effects of multiple chemicals, including endocrine disruptors in human fetuses. *Environ. Health Perspect.*, **111**, 803–9.

Murphy, S. K. and Jirtle, R. L. (2003). Imprinting evolution and the price of silence. *Bioessays*, **25**, 577–88.

Naaz, A., Yellayi, S., Sakroczymski, M. A. *et al.* (2003). The soy isoflavone genistein decreases adipose deposition in mice. *Endocrinology*, **144**, 3315–20.

Nagai, A., Ikeda, Y., Aso, T., Eto, K. and Ikeda, M. A. (2003). Exposure of neonatal rats to diethylstilbestrol affects the expression of genes involved in ovarian differentiation. *J. Med. Dent. Sci.*, **50**, 35–40.

Nakao, M. (2001). Epigenetics: interaction of DNA methylation and chromatin. *Gene*, **278**, 25–31.

Needham, L. L. and Sexton, K. (2000). Assessing children's exposure to hazardous environmental chemicals: an overview of selected research challenges and complexities. *J. Expos. Anal. Environ. Epidemiol.*, **10**, 611–29.

Needleman, H. L., McFarland, C., Ness, R. B., Fienberg, S. E. and Tobin, M. J. (2002). Bone lead levels in adjudicated delinquents. A case control study. *Neurotoxicol. Teratol.*, **24**, 711–17.

Newbold, R. R., Bullock, B. C. and McLachlan, J. A. (1990). Uterine adenocarcinoma in mice following developmental treatment with oestrogens: a model for hormonal carcinogenesis. *Cancer Res.*, **50**, 7677–81.

Newbold, R. R., Banks, E. P., Bullock, B. and Jefferson, W. N. (2001). Uterine adenocarcinoma in mice treated neonatally with genistein. *Cancer Res.*, **61**, 4325–8.

Newbold, R. R., Jefferson, W. J., Padilla-Banks, E. and Haseman, J. (2004). Developmental exposure to diethylstilbestrol (DES) alters uterine response to oestrogens in prepubescent mice: low versus high dose effects. *Rep. Toxicol.* **18**, 399–406.

Novik, K. L., Nimmrich, I., Genc, B. *et al.* (2002). Epigenomics: genome-wide study of methylation phenomena. *Curr. Issues. Mol. Biol.*, **4**, 111–28.

Oken, E. and Gillman, M. W. (2003). Fetal origins of obesity. *Obes. Res.*, **11**, 496–506.

Padmanabhan, V., Evans, E., Taylor, J. A. and Robinson, J. E. (1998). Prenatal exposure to androgens leads to the development of cystic ovaries in the sheep. *Biol. Reprod.* **56** (Suppl. I), 194–9.

Palmer, J. R., Hatch, E. E., Rosenberg, C. L. *et al.* (2002). Risk of breast cancer in women exposed to diethylstilbestrol in utero: preliminary results (United States). *Cancer Causes Control*, **13**, 753–8.

Qiao, D, Seidler, F. J., Tate, C. A., Cousins, M. M. and Slotkin, T. A. (2003). Fetal chlorpyrifos exposure: adverse effects on brain cell development and cholinergic biomarkers emerge postnatally and continue into adolescence and adulthood. *Environ. Health Perspect.*, **111**, 536–44.

Ramos, J. G., Varayoud, J., Sonnenschein, C., Soto, A. M., Munoz de Toro, M. M. and Luque, E. H. (2001). Prenatal exposure to low doses of bisphenol A alters the periductal stroma and glandular cell function in the rat ventral prostate. *Biol. Reprod.*, **65**, 1271–7.

Reik, W., Santos, F. and Dean, W. (2003). Mammalian epigenomics: reprogramming the genome for development and therapy. *Theriogenology*, **59**, 21–32.

Rice, D. C. (1996). Behavioral effects of lead: commonalities between experimental and epidemiologic data. *Environ. Health Perspect.*, **104** (Suppl. 2), 337–51.

Ris, M. D., Dietrich, K. N., Succop, P. A., Berger, O. G. and Bornschein, R. I. (2004). Early exposure to lead and neuropsychological outcome in adolescence. *J. Int. Neuropsychol. Soc.*, **10**, 261–70.

Rogers, I., and the EURO-BLCS Study Group. (2003). The influence of birthweight and intrauterine environment on adiposity and fat distribution in later life. *Int. J. Obes.*, **27**, 755–77.

Rubin, B. R., Murray, M. K., Damassa, D. A., King, J. C. and Soto, A. (2001). Perinatal exposure to low doses of bisphenol A affects body weight, patterns of estrous cyclicity, and plasma LH levels. *Environ. Health Perspect.*, **109**, 675–80.

Sakurai, K., Kawazuma, T., Adachi, T. *et al.* (2004). Bishenol A affects glucose transport in mouse 3T3-F442A adipocytes. *Br. J. Pharmacol.*, **141**, 209–14.

Shuanfang, L, Hansman, R., Newbold, R., Davis, B. and McLachlan, J. A. (2003). Neonatal diethylstilbestrol exposure induces persistent elevation of c-fos expression and hypomethylation in its exon-4 in mouse uterus. *Mol. Carcinog.*, **38**, 78–84.

Silverstone, A. E., Gavalchin, J. and Gasiewicz, T. A. (1998). DES and estradiol potentiate a lupus-like autoimmune nephritis in NZB x SWR (SNF1) mice. *Toxicologist*, **42**, 403.

Stewart, P. W., Reihman, J., Lonky, E. I., Darvill, T. J. and Pagano, J. (2003). Cognitive development in preschool children prenatally exposed to PCBs and Me Hg. *Neurotoxicol. Teratol.*, **25**, 11–22.

Takai, Y., Tsutsumi, O., Ikezuki, Y. *et al.* (2001). Preimplantation exposure to bisphenol A advances postnatal development. *Reprod. Toxicol.*, **15**, 71–4.

Thiruchelvan, M., McCormack, A., Richfield, E. K. *et al.* (2003). Age-related irreversible progressive nigrostriatal dopaminergic neurotoxicity in the paraquat and maneb model of the Parkinson's disease phenotype. *Eur. J. Neurosci.*, **18**, 589–600.

Timms, B. G., Peterson, R. E. and vom Saal, F. S. (2002). 2,3,7,8-tetrachlorodibenzo-p-dioxin interacts with endogenous estradiol to disrupt prostate gland morphogenesis in male rat fetuses. *Toxicol. Sci.*, **67**, 264–74.

Toschke, A. M., Koletzko, B., Slikker, W. Jr., Hermann, M. and von Kries, R. (2002). Childhood obesity is associated with maternal smoking in pregnancy. *Eur. J. Pediatr.*, **161**, 445–8.

Turiel, J. and Wingard, D. L. (1988). Immune response in DES-exposed women. *Fertil. Steril.*, **49**, 928–9.

Uzumcu, M., Suzuki, H. and Skinner, M. (2004). Effect of the anti-androgenic endocrine disruptor vinclozolin on embryonic testis cord formation and postnatal testis development and function. *Reprod. Toxicol.*, **18**, 765–74,

van Driel, R., Fransz, P. F. and Verschure, P. J. (2003). The eukaryotic genome: a system regulated at different hierarchical levels. *J. Cell Sci.*, **116**, 4067–75.

vom Saal, F. S., Timms, B. G., Montano, M. M. *et al.* (1997). Prostate enlargement in mice due to fetal exposure to low doses of estradiol or diethylstilbestrol and opposite effects at high doses. *Proc. Natl. Acad. Sci. USA*, **94**, 2056–61.

Welshons, W. V., Nagel, S. C., Thayer, A., Judy, B. M. and vom Saal, F. S. (1999). Low-dose bioactivity of xenoestrogens in animals: fetal exposure to low doses of methoxychlor and other xenoestrogens increases adult prostate size in mice. *Toxicol. Ind. Health*, **15**, 12–25.

Wideroe, M., Vik, T., Jacobsen, G. and Bakketeig, L. (2003). Does maternal smoking during pregnancy cause childhood overweight? *Pediatr. Perinat. Epidemiol.*, **17**, 171–9.

Williams, C. and Kanagasabai, T. (1984). Maternal adipose tissue response to nicotine administration in the pregnant rat: effects on fetal body fat and cellularity. *Br. J. Nutr.*, **51**, 7–13.

Woodham, C., Birch, L. and Prins, G. S. (2003). Neonatal oestrogen down-regulates prostatic androgen receptor through a proteosome-mediated protein degradation pathway. *Endocrinol.*, **144**, 4841–50.

Younglai, E. V., Foster, W. G., Hughes, E. G., Trim, K. and Farrell, J. F. (2002). Levels of environmental contaminants in human follicular fluid, serum, and seminal plasma of couples undergoing in vitro fertilization. *Arch. Environ. Contam. Toxicol.*, **43**, 121–6.

8

Maternal nutrition and fetal growth and development

Susan M. B. Morton

University of Auckland

Introduction

There has been a great deal of literature devoted to better understanding the determinants of offspring size at birth. Over several decades the importance of maternal size has been acknowledged as a key factor in the fetal development of her offspring and from this association it has followed that maternal nutrition must also be of importance to the growth of her unborn infants. This chapter reviews the extent of the evidence for an association between maternal nutrition and reduced offspring size at birth, as characterised by low birthweight (birthweight of less than 2500 g irrespective of length of gestation). After acknowledging the complexity of the notion of low birthweight (LBW), maternal nutrition is defined in the context of its potential influence on fetal growth and the available evidence is summarised for associations between LBW and maternal anthropometry, nutritional status and diet in pregnancy. The evidence is drawn from both observational studies and from intervention studies (randomised controlled trials, RCTs), the latter of which may avoid the biases that often arise in uncontrolled trials. Where sufficient data are available the effects of nutritional interventions are quantified in terms of their demonstrated effects on fetal size and maturity at birth. The second part of the chapter discusses important limitations in our current understanding of the nature of the association and the potential implications this has for interventions to improve fetal growth.

Why focus on LBW?

While the primary fetal outcome under consideration here is LBW, intrauterine growth retardation (IUGR) and preterm delivery will also be considered as outcomes given that LBW defines a heterogeneous group of infants: some of whom will be growth retarded, some of whom will be born early, and some who will be both early and growth-restricted. Focusing on low birthweight is important as it defines a group of infants born weighing less than 2500 g who are at increased risk of morbidity and mortality both perinatally (Butler and Bonham 1963) and beyond (Goldstein and Peckham 1976). Further, birthweights are the most readily available comparable measure of fetal outcome in different populations, and LBW the commonest measure of comparative poor fetal outcome. It might be argued though that birthweight, whilst relatively simple to measure, is itself a proxy measure for fetal development in its entirety. There are many reasons why an infant may be born LBW, and infants who are born the same absolute size at birth are not a homogeneous group (Metcoff 1994). Birthweight is a measure of both fetal growth rate and length of gestation, so in the crudest sense LBW may

Developmental Origins of Health and Disease, ed. Peter Gluckman and Mark Hanson. Published by Cambridge University Press.
© P. D. Gluckman and M. A. Hanson 2006.

be caused by either reduced gestational duration or reduced intrauterine growth. However, the two contributors are not independent as the primary determinant of birthweight is gestational age. In particular, if gestation is shortened then birthweight will be reduced, although the reverse may not be the case (Dougherty and Jones 1982). Whilst providing a simple classification in terms of perinatal risk, low birthweight, with its associated proximal and distal risks for morbidity and mortality, represents a common final pathway from a complex interaction of biological and social factors acting before and during pregnancy. Birthweight within a population is a continuous measure, so a further concern regarding the comparison of the determinants of LBW (that is according to a defined, fixed cutoff point) across populations is that the proportion of LBW infants in any one population varies according to that population's overall distribution of birthweight (Robinson 1989), and not all LBW infants in different populations carry the same perinatal risk (Wilcox 2001). Wilcox has referred to this as the 'low birthweight paradox', noting that while populations who have higher percentages of LBW infants tend to have higher infant mortality overall, individual LBW infants in populations with high rates of LBW tend to have a lower mortality than LBW babies of the same absolute birthweight in populations with a lower overall rate of LBW. Even within populations infants born to maternal smokers tend to be of lower birthweight on average than their peers born to mothers who are non-smokers, but weight for weight they have a lower mortality than infants born to non-smokers. This paradox is also evident for infants born at high altitude as compared to low altitude, African-American as compared to White US infants, and twins compared to singletons (Wilcox 2001). Essentially considering a fixed cutoff for low birthweight is a crude and often inaccurate way of assessing perinatal mortality risk across populations (Evans and Alberman 1989). Nonetheless much of our knowledge about the determinants of birthweight comes from studies of low birthweight in particular.

Globally, approximately 15% of all babies are estimated to be born LBW (less than 2500 g at delivery). However, the rates vary according to level of development of a country, with the greatest burden of LBW deliveries occurring in developing countries (16.4% of LBW deliveries) compared to developed countries (6.2%) (Mora and Nestel 2000). The underlying broad causation of LBW also tends to differ according to the development status of the country. In developing countries the higher rate of LBW is largely due to intrauterine growth restriction (IUGR), rather than to preterm delivery, which remains the primary cause in developed countries (Kramer 2003). However, assessment of gestational age remains difficult in developing countries.

There has been an attempt to address this heterogeneity in the literature by using body proportions at birth either instead of, or in addition to, absolute size to determine perinatal risk. However few data exist to suggest that these are more informative about the fetal growth trajectory in utero than absolute measures of size and maturity. A common assumption in the past was that body proportionality at birth somehow represented the timing of a nutritional insult that lead to restricted growth (Harding 2001), and a distinction was often made in the literature whereby IUGR infants were divided according to two distinct patterns of growth restriction, symmetrical (an infant proportionately small in all body measurements) and asymmetrical (an infant relatively long and thin for its birthweight), with the presumption that the former infants underwent early nutrient limitation and the latter suffered nutrient limitation late in pregnancy (Barker 1995). However, a careful examination of several large human datasets failed to find support for two distinct subgroups and instead demonstrated a continuum of body proportionality (Kramer et al. 1989), as for other measures of absolute size.

The importance of maternal nutritional status as a determinant of LBW

There is a vast literature on the determinants of size at birth, and LBW in particular, including several extensive reviews of the literature in the last two decades – notably those by Kramer (1987, Kramer *et al.* 2000) and Robinson (1989). Measures of maternal nutritional status have been acknowledged as key parental determinants of fetal growth throughout these reviews.

A comprehensive review of the determinants of low birthweight in 1987, which considered the relevant French and English literature published between 1970 and 1984, concluded that factors with well-established associations with intrauterine growth included infant sex, racial/ethnic origin, maternal height, pre-pregnancy weight, paternal weight and height, maternal birthweight, parity, history of prior low birthweight, gestational weight gain and calorie intake, general morbidity and pregnancy-specific illness, malaria, smoking and alcohol consumption (Kramer 1987). It was acknowledged that it was difficult to ascertain the extent to which factors acted independently. Nevertheless the relative importance of each causal factor was quantified from the available evidence, and an estimate of the aetiological importance of each was made according to whether the population was from a developed or developing country, assuming that for each individual woman within any population the absolute effect of each factor on fetal size was similar regardless of setting, but in different populations the overall prevalence of that factor altered its relative importance. For example in developed countries the greatest contribution to reduced fetal growth was from maternal smoking, which for an individual has a large effect and is responsible for a large proportion of LBW. In contrast, smoking is almost nonexistent in pregnant women in developing countries. In terms of the specific maternal nutritional determinants of LBW in developed countries it was estimated that 25% of the burden of LBW was attributable to low maternal pre-pregnancy weight and poor pregnancy weight gain. The importance of maternal nutritional factors for LBW increased to approximately 33% if the mother's own reduced intrauterine growth and short adult stature were also included as markers of nutritional status. In developing countries approximately 33% of LBW was attributable to maternal low pre-pregnancy weight and low gestational weight gain, and if mother's own LBW and adult short stature

were included the estimated contribution of maternal nutritional status to LBW rose to approximately 50% (Kramer 1987).

Despite the quantity of research reviewed, a major limitation of most of the work was that it failed to distinguish between the different reasons behind an infant being born LBW, in particular between intrauterine growth restriction and prematurity. There was also an inability to establish the temporal ordering of causal sequences because of retrospective data collection, failure to control adequately for potential confounders in observational studies and perhaps most importantly methodological shortcomings that were most pronounced in developing countries so that least was known about LBW in the countries where it occurred at the highest rates.

Kramer produced an updated overview of the epidemiology of adverse pregnancy outcomes, including low birthweight, in 2003. He estimated that the most important determinants of intrauterine growth restriction continue to be related to maternal nutritional status. In particular, low maternal energy intake and gestational weight gain and low pre-pregnancy body mass index and short stature remain important contributors to the burden of LBW, particularly in developing countries (Kramer 2003). Low maternal pre-pregnancy BMI, but not gestational weight gain, was also implicated in preterm delivery, which is the major cause of the majority of LBW in developed countries, but in general the aetiology of preterm delivery remains poorly understood.

Maternal nutrition as it pertains to determinants of fetal growth

In attempting to understand the nature of the association between maternal nutrition and LBW it is necessary to be explicit about what constitutes maternal nutrition in the context of pregnancy. The different aspects of maternal nutrition to be considered with respect to fetal growth include: (a) maternal anthropometry (before and during pregnancy), which acts as a crude proxy of maternal body composition; (b) maternal diet (largely in pregnancy); and (c) specific nutritional deficiencies (especially micronutrient deficiencies). Like fetal growth, measuring maternal nutrition is not straightforward, and cutoff points are often utilised to determine differential risk in what is a continuous measure within a population (e.g. categories of body mass index to define a measure of weight for height). Problems in global comparisons of maternal nutrition are compounded by a lack of consensus regarding appropriate reference standards for the nutritional status of women within different populations, and indeed the appropriate comparative anthropometric measure to be used across populations. For example there are limitations in the use of the Quetelet index (BMI defined as weight in kilograms divided by height in metres squared) to define categories of risk (Nestel and Rustein 2002). However, even with a comparative measure which is appropriate across populations it remains difficult to determine the extent of poor nutrition in women globally, even amongst pregnant women, because there have been few nationally representative samples carried out to assess this (Mora and Nestel 2000).

To evaluate the basis for the effect of measures of maternal nutrition on fetal growth (Kramer 1987, 2003), recent observational studies and where possible intervention studies (RCTs) are considered. A great deal of animal experimental evidence linking maternal nutrition to fetal growth exists, but this will not be reviewed in detail because of problems in extrapolating between species, which will be considered again later in this overview. Ideally the focus should be on the broad classification of maternal nutrition, including not only measures immediately pre-pregnancy or during gestation, but also measures of nutritional status before pregnancy. But in reality there is very limited evidence in humans relating maternal nutritional status measured preconception to pregnancy outcome (Jackson and Robinson 2001).

Maternal anthropometry and LBW

Cross-sectional measures of maternal adult size, adult height and weight, may be thought of as proxy measures for the experience of all the genetic and environmental (including nutritional) influences a

female has been exposed to over her life course up to that point. Kramer (1987) acknowledged the proxy nature of these measures when he classified low pre-pregnancy weight and short maternal height as genetic and constitutional factors in his factors that influence low birthweight, whereas he classified gestational weight gain, caloric intake, energy expenditure (work and physical activity) and specific nutrient status as nutritional factors which influenced pregnancy. Maternal pre-pregnancy weight (either alone or adjusted for height) together with gestational weight gain have been the two anthropometric indicators of maternal status that have shown the most consistent positive associations with birthweight (Neggers and Goldenberg 2003). Most studies that have considered the influence of these maternal anthropometric measures have been limited to considering absolute birthweight or birthweight adjusted for gestational age as their main proxy outcome measure of fetal intrauterine growth. However, a retrospective study of maternal nutritional status and its relationship to infant weight and body proportions from Jamaica found that women with lower BMI measured in early pregnancy tended to give birth to infants who were lighter but also shorter and with smaller head circumferences (Thame *et al.* 1997). These findings concur with other studies in different populations, including the earlier study from the Netherlands (Stein and Susser 1975) and the more recent study from India (Mavalankar *et al.* 1994) in reiterating the importance of maternal anthropometry for measures of fetal growth. Consistently studies have found that women who are underweight tend to deliver infants that are more likely to be LBW or preterm regardless of whether populations are classified as chronically undernourished or assumed to be well nourished (Sebire *et al.* 2001).

In 1990 a large WHO collaborative study quantified the importance of differences in these two aspects of maternal anthropometry, one a proxy for maternal nutrition before pregnancy and the other for nutrition during pregnancy, for fetal outcomes including low birthweight, IUGR and preterm delivery (World Health Organization 1995). The estimates of effect were based on secondary analysis of datasets from 20 countries (developing and developed) representing

Table 8.1 Combined odds ratios for maternal anthropometric indicators and IUGR, LBW and preterm delivery from the WHO Collaborative Study (World Health Organization 1995).

Maternal anthropometric indicator[b]	Combined OR (95% CI)[a]		
	IUGR	LBW	Preterm delivery
Low pre-pregnancy weight	2.5 (2.3, 2.7)	2.3 (2.1, 2.5)	1.4 (1.3, 1.5)
Attained weight at term[c]	3.1 (2.7, 3.4)	2.5 (2.2, 2.9)	—
Low gestational weight gain[d]	2.0 (1.7, 2.4)	1.6 (1.3, 2.1)	—
Low gestational weight gain[d] in mothers of below-average pre-pregnancy weight	5.5 (4.1, 7.4)	2.8 (2.2, 3.5)	—
Low pre-pregnancy BMI	1.8 (1.7, 2.0)	1.8 (1.7, 2.0)	1.3 (1.1, 1.4)
Short stature	1.9 (1.8, 2.0)	1.7 (1.6, 1.8)	1.2 (1.1, 1.2)
Low MUAC[e]	1.6 (1.6, 2.2)	1.9 (1.7, 2.1)	1.2 (1.0, 1.3)

[a] Combined ORs summarise the comparisons within all groups of countries (where groups were defined according to similarities of distributions of individual indicator variables).

[b] The ORs compare fetal outcomes for mothers in the lowest quartile of each maternal anthropometric indicator with those of mothers in the highest quartile.

[c] Maternal weight in the ninth month of gestation (hence no OR for preterm delivery).

[d] Gestational weight gain refers to weight gain between pre-pregnancy weight and 9 months gestation (hence no OR for preterm delivery).

[e] Mean upper arm circumference.

information on over 111 000 births collected in 25 separate studies. Obviously there was much diversity in the extent of these fetal outcomes in the different countries included, with for example a range of only 4% of births classified as LBW in China and the US (Hispanic) study versus 28% of births classified as LBW in Pune, India. Similarly IUGR varied from 5–7% for USA and Ireland to 30–54% for a number of the included Asian countries. In terms of maternal anthropometric measures there was a similar heterogeneity. In general maternal weight patterns tended to follow height patterns, with a few exceptions including China where mean weight was comparatively high for mean maternal height. Estimated odds ratios (OR) were based on a comparison of fetal outcomes in women in the lowest quartile of each anthropometric indicator compared to those of women in the highest quartile within each population. Overall the strongest effects of differences in maternal anthropometric measures were seen in terms of rates of IUGR deliveries, with slightly lower effects on rates of LBW (which included a mixture

of both IUGR and preterm deliveries). A summary of the results are given below and in Table 8.1 for the two indicators most commonly associated with fetal growth. Other maternal measures of anthropometry examined included mean upper arm circumference (MUAC) and maternal height separately from weight-for-height, but these were less strongly associated with fetal size and maturity overall.

Indicators of maternal anthropometry and IUGR

The summary combined odds of an IUGR delivery in women in the lowest quartile of pre-pregnancy weight was estimated as being 2.5 times greater than for women in the highest quartile of pre-pregnancy weight over all the populations. As weight increased during gestation the odds of delivering an IUGR infant increased to threefold for women who were in the lowest quartile of attained weight at full term compared to women in the highest quartile. Women who were of below-average height and below-average pre-pregnancy weight and in the lowest quartile of attained weight had the greatest odds of an IUGR delivery. Being in the lowest quartile for weight gain (that is change in weight during gestation) between early gestation and 5, 7 or 9 months of gestation was associated with a slightly lower odds of IUGR in comparison to absolute attained weight, carrying approximately double the odds of an IUGR infant for women who were in the lowest quartile of weight gain compared to the highest quartile at each measurement point (5, 7 and 9 months gestation). This suggests that the absolute level of pre-pregnancy status is particularly important in determining a woman's relative risk of delivering an IUGR infant, as evidenced by the fivefold increased odds of delivering an IUGR infant in mothers who were of below-average pre-pregnancy weight and subsequently gained the least weight during gestation (Table 8.1).

Indicators of maternal anthropometry and LBW

The summary combined odds for the delivery of a LBW infant for women in the lowest quartile of pre-pregnancy weight was 2.3 times greater than for women in the highest quartile, with lower attained weight during gestation being associated with gradually increasing odds for LBW for the same comparison groups of women (2.5-fold increased odds of LBW for differences in attained weight at 9 months gestation). In particular, women of below-average pre-pregnancy weight who had attained weights in the lowest quartile had the greatest odds of LBW (OR = 2.8 for differences in attained weight at 9 months gestation). Being in the lowest quartile for weight gain (change from pre-pregnancy weight) between early gestation and 5, 7 or 9 months of gestation was associated with a slightly lower odds of an LBW infant than attained weight at each measurement point, carrying approximately a 50% increased odds of delivering an LBW infant compared to women in the highest quartile of weight gain (summary ORs 1.5–1.6). As was the case for IUGR the odds of delivering an LBW infant appeared to be particularly influenced by a woman's absolute pre-pregnancy weight.

Indicators of maternal anthropometry and preterm delivery

Measures of maternal pre-pregnancy weight and gestational weight gain were less important for predicting shortened gestational length than they were for measures of fetal size (IUGR and LBW). Nevertheless having a pre-pregnancy weight in the lowest quartile as compared to the highest quartile did carry an estimated 40% increase in the odds of preterm delivery (before 37 completed weeks of gestation), but there was no evidence that these odds differed according to maternal adult height. Further, mothers in the lowest quartile of attained weight in mid and late pregnancy (at 5 and 7 months gestation) had the same estimated odds of preterm delivery as women who were in the highest quartile of attained weight. Lower gestational weight gain showed contrasting associations with the odds of preterm delivery depending on whether the difference in weight change was in early (5 months) or later (7 months) pregnancy. Mothers in the lowest quartile of gestational weight gain at 5 months gestation appeared to be relatively protected from preterm delivery (summary OR = 0.7), but lower weight gain between 5 and 7 months of gestation was associated with an increased odds of early delivery (OR = 1.4). These results are equivocal but potentially suggest the importance of pre-pregnancy weight, rather than changes in weight during gestation, in influencing length of gestation, but the mechanisms require further consideration and elucidation.

Interestingly, animal experiments have recently demonstrated a significant association between periconceptional nutrition and preterm delivery, whereby modest nutritional restriction around the time of conception in sheep appears to influence fetal maturation rates and result in preterm delivery (Bloomfield *et al.* 2003). In humans a similar result was found from the Dutch famine study, where gestational lengths were shorter among mothers exposed to nutritional deprivation during the first trimester. Evidence to support the importance of maternal pre-pregnancy weight as opposed to weight gain in terms of influence on gestational length has recently emerged from studies of over 1700 deliveries to rural Gambian women where an annual 'hungry season' provides a natural experiment in which to assess the influence of nutritional deprivation on pregnancy outcome. Comparisons of absolute mean maternal weight throughout the year and mean gestational age at delivery of infants show a dramatically similar pattern, whereby the temporal changes in monthly mean maternal weight coincide with the changes in monthly mean length of gestation, with a lag period of nine months (lowest mean absolute maternal weight occurs nine months prior to the shortest mean gestation at delivery). However, there is no similar relationship between maternal weight change and gestational length (Rayco-Solon *et al.* 2005).

Summary of association between maternal anthropometry and fetal growth

The 1990 WHO collaborative study (World Health Organization 1995) was extremely important in terms of summarising and quantifying the association between differences in maternal anthropometric indicators and the risk of poor fetal outcomes (IUGR, LBW and preterm delivery) for diverse populations of women. The summary ORs confirmed the association of low maternal pre-pregnancy weight, low BMI and low attained weight throughout pregnancy with impaired fetal growth. However, the relative strengths of effects of different maternal anthropometric indicators on the risk of LBW was not always uniform across populations. This was particularly true for the strength of the relative effects of maternal height, weight and BMI. For example in the Gambian study absolute maternal weight was a better predictor of infant birthweight than maternal BMI in a population in which women undergo marked changes in their weight according to the season of the year (Cole *et al.* 1995). By contrast in the Colombian study maternal short stature (height < 148 cm) was more strongly associated with risk of LBW in term deliveries than pre-pregnancy weight or BMI, although low pre-pregnancy weight (defined in

this population as < 48 kg) was nevertheless associated with an almost 50% increased risk of LBW compared with women with a weight of 48 kg or above (Rey *et al.* 1995).

The WHO analysis was limited to crude associations between anthropometric measures and pregnancy outcome, irrespective of potential confounding factors, as the authors acknowledged, and it is possible that differences between populations in other factors which influence pregnancy outcome might explain the variation in risk patterns seen for different maternal anthropometric measures. However, disentangling the independent effects of maternal nutritional factors from other associated risk factors is extremely difficult as many of the factors are highly correlated. Additionally population-based studies of sufficient size and power to examine the joint effects often lack sufficient detailed information on all the variables of interest, so that reliable multivariate analyses which might elaborate on the relative effects of maternal nutrition in the light of other environmental influences remain uncommon (Maconochie 1995). For example, recent observational studies have suggested that a low maternal pre-pregnancy BMI may interact with other factors such as smoking and psychosocial stress to increase the risk of adverse fetal outcomes in pregnancy, but the evidence is preliminary (Neggers and Goldenberg 2003).

The aim of the WHO work was to identify which maternal anthropometric measures signalled the greatest risk of a poor pregnancy outcome. Many of the best predictors for fetal growth relied on measures of change in maternal weight or attained weight late in pregnancy when fetal growth trajectories may have already been determined, and it is not surprising that as gestation progressed maternal weight became more strongly related to fetal size, since much of the attained gestational weight in late gestation will be a direct result of fetal weight (Cole *et al.* 1995). However, the differences in odds of reduced fetal growth in women of different pre-pregnancy size did suggest that the ability of a mother to provide nutrition to her growing fetus was to a large extent determined before her pregnancy began.

Pre-pregnancy weight and weight gain in pregnancy are both important

These findings confirmed that maternal pre-pregnant size and gestational weight gain do not act independently on fetal growth, but that maternal pre-pregnancy anthropometry may modify the risks associated with gestational weight gain. Prior to the WHO report the American Institute of Medicine Committee had recognised that pre-pregnancy weight for height appeared to modify the effect of gestational weight gain in women in the United States, using 1980 data collected in the National Perinatal Collaborative Study to reset recommended clinical standards for weight gain in pregnancy (Institute of Medicine 1990). Importantly they also set wide limits for each group, recognising from observational studies that there was considerable variation in the absolute weight gain of individual healthy women who nevertheless produced full-term infants weighing between 3 and 4 kg at birth (King *et al.* 1994).

Evidence from developed countries also supports an interaction between the effects of pre-pregnancy weight and gestational weight gain on length of gestation. In developed countries women who begin pregnancy with a low BMI (measured at <19.5) had a five-times increased risk of a spontaneous preterm delivery if they had a weight gain in the second and third trimesters of less than 0.37 kg on average per week as compared to women with an initial pre-pregnancy BMI of greater than 19.5 (OR = 5.6, 95% CI 2.4, 13.8) (Neggers and Goldenberg 2003). However, comparisons of effects are not widely available for developing countries, where gestational age is more difficult to measure routinely, but where nutritional status of mothers prior to pregnancy may be markedly different to that of women in developed countries. While these studies identify associations between proxy markers of maternal nutritional status and possible interactions between them, they are not able to address the mechanisms that underlie these relationships, nor untangle the effects of maternal nutrition as part of the wider environment in which pregnancy exists within and across populations.

Components of weight gain

Measures of maternal pre-pregnancy weight and gestational weight gain are themselves proxy measures for the different components of weight required to ensure successful fetal development, the three main components of which have been described as energy for fetal, uterine and mammary tissue; energy for maternal fat storage; and energy for the basal metabolism of newly acquired tissues. Maternal fat storage and basal metabolism are not fixed quantifiable energy costs during pregnancy but that they vary widely among healthy women of similar sizes who nevertheless give birth to healthy infants of similar sizes (van Raaij *et al.* 1989, Goldberg *et al.* 1993, Forsum *et al.* 2003). These intensive studies throughout pregnancy suggest an overall absence of an association between absolute energy intake and maternal fat gain in pregnancy and an absence of an association between levels of maternal fat and birthweight of offspring in normal-weight women (King *et al.* 1994) which is contrary to the association found between overall weight gain and fetal size. Similarly for changes in basal metabolic rates in response to pregnancy there are wide individual differences within each of the populations studied. Evidence comparing studies from The Gambia with studies in Europe and the USA suggests that underweight women tend to reduce their overall metabolic expenditure in early pregnancy, only increasing in the second half of pregnancy, whereas in well-nourished women there tends to be a steady increase in expenditure from early pregnancy. This suggests that adaptations to the energy requirements in pregnancy may be setting-dependent according to baseline maternal nutritional status (Poppitt *et al.* 1994). An underweight woman living in a developing country may be unable to increase her food intake in response to pregnancy, given limited food supplies, and may need to continue her level of physical activity for her own survival. Therefore her remaining option is to reduce her basal metabolic energy requirements to allow her to deliver a viable infant. Thus when energy is chronically limited adaptations tend to spare energy for fetal growth (Goldberg *et al.* 1993, Winkvist *et al.* 1994). If energy is abundant, energy requirements appear to be achieved largely via individually variable adjustments in dietary behaviour, basal metabolism and/or fat deposition in normal-weight women (King *et al.* 1994). Longitudinal studies have yet to be carried out on overweight women in developed countries to determine what changes occur in body fat mass during gestation. Pregnancy in general is an anabolic state, and energy tends to be used differently in the hormonally mediated pregnant and non-pregnant state, but it is unclear whether the hormonal changes in pregnancy that facilitate fat deposition in normal-weight women operate in the same manner in women who begin pregnancy with ample fat stores. These individual responses to the energy requirements of pregnancy, which vary according to maternal nutritional status pre-pregnancy and according to individual behaviour and the little-studied but important activity levels, make large-scale population nutritional advice messages or population-based interventions contentious. However, they do provide support for improving the nutritional status of women generally in less-developed countries, preferably prior to pregnancy.

Maternal diet

Despite these findings from intensive longitudinal studies suggesting that there is much individual variation in energy use and adaptation in pregnancy, the broad significant associations between differences in gestational weight gain and in fetal growth suggest it may be reasonable to consider the effect of specific aspects of maternal diet in pregnancy on pregnancy outcome (World Health Organization 1995). Support for the association between maternal diet and fetal growth flourished following reports on reduced birthweight of offspring born to mothers exposed to acute famine in late gestation during the Dutch 'hunger winter' (Stein *et al.* 1975). Subsequent follow-up referred to in other chapters of this book has shown that the effects of acute changes in maternal diet were not always manifested in changes in fetal growth, but there may still be longer-term impacts on the offspring's own later reproductive capacities (Rich-Edwards 2002). In particular, while females born to mothers who were exposed to famine during their first trimester of pregnancy did not have reduced birthweight themselves, their offspring tended to show a reversal of the normally observed increase in mean birthweight with maternal parity (Lumey and Stein 1997a). As reviewed in Chapter 33, it is also reported that individuals exposed to acute maternal malnutrition in early gestation, but not mid or late gestation, are at increased risk of cardiovascular disease later in life (Roseboom *et al.* 2001), that is that biochemical abnormalities may be induced via acute maternal nutritional changes during early pregnancy that persist into adult life without necessarily being mediated by a birthweight effect.

More recent observational studies considering aspects of maternal dietary intake under more normal conditions of food availability that exist today in developed countries have reported equivocal associations between maternal nutrient intake during pregnancy and fetal growth. Two studies that were carried out in similar populations of women (Southampton and Portsmouth in the UK) suggested inconsistent effects of maternal macronutrient intake on fetal growth measured during gestation. Godfrey *et al.* (1997) reported a positive association between high carbohydrate intake in early pregnancy and lower placental and offspring birthweights, associations which were reported to be independent of the mother's own baseline nutritional status. They demonstrated a similar association for low protein in the maternal diet in late pregnancy, finding this was also associated with reduced placental weight and birthweight. By contrast, a study by Matthews *et al.* (1999) which considered dietary intake in the second and third trimester of pregnancy in women in Portsmouth found no evidence of any effect of maternal diet on placental size or offspring birthweight. The measurements of maternal diet were however made at different times during gestation and in each case a cross-sectional assessment acted as a proxy for maternal diet over a much longer time period. These differences found in very similar populations of women highlight how relating nutrient intake at discrete points during pregnancy to size at birth has the potential to produce confounded results, especially in observational studies (Symonds *et al.* 2000), although the studies were based on a small number of women. In support of the importance of time of measurement of dietary intake, a further relatively small study which considered the influence of maternal dietary supplementation in a socially disadvantaged population in the United Kingdom reported that whilst first-trimester maternal dietary supplementation was associated with a modest increase in offspring birthweight, supplementation in the second and third trimesters failed to reduce the incidence of LBW (Doyle *et al.* 1990, 1992).

In contrast to the equivocal evidence for an effect of macronutrient intake during gestation in developed countries, there is a growing body of evidence from observational studies that suggests that micronutrients in particular may have an important effect on fetal growth, especially in underweight women. In a recent prospective study carried out in India (mean pre-pregnancy BMI = 18.2), higher infant birthweights were associated with maternal consumption of green leafy vegetables, fruits or milk products (foods rich in micronutrients including vitamins A and C, folate and iron) at least three times a week as compared to once or less during pregnancy, whereas energy and protein intake alone was not associated with birth size (Rao *et al.* 2001). Higher fat intake at week 18 of gestation was also significantly positively associated with infant birth length and infant triceps fold thickness in addition to birthweight.

However, estimates from observational studies are likely to be confounded by the effect of other covariates that tend to coexist in populations under nutritional stress. This is particularly the case for developing countries where nutritional deficiencies tend to be most common. These largely observational studies do nonetheless suggest that the frequency and severity of adverse pregnancy outcomes, including LBW, may be reduced via improvement in the macro- or micronutrient status of the mother (Keen *et al.* 2003).

Macro- and micronutrient intervention studies

In an attempt to measure the effect of dietary interventions on fetal size and maturity at birth, evidence was reviewed from randomised controlled trials (RCTs) that largely sought to address specific macro- and micronutrient deficiencies through maternal dietary manipulation during pregnancy (although some studies were also carried out in non-deficient populations) to attempt to measure the effect of these dietary interventions on fetal size and maturity at delivery. The results of RCTs are often preferred over observational studies because they generally provide a less biased estimate of the true effect of an intervention, although they have been criticised because of the sometimes artificial conditions under which an intervention is tested. In the case of the effect of maternal nutritional status on fetal outcomes, there has been much work in collating evidence from studies carried out in this area, including several Cochrane reviews and most recently the substantive overview by Merialdi *et al.* (2003) of the RCTs that tested nutritional interventions for evidence of an ability to treat or prevent impaired fetal growth, and the related overview by Villar *et al.* (2003a) of evidence for the ability of nutritional interventions during pregnancy to prevent preterm delivery. These overviews included an evaluation of the results of 13 systematic reviews included in the *Cochrane Database of Systematic Reviews* (2002, issue 4) as well as nine further trials up until October 2002 not included in those reviews. There were 65 randomised controlled trials included in these reviews, full details of which were provided, including a description of the intervention, participants and setting and additional comments by which to evaluate the quality of the evidence, in a related publication by the same group of authors (Villar *et al.* 2003b).

The summary of findings of the effects of maternal dietary manipulation on fetal growth from RCTs presented below draws heavily on this substantial work, together with additional evidence from the Cochrane reviews and the studies to which they refer. The overview is presented according to the type of nutritional intervention under consideration, and its effect on birthweight and on the incidence of small for gestational age (SGA) and prematurity.

Nutritional advice

Given that observational studies have previously reported that gestational weight gain is positively associated with fetal growth and potentially with a reduced risk of preterm birth (Kramer 1987), evidence was assessed for the effects of advising women to increase their energy and protein intakes in randomized controlled trials (Kramer 1996a).

This Cochrane review of nutritional advice in pregnancy included four trials involving 1108 women. The major conclusions reached were that whilst nutritional advice to women does tend to increase their intake of energy and protein the effects on pregnancy outcome are at best modest. Only one trial, carried out in Greece, which randomised clinics to give either no counselling or counselling to improve the 'quality' of maternal diet during pregnancy, specifically evaluated the effect on fetal growth (Kafatos et al. 1989). That trial found no evidence that nutritional advice alone was beneficial in reducing the proportion of infants born growth-restricted (SGA). They did however, suggest that there was a reduction in preterm deliveries, but this was inconsistent with their finding of an absence of effect on mean gestational age. However, caution is required in extrapolating the findings from this study more widely as there were methodological concerns. Whilst the randomisation was carried out by clinic (cluster randomisation) the analyses were carried out for individual women, thereby not accounting for the similarities between women from the same clinic, which may lead to an overestimate of the variance and potentially biased estimates (Merialdi et al. 2003). The conclusion from the evidence available from intervention trials of nutritional advice in pregnancy is that whilst advice may have a positive effect

on maternal gestational weight gain in the mother the benefits for fetal growth remain limited.

Balanced protein/energy supplementation

Based on the same evidence from observational studies that gestational weight gain and energy intake are strongly linked with fetal growth and possibly with preterm delivery, the evidence for this was assessed from randomised controlled trials of energy/protein supplementation (protein content less than 25% of total energy content) (Kramer 2000).

The evidence for the potential benefits of balanced protein/energy supplementation for improving fetal growth was more positive than for nutritional advice alone. There were 13 trials included in the Cochrane review and overall balanced protein/energy supplementation was associated with modest maternal weight gain increases (weighted mean difference of +17 g/week, 95% CI 5 g, 29 g). Of the 13 trials, 11 reported birthweight as an outcome, with the overall finding being that infants born to supplemented mothers tended to have a higher mean absolute birthweight than those born to non-supplemented mothers; however, the overall difference was small and statistically non-significant at approximately 25 g (95% CI −3.6 g, 54.5 g). The Cochrane review also conducted a stratified analysis of the effects of balanced protein/energy supplementation on mean offspring birthweight according to the presumed nutritional status of mothers prior to pregnancy, as observational studies have suggested that there may be a threshold effect of weight gain according to whether the mother is well nourished or undernourished prior to pregnancy. There was, however, no evidence that the increases in fetal growth were conditional on the mothers' pre-pregnancy nutritional status after dividing study populations according to their presumed pre-pregnancy nutritional status (dichotomised into under- or adequately nourished groups) (Kramer 2000). Six of the 13 trials reported the effects of balanced protein/energy supplementation on rates of SGA and all showed a protective effect of this intervention, although only in one large trial in rural Gambia was the difference in rates of SGA delivery between supplemented and non-supplemented mothers statistically significant. This trial though was conducted amongst women who had prior chronic marginal nutritional status and who received a much higher energy supplement in pregnancy than in other similar studies (Ceesay *et al.* 1997). This study also found a small positive effect on head circumference of infants born to supplemented mothers (3.1 mm difference). The overall effect of providing balanced protein/energy supplementation was estimated as leading to a 32% reduction in SGA deliveries among mothers who received the supplement (RR = 0.68, 95% CI 0.57, 0.80) (Merialdi *et al.* 2003). No significant effects of supplementation were however detected for mean gestational age at delivery (Kramer 2000).

Overall there appeared to be a modest effect on fetal growth via maternal balanced protein/energy supplementation during pregnancy, which appeared to operate by improving rates of fetal growth rather than by extending gestation. Beyond the immediate period of birth, however, the few trials that have followed these mothers and infants after birth have found little or no evidence of longer-lasting benefits which might be expected to follow from a decreased rate of LBW and SGA deliveries. Maternal weight did not remain increased postpartum, nor was there any significant increase in breast-milk output at 2–3 months (Kardjati *et al.* 1988), nor any improvement in neurocognitive tests for the infants themselves at 12 months of age (Blackwell *et al.* 1973). An early study of supplementation of pregnant women in East Java suggested that there might be a beneficial effect on postnatal growth for the infants of mothers who received high-energy supplementation (Kusin *et al.* 1992), but recent follow-up of the larger Gambian study has not shown any similar effect on childhood growth to 5 years of age, beyond a slight advantage in the immediate perinatal period (A. M. Prentice, personal communication). The review was also unable to assess whether there might be any adverse effects relating to increased birthweight such as labour difficulties, although three studies did provide evidence in support of a reduced perinatal mortality risk in infants born to supplemented

mothers, including the large Gambian study (Ceesay *et al.* 1997, Kramer 2000). This is not a trivial matter, however, as the benefits of interventions which result in increased size at birth and in particular larger head size will need to be carefully assessed in the light of a potentially greater risk of obstructed labour and the resultant maternal and infant morbidity.

Isocaloric balanced protein

Isocaloric supplementation denotes a supplement in which the protein content is 'balanced', i.e. provides less than 25% of its total energy content, and replaces an equivalent amount of energy in the diet. Trials to date have not compared such a replacement diet with 'usual' diet, but have rather compared them to supplements with the same total energy content but differing amounts of protein. Assessment of the evidence is therefore limited to these trials (Kramer 1996b). Three reviews in total reported effects on birthweight, each demonstrating a reduction in mean birthweight of infants born to supplemented mothers compared to the control group, with an average difference of −63.5 g (95% CI −124.3 g, −2.9 g). Two of the studies were however based on a relatively small number of Asian females living in Birmingham, Alabama (Viegas *et al.* 1982a, 1982b). The third study, in low-income Chilean women who had low weight-for-height (measured at their first antenatal visit, which took place before 20 weeks gestation) (Mardones-Santander *et al.* 1998), also reported effects on rates of SGA deliveries in supplemented versus control groups. In contrast to the effects on fetal growth seen for balanced protein/energy supplementation, isocaloric balanced protein supplementation had an overall adverse effect on SGA, based on this one trial. None of the three studies provided any evidence for an effect of high-protein supplementation on mean gestational age or preterm delivery (Kramer 1996b). Overall there is no evidence to suggest that isocaloric balanced protein supplementation has any beneficial effect on fetal growth and rates of LBW in particular, with limited evidence that the effect on birthweight may even be adverse.

High protein

Similarly, high-protein supplemented diets lead to a non-significant decrease in mean birthweight (−58.4 g, 95% CI −146.2 g, 29.5 g) (Merialdi *et al.* 2003), despite a small, non-significant weekly maternal weight increase (Kramer 1996c). This evidence, though, was based largely on one trial which considered outcomes in women of low socioeconomic status in the United States (Rush *et al.* 1980). This study also provided evidence of an increased risk of delivering an SGA infant in supplemented mothers. However, there was considerable loss to follow-up post-randomisation in this study, which means the results should be interpreted with some caution. Follow-up of the infants at 1 year of age found that high-protein supplementation was also not associated with any later detectable difference in infant growth (height, weight or head circumference) or neurocognitive development (Bayley mental score) (Kramer 1996c). A smaller study in India several decades earlier had found no evidence of any significant difference in the mean birthweight of infants born to mothers who received high-protein supplements compared to those who did not, although this was based on late hospitalisation at 36 weeks gestation and considered only a small number ($n = 25$) of selected, low-socioeconomic-status women (Iyenger 1967). It is possible that supplementation at this late stage in pregnancy may have been too late to have changed the established growth trajectory in either direction. Overall, while there is limited evidence to assess the benefits or risks of high-protein supplementation in pregnancy, the available evidence provides no justification for prescribing such a nutritional supplement, either for size-at-birth effects or for later developmental gains, and there is some evidence to suggest it may reduce birthweight, making any further studies difficult to justify (Kramer 1996c).

Energy/protein restriction

Excessive weight gain during pregnancy has previously been associated with increased risks of pre-eclampsia in observational studies. Evidence from intervention trials was therefore examined to determine whether there was any benefit to selected mothers and their infants of energy/protein restriction, primarily in terms of pre-eclampsia but secondarily because of the effect gestational hypertension may have on growth restriction (Kramer 1996d). The effect of energy/protein restriction amongst women who either were classified as obese pre-pregnancy or had rapid early gestational weight gain was available from three trials, two relating to obese women and the third pertaining to early gestational weight gain. However, only the former two reported effects of energy/protein restriction on mean birthweight (LBW and SGA were not reported separately as outcomes). Energy/protein restriction in women who were classified as obese at the beginning of pregnancy was associated with a fall in mean birthweight, which was large and significant in an Egyptian study ($n = 100$) (difference of −450 g, 95% CI −625 g, −275 g) (Badrawi *et al.* 1992), but in a larger Scottish study ($n = 153$) was associated with a non-significant small negative difference in mean birthweight (Campbell and MacGillivray 1975). With respect to other outcomes associated with birthweight, there was no evidence of an effect on gestational length and also no effect on rates of pre-eclampsia in the energy/protein-restricted mothers (Kramer 1996d). Given the few studies that have considered this intervention it is difficult to determine its effect, but the studies to date suggest that such a dietary restriction in pregnancy is unlikely to be beneficial in terms of fetal growth and may potentially have detrimental effect in terms of fetal growth restriction.

Salt restriction

Two randomised controlled trials which sought evidence of an effect of salt restriction during pregnancy were available. The primary aim of this intervention also appeared to be the prevention of pregnancy-induced hypertension, but given the association of pre-eclampsia with restricted fetal growth both trials reported on offspring size at birth. In one trial there was a weak but non-significant trend towards a decreased rate of LBW in the salt-restricted group (Merialdi *et al.* 2003). The second trial reported on SGA as the outcome and also showed no significant effect of the salt restriction on intrauterine growth, although the trend was towards a slightly greater risk of SGA. Hence, given the limited studies and the opposite trends in effects on fetal growth rates, it remains difficult to draw any conclusions about this intervention, but given that salt restriction did not appear to prevent pre-eclampsia it seems reasonable that salt restriction during pregnancy should not be routinely recommended (Duley and Henderson-Smart 1999).

Calcium supplementation

Calcium supplementation was also largely used as a potential preventive measure against hypertensive disorders in pregnancy, but there was some evidence from observational studies that it might also prevent preterm labour (Atallah *et al.* 2002). There were 11 randomised controlled trials relating to this intervention, nine of which assessed fetal growth as an outcome. Supplementation trials were carried out in populations who were considered to be at high risk of developing hypertension in pregnancy (Niromanesh *et al.* 2001) and in previously healthy women (Levine *et al.* 1997), including those with normally low calcium intakes (Lopez-Jamarillo *et al.* 1997). Over half of the trials presented data on LBW and tended to show a protective effect of calcium supplementation on fetal growth, although there was significant heterogeneity in the risk reduction estimate according to the size of the trial and the baseline risks and calcium status of the participants. Overall there was an estimated 17% reduction in LBW in the supplemented groups (Merialdi *et al.* 2003), but in women considered to be at high risk of hypertension at baseline there was an estimated 50% reduction in the risk of LBW. There was no overall effect of calcium supplementation on preterm delivery, but there was a reduction in risk of shortened gestation amongst women at highest risk of hypertension at baseline (RR = 0.45, 95% CI 0.24, to 0.83) (Atallah *et al.* 2002). These effects on reduction of LBW delivery may

have been due in part to the reduced risk of gestational hypertension and pre-eclampsia generally via calcium supplementation in normal women but of greatest impact in women either at pre-existing high risk of pre-eclampsia or with baseline low calcium intake. However the largest trial, which was carried out in 4589 healthy nulliparous women in early pregnancy, showed no benefit on reducing the incidence of pre-eclampsia or any reduction in preterm or SGA deliveries (Levine *et al.* 1997). Importantly however, it did not report any adverse effects on other measured fetal or maternal outcomes. Overall there is some evidence, although inconsistent, that calcium supplementation may be beneficial in improving fetal growth and reducing rates of LBW, especially in women who are at high risk of developing pre-eclampsia or in populations with low baseline calcium intakes. It has been hypothesised that calcium supplementation may lengthen gestation and therefore provide extra time for growth in utero, but the mechanism remains to be elucidated. Further, the optimum dosage and duration of treatment requires further investigation and the lack of effect in the largest trial in women who were not nutrient-deficient or at increased risk of gestational hypertension needs further investigation in other large studies to determine an appropriate target population for this intervention. Currently there are ongoing large trials of calcium supplementation during pregnancy in several low-intake populations which have recently completed follow-up and which should be able to add their findings to this literature in the near future (WHO controlled trials register).

Iron supplementation

In the course of normal pregnancy most women develop haematological changes in the latter stages of pregnancy that suggest iron-deficiency as the fetus utilises iron stores and plasma volume expands. In developed countries overt iron deficiency anaemia is relatively rare but it has been common practice in many of those countries to routinely prescribe iron supplements in pregnancy (Mahomed 1999). However, in developing countries, where nutritional deficiencies and infections such as malaria and other parasitic infections commonly lead to anaemia, there is a particular concern that the amount of iron available from dietary sources may not be sufficient to meet the additional demands placed on maternal iron stores by the growing fetus. Therefore two separate Cochrane reviews were conducted firstly to consider evidence for an effect of iron supplementation in women with normal haemoglobin levels (Hb $\geq$ 11 g/dl) (Mahomed 1999) and secondly to consider evidence of an effect of iron therapy for women classified as having anaemia in pregnancy (Hb < 11 g/dl) (Cuervo and Mahomed 2001). However, there is little consistency in the point at which haemoglobin was measured during pregnancy in different studies, which complicates the comparative process as concentrations are gestation-dependent (Rasmussen 2001). Previously it has been noted that the association between maternal haemoglobin concentration (measured in the latter half of gestation) and fetal size and maturity at delivery is in fact U-shaped in several different ethnic groups, with the highest rates of LBW and preterm infants born to mothers whose haemoglobin concentration is either less than 8.5 g/dl or greater than 12.5 g/dl (Steer *et al.* 1995). It has been suggested that the shape of the curve may represent the overlap of two different underlying processes. While the low haemoglobin concentrations may be indicative of underlying maternal anaemia, the association of increased rates of reduced intrauterine growth and preterm delivery at high maternal haemoglobin concentrations more probably represents failure of maternal plasma expansion, which may be a consequence of other maternal or fetal problems (Rasmussen 2001).

There were 20 studies available that compared routine iron supplementation versus no iron or placebo, conventional versus slow-release iron and selective versus routine iron in pregnancy, but data for fetal outcomes were limited (Mahomed 1999, Merialdi *et al.* 2003). Only one trial reported effects of routine iron supplementation on fetal growth in women without pre-existing anaemia, and that trial showed no differences in fetal growth rates for supplemented versus non-supplemented women (Hemminki and Rimpela 1991).

Secondly, despite many small trials considering the effect of iron therapy in iron-deficient mothers, there is little evidence regarding its effects on fetal outcomes and what evidence exists is of relatively poor quality (Cuervo and Mahomed 2001). Only one study reported differences in mean birthweight between women treated with either intravenous or oral iron, finding a negative but non-significant effect on size at birth in the intravenous group. However, the sample size was small and the confidence intervals wide, and there was no comparison group (Mahomed 1999). Severe maternal iron-deficiency anaemia is common in developing countries, but on the basis of these reviews it is not possible to determine whether treatment for severe or even mild anaemia has any beneficial effects on fetal growth. Supplementation may well improve maternal health, during gestation and postnatally, but there is also a lack of evidence to support this hypothesis from developing countries where the problem is of greatest concern (Rasmussen 2001). In terms of routine iron treatment for women in developed countries, where iron-deficiency anaemia is uncommon, there is also little evidence that this is beneficial in terms of fetal growth, but studies reporting relevant fetal outcomes are also rare.

Folate supplementation

In well-nourished populations demands for folic acid are usually met by dietary intake, but under starvation conditions or in areas where malaria or sickle cell disease are endemic, deficiencies may lead to anaemia during pregnancy. Recently the role of periconceptional folic acid has been reviewed in its capacity to reduce the risk of neural tube defects (Lumley *et al.* 2001), but the focus in that review was not on fetal growth. There were, however, 21 trials of varying quality included in a separate Cochrane review of folate supplementation more generally in pregnancy (Mahomed 1997a). Most of the trials though were concerned with effects on maternal serum folate and red cell folate, with few reporting outcomes related to fetal growth. In the five trials which reported data on LBW there was considerable heterogeneity in the results (Merialdi *et al.* 2003). While there was some evidence from these five trials involving nearly 1500 women that there may be a trend towards a reduction in LBW with folate supplementation (RR = 0.73, 95% CI 0.47, 1.13) (Mahomed 1997a), this needs further evaluation because of inconsistencies in findings. Overall, while the effect of folate supplementation on maternal haematological indices is well established, there remains the need to assess its effect on fetal growth in better controlled trials, especially in populations where folate deficiency is common, and in areas where malaria is endemic (Fleming *et al.* 1986). In poorly nourished populations who are folate-deficient, appropriate strategies for the prevention of folate as well as iron deficiencies prior to pregnancy are also required.

Iron and folate supplementation

There were eight trials which reviewed iron and folate supplementation together in pregnancy which were included in a Cochrane review (Mahomed 1997b). However, few had any information on fetal growth and few were conducted in areas where iron and folate deficiency was common and maternal anaemia a serious problem. Only one study had information on LBW, but the sample size was small and although it suggested an increased risk of LBW the confidence intervals were very wide (Merialdi *et al.* 2003). Therefore it remains difficult to assess whether iron and folate together are beneficial for fetal growth, in addition to improving maternal haemoglobin levels.

Magnesium

Magnesium is an essential mineral and it is usually available in adequate quantities for women who eat a varied diet. However, women from disadvantaged socioeconomic backgrounds have been found to have intakes of magnesium below the recommended level (Makrides and Crowther 2001). A cross-sectional study of dietary intake in early

pregnancy had suggested that higher magnesium intake might be associated with increased birthweight (Doyle *et al.* 1989). Several randomised controlled intervention trials of magnesium supplementation were subsequently undertaken to assess the effects on fetal growth as well as on maternal and paediatric outcomes, the effects of which were evaluated in a recent Cochrane review (Makrides and Crowther 2001). There were seven trials included in the review where results were available for rates of LBW, SGA and preterm deliveries. The collective results from all the trials in which oral magnesium was begun before the 25th week of gestation showed that this was associated with a lower frequency of LBW (RR = 0.76, 95% CI 0.46, 0.96), fewer SGA infants (RR = 0.70, 95% CI 0.53, 0.93) and a lower rate of preterm delivery (RR = 0.70, 95% CI 057, 0.94) in supplemented mothers. However the largest trial in this group (*n* = 985) used medical centres as their units for cluster randomisation but analysed the results as if the women were randomised individually. Removing this study from the combined analysis because of this methodological concern of bias in the estimates of effect, resulted in an attenuation of each of the protective effects with the results for each fetal outcome becoming statistically non-significant, although the protective trends remained for each of the fetal growth outcomes (Merialdi *et al.* 2003). Therefore, while overall there remains a lack of high-quality evidence to show that magnesium supplementation is beneficial for fetal growth, further high-quality trials are indicated given the promising trends in improved fetal outcome (in terms of both growth rate and length of gestation) reported to date.

Fish oil

Fish oil has been mooted as being responsible for prolonging gestation in Nordic countries (Olsen *et al.* 1992), but trials of fish-oil supplements in pregnancy either for prevention or treatment purposes appear to have had no significant effect on rates of intrauterine growth retardation. The most recent Cochrane review was updated in 1995 (Duley 1995), but three later trials of fish oil in pregnancy were identified by Merialdi *et al.* (2003).The earlier Cochrane review had found a trend towards an increased risk of LBW in women who received fish-oil supplements in otherwise uncomplicated pregnancies (Duley 1995). However, the later trials, which tended to concentrate on either prevention of IUGR in women with a poor reproductive history, including a previous IUGR delivery, or fish oil for the treatment of suspected intrauterine growth retardation (following ultrasound assessment), found no difference in the mean birthweight adjusted for gestational age in infants born to either the preventive or treated groups of women, based on a large multicentre European study (FOTIP Team 2000). They did however find evidence that fish oil (as compared to olive oil) reduced the risk of subsequent preterm delivery in women with a previous preterm birth. Similarly, a Dutch trial amongst women with a previous history of IUGR delivery found no evidence of an effect of fish oil on birthweight below the third centile in subsequent deliveries (Onwude *et al.* 1995). Hence overall there is no evidence from intervention studies to support a beneficial effect of fish-oil supplements for either the prevention or treatment of IUGR in women at risk of retarded fetal growth. The earlier Cochrane review suggested that there may be a slight negative impact on birthweight in women without any pre-existing risk factors for LBW, but this was based on limited evidence. The hypothesised effects on length of gestation may require further evaluation, especially in women with a prior history of preterm delivery.

Zinc

Zinc deficiency is known to limit growth in young children, and it has been shown in animal models to limit fetal growth. However, there have been equivocal findings from epidemiological and controlled trials of zinc supplementation during pregnancy in humans (Castillo-Durán and Weisstaub 2003). The Cochrane review evaluated the role of routine zinc supplementation in pregnancy and included seven trials, mostly from developed countries. Overall they failed to find a significant effect either on rates of

LBW (summary RR = 0.75, 95% CI 0.52, 1.07) or rates of SGA deliveries of infants born to supplemented mothers compared to mothers who received a placebo or no supplement (summary RR = 0.89, 95% CI 0.61, 1.30). However, there did appear to be an overall protective effect on preterm delivery, though the significance was marginal (summary RR = 0.73, 95% CI 0.54, 0.98) (Mahomed 1997c). Further trials have been conducted in developing countries since this review was published (Merialdi *et al.* 2003), although the nutritional status of the mothers in each varied widely (Osendarp *et al.* 2003). However, they also failed to find an association between zinc supplementation and birthweight. Only one study in Chile found a small increase in birthweight amongst women who received zinc supplements during pregnancy, but this appeared to be due to a lengthened gestation rather than an improved rate of fetal growth (Osendarp *et al.* 2003). The evidence that is currently available does not support the hypothesis that maternal zinc supplementation enhances fetal growth, even though there is limited evidence that it might protect against preterm delivery. However, most of the evidence to date is based on studies carried out in countries where primary zinc deficiency is likely to be rare (Osendarp *et al.* 2003). More research is required to determine whether there are potential benefits for rates of fetal growth in less-developed countries where zinc deficiency may be part of a wider nutritionally deficient state or may be secondary to other disease states (Keen *et al.* 2003). The evidence for a lack of effect of zinc supplementation on fetal and indeed early infant growth is in contrast to the previously shown detrimental effect of zinc deficiency on childhood growth (Brown *et al.* 2002), and despite its biologically demonstrated effect on altering resistance to infection (Shankar and Prasad 1998). However, this highlights issues regarding the appropriate timing of interventions, in that supplementation with zinc, or other micronutrients, beginning in mid-pregnancy may be too late to affect fetal growth, although it may be plausible that it might help to prevent infections that could initiate preterm labour. It also highlights issues of the combined effects of multiple micronutrient deficiencies on fetal growth, as the effect of zinc supplementation on other micronutrients has not been adequately studied (Osendarp *et al.* 2003).

Other vitamins and multivitamins

Several vitamins and multivitamins have been recommended for pregnant women, and in many developed countries they are routinely suggested for pregnant women (King 2001), but not all have been hypothesised to have an effect on fetal growth. A Cochrane review of vitamin-A supplementation in pregnancy, in terms of its effects on maternal morbidity and mortality, for example reported no effects on fetal growth (van den Broek *et al.* 2002). However, of two trials of vitamin-D supplementation in pregnancy, one reported a non-significantly lower number of LBW infants. But the small numbers of women included mean that any potential effect remains speculative (Mahomed and Gülmezoglu 1999). One trial of vitamin-C and vitamin-E supplementation among women who were at risk of preeclampsia reported a non-significant reduced risk of SGA delivery associated with vitamin supplementation (Merialdi *et al.* 2003). Hence there is limited evidence to support any beneficial effect of maternal single-vitamin supplementation in pregnancy on fetal growth from the studies to date.

However, the role of multivitamins needs further assessment, particularly in poorly nourished populations where multiple deficiencies are common. Several studies have been carried out in the past but there are methodological issues that make interpretation of results difficult (Fall *et al.* 2003) and many have been in developed countries, albeit in disadvantaged subgroups. A prospective observational study conducted in low-income urban teenage women in the United States between 1985 and 1995 found that early multivitamin supplementation was associated with a significant reduction in both LBW and preterm deliveries (Scholl *et al.* 1997). Retrospective evaluation of data from the US Federal Women, Infants and Children's (WIC) Program, which provided food vouchers for specific foods to low-income mothers, suggested that supplementing maternal diets with

foods rich in vitamins and minerals might be beneficial for fetal growth, with infants born to supplemented mothers having marginally higher birthweight and a larger mean head circumference, with a trend towards reduced preterm delivery. However, these interventions have not yet been fully assessed in a controlled, randomised trial so results may be biased by differences in other factors that also influence pregnancy outcome (Fall *et al.* 2003). Similarly in developing countries the evidence tends to be fragmentary, although suggestive that multivitamin supplementation may be beneficial, with the most promising results from studies in The Gambia (Ceesay *et al.* 1997) and Guatemala (Villar and Rivera 1988). However, in the latter trial the micronutrients were given incidentally and to both supplemented and unsupplemented groups, and in The Gambia they were given with balanced protein/energy supplements, so that overall assessing the benefit of multiple micronutrient supplementation remains a challenge (Fall *et al.* 2003).

A more recent randomised controlled clinical trial was conducted in a semirural community in Mexico to consider if there was any differential effect of multiple micronutrient supplementation as compared to iron-only on infant size at birth, but there was no evidence that this was the case from this study (Ramakrishnan *et al.* 2003), even though supplementation began during the first trimester in most women. A large, randomised controlled trial of multivitamin and/or vitamin-A supplementation was also carried out in Tanzania on HIV-1-infected pregnant women ($n = 1075$) by Fawzi *et al* (1998). Poor micronutrient status had previously been associated with both faster progression of disease status and adverse pregnancy outcomes in HIV-infected women, including fetal growth retardation (Tang *et al.* 1996). In this trial multivitamin supplementation significantly decreased the risk of LBW by 44% (RR = 0.56, 95% CI 0.38, 0.82), early preterm delivery, defined by the authors as less than 34 completed weeks gestation, by 39% (RR = 0.61, 95% CI 0.38, 0.96) and SGA by 43% (RR = 0.57, 95% CI 0.39, 0.82), whereas vitamin A alone had no significant effect on these fetal outcomes. In addition, multivitamins did appear to slow the progression of maternal disease (CD3, CD4 and CD8 counts all showed a significant increase) (Fawzi *et al.* 1998). This trial was particularly promising in terms of demonstrating the benefits of multivitamin supplementation during pregnancy for improving fetal growth, but it was not generalisable beyond mothers who were HIV positive, although this is the case for an increasing proportion of the reproductive population in Asia and sub-Saharan Africa. Further trials of multivitamin and multinutrient supplementation in pregnancy are ongoing, with eight studies in Asia and three in Africa and efficacy studies taking place in Bangladesh, China, India, Indonesia and Pakistan under the UNICEF framework which focuses on integrated interventions, including food-based approaches, to prevent LBW. Of particular note is that the trials are being conducted using comparable protocols and methodology so that results may be pooled and meta-analysis of the effects of supplementation using large numbers of mother–infant pairs in different populations will be possible. The results from these trials are eagerly awaited before firm conclusions regarding the benefit or otherwise of multinutrient supplementation can be reached.

Summary of effects of maternal dietary interventions on fetal growth

Despite numerous observational studies and pooled analysis of intervention studies considering the effects of maternal dietary manipulation in pregnancy the overall effects of macronutrient and specific micronutrient supplements during pregnancy on proxy measures of fetal growth, and rates of LBW in particular, tend to be modest at best (Table 8.2). However, it is important to bear in mind the methodological difficulties in pooling results from heterogeneous studies to reach these summary conclusions. Authors have rightly cautioned that meta-analyses of many small studies are not a substitute for large, well-conducted clinical trials (Levine *et al.* 1997).

In terms of maternal macronutrient status there is evidence that balanced protein/energy supplementation may be beneficial for decreasing rates of LBW and SGA deliveries, especially in populations where women have chronic marginal nutritional status prior to pregnancy (De Onis *et al.* 1998). This benefit will need to be carefully balanced against the potential risks of obstructed labour, which have not been thoroughly investigated, although the trial in The Gambia reported only a small increase in head circumference which was felt to be unlikely to result in increased rates of cephalopelvic disproportion (Ceesay *et al.* 1997). The longer-term benefits and/or risks of supplementation also require further study, although the immediate perinatal mortality risk to infants born to supplemented mothers was decreased in the few follow-up studies of infants born following maternal energy/protein supplementation who were followed up in the postnatal period. Maternal supplementation with an isocaloric balanced protein or high-protein diet, however, had no beneficial effect on fetal growth and there was limited evidence that it adversely affected fetal growth rate (as measured by mean birthweight) and therefore potentially increased the rates of LBW deliveries. In women who were obese before pregnancy there have been no benefits with respect to fetal growth by restricting energy and protein during gestation, although evidence from controlled trials is limited.

In terms of specific micronutrients, maternal calcium supplementation may have a beneficial effect on fetal growth, particularly in women with low calcium status at the outset of pregnancy or who were classified as being at high risk of gestational hypertension. The effects on fetal growth appeared to act partly via a reduction in pre-eclampsia in mothers and a lengthened gestation. Maternal magnesium and zinc supplementation both appeared to be potentially beneficial in terms of lengthening gestation and improving fetal growth rates. However, further high-quality studies are required, addressing some of the methodological concerns, to evaluate these specific micronutrient effects, particularly in populations who are chronically deficient. Although biological mechanisms exist by which magnesium,

Table 8.2 Summary effects of dietary interventions on birthweight, rates of small for gestational age (SGA) and preterm deliveries in supplemented compared to non-supplemented mothers (derived from RCTs).

Nutritional supplement	Summary effect on fetal outcome			Overall evidence of beneficial effect on LBW[c]
	Birthweight: mean change[a] (95% CI)	SGA: RR[b] (95% CI)	Preterm delivery: RR[b] (95% CI)	
Balanced protein/energy	+25g (−4g, +55g)	0.68 (0.57, 0.80)	No significant effect	++
Isocaloric balanced protein	−64g (−124g, −3g)	Increase?	No significant effect	−
High protein	−58g (−146g, +30g)	Increase?	Not reported	−
Energy/protein restriction	Decrease	Not reported	No significant effect	−
Salt restriction	Increase?	Increase?	Not reported	Inconclusive
Calcium	Increase?	No sig. effect	Decrease?	+
Iron	No sig. effect	No sig. effect	No sig. effect	No[d]
Folate	Increase?	Not reported	Not reported	+
Iron and folate	Decrease?	Not reported	Not reported	Inconclusive[d]
Magnesium	0.76 (0.46, 0.96)[e]	0.70 (0.53, 0.93)	0.70 (0.57, 0.94)	++
Fish oil	No significant effect	No significant effect	Decrease??	No
Zinc	0.75 (0.52, 1.07)[e]	0.89 (0.61, 1.30)	0.73 (0.54, 0.98)	+

[a] Mean change refers to mean difference in absolute birthweight for supplemented compared to non-supplemented mothers.

[b] RR refers to the relative risk of outcome in supplemented compared to non-supplemented mothers.

[c] Overall evidence based on strength of summary effect and quality of studies. + suggests weak evidence of benefit and ++ moderately strong evidence; − suggests weak evidence of adverse effects.

[d] Studies largely limited to women without pre-existing deficiency.

[e] Refers to RR of LBW in supplemented compared to non-supplemented mothers.

? Weak evidence of an effect, either due to methodological concerns, too few studies or equivocal findings between studies.

?? Limited evidence of reduction of risk of a subsequent preterm delivery in high-risk mothers.

calcium and zinc might potentially affect the initiation of labour, further understanding and testing of hypotheses regarding the mechanisms by which these micronutrients provided to the mother might affect either fetal growth rate or gestational duration will also be essential for the appropriate targeting of interventions. Other micronutrients such as B-complex vitamins, copper and selenium may also have an as yet unexplained role in the association between maternal nutrition and fetal growth, but too few experimental studies have been conducted to date to consider evidence for or against their roles (Ramakrishnan et al. 1999).

There have been few studies published which have examined whether multiple micronutrient supplements might be more beneficial than single micronutrients, although there is much current research in this area, and the results of large trials are awaited in the light of some promising effects in HIV-1-infected mothers (Fawzi et al. 1998). Also, whilst there is evidence of the interactions of several micronutrients at the metabolic level, little is yet known about the significance of these interactions for pregnancy outcomes, especially in developing countries, where nutrient deficiencies rarely occur in isolation and multiple micronutrient deficiencies are common (Ramakrishnan et al. 1999).

In general, the findings to date question the underlying assumption of causality that these intervention studies are based on, namely that altering maternal nutrition in pregnancy will have a direct effect on fetal growth. While there is evidence that maternal dietary interventions and even nutritional advice have a positive effect on maternal gestational weight gain the associated gain in fetal weight is comparatively small and at times non existent. The nature of the causal pathway linking maternal and fetal nutrition in human pregnancy requires further elucidation if interventions are to be appropriately targeted to improving fetal outcome.

Limitations in current knowledge of the association between maternal nutrition and LBW

Understanding the association: is it causal?

While maternal nutritional deficiencies do often arise from low dietary intakes of essential nutrients, nutritional deficiencies at the level of the fetus may arise through several different mechanisms, including genetic, maternal disease, placental dysfunction, toxicant insults and physiological stressors (Keen et al. 2003). In 1991 Susser called into question the causal sequence of maternal nutrition leading to maternal weight gain leading to infant birthweight, suggesting that it was not sustained by the evidence available at that time (Susser 1991). He suggested, after examining the results of several studies under different conditions, that the complete sequence of association had only been proven in times of acute famine, such as the Dutch 'hunger winter', and that outside of famine the association was modified by baseline nutritional status. The essential question that arises, therefore, is: how are the associations between maternal nutritional intake and fetal growth understood?

The human fetus grows at the end of what has been described by Harding (2001) as a 'long and sometimes precarious supply line', which links maternal diet at one end with fetal uptake of nutrients at the other. Between these two points are maternal nutrient uptake, maternal metabolism, uterine blood flow, placental transport and metabolism and umbilical blood flow. There may be large changes in maternal diet which have very small or negligible effects on fetal nutrition if the steps in the fetal 'supply line' allow for a large margin of safety for fetal growth (Harding 2001). Conversely, maternal diseases such as gestational hypertension which are associated with reduced uterine blood flow or placental pathology may severely limit the transfer of nutrients to the fetus, and thus limit fetal growth, without any change in maternal nutrition. Harding also comments that there has been a great deal of confusion and debate in the literature because a distinction is not made between maternal and fetal nutrition. Whilst maternal nutrition may be relatively straightforward to measure, measuring fetal nutrition is much more problematic but it is extremely important in terms of fetal growth whereas maternal nutrition overall may be much less important. Much of our knowledge regarding the association between maternal nutrition and fetal nutrition comes from animal experiments, but there are essential differences between placental function and metabolic responses to different maternal nutritional states between humans and the animals which are commonly used in experimental models (Harding 2001). Animal experiments also tend to focus on a single acute insult to the mother and/or fetus at a clearly defined point, when the reality of human experience (both within and outside of pregnancy) is that insults are more likely to be chronic and may involve several triggering factors acting over several periods of development (Gluckman and Hanson 2005). Therefore cautious extrapolation of results is required from animal experiments to the human condition.

Incorporating the temporal dimension

There are also important questions regarding the timing of interventions which remain unanswered by studies to date. The timing (length and dose) of nutrient intervention and the association between the timing of nutrient deposition in the mothers and the effect on the fetal trajectory of growth needs fuller exploration, particularly in populations with long-standing nutritional deprivation (De Onis et al. 1998). Observational studies in particular have suggested that achieved fetal growth is highly dependent on maternal pre-pregnancy weight or nutritional status and that gestational weight gain may have an effect which is conditional on this starting point, but the limited assessment of this phenomenon using evidence from intervention studies has not supported this.

Maternal diet in pregnancy is often measured over a limited time period as a proxy for her general dietary intake, and in many studies, observational and RCTs, pre-pregnancy weight or BMI are based on measurements made in early gestation rather than measurements made prior to conception, as the former are more readily attainable and many pregnancies are unplanned (Thame et al. 1997). These proxy measures of pre-pregnancy status may, however, dilute the associations between maternal pre-pregnancy nutritional status and her offspring's intrauterine growth, depending on the timing of measurement and the degree of placental and fetal growth up to that point. There is evidence from studies in sheep that the fetal growth trajectory is set by periconceptional maternal nutrition and that the nutritional status of the mother leading up to pregnancy determines the ability of the fetus to respond to acute maternal nutritional challenges whilst in utero (Harding 1997). Hence measuring maternal nutritional or dietary status in early pregnancy may not be the most appropriate point at which to assess the impact of nutritional status on final fetal size at birth. Within any one pregnancy there are also unresolved issues regarding the timing of gestational weight gain, patterns of fat and fat-free mass and their locations and how differences in the timings may influence nutrient transfer to the growing fetus (Villar et al. 2003a). It has been suggested that birthweight is associated more with maternal changes in skinfold thickness and early gestational fat gain than with changes in other body sites or other gestational weight gain (Villar et al. 1992, Mardones-Santander et al. 1998, Lederman et al. 1999), but this has yet to be proven in different populations. Few studies, if any in humans, have been able to examine the trajectory of fetal growth throughout gestation in the context of repeated assessments of maternal nutritional status.

It is also relatively rare for studies to follow women through the course of more than one pregnancy to determine the impact of a mother's nutritional status on her ability to grow and nourish successive infants. This may be of particular importance to reduced fetal growth as short pregnancy intervals have been acknowledged to be associated with an increased risk of LBW and preterm delivery in the subsequent pregnancy in several different populations irrespective of their underlying maternal nutritional status (Ramachandran 2002). One potential explanation for this phenomenon is that women who either have closely spaced pregnancies or who become pregnant as adolescents (while they are still growing) may enter a reproductive cycle with reduced nutritional reserves (King 2003), but this hypothesised maternal nutritional depletion over the course of several reproductive cycles remains a little-studied phenomenon (Kusin et al. 1994).

An attempt to address the shortcomings of failure to include the temporal dimension in studies that considered the effects of maternal nutritional status and supplementation over a complete reproductive cycle of two pregnancies and a period of lactation was addressed by two studies using subsets of data collected from a nutritional supplementation trial conducted by the Institute of Nutrition of Central America and Panama (INCAP) in Guatemala (1969–77) (Villar and Rivera 1988, Winkvist et al. 1998), where women were assumed to be chronically but not severely malnourished. The earlier study compared the birthweights of infants born over two successive pregnancies to 169 mothers who received either of two caloric supplements (high or low) during both pregnancies and the intervening period or only during the second pregnancy. Overall the study found greater benefits in terms of higher mean birthweights of infants born to mothers who received high caloric supplementation over the period of both pregnancies and during lactation, than in mothers who received the high caloric supplement only during the second pregnancy (Villar and Rivera 1988). The later study analysed data on 176 complete reproductive cycles from the same database and considered effects of the different levels of caloric supplementation on maternal and infant weight change during both pregnancies according to initial maternal nutritional status (greater than or less than 50 kg). The authors concluded that the effect of maternal high caloric supplementation over both pregnancies on change in sibling birthweight was most marked in women who were classified as being undernourished prior to pregnancy (using a cut off of less than 50 kg), whereas there was little evidence of any benefit of either supplementation on change in sibling birthweight in the group of women originally classified as being of normal weight (not less than 50 kg) (Winkvist *et al.* 1998).

The earlier study suggested that the ability of a mother to nourish her growing fetus was greatest when maternal energy supplementation was provided at sufficient levels before pregnancy began, rather than only once gestation was established, in a population of women who were classified as chronically undernourished. The later study, although reliant on small numbers in each subgroup of women and having multiple exclusions, supports the concept of a differential partitioning of nutrients between mothers and their offspring over the course of a reproductive career, according to initial maternal nutritional status. It also reinforces the results of supplementation studies which have found little or no effect of dietary supplementation on fetal growth of infants born to women who were previously well nourished, and suggests that this was not just a feature of supplements being provided too late in gestation. Overall, the studies, though small, support calls for wider interventions to improve the nutrition of all women, regardless of their reproductive status, since the effects of dietary manipulation may be delayed rather than immediate, as many current intervention trials assume.

Beyond the immediate periconceptional period

The traditional preoccupation in perinatal epidemiology has been to examine offspring size at birth in the context of concurrently measured adult maternal characteristics and the specific pregnancy course in particular. This ignores the more distal temporal influences on determinants of size at birth and lim-

its the studies' ability to address the temporal ordering in the associated measures. Recently, however, there has been a renewed interest in the intergenerational influences on offspring size at birth and a further growing body of literature taking a life-course (sometimes called a life-cycle) approach to health outcomes including reproduction and offspring size at birth (Rich-Edwards 2002). It is now well established that there is a tendency to repeat birthweight across generations, and it has been estimated that approximately 12% of fetal growth restriction in the developed world is attributable to the effect of the mother's own birthweight on that of her offspring (Emanuel 1997). In particular, mothers in a UK intergenerational study who were born LBW themselves had an estimated two fold increased risk of delivering an LBW infant during their own reproductive life (Hennessy and Alberman 1998). An adult follow-up study of females born during the Dutch 'hunger winter' (1944–5) traced 700 of the infants into adulthood to examine the intergenerational effects of maternal intrauterine exposure to famine (Lumey and Stein 1997b). Mothers whose own birthweights were depressed by intrauterine famine exposure also tended to bear offspring of reduced birthweight, that is the nutrition of the first-generation mothers during the famine appeared to have a far-reaching influence on the fetal growth of the third generation, potentially mediated by the reduced birthweight of the second (Rich-Edwards 2002). Most studies, though, even those that take an intergenerational approach, focus on attained maternal adult size (as a proxy for maternal nutritional status) and maternal size at birth, and there is less evidence to support any influence of differential maternal lifetime growth and development on her offspring's size at birth. Some indirect evidence comes from the 1958 British birth cohort study, in which early age at menarche was noted to be a predictor of offspring size (Hennessy and Alberman 1998). Age at menarche is associated with childhood growth, which in turn has been associated with early-life nutrition. Age at menarche was used as a proxy for early maternal development in this study, having previously been found to be associated with weight at the age of

7 years and in turn with adult weight (Cooper *et al.* 1996) in the earlier 1946 British birth cohort. Recent work using a revitalised Aberdeen intergenerational cohort, though, has shown the importance of maternal growth throughout her life-course (intrauterine through childhood to achieved adult size), rather than just at discrete points, on the growth of her offspring, with the most enduring effects arising directly and indirectly from her own intrauterine growth (Morton 2002).

The intergenerational and life-course influence of maternal growth on her offspring's growth highlights that whilst studies usually describe associations between maternal adult anthropometric measures and fetal growth, the adult measures act as proxy measures for a woman's life-course development to that point in time. Her body composition and ability to nourish a growing fetus at the time of pregnancy may be associated with her current (adult) nutritional status, but changing her capacity to do so may be dependent as much on her early-life growth and development as on her immediate nutritional environment.

Implications for targeting interventions to improve fetal growth

Timescale for action

Consideration of the temporal issues in determining whether a mother is able to adequately nourish her fetus raises issues of the appropriate timing of any nutritional interventions with this outcome in mind. Intrauterine growth retardation may be viewed as a downstream marker of pregnancy complications, which once in existence are difficult to treat. Diagnosis in mid to late pregnancy may have important implications for delivery and perinatal risk, which might be managed in the appropriate clinical situation, but in terms of preventing growth restriction it may be a late marker in the causal chain of events that lead ultimately to reduced fetal growth. It is becoming increasingly clear that interventions during or late in pregnancy are less likely to exert significant

effects on pregnancy outcome than interventions either early in pregnancy or even prior to conception (Jackson *et al.* 2003).

What is feasible based on the evidence to date?

Given the availability of the current evidence for the effectiveness of nutritional interventions during pregnancy (some of which are routine and widespread in women without overt deficiencies, for example routine iron–folate administration), the only immediate intervention which is consistently supported by evidence from observational and intervention studies is energy/protein supplementation in women who are considered to be undernourished (either in developing or developed countries). However, although based on more limited evidence, this supplementation too may be most beneficial if it is provided in the pre-conception period or over more than one reproductive cycle. Potentially providing supplementation prior to pregnancy may also be more cost-effective but there is almost a complete absence of any formal cost-effectiveness analysis in developing countries on which to assess this (Rouse 2003). There may also be a place for short-term solutions to address specific maternal nutritional deficiencies, particularly related to iron-deficiency, but evidence is lacking on interventions that are best able to tackle the multiple nutrient deficiencies that frequently coexist in populations who have the highest burden of LBW. Overall it seems unlikely that there will be short-term nutritional interventions or advice that will quickly lessen the burden of LBW; rather, nutritional status may need to be improved over more than one generation before changes are seen at the population level.

Previous large-scale nutritional interventions

Widespread public health interventions have been few with respect to improving fetal growth, although guidelines for care in pregnancy, including nutritional advice, are widely available, particularly in developed countries. There is, however, an ongoing nationwide nutrition project in Bangladesh which was launched in 1995 with support from the World Bank and UNICEF. The Bangladesh Integrated Nutrition Project (BINP) aims to achieve a substantial and sustainable improvement in the nutritional status of women and children through the improved practice of dietary behaviours and appropriate use of nutrition services which will be increasingly managed and financed by communities themselves. The objective of the project is to break the intergenerational cycle of malnutrition through reductions in the incidence of low birthweight as well as reductions in rates of malnutrition in children and women of reproductive age. The project runs for 10 years and includes vitamin-A supplementation, iodisation of salt, food fortification and promotion of breast-feeding as well as area, school and national programmes to support and evaluate the different components of the wide-ranging scheme. The results of the project are eagerly awaited.

Two major strategies related more specifically to pregnancy outcomes that have been widely implemented are iodine supplementation to prevent cretinism and periconceptional folic acid for the prevention of neural tube defects. In populations where these policies have been implemented there has been a large reduction in both of these adverse pregnancy outcomes, but neither of these interventions has a specific effect on fetal growth per se. It is also salient to note that despite sound evidence that these strategies have reduced adverse events they have not completely eliminated them, because as with fetal growth retardation the underlying causes of the problems are multidimensional and not just related to a single nutrient deficiency. Additionally, new cases of cretinism and neural tube defects continue to arise in populations who remain unsupplemented, despite the available evidence of the association and the effectiveness of the intervention, highlighting the gap which often exists between knowledge and action – a gap that is also multidimensional, particularly for developing countries, with limited resources for health promotion or service provision. While it is anticipated that the greatest benefit of nutritional supplementation on pregnancy outcome will be seen in developing

countries, research is most limited in those countries and delivery of interventions is also most difficult (Goldenberg 2003). There are important cost-effectiveness and risk–benefit analyses required to consider the advantages of food-based versus pharmacologic interventions, particularly in populations under nutritional stress. There may be potential benefits in utilising food-based supplements instead of pharmacologic supplements because of the potential for toxicity of the latter (in accidental overdose) and in terms of their relative acceptability and sustainability over time. There is evidence from the Pune Maternal Nutritional Study that compliance may be low in trials of pharmacologic supplements, because women prefer a good diet for themselves and their families to tablets (Fall *et al.* 2003). This potential wastage of pharmacologic agents has important implications for the cost-effectiveness of different interventions (Rouse 2003).

The challenge of translating evidence into practice

Currently questions arise as to whether nutritional interventions should be targeted at whole populations who are nutritionally deficient, or whether interventions are also potentially of benefit for populations for whom nutrition either at the level of macro- or micronutrients is adequate, as the effect of supplementation on fetal growth appears to differ in these groups. Most nutritional supplementation currently occurs in populations who are well nourished and there is little evidence to support any benefits of intervention for fetal growth in these groups of women. With respect to nutritional interventions aimed at reducing the rates of LBW there remains a lack of information regarding the specific optimal level of supplementation that might be associated with nutritional benefit and not with harm, and also with the timing of the supplementation and the duration of 'treatment'. Any intervention must not be harmful either in the short term or in the longer term. In some cases there is evidence that providing women with a supplement in the absence of a background nutritional deficiency may have the opposite effect on birthweight to that anticipated (Rush *et al.* 1980). Improving fetal growth will only be an important goal if it is associated with better health of infants in the long term as well as in the immediate perinatal period, but few studies have followed up their cohorts of supplemented mothers or infants to determine whether any early benefit seen with respect to reduction of rates of LBW is maintained throughout their early development and in terms of their own adult reproductive and later health (Belizán *et al.* 1997), particularly in the light of the increasing evidence of a line between size at birth and later adult chronic disease (Barker 1997). There are potential concerns relating to later adult disease that need to be carefully considered if women in developing countries are to be routinely supplemented with food or pharmacologic agents during pregnancy. The fetal origins of adult disease hypothesis originally suggested that nutritional perturbations during gestation resulted in adaptations by the fetus that altered the metabolic and physiologic functioning of the infant postnatally so that infants who were born small were at increased risk of chronic diseases, particularly diabetes and the metabolic syndrome, in later life (Barker 1998). More recently it appears that disharmony between reduced fetal growth and accelerated postnatal growth may be more important for later disease risk than small size alone (Eriksson *et al.* 1999). A study which compared the neonatal anthropometry of babies born in Pune, India, with those born in Southampton, England, found that infants in Pune were generally born lighter (mean 2.7 kg versus 3.5 kg) and thinner (smaller abdominal circumference and upper arm circumference) but relatively fatter, especially in terms of measures of central adiposity, than their Southampton counterparts. It has been hypothesised that this body composition may persist postnatally and predispose them to an insulin-resistant state in later life. Indian mothers also tend to be small (mean height of 1.52 m) and thin (mean BMI 18 kg m^2), but relatively centrally obese (as measured by subscapular skinfolds) (Yajnik *et al.* 2002). With mothers who are small but relatively centrally obese, maternal con-

straint no doubt acts as an important determinant of small infant size, to avoid the problems of delivering an inappropriately large infant. If interventions are directed towards feeding these mothers with the aim of increasing fetal growth, there may be short-term problems with respect to increased problems at delivery but in the longer term the potential augmentation of fetal growth may be out of harmony with the infants innately determined growth patterns, which may increase rather than ameliorate their disease risk in adult life (Prentice 2003). Therefore there are issues about whether targeting reductions in LBW will necessarily lead to reductions in what have been assumed to be associated later health risks.

There is also some evidence that nutritional supplements may confer benefit without having an effect on birthweight or duration of gestation. For example a trial of maternal zinc supplementation in Peru (25 mg/day) produced a short-term benefit in fetal femur growth without a specific effect on birthweight (Villar *et al.* 2003a). Follow-up is required to determine if increased leg-length in these infants is firstly apparent and secondly maintained in extrauterine life, and whether this confers later health benefits, as other studies suggest it might (Gunnell *et al.* 1998).

Throughout discussions considering interventions to optimise fetal growth it is important to remember the multi causal nature of LBW beyond the consideration of subgroups of IUGR and preterm deliveries. To implement effective interventions requires a fuller understanding of the many different underlying processes that lead to reduced intrauterine growth (Jackson *et al.* 2003), both their nature and their timing, beyond a general association with proxy measures of maternal anthropometry or nutrition which may merely represent summary measures of previous insults or mediating factors in the pathway of risk.

Whilst it may be biologically plausible to consider a pathway of causation between maternal nutrition (anthropometry and diet) and fetal growth, it may be less intuitive to consider a plausible causal sequence between maternal nutrition and preterm delivery. However, there is emerging evidence that both infectious and non-infectious pre-term delivery may be more intimately connected to maternal nutrition than previously anticipated. Recent evidence from sheep and in humans suggests that periconceptional undernutrition may be associated with an increased risk of non-infectious preterm delivery (Bloomfield *et al.* 2003, Rayco-Solon *et al.* 2005). With respect to infectious preterm delivery it is known that impaired immune function is a common result of malnutrition. Therefore a biologically plausible pathway may exist between chronic maternal malnutrition, evidenced through low pre-pregnancy BMI or weight, and an increased risk of preterm delivery via maternal infection, but there has been virtually no literature that relates micronutrient deficiencies to infections that are clearly related to pregnancy outcomes, such as those pertaining to the genitourinary tract (Goldenberg 2003). This may well be of particular relevance in developing countries, where nutritional deficiencies and infections tend to coexist in women of child-bearing age (Villar *et al.* 2003a).

Maternal nutrition in its wider context

A successful pregnancy negotiates a complex partitioning of energy and nutrients between the mother, the placenta and the fetus (Harding 2001). There is an essential need for the mother to be able to transfer appropriate nutrients to the fetus at the appropriate time during gestation, but it is overly simplistic to assume that this may only be constrained by the immediate dietary intake or overall nutritional status of the mother (Jackson *et al.* 2003).

An individual's nutritional status is in reality influenced by numerous factors in addition to diet, including genetics, environment, lifestyle habits, the presence of disease and/or exposures to drugs or toxicants (Keen *et al.* 2003). Further, it is a product of the complex interplay of biological, social, cultural, behavioural and health-related factors throughout a woman's entire life-course (Mora and Nestel 2000) and for this reason it is often extremely difficult to separate the nutritional causation from the socio-economic disparities we see in size at birth. It is probably rare that poor maternal diet is the sole insult that

occurs in women with poor pregnancy outcomes. An alternative possibility is that the compromised nutritional status of an individual potentiates the effect of other reproductive hazards that may coexist in a particular population at risk (Keen *et al.* 2003), including the risk of severe infection and the impact of strenuous physical work during pregnancy (Scholl and Hediger 1994, Shaw 2003).

While the role of maternal nutrition may be considered central to maternal well being and therefore to optimal pregnancy outcomes, the role of nutrition can really only be fully understood in the context of the behavioural and social environment in which the mother finds herself not only during pregnancy but also during her growth to adult reproductive life. Globally the initiatives that have the most potential benefit for improving fetal nutrition and fetal growth are likely to be longer-term and will address the nutritional deficiencies in the light of the social, political and cultural contexts in which they occur over several generations. Strategies to improve maternal nutrition and potentially fetal growth need to go beyond the conventional approach of providing periconceptional and pregnancy-care services to embrace the life-course approach that seeks to address risk factors present well before pregnancy, ideally beginning in the early life of all potential mothers (Mora and Nestel 2000).

Summary

There has been a large quantity of research, both observational and intervention studies, which have allowed the effects of maternal adult anthropometric indices, dietary intake in pregnancy and nutritional supplements to be quantified with respect to the measures of fetal size and maturity at birth. Overall they suggest a strong positive association between maternal pre-pregnancy nutritional status in particular and the ability of a mother to nourish her growing fetus, mostly through defining rates of fetal growth, but recent evidence also suggests that periconceptional undernutrition may also be important in setting gestational length. Gestational weight gain and nutritional interventions during pregnancy appear able to modify this association by altering the rate of fetal growth, although the extent of the modification appears dependent on maternal baseline nutritional status, and it is always modest. Despite the overall positive association between maternal nutritional status and fetal growth across populations, within populations there is much individual variation in adaptation to the energy requirements of pregnancy, even in women of normal pre-pregnancy weight and with pre-existing adequate nutritional status. These variations are not always evident from anthropometric measures or cross-sectional dietary documentation.

The association that has been repeatedly found between maternal nutrition (however it is measured) and fetal growth has led to the trialling of nutritional interventions during gestation in an attempt to address the burden of reduced intrauterine growth (as manifest primarily in low birthweight), especially in developed countries. However, overall the results of dietary-intervention trials have been modest at best and occasionally detrimental in terms of birthweight in particular. Most trials have focused on single micronutrients when in reality it is multi-nutrient deficiencies that are prevalent in under-nourished women. There is emerging evidence from developing countries that diets that are dense in multiple micronutrient foods may be a more viable and appropriate solution to improving fetal growth than pharmacologic interventions but this requires further investigation, in terms of cost-effectiveness, sustainability and longer-term benefits. Whilst there is little doubt that maternal supplementation may have benefits for maternal health there has been little evidence that supplementation during pregnancy is able to affect fetal growth, although whether maternal nutritional interventions are able to positively affect infant health independently of an effect on absolute size at delivery also requires further assessment. Problems in understanding the reason for this limited impact of dietary modifications include our as yet incomplete unravelling of the causal pathway between maternal nutrition (whether cumulative or dietary) and fetal nutrition. It is possible that the determinants of fetal growth are largely established prior to pregnancy, either in the immediate pericon-ceptional period or during the life-course development of the mother (including her own intrauterine development) so that interventions during gestation, particularly in the latter half of pregnancy, are only able to have a limited effect because the fetal growth trajectory is largely established by her nutritional status at the outset of pregnancy, except perhaps under conditions of acute and severe food restriction.

The burden of low birthweight in the world remains high, with the greatest contribution from developing countries, where the bulk of the cause of low birthweight at delivery is reduced growth rate in utero. Being born LBW exposes an infant to immediate perinatal risks, increased risks of adult disease in later life, and contributes to the perpetuation of the cycle of LBW into the next generation. Addressing this problem in the long term may have more to do with improving the nutritional status and food availability to women globally, throughout their entire life-course development, rather than with short-term pregnancy interventions. Focusing only on nutritional solutions, though, ignores the social and cultural context in which maternal dietary deficiencies have arisen and the coexisting problems, including poverty and infection, that allow them to proliferate.

REFERENCES

Atallah, A. N., Hofmeyr, G. and Duley, L. (2002). Calcium supplementation during pregnancy for preventing hypertensive disorders and related problems. *Cochrane Database Syst. Rev.*, **2002** (1).

Badrawi, H., Hassanein, M. K., Badroui, M. H. H., Wafa, Y. A. and Badrawi N. (1992). Pregnancy outcome in obese pregnant mothers. *J. Perinat. Med.*, **20**, 1–203.

Barker, D. J. P. (1995). Fetal origins of coronary heart disease. *BMJ*, **311**, 171–4.

  (1997). Intrauterine programming of coronary heart disease and stroke. *Acta Paediatr. Suppl.*, **423**, 178–82.

  (1998). *Mothers, Babies and Health in Later Life*. Edinburgh: Churchill Livingstone.

Belizán, J. M., Villar, J., Bergel, E. *et al.* (1997). Long term effect of calcium supplementation during pregnancy on the blood pressure of the offspring: follow up of a randomised controlled trial. *BMJ*, **315**, 281–5.

Blackwell, R. Q., Chow, B. F., Chinn, K. S. K., Blackwell, B. N. and Hsu, S. C. (1973). Prospective maternal nutrition study in Taiwan: rationale, study design, feasibility and preliminary findings. *Nutr. Rep. Int.*, **7**, 517–32.

Bloomfield, F. H., Oliver, M. H., Hawkins, P. *et al.* (2003). A peri-conceptional nutritional origin for non-infectious preterm birth. *Science*, **300**, 606.

Brown, K. H., Peerson, J. M. and Allen, L. H. (2002). Effect of zinc supplementation on the growth and serum zinc concentrations of pre-pubertal children: a meta-analysis of randomized controlled trials. *Am. J. Clin. Nutr.*, **75**, 1062–71.

Butler, N. R. and Bonham, D. G. (1963). *Perinatal Mortality*. London: Livingstone.

Campbell, D. M. and MacGillivray, I. (1975). The effect of a low calorie intake or a thiazide diuretic on the incidence of pre-eclampsia and on birthweight. *Br. J. Obstet. Gynaecol.*, **82**, 572–7.

Castillo-Durán, C. and Weisstaub, G. (2003). Zinc supplementation and growth of the fetus and low birth weight infant. *J. Nutr.*, **133**, 1494–7S.

Ceesay, S. M., Prentice, A. M., Cole, T. J. *et al.* (1997). Effects on birthweight and perinatal mortality of maternal dietary supplements in rural Gambia: 5 year randomised controlled trial. *BMJ*, **315**, 786–90.

Cole, T. J., Foord, F. A., Watkinson, M., Lamb, W. H. and Whitehead, R. G. (1995). The Keneba pregnancy supplementation study. *Bull. World Health Organ.*, **73**, 72–6.

Cooper, C., Kuh, D., Egger, P., Wadsworth, M. and Barker, D. J. P. (1996). Childhood growth and age at menarche. *Br. J. Obstet. Gynaecol.*, **103**, 814–17.

Cuervo, L. G. and Mahomed, K. (2001). Treatments for iron deficiency anaemia in pregnancy. *Cochrane Database Syst. Rev.*, **2001** (2).

De Onis, M., Villar, J. and Gülmezoglu, A. M. (1998). Nutritional interventions to prevent intrauterine growth retardation: evidence from randomized controlled trials. *Eur. J. Clin. Nutr.*, **52**, S83–93.

Dougherty, C. R. and Jones, A. D. (1982). The determinants of birthweight. *Am. J. Obstet. Gynecol.*, **144**, 190–200.

Doyle, W., Crawford, M. A., Wynn, A. H. and Wynn, S. W. (1989). Maternal magnesium intake and pregnancy outcome. *Magnes. Res.*, **2**, 205–10.

(1990). The association between maternal diet and birth dimensions. *J. Nutr. Med.*, **1**, 9–17.

(1992). Nutritional counselling and supplementation in the second and third trimester of pregnancy. *J. Nutr. Med.*, **3**, 249–56.

Duley, L. (1995). Prophylactic fish oil in pregnancy. In *Pregnancy and Childbirth Module of the Cochrane Database of Systematic Reviews* (ed. M. Enkin, M. Keirse, M. Renfrew

and J. Nelson). London: British Medical Journal Publishing Group.

Duley, L. and Henderson-Smart, D. (1999). Reduced salt intake compared to normal dietary salt, or high intake, in pregnancy. *Cochrane Database Syst. Rev.*, **1999** (3).

Emanuel, I. (1997). Invited commentary: an assessment of maternal intergenerational factors in pregnancy outcome. *Am. J. Epidemiol.*, **146**, 820–5.

Eriksson, J. G., Forsén, T. J., Tuomilehto, J., Winter, P. D., Osmond, C. and Barker, D. J. P. (1999). Catch-up growth in childhood and death from coronary heart disease: longitudinal study. *BMJ*, **318**, 427–31.

Evans, S. and Alberman, E. (1989). International Collaborative Effort (ICE) on Birthweight, Plurality, and Perinatal and Infant Mortality. II. Comparisons between birthweight distributions in member countries from 1970 to 1984. *Acta Obstet. Gynecol. Scand*, **68**, 11–17.

Fall, C. H. D., Yajnik, C. S., Rao, S., Davies, A. A., Brown, N. and Farrant, H. J. W. (2003). Micronutrients and fetal growth. *J. Nutr.*, **133**, 1747–56S.

Fawzi, W. W., Msamanga, G. I., Spiegelman, D. *et al.* (1998). Randomised trials of effects of vitamin supplements on pregnancy outcomes and T cell counts in HIV-1-infected women in Tanzania. *Lancet*, **351**, 1477–82.

Fish Oil Trials In Pregnancy (FOTIP) Team. (2000). Randomised controlled trials of fish oil supplementation in high risk pregnancies. *Br. J. Obstet. Gynaecol.*, **107**, 382–95.

Fleming, A. F., Ghatoura, G. B. S., Harrison, K. A., Briggs, N. D. and Dunn, D. T. (1986). The prevention of anaemia in pregnancy in primigravidae in the Guinea savannah of Nigeria. *Ann. Trop. Med. Parasitol.*, **80**, 211–33.

Forsum, E., Sadurskis, A. and Wager, J. (2003). Resting metabolic rate and body composition of healthy Swedish women during pregnancy. *Am. J. Clin. Nutr.*, **47**, 942–7.

Gluckman, P. D. and Hanson, M. A. (2005). *The Fetal Matrix*. Cambridge: Cambridge University Press.

Godfrey, K., Robinson, S. and Barker, D. J. P. (1997). Maternal nutrition in early and late pregnancy in relation to placental and fetal growth. *BMJ*, **312**, 410–14.

Goldberg, G. R., Prentice, A. M. and Coward, W. A. (1993). Longitudinal assessment of energy expenditure in pregnancy by the doubly labelled water method. *Am. J. Clin. Nutr.*, **57**, 494–505.

Goldenberg, R. L. (2003). The plausibility of micronutrient deficiency in relationship to perinatal infection. *J. Nutr.*, **133**, 1645–8S.

Goldstein, H. and Peckham, C. (1976). Birthweight, gestation, neonatal mortality and child development. In *The Biology of Human Fetal Growth* (ed. D. F. Roberts and A. M. Thomson). London: Taylor & Francis, pp. 81–102.

Gunnell, D. J., Davey Smith, G., Frankel, S. J., Kemp, M. and Peters, T. J. (1998). Socio-economic and dietary influences on leg and trunk length in childhood: a reanalysis of the Carnegie (Boyd Orr) survey of diet and health in pre-war Britain (1937–39). *Paediatr. Perinat. Epidemiol.*, **12**, 96–113.

Harding, J. E. (1997). Periconceptual nutrition determines the fetal growth response to acute maternal undernutrition in fetal sheep of late gestation. *Prenat. Neonat. Med.*, **2**, 310–19.

(2001). The nutritional basis of the fetal origins of adult disease. *Int. J. Epidemiol.*, **30**, 15–23.

Hemminki, E. and Rimpela, U. (1991). Iron supplementation, maternal packed cell volume, and fetal growth. *Arch. Dis. Child.*, **66**, 422–5.

Hennessy, E. and Alberman, E. (1998). Intergenerational influences affecting birth outcome. I. Birthweight for gestational age in the children of the 1958 British birth cohort. *Paediatr. Perinat Epidemiol.*, **12** (Suppl. 1), 45–60.

Institute of Medicine (1990). *Nutrition During Pregnancy. Part I. Weight Gain. Part II. Nutrient Supplements.* Washington, DC: National Academy Press.

Iyenger L. (1967). Effects of dietary supplements late in pregnancy on the expectant mother and her newborn. *Indian J. Med. Res.*, **55**, 85–9.

Jackson, A. A. and Robinson. S. M. (2001). Dietary guidelines for pregnancy: a review of current evidence. *Public Health Nutr.*, **4**, 625–30.

Jackson, A. A., Bhutta, Z. A. and Lumbiganon, P. (2003). Nutrition as a preventive strategy against adverse pregnancy outcomes. *J. Nutr.*, **133**, 1589–91S.

Kafatos, A. G., Vlachonikolis, I. G. and Codrington, C. A. (1989). Nutrition during pregnancy: the effects of an educational intervention program in Greece. *Am. J. Clin. Nutr.*, **50**, 970–9.

Kardjati, S., Kusin, J. A. and De With, C. (1988). Energy supplementation in the last trimester of pregnancy in East Java. I. Effect on birthweight. *Br. J. Obstet. Gynaecol*, **95**, 783–94.

Keen, C. L., Clegg, M. S., Hanna, L. A. *et al.* (2003). The plausibility of micronutrient deficiencies being a significant contributing factor to the occurrence of pregnancy complications. *J. Nutr.*, **133**, 1597–605S.

King, J., Butte, N., Bronstein, M., Kopp, L. and Lindquist, S. (1994). Energy metabolism during pregnancy: influence of maternal energy status. *Am. J. Clin. Nutr.*, **59**, 439–45S.

King, J. C. (2001). Effect of reproduction on the bioavailability of calcium, zinc and selenium. *J. Nutr.*, **131**, 1355–8S.

(2003). The risk of maternal nutritional depletion and poor outcomes increases in early or closely spaced pregnancies. *J. Nutr.*, **133**, 1732–6S.

Kramer, M. S. (1987). Determinants of low birthweight: methodological assessment and meta-analysis. *Bull. World Health Organ.*, **65**, 663–737.

(1996a). Nutritional advice in pregnancy. *Cochrane Database Syst. Rev.*, **1996** (2).

(1996b). Isocaloric balanced protein supplementation in pregnancy. *Cochrane Database Syst. Rev.*, **1996** (2).

(1996c). High protein supplementation in pregnancy. *Cochrane Database Syst. Rev.*, **1996** (2).

(1996d). Energy/protein restriction for high weight-for-height or weight gain during pregnancy. *Cochrane Database Syst. Rev.*, **1996** (2).

(2000). Balanced protein/energy supplementation in pregnancy. *Cochrane Database Syst. Rev.*, **2000** (2).

(2003). The Epidemiology of adverse pregnancy outcomes: an overview. *J. Nutr.*, **133**, 1592–6S.

Kramer, M. S., McLean, F. H., Olivier, M., Willis, D. M. and Usher, R. H. (1989). Body proportionality and head and length 'sparing' in growth-retarded neonates: a critical reappraisal. *Pediatrics*, **84**, 717–23.

Kramer, M. S., Seguin, L., Lydon, J. and Goulet, L. (2000). Socio-economic disparities in pregnancy outcome: why do the poor fare so poorly? *Paed. Perinat. Epidemiol.*, **14**, 194–210.

Kusin, J. A., Kardjati, S., Houtkooper, J. M. and Renqvist, U. H. (1992). Energy supplementation during pregnancy and postnatal growth. *Lancet*, **340**, 623–6.

Kusin, J. A., Kardjati, S. and Renqvist, U. H. (1994). Maternal body mass index: the functional significance during reproduction. *Eur. J. Clin. Nutr.*, **48**, S56–67.

Lederman, S. A., Paxton, A., Heymsfield, S. B., Wang, J., Thornton, J. and Pierson, R. N. J. (1999). Maternal body fat and water during pregnancy: do they raise infant birth weight? *Am. J. Obstet. Gynecol.*, **180**, 235–40.

Levine, R. J., Hauth, J. C., Sibai, B. M. *et al.* (1997). Trial of calcium to prevent pre-eclampsia. *N. Engl. J. Med.*, **337**, 69–76.

Lopez-Jamarillo, P., Delgado, F., Jacome, P., Teran, M., Ruano, C. and Rivera, J. (1997). Calcium supplementation and the risk of pre-eclampsia in Ecuadorian pregnant teenagers. *Obstet. Gynecol.*, **90**, 162–7.

Lumey, L. H. and Stein, A. D. (1997a). Offspring birthweights after maternal intrauterine undernutrition: a comparison within sibships. *Am. J. Epidemiol.*, **146**, 810–19.

(1997b). In utero exposure to famine and subsequent fertility: the Dutch Famine Birth Cohort Study. *Am. J. Public Health*, **87**, 1962–6.

Lumley, J., Watson, L., Watson, M. and Bower, C. (2001). Periconceptual supplementation with folate and/or multivitamins for preventing neural tube defects. *Cochrane Database Syst. Rev.*, **2001** (3).

Maconochie, N. (1995). Abnormal fetal growth: a longitudinal analysis of women and their pregnancies. Unpublished Ph.D. thesis, University of London.

Mahomed, K. (1997a). Folate supplementation in pregnancy. *Cochrane Database Syst. Rev.*, **1997** (3).

(1997b). Iron and folate supplementation in pregnancy. *Cochrane Database Syst. Rev.*, **1997** (4).

(1997c). Zinc supplementaion in pregnancy. *Cochrane Database Syst. Rev.*, **1997** (3).

(1999). Iron supplementation in pregnancy. *Cochrane Database Syst. Rev.*, **1999** (4).

Mahomed, K. and Gülmezoglu, A. M. (1999). Vitamin D supplementation in pregancy. *Cochrane Database Syst. Rev.*, **1999** (1).

Makrides, M. and Crowther, C. (2001). Magnesium supplementation in pregnancy. *Cochrane Database Syst. Rev.*, **2001** (4).

Mardones-Santander, F., Salazar, G., Rosso, P. and Villaroel, L. (1998). Maternal body composition near term and birthweight. *Obstet. Gynecol.*, **91**, 873–7.

Matthews, F., Yudkin, P. and Neil, A. (1999). Influence of maternal nutrition on outcome of pregnancy: prospective cohort study. *BMJ*, **319**, 339–43.

Mavalankar, D. V., Gray, R. H., Triedi, C. R. and Parkh, V. C. (1994). Risk factors for small for gestational age births in Ahmedadab, India. *J. Trop. Pediatr.*, **40**, 285–90.

Merialdi, M., Carroli, G., Villar, J. *et al.* (2003). Nutritional interventions during pregnancy for the prevention or treatment of impaired fetal growth: an overview of randomized controlled trials. *J. Nutr.*, **133**, 1626–31S.

Metcoff, J. (1994). Clinical assessment of nutritional status at birth: fetal malnutrition and SGA are not synonymous. *Pediatr. Clin. North Am.*, **41**, 875–91.

Mora, J. O. and Nestel, P. E. (2000). Improving prenatal nutrition in developing countries: strategies, prospects and challenges. *Am. J. Clin. Nutr.*, **71**, 1353–63S.

Morton, S. M. B. (2002). Lifecourse determinants of offspring size at birth: an intergenerational study of Aberdeen women. Unpublished Ph.D. thesis, University of London.

Neggers, Y. and Goldenberg, R. L. (2003). Some thoughts on body mass index, micronutrient intakes and pregnancy outcome. *J. Nutr.*, **133**, 1737–40S.

Nestel, P. E. and Rutstein, S. O. (2002). Defining nutritional status of women in developing countries. *Public Health Nutr.*, **5**, 17–27.

Niromanesh, S., Laghaii, S. and Mosavi-Jarrahi A. (2001). Supplementary calcium in the prevention of pre-eclampsia. *Int. J. Gynaecol. Obstet*, **74**, 17–21.

Olsen, S. F., Sorensen, J. D., Secher, N. J. *et al.* (1992). Randomised controlled trial of effect of fish-oil supplementation on pregnancy duration. *Lancet*, **339**, 1003–7.

Onwude, J. L., Lilford, R. J., Hjartardottir, H., Staines, A. and Tufnell, D. (1995). A randomised double blind placebo trial of fish oil in high risk pregnancy. *Br. J. Obstet. Gynaecol.*, **102**, 95–100.

Osendarp, S. J. M., West, C. E. and Black, R. E. (2003). The need for maternal zinc supplementation in developing countries: an unresolved issue. *J. Nutr.*, **133**, 817–27S.

Poppitt, S. D., Prentice, A. M., Goldberg, G. R., Roger, S. and Whitehead, R. G. (1994). Energy-sparing strategies to protect human fetal growth. *Am. J. Obstet. Gynecol.*, **171**, 118–25.

Prentice, A. M. (2003). Intrauterine factors, adiposity and hyperinsulinaemia. *BMJ*, **327**, 880–1.

Ramachandran, P. (2002). Maternal nutrition: effect on fetal growth and outcome of pregnancy. *Nutr. Rev.*, **60**, S26–34.

Ramakrishnan, U., Manjrekar, R., Rivera, J., Gonzáles-Cossio, T. and Martorell, R. (1999). Micronutrients and pregnancy outcome: a review of the literature. *Nutr. Res.*, **19**, 103–59.

Ramakrishnan, U., Gonzáles-Cossio, T., Neufield, L. M., Rivera, J. and Martorell, R. (2003). Multiple micronutrient supplementation during pregnancy does not lead to greater infant birth size than does iron-only supplementation: a randomized controlled trial in a semirural community in Mexico. *Am. J. Clin. Nutr.*, **77**, 720–5.

Rao, S., Yajnik, C. S., Kanade, A. *et al.* (2001). Intake of micronutrient-rich foods in rural Indian mothers is associated with the size of their babies at birth: Pune maternal nutritional study. *J. Nutr.*, **131**, 1217–24.

Rasmussen, K. M. (2001). Is there a causal relationship between iron deficiency or iron-deficiency anaemia and weight at birth, length of gestation and perinatal mortality. *J. Nutr.*, **131**, 590–603S.

Rayco-Solon, P., Fulford, A. J. and Prentice, A. M. (2005). Maternal preconceptional weight and gestational length. *Am. J. Obstet. Gynecol.*, **192**, 1133–6.

Rey, H., Ortiz, E. I., Fajardo, L. and Pradilla, A. (1995). Maternal anthropometry: its predictive value for pregnancy outcome. *Bull. World Health Organ.*, **73**, 70–1.

Rich-Edwards, J. (2002). A life course approach to women's reproductive health. In *A Life Course Approach to Women's Health* (ed. D. Kuh and R. Hardy). Oxford: Oxford University Press, pp. 23–34.

Robinson, J. S. (1989). Fetal growth. In *Obstetrics* (ed. A. Turnbull and G. Chamberlain) London: Churchill Livingstone, pp. 141–50.

Roseboom, T. J., van der Meulen, J. H. P., Ravelli, A. C., Osmond, C., Barker, D. J. and Bleker, O. P. (2001). Effects of prenatal exposure to the Dutch famine on adult disease in later life: an overview. *Twin Res.*, **4**, 293–8.

Rouse, D. J. (2003). Potential cost-effectiveness of nutrition interventions to prevent adverse pregnancy outcomes in the developing world. *J. Nutr.*, **133**, 1640–4S.

Rush, D., Stein, Z. and Susser M. (1980). A randomized controlled trial of prenatal nutritional supplementation in New York City. *Pediatrics*, **65**, 683–97.

Scholl, T. O. and Hediger, M. L. (1994). Anaemia and iron-deficiency anaemia: compilation of data on pregnancy outcome. *Am. J. Clin. Nutr.*, **59**, 492–501S.

Scholl, T. O., Hediger, M. L., Bendich, A., Schall, J. I., Smith, W. K. and Krueger, P. M. (1997). Use of multivitamin/mineral prenatal supplements: influence on outcome of pregnancy. *Am. J. Epidemiol.*, **146**, 134–41.

Sebire, N., Jolly, M., Harris, J., Regan, L. and Robinson, S. (2001). Is maternal underweight really a risk factor for adverse pregnancy outcome? A population-based study in London. *Br. J. Obstet. Gynaecol.*, **108**, 61–6.

Shankar, A. H. and Prasad, A. S. (1998). Zinc and immune function: the biological basis of altered immune function. *Am. J. Clin. Nutr.*, **68**, 447–63S.

Shaw, G. M. (2003). Strenuous work and nutrition and adverse pregnancy outcomes. *J. Nutr.*, **133**, 1718–21S.

Steer, P., Alam, M. A., Wadsworth, J. and Welch, A. (1995). Relation between maternal haemoglobin concentration and birthweight in different ethnic groups. *BMJ*, **310**, 489–91.

Stein, Z. A. and Susser M. W. (1975). The Dutch famine 1944–45 and the reproductive process. I. Effects on six indices at birth. *Pediatr. Res.*, **9**, 70–6.

Stein, Z. A., Susser, M., Saenger, G. and Marolla, F. (1975). *Famine and Human Development: the Dutch Hunger Winter of 1944–1945*. New York, NY: Oxford University Press.

Susser, M. (1991). Maternal weight gain, infant birthweight, and diet: causal sequences. *Am. J. Clin. Nutr.*, **53**, 1384–96.

Symonds, M. E., Budge, H., Stephenson, T. (2000). Limitations of models used to examine the influence of nutrition during pregnancy and adult disease. *Arch. Dis. Child.*, **83**, 215–19.

Tang, A. M., Graham, N. M. H. and Saah, A. J. (1996). Effects of micronutrient intake on survival in human immunodeficiency virus type 1 infection. *Am. J. Epidemiol.*, **143**, 1244–56.

Thame, M., Wilks, R. J., McFarlane-Anderson, N., Bennett, F. I. and Forrester, T. E. (1997). Relationship between maternal nutritional status and infant's weight and body proportions at birth. *Eur. J. Clin. Nutr.*, **51**, 134–8.

van den Broek, N., Kulier, R., Gülmezoglu, A. M. and Villar, J. (2002). Vitamin A supplementation during pregnancy. *Cochrane Database Syst. Rev.*, **2002** (4).

van Raaij, J. M. A., Schonk, C. M., Vermaat-Miedema, S. H., Peek, M. E. M. and Hautvast, J. G. A. J. (1989). Body fat mass and basal metabolic rate in Dutch women before, during, and after pregnancy: a reappraisal of the energy cost of pregnancy. *Am. J. Clin. Nutr.*, **49**, 765–72.

Viegas, O. A., Scott, P. H., Cole, T. J. *et al.* (1982a). Dietary protein energy supplementation of pregnant Asian mothers at Sorrento, Birmingham. I. Unselective during second and third trimesters. *BMG*, **285**, 589–92.

Viegas, O. A., Scott, P. H., Cole, T. J., Eaton, P., Needham, P. G. and Wharton, B. A. (1982b). Dietary protein energy supplementation of pregnant Asian mothers at Sorrento, Birmingham. II. Selective during third trimester only. *BMJ*, **285**, 592–5.

Villar, J. and Rivera, J. (1988). Nutritional supplementation during two consecutive pregnancies and the interim lactation period: effect on birth weight. *Pediatrics*, **81**, 51–7.

Villar, J., Cogswell, M. E., Kestler, E., Castillo, P., Menendez, R. and Repke, J. (1992). Effect of fat and fat-free mass deposition during pregnancy on birth weight. *Am. J. Obstet. Gynecol.*, **167**, 1344–52.

Villar, J., Merialdi, M., Gülmezoglu, A. M. *et al.* (2003a). Nutritional interventions during pregnancy for the prevention or treatment of maternal morbidity and preterm delivery: an overview of randomized controlled trials. *J. Nutr.*, **133**, 1606–25S.

(2003b). Characteristics of randomized controlled trials included in systematic reviews of nutritional interventions reporting maternal morbidity, mortality, preterm delivery, intrauterine growth restriction and small for gestational age and birthweight outcomes. *J. Nutr.*, **133**, 1632–9S.

Wilcox, A. J. (2001). On the importance – and the unimportance – of birthweight. *Int. J. Epidemiol.*, **30**, 1233–41.

Winkvist, A., Jalil, F., Habicht, J. P. and Rasmussen, K. M. (1994). Maternal energy depletion is buffered among malnourished women in Punjab, Pakistan. *J. Nutr.*, **124**, 2376–85.

Winkvist, A., Habicht, J. P. and Rasmussen, K. M. (1998). Linking maternal and infant benefits of a nutritional supplement during pregnancy and lactation. *Am. J. Clin. Nutr.*, **68**, 656–61.

World Health Organization (1995). Maternal Anthropometry and Pregnancy Outcomes: a WHO Collaborative Study. *Bull. World Health Organ.*, **73**, 1–98.

Yajnik, C. S., Fall, C. H., Coyaji, K. J. *et al.* (2002). Neonatal anthropometry: the thin-fat Indian baby. The Pune Maternal Nutrition Study. *Int. J. Obes.*, **27**, 173–80.

9

Placental mechanisms and developmental origins of health and disease

Leslie Myatt and Victoria Roberts

University of Cincinnati

Introduction

The placenta plays a unique role in supporting the fetal allograft throughout gestation, protecting against immune rejection whilst also serving to supply oxygen and nutrients to, and remove carbon dioxide and waste products from, the fetus. As the nutrient interface between mother and fetus, the placenta may passively or actively transfer nutrients to the fetus or metabolise them en route. In addition the placenta produces a variety of peptide and steroid hormones that affect placental, maternal and fetal metabolism and development. The developmental origins of health and adult disease hypothesis proposes that alterations in fetal development, or adaptations of the fetus to alterations in the normal amount or pattern of substrate supply across the placenta, lead somehow to cardiovascular and metabolic disease in adult life. There is now abundant evidence both from human epidemiological studies and from animal studies that maternal nutrition may 'programme' the offspring for adult disease. This effect may be direct but it is more likely to be mediated in some manner by placental structure and/or function regulating the amount or composition of nutrients transferred. Does the placenta therefore play an active or a pas-

sive role in programming? Reduced fetal and placental weights are both associated with fetal programming. However, it is argued that, rather than reduced placental weight (and function) being linked to reduced fetal weight in a cause-and-effect relationship, reduced weight(s) might be a surrogate marker for an adverse intrauterine experience. The fact that several manipulations that alter placental structure/function and reduce placental (and fetal) weight lead to programming effects does however point to a more central role for the placenta. There is now a great deal of associative data from human studies that demonstrate changes in placental structure/function in conditions such as diabetes and intrauterine growth restriction (IUGR) where fetal programming occurs. Animal studies are also beginning to investigate the mechanism and cause-and-effect relationships responsible. Genetically manipulated mouse models are being and will continue to be useful in this reductionist approach, highlighting those aspects of placental structure/function that might impact on fetal growth and possibly underlie programming.

The aim of this chapter is to review data from human and animal studies that support a role for the placenta as a mediator of fetal programming, and to describe the potential mechanisms that exist.

Developmental Origins of Health and Disease, ed. Peter Gluckman and Mark Hanson. Published by Cambridge University Press.
© P. D. Gluckman and M. A. Hanson 2006.

Mechanisms of placental involvement in programming

Conceivably there are several ways in which placental structure/function or the placental supply of substrate may be altered to yield an adverse in-utero environment which programmes the fetus (Table 9.1). These include:

(1) a normal placenta with inadequate/inappropriate substrate supply from the mother

(2) abnormal trophoblast invasion leading to altered/abnormal maternal blood flow to the placenta and nutrient supply to the fetus

(3) deficiencies/alterations in placental vasculogenesis leading to altered perfusion of the fetal placenta and nutrient supply to the fetus

(4) abnormal trophoblast differentiation/function leading to altered placental barrier thickness and expression of transport proteins

(5) abnormal trophoblast differentiation/function leading to altered placental hormone synthesis which alters the sequence of fetal developmental milestones

(6) insults, e.g. hypoxia/oxidative stress, occurring at critical times in gestation which alter placental function, e.g. hormone synthesis, expression of transporter proteins

Table 9.1 Structural and functional determinants that may mediate the role of the placenta in programming.

Maternal/uterine factors	Inadequate trophoblast invasion
	Uteroplacental blood flow/oxygenation
	Maternal substrate amount and composition
	Maternal hormone production and action
Placental factors	Trophoblast growth and differentiation
	Transporter expression and activity
	Hormone production and metabolism
	Vasculogenesis
Fetal/placental factors	Angiogenesis
	Altered fetal–placental blood flow/oxygenation
	Nutrient extraction/delivery

Placental growth and development throughout gestation

Fetal growth occurs at an exponential rate throughout gestation, rather than in a linear manner. To support this growth the placenta undergoes in parallel a differential growth of its vasculature and trophoblast layers that increases its efficiency for transport of nutrients. Fetal/placental weight (a measure of placental efficiency) increases from a ratio of 0.18 at 6 weeks gestation to 7.23 at term (Benirschke and Kaufmann 2000). Over this time the trophoblast surface area increases from 0.08 to 12.5 m^2, mean trophoblastic thickness decreases from 18.9 to 4.1 μm and maternofetal diffusion distance decreases from 55.9 to 4.8 μm, whereas there is an increase in the percentage of villous volume occupied by vessels from 2.7% to 28.4%. The net result is an increase in trophoblast surface area available for nutrient transfer and placental blood flows to transport oxygen and nutrients to and from the trophoblast surface.

As blood flows in the uteroplacental and umbilical circulations are clearly shown to be reduced in pregnancies complicated by IUGR (Harrington *et al.* 1991), the adequacy of this blood flow has been traditionally thought of as a major determinant of transfer of nutrients (particularly oxygen) across the placenta. There has been limited evidence of the rate-limiting role of the placental exchange barrier per se in nutrient transfer and fetal growth. This view is now being challenged with the emergence of data on altered expression and activity of transporters in the trophoblast from human studies, and on regulation of placental structure/function from genetically manipulated mouse models, as summarised in Fig. 9.1 and discussed below.

Placental blood flows and regulation of growth

Trophoblast invasion and uteroplacental perfusion

In severe pre-eclampsia and IUGR the size of the placenta is reduced due to either a primary defect

UTERUS

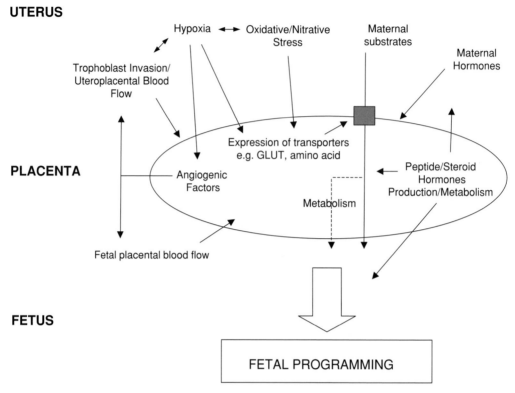

Figure 9.1 Placental involvement in fetal programming.

in placental angiogenesis/growth mechanisms or inadequate trophoblast invasion into the uterine wall leading to failure to establish an adequate maternal vascular supply line to support placental and fetal growth. At the placental–maternal interface, villous cytotrophoblast stem cells differentiate to extravillous trophoblasts that invade the maternal decidua and myometrium. Trophoblast invasion converts spiral arteries to flaccid low-resistance uteroplacental arteries. In both IUGR and pre-eclampsia, a defect in endovascular trophoblast invasion of the spiral arteries has been clearly described (Brosens *et al.* 1970, Sheppard and Bonnar 1976), with superficial invasion leading to a lack of the normal adaptation or physiological change of uteroplacental vessels. The net result may

be reduced blood flow into the intervillous space of the placenta which, if severely compromised, may lead to decreased transport of flow-limited substrates, e.g. oxygen, such that a relative hypoxia with consequent metabolic derangement and oxidative stress may ensue.

Invasion of the decidua and myometrium by extravillous trophoblast occurs in an orchestrated manner in which these cells express specific markers defining their stage in the differentiation process and their role in invasion. These include vascular endothelial growth factor (VEGF) and VEGF receptors (Zhou *et al.* 2002), and insulin-like growth factor 2 (IGF2) (Irwin *et al.* 1999) which interacts with decidual IGF binding protein1 (IGFBP1). The repertoire of biochemical changes known to be involved in trophoblast differentiation/invasion has grown in recent years (Myatt 2002), with oxygen appearing to be a major regulatory factor.

Hypoxia and placental function

Prior to 12 weeks gestation the villous tissue is separated from maternal blood by a continuous layer of trophoblast cells. The villous placenta thus develops by histiotrophic nutrition during the first trimester (Burton *et al.* 2001) and is in a hypoxic environment. Low oxygen tension is physiological for organogenesis and is also a key regulator of a variety of cellular events in early trophoblast differentiation (Genbacev *et al.* 1997). At around 10–12 weeks of gestation the trophoblastic shell is disrupted and the maternal circulation is established into the intervillous space (Jauniaux 1996). The rapid increase in oxygen tension at this time, often referred to as the oxygen 'switch', subjects the placenta to oxidative stress and the potential for complications (Jauniaux *et al.* 2000) (see later). The local partial pressure of oxygen increases from around 20 mm Hg at 8 weeks to >50 mm Hg at 12 weeks (Jauniaux *et al.* 2000). The premature onset of maternal blood flow to the intervillous space and the accompanying oxidative damage to the trophoblast is a key factor in early pregnancy loss (Jauniaux *et al.* 2003).

This switch in oxygen tension may also regulate trophoblast invasion, with low oxygen tension prior to 10–12 weeks appearing to prevent trophoblast differentiation towards the invasive extravillous trophoblast (EVT) cell type. One mechanism by which oxygen modulates placental development involves the transcription factor hypoxia-inducible factor 1 (HIF1). This molecule activates the transcription of genes in response to varying oxygen concentration of cells. In a mouse model, the central role of HIF-mediated hypoxic responses in determining placental cell differentiation has been clearly shown (Adelman *et al.* 2000). Animals with placentas null for Arnt, a HIF1 subunit, show reduced labyrinthine and spongiotrophoblast layers in the placenta.

The defective trophoblast invasion of IUGR and pre-eclampsia is thought also to give rise to a relatively hypoxic placenta. In placental tissues collected at term, protein expression of HIF2α but not HIF1α or 1β was found to be increased in the pre-eclamptic placenta (Rajakumar *et al.* 2001). The relationship of this finding to events earlier in pregnancy when trophoblast invasion is occurring is unclear. However, hypoxia is reported to alter trophoblast differentiation/invasion in vitro and mimic the changes seen in pre-eclampsia (Genbacev *et al.* 1996).

Oxidative and nitrative stress

The increasing metabolic activity of placental mitochondria throughout gestation imposes increasing oxidative stress. In pregnancies complicated by pre-eclampsia or pregestational diabetes this oxidative stress is increased further (Wang *et al.* 1992, Giugliano *et al.* 1996), as measured indirectly by production of reactive oxygen species and consumption of antioxidant defences. Amongst the reactive oxygen species produced are superoxide and nitric oxide. When produced in increasing quantities such as with oxidative stress these radicals interact to produce the much more potent pro-oxidant peroxynitrite, the characteristic action of which is nitration of tyrosine residues on proteins, a covalent modification that can give either loss or gain of protein function. We have presented evidence that nitrotyrosine residues are present in the placentas of pregnancies complicated by either pre-eclampsia (Myatt *et al.* 1996) or pregestational diabetes (Lyall *et al.* 1998) and are associated with altered vascular reactivity (Kossenjans *et al.* 2000). In-vitro treatment of the placental vasculature with exogenous peroxynitrite alters vascular reactivity and deposits nitrotyrosine residues, suggesting a cause-and-effect relationship (Kossenjans *et al.* 2000). We have shown using a proteomics approach that there is increased abundance of nitrated proteins in the pre-eclamptic placenta, which include p38MAP kinase (R. Webster, unpublished observations). Nitration of p38MAP kinase reduces its catalytic activity. As p38MAP kinase is a critical signal transduction molecule, with the p38-null mouse exhibiting embryonic lethality with decreased labyrinthine and spongiotrophoblast layers and a lack of vascularisation in the labyrinth (Adams *et al.* 2000, Mudgett *et al.* 2000), this finding suggests that oxidative stress via protein nitration may also regulate placental development/function with potential programming effects.

Control of villous vascular development

Oxygen is a major regulator not only of extravillous trophoblast invasion, but also of development of the villous vascular tree and villous trophoblast proliferation, which seems to mount a response to low oxygen. In all pathological conditions where the placenta is hypoxic, the amount of villous cytotrophoblast is increased, whereas strong oxygenation of villi reduces the rate of proliferation (Kingdom and Kaufmann 1997). The villous vasculature responds to hypoxia with hypercapillarisation (arising from branching angiogenesis) (Kingdom and Kaufmann 1997), resulting in a similar appearance to placentas from high altitude and with maternal anaemia. Angiogenic factors mediating the hypoxic signal include platelet-derived growth factor, acidic and basic fibroblast growth factor (FGF), VEGF, placental growth factor (PLGF) and angiopoietins (Ang) 1 and 2 (Charnock-Jones *et al.* 2004, Kaufmann *et al.* 2004). Oxygen may regulate the balance between VEGF and PLGF, with hypoxia up-regulating expression of VEGF and its receptors but down-regulating PLGF (Shore *et al.* 1997), suggesting changing oxygen tensions throughout gestation control the switch from VEGF to PLGF effects.

The mRNA for Ang1 and Ang2 are found in the placenta, with Ang2 abundant on syncytiotrophoblast. Placentas from women with pre-eclampsia have reduced Ang2 mRNA with no difference in Ang1. In

vitro hypoxia has opposite effects on the molecules, increasing Ang2 mRNA but reducing stability of Ang1 mRNA (Zhang *et al.* 2001). This again highlights the potential role of oxygen tension in regulating placental angiogenesis. In pre-eclampsia decreases (Cooper *et al.* 1996), increases (Ahmed and Khaliq 1997), and no change (Ranheim *et al.* 2001) in placental VEGF mRNA with reduced PLGF mRNA have all been reported. These differences in findings may represent the heterogeneity of fetoplacental angiogenesis seen in pre-eclampsia (Kingdom and Kaufmann 1997).

Placental vascular development and fetal programming

In adolescents, who are still growing at the time of conception, poor pregnancy outcomes including increased risk of spontaneous miscarriage, prematurity and IUGR are seen. This can be modelled in overnourished adolescent sheep (Wallace *et al.* 2004). The placentas of these animals exhibit less proliferation of fetal trophectoderm and reduced expression in the placenta of angiogenic factors. Later in pregnancy these animals have reduced placental mass, reduced uterine and umbilical blood flows and reduced fetal oxygen, glucose and amino acid concentrations. However, transporter activity is normal when adjusted to placental mass. This suggests that placental size per se, rather than transporter activity, limits fetal growth in this model. High nutrient intakes in the second two-thirds of gestation are most detrimental to pregnancy outcomes (Wallace *et al.* 2001), times when development of the fetal–placental vasculature is occurring. In a sheep model of IUGR Regnault *et al.* (2003) have reported that changes in expression of VEGF, PLGF and their receptors may be stimulated by an altered transplacental oxygen gradient.

The role of placental angiogenesis in the control of placental/fetal growth is illustrated further by observations from animal studies. Fetal growth in the Yorkshire breed of pig from mid to late gestation is associated with an increasing surface area of endometrial attachment, i.e. a larger exchange area. However, growth of the Chinese Meishan pig fetus at this time is associated with an increase in the density of placental blood vessels (Vonnahme and Ford 2004) such that placental efficiency (fetal/placental weight) is greater in the Meishan conceptus. Accompanying this increased vascularity is increased expression of VEGF mRNA in the placenta and VEGF concentrations in fetal blood and allantoic fluid of the Meishan. Development of the placental vasculature therefore has profound effects on the capacity of the placenta to support growth.

Placental transport/barrier function and fetal growth

Glucose transport

The primary substrate for fetal oxidative metabolism is glucose, so its efficient placental transfer is essential for normal growth and development (Hahn *et al.* 1999). Members of the glucose transporter (GLUT) family facilitate glucose transfer, and in the human trophoblast the GLUT1 isoform is the predominant transporter (Illsley 2000). GLUT1 expression at the microvillous membrane (MVM) is approximately fivefold greater than at the basal membrane (BM). Thus GLUT1 on the BM is the rate-limiting step for glucose transfer across the syncytiotrophoblast. Normal pregnancy is a state of insulin resistance, to increase glucose availability for the fetus, and this is exacerbated during diabetic pregnancy, where the mother becomes hyperglycaemic, leading to fetal hyperglycaemia. The effects of fetal hyperglycaemia include the increased production of insulin, IGFI and leptin, which are all factors that stimulate fetoplacental growth.

We suggest that the timing of an 'insult' during gestation may affect placental function in a particular manner and lead to a programming effect. The regulation of GLUT transporter activity depends on

blood glucose levels and the maternal–fetal glucose gradient. For example, glucose transport and expression of the GLUT1 transporter in basement membrane of trophoblast is found to be up-regulated in pregnancies complicated by insulin-dependent diabetes mellitus and a large-for-gestational-age fetus (Jansson *et al.* 1999) but not in pregnancies complicated by gestational diabetes and a large-for-gestational-age fetus at term (Jansson *et al.* 2001). These data could be interpreted as placental glucose transporters being susceptible to up-regulation by hyperglycaemia in the first trimester, which leads to accelerated fetal growth in late gestation. In contrast, activity of system A amino acid transporters appears to be up-regulated in both groups (Jansson *et al.* 2002). Additional work by this group has shown that system A amino acid transporters can be regulated late in gestation but not in the first trimester (Jansson *et al.* 2003). Impaired expression and function of the GLUT transporters can also occur after exposure to glucocorticoids, which are regulated by 11β-hydroxysteroid dehydrogenase (11β-HSD) (Hahn *et al.* 1999), suggesting hormonal regulation.

Amino acid transport

The requirement by the fetus for amino acids is related to protein synthesis and the interconversion to other substrates. There are approximately 15 amino acid transporters in the trophoblast of the human placenta, and their activity is classed as sodium-dependent or sodium-independent (Jansson and Powell 2000). System A is a sodium-dependent system which transports neutral amino acids such as alanine, serine, proline and glycine (Cetin 2003) and is the most-studied amino acid transport system in the human placenta. Although regulation of amino acid transport function is not completely understood, it is known that hypoxia diminishes the expression and transport of system A in human trophoblast, and this may be the primary regulator of amino acid transport across the syncytiotrophoblast (Nelson *et al.* 2003). In IUGR system A activity has been shown to be reduced in the MVM of the syncytiotrophoblast (Mahendran *et al.* 1993, Cetin 2003), whereas in pregnancies complicated by diabetes, where accelerated fetal growth is common, the activity of system A is increased (Jansson *et al.* 2002). In humans there is an inverse relationship between system A amino acid transporter activity in placental microvillous membranes and size at birth (Godfrey 1998), i.e. there is up-regulation of this transporter to maintain transport in the placenta. Inhibition of system A transporter in rats results in fetal growth restriction (Cramer *et al.* 2002). In the placenta-specific *Igf2* knockout mouse (Constancia *et al.* 2002) where there is growth restriction, a small placenta with abnormal barrier thickness and altered passive permeability but up-regulation of amino acid transport is found (Sibley *et al.* 2004). These data suggest that in addition to blood flows modulating fetal growth, the barrier function of the placenta is also important and, more so, also adaptive. Not all transporters may be regulated in the same manner. For example, whereas system A transport is altered in IUGR, system y^+ activity is unaltered (Jansson *et al.* 1998, Ayuk *et al.* 2002).

Fatty acid transport

The placenta has a considerable capacity for fat uptake and transport of fatty acids, especially in diabetes. This transport involves the breakdown of triglycerides to free fatty acids and glycerol and re-esterification with intracellularly generated glycerol phosphate on the fetal side (Hauguel-de Mouzon and Shafrir 2001), and is mediated by lipase activity. Several triglyceride lipases have been identified in human placenta, including pH 4 lipase. The activity of pH 4 lipase is increased in diabetes, where the maternal–fetal lipid gradient is elevated, leading to increased fat uptake (Kaminsky *et al.* 1991a). Conversely, pH 4 lipase activity decreases with fetal growth restriction (Kaminsky *et al.* 1991b).

Fatty acids act in an autocrine manner to regulate their metabolism, uptake and transport. This autocrine effect is facilitated by nuclear hormone receptors of the peroxisome proliferators-activated receptor (PPAR) family (Wang *et al.* 2002). There are three isoforms, α, β and γ, each of which performs a different function. It has been demonstrated in knockout mice that PPARγ is a key factor which regulates placental vascular function. At the whole-tissue level the vascular structures of PPARγ-null mice are disarrayed and fetal vessels do not fully penetrate the labyrinth or the maternal blood pools, which compromises maternal–fetal exchange. These vascular defects are trophoblast-derived, as PPARγ expression is restricted to the trophoblast (Barak *et al.* 1999).

Placental endocrine function and programming

The placenta is not innervated, hence any communication between it, the mother and the fetus must involve humoral agents. As an endocrine organ the placenta produces a large number of hormones that can be secreted into both the fetal and maternal circulations. The principal function of these hormones is to adapt maternal metabolism to the specific metabolic requirements of pregnancy. Many receptors for the signalling molecules secreted by the placenta are expressed on the syncytiotrophoblast, which is compatible with autocrine and paracrine actions. This raises the possibility that the placenta regulates its own function in response to the conditions of the uterine environment (Jansson *et al.* 2003).

Peptide hormones

The placenta synthesises and releases a wide variety of peptide hormones during gestation, mainly from syncytiotrophoblast. Altered production of these hormones (usually increased), including activin, inhibin (Muttukrishna *et al.* 1997), corticotrophin-releasing hormone (Laatikainen *et al.* 1991), neurokinin B (Page *et al.* 2000), leptin (Lepercq *et al.* 2003) and hCG (Bartha *et al.* 2003), is seen in pregnancies complicated by IUGR or pre-eclampsia. These increases may be taken as a sign of placental dysfunction related to altered trophoblast function that is perhaps the result of oxidative stress associated with this disease. The local or systemic roles of these raised peptide levels in altering maternal metabolism or placental function, and whether this mediates programming, remains to be determined.

Insulin-like growth factors and their binding proteins regulate cellular proliferation, differentiation and function, and play an important role in placental development (Gratton *et al.* 2002). During implantation the cell-to-cell communication between fetal trophoblast and maternal decidua is mediated by IGF2 and IGFBP1. IGF2 regulates IGFBP1 in a biphasic manner: low concentrations stimulate production whereas high concentrations inhibit it. In pre-eclamptic placentas IGF2 expression is decreased whilst IGFBP1 is increased (Shin *et al.* 2003).

Recently the role played by the IGFs in normal fetal growth and development has become a rapidly expanding field of interest. Constancia *et al.* (2002) deleted the placental labyrinth-specific P0 transcript of the paternally imprinted *Igf2* gene in mice. This led to reduced growth of the placenta and subsequent fetal growth retardation and an increased fetal/placental ratio (placental efficiency). Placental nutrient permeability was reduced but initially there was up-regulation of amino acid transport (system A) to compensate for the decrease in passive permeability. A role of the *Igf2* gene in the control of the placental supply and the genetic demand for nutrients to the fetus was proposed (Constancia *et al.* 2002).

Glucocorticoid action and metabolism

Glucocorticoids have critical roles in regulation of organ development and maturation but excessive exposure of the fetus to maternal glucocorticoids or administration of exogenous glucocorticoids causes growth restriction and hypertension in later life. Exposure of the fetus in utero to glucocorticoids occurs in a temporally defined window that is regulated by the activity of the 11β hydroxy steroid dehydrogenase enzymes which catalyse reduction (11β-HSD1) or oxidation (11β-HSD2) of glucocorticoids. One key role of the syncytiotro-

phoblast as the transporting epithelia of the placenta is to act as a protective barrier (both physical and metabolic) to the fetus. Therefore 11β-HSD2 is an important example of a metabolic barrier mechanism, being localised extensively to the syncytiotrophoblast layer of floating villi, where it converts cortisol to inactive cortisone and thus may prevent exposure of the fetus to high levels of maternal cortisol (Krozowski *et al.* 1995).

In the human, 11β-HSD2 expression rises with gestational age (Murphy and Clifton 2003), and a significant increase in expression is observed around the time of the 'oxygen switch' at 10–12 weeks. Changes in oxygen tension alter the expression and activity of placental 11β-HSD2 (Alfaidy *et al.* 2002), raising the possibility that sustained low placental oxygenation after the first trimester might be the cause of reduced 11β-HSD2 expression and activity in pre-eclampsia.

Expression and activity of 11β-HSD2 in the placenta is regulated in a cell-specific and gestational-age-specific manner in both the human and baboon (Pepe *et al.* 2001). An increase in the ratio of 11β-HSD2 to 11β-HSD1 in placental membranes near term is associated with a switch in transplacental glucocorticoid metabolism, from reduction at mid gestation to oxidation late in gestation, and may be responsible for the maturation of the fetal hypothalamic–pituitary–adrenal (HPA) axis (Pepe *et al.* 2001). In rats prenatal exposure to dexamathasone, which is not metabolised by 11β-HSD, or to carbenoxolone, an inhibitor of 11β-HSD2, reduces birthweight and results in hypertension, hyperglycaemia, increased activity of the HPA axis and anxiety-like behaviour in aversive situations (Lindsay *et al.* 1996; Welberg *et al.* 2000). In humans mutations in the 11β-HSD2 gene have been reported to produce low birthweight and reduced placental 11β-HSD2 activity and increased fetal cortisol levels in association with IUGR (reviewed by Seckl *et al.* 2000). Similarly, the expression of 11β-HSD2 has been reported to be reduced with hypoxaemia and in placentas from women with pre-eclampsia (Challis *et al.* 2002). The mechanisms that lead to alterations in 11β-HSD2 are as yet not established.

In a model of maternal protein restriction in rats, changes in maternal levels of steroid and peptide hormones derived from the placenta were seen (Fernandez-Twinn *et al.* 2003). Similarly, in a sheep model of nutritional restriction, restriction for more than 45 consecutive days significantly decreased placental 11β-HSD activities in addition to causing IUGR (McMullen *et al.* 2004). Several factors regulate 11β-HSD mRNA expression and activity: cAMP activation increases activity while nitric oxide, progesterone and oestrogens decrease it (Sun *et al.* 1998). However, the mechanism linking altered nutrient status to placental steroid metabolism is not yet understood.

Imprinted genes

To date at least 60 imprinted genes have been described in mice which are also found to be conserved in humans. Gene knockout studies have shown that the function of paternally expressed imprinted genes is to enhance fetal growth, whereas maternally imprinted genes suppress it (reviewed in Reik *et al.* 2003). All imprinted genes are found in the placenta, where they affect the growth of placental cell types including the labyrinthine trophoblast and spongiotrophoblast. Knockout of the paternally expressed genes (e.g. *Igf2*) reduces placental growth whereas knockout of maternally expressed genes (e.g. *p57Kip2*) results in placental hyperplasia. In addition, imprinted genes may also regulate expression of placental transporters, including the paternally expressed gene *Ata3*, which encodes a component of the system A amino acid transporter (Mizuno *et al.* 2002), and the maternally imprinted *Impt1/Slc22a11* gene, which encodes an organic cation transporter (Dao *et al.* 1998). Imprinted genes therefore regulate overall placental growth, growth of specific cell types and activity of specific transporters. At the fetal level they appear to control growth and hence the demand for nutrients from the placenta. Overall they therefore may control supply (placenta) and demand (fetus) for nutrients.

Igf2 lies on chromosome 7 and is surrounded by a cluster of other imprinted genes (reviewed by Reik *et al.* 2003). This cluster contains demand promoters, supply promoters and supply suppressors which balance each other. Recent evidence suggests that the *Ata3* gene is also paternally expressed and imprinted in a cluster on chromosome 15 (Mizuno *et al.* 2002). Obviously regulation of the imprinted genes may be crucial to programming of the fetus. Imprinting is controlled epigenetically by DNA methylation and chromatin modifications under the control of environmental factors and nutrition (Reik *et al.* 2003). This suggests a link between maternal nutrition and fetoplacental growth via imprinted genes acting in the placenta, which potentially balances the supply and demand for nutrients in utero.

Summary

Programming is said to occur when an abnormal stimulus or insult is applied during a critical stage of development (Fig. 9.2), causing long-term effects on the structure/function of certain organs. In this chapter we have described the key stages of placental development, alterations during pathological pregnancies and the manner in which the placenta may participate in programming. Determinants of the supply of oxygen and nutrients to the fetus are blood flows in the uteroplacental and fetoplacental circulations and, as we are increasingly becoming aware, the physical structure of and expression and activity of transporters on the trophoblast, the placental barrier. The participation of these factors is being dissected using animal models. How they are regulated is less clear, but we are gaining knowledge of the ontogeny of placental development and its relationship to function. Evidence is accruing that disturbance of the normal gestational-age-specific developmental pathways of the vasculature or the trophoblast barrier by hormonal, nutritional, hypoxic or oxidative stress 'insults' changes placental structure/function in a manner that can lead to programming. Increased understanding of the role of imprinted genes illustrates the integrative nature of events at the placental/fetal interface. What is

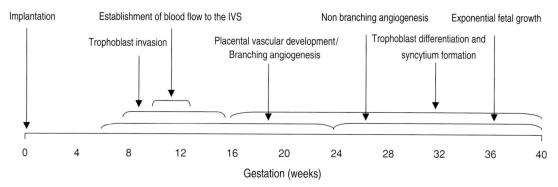

Figure 9.2 Critical periods during human placental development potentially related to fetal programming.

abundantly clear is that the placenta is not simply an innocent bystander in programming, but itself undergoes adaptive responses to the environment which may then influence the fetus.

REFERENCES

Adams, R. H., Porras, A., Alonso, G. *et al.* (2000). Essential role of p38alpha MAP kinase in placental but not embryonic cardiovascular development. *Mol. Cell*, **6**, 109–16.

Adelman, D. M., Gertsenstein, M., Nagy, A., Simon, M. C. and Maltepe, E. (2000). Placental cell fates are regulated in vivo by HIF-mediated hypoxia responses. *Genes Dev.*, **14**, 3191–203.

Ahmed, A. W. M. and Khaliq, A. (1997). *J. Soc. Gynecol. Investig.*, **4**, A663.

Alfaidy, N., Gupta, S., DeMarco, C., Caniggia, I. and Challis, J. R. (2002). Oxygen regulation of placental 11 beta-hydroxysteroid dehydrogenase 2: physiological and pathological implications. *J. Clin. Endocrinol. Metab.*, **87**, 4797–805.

Ayuk, P. T., Theophanous, D., D'Souza, S. W., Sibley, C. P. and Glazier, J. D. (2002). L-arginine transport by the microvillous plasma membrane of the syncytiotrophoblast from human placenta in relation to nitric oxide production: effects of gestation, preeclampsia, and intrauterine growth restriction. *J. Clin. Endocrinol. Metab.*, **87**, 747–51.

Barak, Y., Nelson, M. C., Ong, E. S. *et al.* (1999). PPAR gamma is required for placental, cardiac, and adipose tissue development. *Mol. Cell*, **4**, 585–95.

Bartha, J. L., Romero-Carmona, R., Escobar-Llompart, M., Paloma-Castro, O. and Comino-Delgado, R. (2003). Human chorionic gonadotropin and vascular endothelial growth factor in normal and complicated pregnancies. *Obstet. Gynecol.*, **102**, 995–9.

Benirschke, K. and Kaufmann, P. (2000). *Pathology of the Human Placenta*. New York, NY: Springer.

Brosens, I. A., Robertson, W. B. and Dixon, H. G. (1970). The role of the spiral arteries in the pathogenesis of pre-eclampsia. *J. Pathol.*, **101**, Pvi.

Burton, G. J., Hempstock, J. and Jauniaux, E. (2001). Nutrition of the human fetus during the first trimester: a review. *Placenta*, **22** (Suppl. A) S70–7.

Cetin, I. (2003). Placental transport of amino acids in normal and growth-restricted pregnancies. *Eur. J. Obstet. Gynecol. Reprod. Biol.*, **110** (Suppl. 1), S50–4.

Challis, J. R., Sloboda, D. M., Alfaidy, N. *et al.* (2002). Prostaglandins and mechanisms of preterm birth. *Reproduction*, **124**, 1–17.

Charnock-Jones, D. S., Kaufmann, P. and Mayhew, T. M. (2004). Aspects of human fetoplacental vasculogenesis and angiogenesis. I. Molecular regulation. *Placenta*, **25**, 103–13.

Constancia, M., Hemberger, M., Hughes, J., *et al.* (2002). Placental-specific IGF-II is a major modulator of placental and fetal growth. *Nature*, **417**, 945–8.

Cooper, J. C., Sharkey, A. M., Charnock-Jones, D. S., Palmer, C. R. and Smith, S. K. (1996). VEGF mRNA levels in placentae from pregnancies complicated by pre-eclampsia. *Br. J. Obstet. Gynaecol.*, **103**, 1191–6.

Cramer, S., Beveridge, M., Kilberg, M. and Novak, D. (2002). Physiological importance of system A-mediated amino acid transport to rat fetal development. *Am. J. Physiol. Cell Physiol.*, **282**, C153–60.

Dao, D., Frank, D., Qian, N. *et al.* (1998). IMPT1, an imprinted gene similar to polyspecific transporter and multi-drug resistance genes. *Hum. Mol. Genet.*, **7**, 597–608.

Fernandez-Twinn, D. S., Ozanne, S. E., Ekizoglou, S. *et al.* (2003). The maternal endocrine environment in the low-protein model of intra-uterine growth restriction. *Br. J. Nutr.*, **90**, 815–22.

Genbacev, O., Joslin, R., Damsky, C. H., Polliotti, B. M. and Fisher, S. J. (1996). Hypoxia alters early gestation human cytotrophoblast differentiation/invasion in vitro and models the placental defects that occur in preeclampsia. *J. Clin. Invest.*, **97**, 540–50.

Genbacev, O., Zhou, Y., Ludlow, J. W. and Fisher, S. J. (1997). Regulation of human placental development by oxygen tension. *Science*, **277**, 1669–72.

Giugliano, D., Ceriello, A. and Paolisso, G. (1996). Oxidative stress and diabetic vascular complications. *Diabetes Care*, **19**, 257–67.

Godfrey, K. M. (1998). Maternal regulation of fetal development and health in adult life. *Eur. J. Obstet. Gynecol. Reprod. Biol.*, **78**, 141–50.

Gratton, R. J., Asano, H. and Han, V. K. (2002). The regional expression of insulin-like growth factor II (IGF-II) and insulin-like growth factor binding protein-1 (IGFBP-1) in the placentae of women with pre-eclampsia. *Placenta*, **23**, 303–10.

Hahn, T., Barth, S., Graf, R. *et al.* (1999). Placental glucose transporter expression is regulated by glucocorticoids. *J. Clin. Endocrinol. Metab.*, **84**, 1445–52.

Harrington, K. F., Campbell, S., Bewley, S. and Bower, S. (1991). Doppler velocimetry studies of the uterine artery in the early prediction of pre-eclampsia and intra-uterine growth retardation. *Eur. J. Obstet. Gynecol. Reprod. Biol.*, **42** (Suppl.) S14–20.

Hauguel-de Mouzon, S. and Shafrir, E. (2001). Carbohydrate and fat metabolism and related hormonal regulation in normal and diabetic placenta. *Placenta*, **22**, 619–27.

Illsley, N. P. (2000). Placental glucose transport in diabetic pregnancy. *Clin. Obstet. Gynecol.*, **43**, 116–26.

Irwin, J. C., Suen, L. F., Martina, N. A., Mark, S. P. and Giudice, L. C. (1999). Role of the IGF system in trophoblast invasion and pre-eclampsia. *Hum. Reprod.*, **14** (Suppl. 2), 90–6.

Jansson, T. and Powell, T. L. (2000). Placental nutrient transfer and fetal growth. *Nutrition*, **16**, 500–2.

Jansson, T., Scholtbach, V. and Powell, T. L. (1998). Placental transport of leucine and lysine is reduced in intrauterine growth restriction. *Pediatr. Res.*, **44**, 532–7.

Jansson, T., Wennergren, M. and Powell, T. L. (1999). Placental glucose transport and GLUT 1 expression in insulin-dependent diabetes. *Am. J. Obstet. Gynecol.*, **180**, 163–8.

Jansson, T., Ekstrand, Y., Wennergren, M. and Powell, T. L. (2001). Placental glucose transport in gestational diabetes mellitus. *Am. J. Obstet. Gynecol.*, **184**, 111–16.

Jansson, T., Ekstrand, Y., Bjorn, C., Wennergren, M. and Powell, T. L. (2002). Alterations in the activity of placental amino acid transporters in pregnancies complicated by diabetes. *Diabetes*, **51**, 2214–19.

Jansson, N., Greenwood, S. L., Johansson, B. R., Powell, T. L. and Jansson, T. (2003). Leptin stimulates the activity of the system A amino acid transporter in human placental villous fragments. *J. Clin. Endocrinol. Metab.*, **88**, 1205–11.

Jauniaux, E. (1996). Intervillous circulation in the first trimester: the phantom of the color Doppler obstetric opera. *Ultrasound Obstet. Gynecol.*, **8**, 73–6.

Jauniaux, E., Watson, A. L., Hempstock, J., Bao, Y. P., Skepper, J. N. and Burton, G. J. (2000). Onset of maternal arterial blood flow and placental oxidative stress: a possible factor in human early pregnancy failure. *Am. J. Pathol.*, **157**, 2111–22.

Jauniaux, E., Greenwold, N., Hempstock, J. and Burton, G. J. (2003). Comparison of ultrasonographic and Doppler mapping of the intervillous circulation in normal and abnormal early pregnancies. *Fertil. Steril.*, **79**, 100–6.

Kaminsky, S., Sibley, C. P., Maresh, M., Thomas, C. R. and D'Souza, S. W. (1991a). The effects of diabetes on placental lipase activity in the rat and human. *Pediatr. Res.*, **30**, 541–3.

Kaminsky, S., D'Souza, S. W., Massey, R. F., Smart, J. L. and Sibley, C. P. (1991b). Effects of maternal undernutrition and uterine artery ligation on placental lipase activities in the rat. *Biol. Neonate*, **60**, 201–6.

Kaufmann, P., Mayhew, T. M. and Charnock-Jones, D. S. (2004). Aspects of human fetoplacental vasculogenesis and angiogenesis. II. Changes during normal pregnancy. *Placenta*, **25**, 114–26.

Kingdom, J. C. and Kaufmann, P. (1997). Oxygen and placental villous development: origins of fetal hypoxia. *Placenta*, **18**, 613–21; discussion 623–6.

Kossenjans, W., Eis, A., Sahay, R., Brockman, D. and Myatt, L. (2000). Role of peroxynitrite in altered fetal–placental vascular reactivity in diabetes or preeclampsia. *Am. J. Physiol. Heart. Circ. Physiol.*, **278**, H1311–19.

Krozowski, Z., MaGuire, J. A., Stein-Oakley, A. N., Dowling, J., Smith, R. E. and Andrews, R. K. (1995). Immunohistochemical localization of the 11 beta-hydroxysteroid dehydrogenase type II enzyme in human kidney and placenta. *J. Clin. Endocrinol. Metab.*, **80**, 2203–9.

Laatikainen, T., Virtanen, T., Kaaja, R. and Salminen-Lappalainen, K. (1991). Corticotropin-releasing hormone in maternal and cord plasma in pre-eclampsia. *Eur. J. Obstet. Gynecol. Reprod. Biol.*, **39**, 19–24.

Lepercq, J., Guerre-Millo, M., Andre, J., Cauzac, M. and Hauguel-de Mouzon, S. (2003). Leptin: a potential marker of placental insufficiency. *Gynecol. Obstet. Invest.*, **55**, 151–5.

Lindsay, R. S., Lindsay, R. M., Waddell, B. J. and Seckl, J. R. (1996). Prenatal glucocorticoid exposure leads to offspring hyperglycaemia in the rat: studies with the 11 beta-hydroxysteroid dehydrogenase inhibitor carbenoxolone. *Diabetologia*, **39**, 1299–305.

Lyall, F., Gibson, J. L., Greer, I. A., Brockman, D. E., Eis, A. L. and Myatt, L. (1998). Increased nitrotyrosine in the diabetic placenta: evidence for oxidative stress. *Diabetes Care*, **21**, 1753–8.

Mahendran, D., Donnai, P., Glazier, J. D., D'Souza, S. W., Boyd, R. D. and Sibley, C. P. (1993). Amino acid (system A) transporter activity in microvillous membrane vesicles from the placentas of appropriate and small for gestational age babies. *Pediatr. Res.*, **34**, 661–5.

McMullen, S., Osgerby, J. C., Thurston, L. M. *et al.* (2004). Alterations in placental 11 beta-hydroxysteroid dehydrogenase (11 betaHSD) activities and fetal cortisol: cortisone ratios induced by nutritional restriction prior to conception and at defined stages of gestation in ewes. *Reproduction*, **127**, 717–25.

Mizuno, Y., Sotomaru, Y., Katsuzawa, Y., *et al.* (2002). Asb4, Ata3, and Dcn are novel imprinted genes identified by high-throughput screening using RIKEN cDNA microarray. *Biochem. Biophys. Res. Commun.*, **290**, 1499–505.

Mudgett, J. S., Ding, J., Guh-Siesel, L. *et al.* (2000) Essential role for p38alpha mitogen-activated protein kinase in placental angiogenesis. *Proc. Natl. Acad. Sci. USA*, **97**, 10454–9.

Murphy, V. E. and Clifton, V. L. (2003). Alterations in human placental 11beta-hydroxysteroid dehydrogenase type 1 and 2 with gestational age and labour. *Placenta*, **24**, 739–44.

Muttukrishna, S., Knight, P. G., Groome, N. P., Redman, C. W. and Ledger, W. L. (1997). Activin A and inhibin A as possible endocrine markers for pre-eclampsia. *Lancet*, **349**, 1285–8.

Myatt, L. (2002) Role of placenta in preeclampsia. *Endocrine*, **19**, 103–11.

Myatt, L., Rosenfield, R. B., Eis, A. L., Brockman, D. E., Greer, I. and Lyall, F. (1996). Nitrotyrosine residues in placenta. Evidence of peroxynitrite formation and action. *Hypertension*, **28**, 488–93.

Nelson, D. M., Smith, S. D., Furesz, T. C. *et al.* (2003). Hypoxia reduces expression and function of system A amino acid transporters in cultured term human trophoblasts. *Am. J. Physiol. Cell Physiol.*, **284**, C310–15.

Page, N. M., Woods, R. J., Gardiner, S. M. *et al.* (2000). Excessive placental secretion of neurokinin B during the third trimester causes pre-eclampsia. *Nature*, **405**, 797–800.

Pepe, G. J., Burch, M. G. and Albrecht, E. D. (2001). Localization and developmental regulation of 11beta-hydroxysteroid dehydrogenase-1 and -2 in the baboon syncytiotrophoblast. *Endocrinology*, **142**, 68–80.

Rajakumar, A., Whitelock, K. A., Weissfeld, L. A., Daftary, A. R., Markovic, N. and Conrad, K. P. (2001). Selective over-expression of the hypoxia-inducible transcription factor, HIF-2alpha, in placentas from women with preeclampsia. *Biol. Reprod.*, **64**, 499–506.

Ranheim, T., Staff, A. C. and Henriksen, T. (2001). VEGF mRNA is unaltered in decidual and placental tissues in preeclampsia at delivery. *Acta Obstet. Gynecol. Scand.*, **80**, 93–8.

Regnanlt, T.R., de Vrijer, B.,Galan, H.L. *et al.* (2003). The relationship between transplacental O_2 diffusion and placental expression of PIGF, VEGF and their receptors in a placental insufficiency model of fetal growth restriction. *J. Physiol.*, **550**, 641–56.

Reik, W., Constancia, M., Fowden, A. *et al.* (2003). Regulation of supply and demand for maternal nutrients in mammals by imprinted genes. *J. Physiol.*, **547**, 35–44.

Seckl, J. R., Cleasby, M. and Nyirenda, M. J. (2000). Glucocorticoids, 11beta-hydroxysteroid dehydrogenase, and fetal programming. *Kidney Int.*, **57**, 1412–17.

Sheppard, B. L. and Bonnar, J. (1976). The ultrastructure of the arterial supply of the human placenta in pregnancy complicated by fetal growth retardation. *Br. J. Obstet. Gynaecol.*, **83**, 948–59.

Shin, J. C., Lee, J. H., Yang, D. E., Moon, H. B., Rha, J. G. and Kim, S. P. (2003). Expression of insulin-like growth factor-II and insulin-like growth factor binding protein-1 in the placental basal plate from pre-eclamptic pregnancies. *Int. J. Gynaecol. Obstet.*, **81**, 273–80.

Shore, V. H., Wang, T. H., Wang, C. L., Torry, R. J., Caudle, M. R. and Torry, D. S. (1997). Vascular endothelial growth factor, placenta growth factor and their receptors in isolated human trophoblast. *Placenta*, **18**, 657–65.

Sibley, C. P., Coan, P. M., Ferguson-Smith, A. C. *et al.* (2004). Placental-specific insulin-like growth factor 2 (Igf2) regulates the diffusional exchange characteristics of the mouse placenta. *Proc. Natl. Acad. Sci. USA*, **101**, 8204–8.

Sun, K., Yang, K. and Challis, J. R. (1998). Glucocorticoid actions and metabolism in pregnancy: implications for placental function and fetal cardiovascular activity. *Placenta*, **19**, 353–60.

Vonnahme, K. A. and Ford, S. P. (2004). Differential expression of the vascular endothelial growth factor-receptor system in the gravid uterus of Yorkshire and Meishan pigs. *Biol. Reprod.*, **71**, 163–9.

Wallace, J., Bourke, D., Da Silva, P. and Aitken, R. (2001). Nutrient partitioning during adolescent pregnancy. *Reproduction*, **122**, 347–57.

Wallace, J. M., Aitken, R. P., Milne, J. S. and Hay, W. W. (2004). Nutritionally mediated placental growth restriction in the growing adolescent: consequences for the fetus. *Biol. Reprod.*, **71**, 1055–62.

Wang, Q., Fujii, H. and Knipp, G. T. (2002). Expression of PPAR and RXR isoforms in the developing rat and human term placentas. *Placenta*, **23**, 661–71.

Wang, Y., Walsh, S. W. and Kay, H. H. (1992). Placental lipid peroxides and thromboxane are increased and prostacyclin is decreased in women with preeclampsia. *Am. J. Obstet. Gynecol.*, **167**, 946–9.

Welberg, L. A., Seckl, J. R. and Holmes, M. C. (2000). Inhibition of 11beta-hydroxysteroid dehydrogenase, the foetoplacental barrier to maternal glucocorticoids, permanently programs amygdala GR mRNA expression and anxiety-like behaviour in the offspring. *Eur. J. Neurosci.*, **12**, 1047–54.

Zhang, E. G., Smith, S. K., Baker, P. N. and Charnock-Jones, D. S. (2001). The regulation and localization of angiopoietin-1, -2, and their receptor Tie2 in normal and pathologic human placentae. *Mol. Med.*, **7**, 624–35.

Zhou, Y., McMaster, M., Woo, K. *et al.* (2002). Vascular endothelial growth factor ligands and receptors that regulate human cytotrophoblast survival are dysregulated in severe preeclampsia and hemolysis, elevated liver enzymes, and low platelets syndrome. *Am. J. Pathol.*, **160**, 1405–23.

10

Control of fetal metabolism: relevance to developmental origins of health and disease

Abigail L. Fowden, Janelle W. Ward and Alison J. Forhead

University of Cambridge

Introduction

Epidemiological observations in several human populations have shown that impaired growth in utero is associated with an increased risk of cardiovascular, metabolic and other diseases in later life (Barker 2001). Since the major determinant of fetal growth is the supply of nutrients to the fetus (Harding and Johnson 1995), these epidemiological associations have led to the hypothesis that adult disease originates in utero as a result of nutritional programming of tissues during early life. This hypothesis has been investigated experimentally in a number of species using a range of techniques to manipulate nutrient availability in the fetus (Table 10.1). These studies all support the hypothesis and show that the prenatal nutritional environment has long-term consequences for the offspring, even when there is little change in body weight. Hence, the factors controlling the fetal supply and utilisation of nutrients are important in the aetiology of adult disease. However, compared to postnatal metabolism, little is known about the programming of fetal metabolism per se. The aims of this review are, therefore, threefold: first, to consider the effects of varying nutrient availability on fetal metabolism; second, to examine the role of hormones in mediating these effects; and, finally, to discuss the mechanisms by which metabolic programming may occur in utero.

Nutritional regulation of fetal metabolism

The effects of varying nutrient availability on fetal metabolism depend on the specific nature of the nutritional challenge and on the duration, severity and gestational age at onset of the insult. Deprivation of oxidative substrates, such as glucose, produces a different metabolic response in the fetus to that seen during oxygen deprivation alone or when there is combined oxygen and substrate deficiency. These different nutritional challenges also have different effects on the uteroplacental tissues and on the fetal hormonal environment, both of which influence the availability and metabolic fate of specific nutrients in the fetus (Fowden 1995, Fowden and Forhead, 2001).

Altered substrate availability

In sheep, reducing maternal calorific intake for 2–7 days reduces fetal glucose concentrations but has no effect on fetal arterial oxygen content or plasma lactate levels (Hay *et al.* 1984, Leury *et al.* 1990, Jones 1991, Dalinghaus *et al.* 1991, Fowden *et al.* 1998a). In contrast, fetal concentrations of urea and several gluconeogenic amino acids increase (Simmons *et al.* 1974, Lemons and Schreiner 1983, Liechty and Lemons 1984). These changes in metabolite concentration are accompanied by alterations in glucose and amino acid metabolism but not in O_2 consumption by the fetus (Hay *et al.* 1984, Harding and

Developmental Origins of Health and Disease, ed. Peter Gluckman and Mark Hanson. Published by Cambridge University Press.
© P. D. Gluckman and M. A. Hanson 2006.

Table 10.1 Postnatal consequences of varying nutritional availability in the fetus.

Procedure	Species	Postnatal outcome
Maternal origin		
Calorie deprivation	Rat	Hypertension, hypercholesterolaemia, obesity, glucose intolerance
	Guinea pig	Hypertension, insulin resistance, obesity
	Sheep	Hypertension, altered hypothalamic–pituitary–adrenal axis
Protein deprivation	Rat	Hypertension, glucose intolerance, insulin resistance
Salt deficiency	Rat	Hypertension, altered renin–angiotensin system
Iron deficiency	Rat	Hypertension
Diabetes	Rat	Glucose intolerance, insulin deficiency
Placental origin		
Increased litter size	Guinea pig	Glucose intolerance, insulin deficiency
	Pig	Hypertension, glucose intolerance, insulin resistance, obesity
Restricted blood flow	Rat	Glucose intolerance, insulin deficiency and resistance
	Guinea pig	Hypertension
	Sheep	Altered blood pressure and lung compliance
Decreased size	Sheep	Altered glucose tolerance, blood pressure
	Horse	Altered sympathoadrenal function
Increased size	Horse	Increased insulin secretion

Data from Fowden and Forhead (2004), Forhead *et al.* (2004).

Johnson 1995, Hay 1995). Short-term maternal fasting reduces the fetal rates of umbilical uptake, utilisation and oxidation of glucose (Hay *et al.* 1984, Fowden *et al.* 1998b). Similar changes in fetal glucose metabolism are observed when glucose availability is reduced by maternal insulin infusion for 20 days (DiGiacomo and Hay 1990). Fetal glucose production is activated by both maternal undernutrition and insulin treatment, and accounts for 20–30% of the glucose used by the fetus in these circumstances (Hay *et al.* 1984, DiGiacomo & Hay 1990). The ability of the fetus to produce glucose endogenously increases towards term as the fetal glucogenic capacity rises (Fowden *et al.* 1998b). Short periods of undernutrition can, therefore, evoke glucogenesis close to term but not earlier in gestation (Fowden *et al.* 1998a). This helps to ameliorate the fall in umbilical glucose uptake during maternal hypoglycaemia.

The fetal liver appears to be the main site of glucose production as hepatic glucose output, gluconeogenesis and gluconeogenic enzyme activitites all rise in response to undernutrition (Lemons *et al.* 1986, Dalinghaus *et al.* 1991). Before term, the glyco-

gen content of the fetal liver is unaffected by undernutrition and glucose is derived primarily by gluconeogenesis (Dalinghaus *et al.* 1991, Kaneta *et al.* 1991). However, at term, hepatic glycogen levels are significantly lower in fetuses from fasted than fed ewes, which suggests that either glycogenolysis contributes significantly to glucogenesis or that the amino acid carbon normally used for glycogen deposition is diverted into hepatic glucogenesis during hypoglycaemic conditions (Levitsky *et al.* 1988, Fowden *et al.* 1998a). However, despite the increase in glucose production, glucose utilisation falls and less glucose carbon is oxidised during maternal undernutrition (Hay 1995, Aldoretta and Hay 1999). Since fetal O_2 consumption is maintained in these circumstances (Hay 1995, Fowden *et al.* 1998a), substrates other than glucose must be used for oxidative metabolism.

Maternal undernutrition for 2–7 days has little effect on the umbilical uptake of amino acids overall but alters amino acid flux into the fetal liver, skeletal muscle and placenta (Lemons and Schreiner 1983, 1984, Levitsky *et al.* 1993). In fetal skeletal muscle, maternal fasting leads to an increased uptake of branched chain amino acids and an enhanced efflux of the gluconeogenic amino acids alanine and glutamine (Liechty and Lemons 1984). In fetal liver and placenta, there are increases in the activities of the aminotransaminases and urea cycle enzymes during maternal undernutrition, which increase amino acid turnover and the inter-organ shuttling of specific amino acids (Lemons and Schreiner 1983, Liechty *et al.* 1987). These changes are accompanied by a decrease in whole-body protein synthesis, a 30% increase in leucine oxidation and a doubling of the fetal production rate of urea, the main deamination product of amino acid catabolism (Simmons *et al.* 1974, Liechty *et al.* 1992). More amino acid carbon is, therefore, used for fetal oxidation as well as for *de novo* glucose production when glucose availability is limited by maternal undernutrition. This will reduce amino acid availability for protein synthesis and may programme muscle and liver development during suboptimal nutritional conditions in utero.

When nutrient restriction is prolonged beyond seven days in sheep, the changes in fetal metabolism are exaggerated and fetal hypoglycaemia becomes profound (DiGiacomo and Hay 1990, Carver and Hay 1995, Aldoretta and Hay 1999). The fall in fetal glucose levels will maximise the transplacental glucose concentration gradient and help maintain umbilical glucose uptake in conditions when maternal glucose levels are low. Nevertheless, umbilical uptake, utilisation and oxidation of glucose all fall by 50% or more and fetal glucose production rises to account for 50% of the glucose used by fetal tissues (Carver and Hay 1995). For periods of maternal hypoglycaemia up to 20 days, the uteroplacental tissues appear to share equally in the glucose deprivation but, after 40 days of insulin treatment, glucose partitioning appears to change in favour of the placenta (DiGiacomo and Hay 1990, Carver and Hay 1995). In part, this is due to the increased dependence on fetal glucogenesis as the source of glucose for both the fetal and uteroplacental tissues but it may also reflect changes in uteroplacental metabolism associated with maintaining pregnancy during sustained hypoglycaemia (Ward *et al.* 2004). The substrates used for glucose

production in these circumstances remain obscure as fetal urea production returns to normal values after seven days of maternal fasting (Simmons *et al.* 1974). Short-term nutrient deprivation may, therefore, lead to proteolysis of existing protein to maintain the fetoplacental metabolic balance, particularly during late gestation when the absolute demand for nutrients is high. Chronic undernutrition, on the other hand, appears to reduce the rate of protein accretion and, hence, lowers the demand for nutrients by the smaller fetal mass (Johnson and Dunham 1988). With no evidence of sustained amino acid catabolism, and a lower weight-specific rate of glucose oxidation during chronic undernutrition (Hay 1995), fetoplacental metabolic balance and the weight-specific rate of fetal O_2 consumption must be maintained by unidentified sources of oxidative substrates, such as lipid.

Oxygen deprivation

Fetal hypoxaemia has been induced experimentally by maternal inhalation of gases low in O_2 at sea level (normobaric hypoxia) or of gases at low partial pressure at high altitude (hypobaric hypoxia). In fetal sheep during the second half of gestation, acute isocapnic hypoxaemia induced by maternal-inhalation normobaric hypoxia is accompanied by fetal hyperglycaemia, hyperlactacidaemia and by increased O_2 extraction, which maintains the rate of oxygen consumption by the fetal tissues, provided the fall in O_2 delivery is less than 50% (Jones 1991, Richardson and Bocking 1998). There is also a decrease in the umbilical uptake and fetal utilisation of glucose, and an increase in fetal glucose production (Jones 1991). The fetal hyperglycaemic and lactacidaemic responses to acute hypoxaemia increase towards term in parallel with the rise in muscle mass and hepatic glucogenic capacity (Fletcher *et al.* 2003). Acute isocapnic hypoxaemia also reduces umbilical amino acid uptake by 17% and lowers protein accretion by 20% by decreasing protein synthesis rather than by enhancing proteolysis in fetal sheep (Milley 1987). These changes in protein metabolism reduce the O_2 requirement by about 30% and would eventually lead to fetal growth retardation. Fetal energy requirements are also lowered during fetal hypoxaemia by reducing fetal breathing and other movements (Richardson and Bocking 1998). However, other metabolic costs must rise to compensate for these decreases since fetal O_2 consumption is maintained during moderate fetal hypoxaemia. Less is known about the metabolic effects of chronic hypobaric hypoxaemia. In sheep, exposure to low pO_2, equivalent to high altitude, for 20–40 days retards fetoplacental growth and increases fetal concentrations of lactate and alanine but not glucose (Jacobs *et al.* 1988a, 1988b). In rats, chronic hypoxaemia leads to increased glucose uptake by the fetal heart, lung and kidney, probably as a result of the increased glycolysis required to meet fetal ATP requirements anaerobically (Lueder *et al.* 1995).

Combined oxygen and substrate deficiency

Combined fetal hypoxaemia and nutrient deprivation has been induced by restricting uterine or umbilical blood flow via injection of microspheres or mechanical constriction of the uterine artery or umbilical cord. These procedures produce a sustained reduction in fetal arterial pO_2 but, due to increased O_2 extraction, have little effect on the rate of fetal O_2 consumption, unless the reduction in pO_2 is severe or prolonged (Richardson and Bocking 1998). In fetal sheep, there is a transient increase in glucose concentration in response to constriction of either the uterine or umbilical arteries which is not sustained for more than 8 hours even when blood flow is reduced for 24 hours or more (Hooper *et al.* 1995, Gardner *et al.* 2001a). Moderate reductions in uterine blood flow have no effect on umbilical glucose uptake even after 24 hours but more severe restriction lowers glucose uptake by 25% at 4 hours (Boyle *et al.* 1992, Hooper *et al.* 1995). These observations suggest that there is a decrease in fetal glucose utilisation and possibly also a transient rise in fetal glucose production when the delivery of O_2 and glucose are both compromised (Rudolph *et al.* 1989, Jones 1991). Certainly, there is a reduction in the glycogen content of the fetal liver by 4 hours after restricting uterine blood flow (Stratford and Hooper 1997).

Combined reductions in the delivery of O_2 and nutrients to fetal sheep are invariably associated with fetal lactacidaemia which is sustained throughout the insult and for several hours thereafter (Gardner *et al.* 2001a, Hooper *et al.* 1995). The normal output of lactate from the fetal hind limbs increases in these circumstances, presumably as a result of anaerobic metabolism (Boyle *et al.* 1992, Gardner *et al.* 2003). The fetal liver also takes up less lactate during cord constriction, which will contribute to the lactacidaemia (Rudolph *et al.* 1989). Umbilical lactate uptake ceases during restriction of uterine blood flow and the uteroplacental tissues switch from producing to clearing lactate from the fetal circulation (Hooper *et al.* 1995). There are, therefore, major changes in the production and distribution of lactate during hypoxaemia conditions, but not in response to deprivation of nutrients alone.

Endocrine regulation of fetal metabolism

Many of the nutritionally induced alterations in fetal metabolism and growth are likely to be mediated by hormonal changes in either the mother or the fetus. Dietary restriction is known to alter maternal concentrations of growth hormone (GH), insulin-like growth factors (IGFs), insulin, glucocorticoids, leptin, thyroid hormones and placental lactogen (Bauer *et al.* 1995, Harding *et al.* 1997, Rae *et al.* 2002, Bispham *et al.* 2003). These hormones all alter maternal metabolite concentrations, which, in turn, will influence fetal substrate availability, particularly for those metabolites crossing the placenta down a concentration gradient. Some of the maternal hormonal changes also affect the morphology, metabolism and nutrient transfer capacity of the placenta (Bauer *et al.* 1998, Jenkinson *et al.* 1999). For instance, maternal treatment with GH for 10 days increases lactate production and the urea diffusing capacity of ovine placental tissues (Harding *et al.* 1997). Similarly, treatment of pregnant ewes with IGF1 increases placental lactate production and amino-nitrogen uptake with consequences for the delivery of substrates to the fetus (Liu *et al.* 1994, Bauer *et al.* 1998). Neither GH nor IGF1 are transported across the ovine placenta but other nutritionally sensitive hormones, such as cortisol, can cross the placenta and lead to direct changes in the fetal endocrine environment (Jensen *et al.* 2002). Hence, nutritionally induced hormonal changes in the fetus reflect both maternal endocrine changes and the responses of the fetal endocrine glands themselves (Fowden and Forhead 2001).

The precise nature of the fetal hormonal response to undernutrition depends on the type of nutrient deficit and on the duration, severity and gestational age at onset of the nutritional insult. In general, reducing fetal delivery of O_2 and nutrients lowers anabolic hormones (e.g. insulin, IGFs, thyroid hormones) and increases catabolic hormone concentrations (e.g. cortisol, catecholamines, glucagon, GH). However, the specific pattern of endocrine changes in the fetus is determined by whether hypoglycaemia and hypoxaemia occur simultaneously or alone. For instance, catecholamine and glucagon levels are raised in response to hypoxaemia but not hypoglycaemia whereas prostaglandin E_2 concentrations are increased by hypoglycaemia but not by hypoxaemia (see Fowden and Forhead 2001). In contrast, anabolic hormones like insulin and IGF1 are invariably reduced in concentration, irrespective of the nutrient deficit (Fowden 1995).

The effects of the nutritionally sensitive hormone on fetal metabolism are summarised in Table 10.2. The anabolic hormones tend to increase the uptake and utilisation of glucose and reduce the oxidative use of amino acid carbon. They also enhance protein accretion either by stimulating protein synthesis or by reducing protein proteolysis or both. The catabolic hormones are generally hyperglycaemic and tend to increase fetal glucose production by activating hepatic glucogenesis. They also tend to reduce protein accretion and the umbilical uptake of amino acids. None of the nutritionally sensitive hormones has a major effect on fetal O_2 consumption, apart from the thyroid hormones.

Many of the hormonal effects on fetal metabolism are interrelated. For instance, the catecholamine-induced rise in fetal glucose levels is a combined effect of direct activation of hepatic glucogenesis and indirect suppression of fetal glucose utilisation by catecholamine-mediated hypoinsulinaemia (Sperling *et al.* 1984, Jones 1991). Similarly, the IGF1-induced fall in fetal plasma insulin may mask any effect of IGF1 on fetal glucose metabolism (Liechty *et al.* 1996). Furthermore, hormone-stimulated reductions in umbilical glucose uptake may be the cause or consequence of fetal glucose production depending on the nature of the nutrient deficit. In hypoglycaemic conditions, decreased umbilical uptake probably precedes initiation of glucogenesis whereas, in hypoxaemic conditions, activation of fetal glucose production lowers the umbilical glucose delivery to the fetus by inducing fetal hyperglycaemia and reducing the transplacental glucose concentration gradient (Jones 1991, Fowden *et al.* 1998a, Ward *et al.* 2004).

The metabolic actions of hormones in the fetus are also dependent on the duration of hormone exposure. Cortisol has little effect on fetal glucose metabolism during short-term infusion (<48 h, Milley 1995) but significantly reduces the umbilical uptake of glucose during longer infusions or when concentrations rise naturally over the last 10–15 days of gestation (Fig. 10.1). Conversely, catecholamines become less effective at raising fetal glucose levels with prolonged exposure as the mobilisable glycogen stores in the liver are rapidly depleted (Stratford and Hooper 1997, Bassett and Hanson 1998). Hormones, therefore, act as qualitative, quantitative and temporal signals of nutrient and O_2 availability to the fetal tissues and modify fetal metabolism and growth in relation to the prevailing nutritional condition in utero.

Mechanisms of metabolic programming in utero

While the effects of undernutrition and hormone manipulation on fetal metabolism *during* the

Table 10.2 Effects of fetal administration of hormones on the metabolism of carbohydrate, amino acids and oxygen by the fetus.

Hormone	Duration of treatment	Carbohydrate	Amino acids	Oxygen
Insulin	4–10 h	Hypoglycaemia ↑ umbilical glucose uptake ↑ glucose utilisation ↑ glucose oxidation	↓ amino acid concentrations ↓ proteolysis ↑ protein synthesis ↓ urea production ↓ amino acid oxidation	Small ↑ O_2 consumption
Thyroid hormones	4 h–120 h	↑ glucose oxidation ↑ gluconeogenic enzyme activities	↑ tissue amino acid uptake ↑ protein synthesis	↑ O_2 consumption
IGF-I	2–4 h	Hypoglycaemia Hyperlactaemia No Δ umbilical glucose uptake ↓ umbilical lactate uptake	↓ amino acid concentrations ↓ amino acid oxidation ↓ urea production ↓ proteolysis	No Δ O_2 consumption
Glucagon	3–20 h	Hyperglycaemia ↑ fetal glucose production ↑ hepatic gluconeogenesis ↑ hepatic PEPCK activity ↓ umbilical glucose uptake	↓ gluconeogenic amino acid levels ↓ umbilical uptake of specific amino acids	No Δ O_2 consumption
Catecholamines	3–4 h	Hyperglycaemia ↑ glucose production ↓ glucose utilisation ↓ umbilical glucose uptake ↑ hepatic glucogenesis ↓ glycogen accumulation ↓ umbilical lactate uptake	↓ umbilical amino acid uptake ↓ proteolysis ↓ protein synthesis ↓ protein accretion ↓ amino acid oxidation	Small ↑ O_2 consumption
Cortisol	4h–120 h	↓ umbilical glucose uptake ↑ hepatic glycogen deposition ↑ gluconeogenic enzyme activities ↑ hepatic glucogenesis ↓ umbilical lactate uptake	↓ umbilical amino acid uptake ↑ proteolysis No Δ protein synthesis ↓ protein accretion	No Δ to small ↑ in O_2 consumption
GH	10 days	↓ umbilical glucose uptake No Δ umbilical lactate uptake	↓ urea concentration ↓ umbilical amino acid uptake	No Δ O_2 consumption

Data from Barnes *et al.* (1978), Lorijn *et al.* (1980), Young *et al.* (1982), Devaskar *et al.* (1984), Milley (1988, 1994, 1995, 1996, 1997, 1998), Hay *et al.* (1989), Phillips *et al.* (1990), Apatu and Barnes (1991), Townsend *et al.* (1991), Liechty *et al.* (1992, 1996), Rosato *et al.* (1992), Harding *et al.* (1994), Fowden and Silver (1995), Hendrich and Porterfield (1996), Bassett and Hanson (1998), Jensen *et al.* (1999), Bauer *et al.* (2000), Walker *et al.* (2000), Teng *et al.* (2002).

challenge have been well documented, much less is known about the metabolic consequences of these challenges *after* restoration of normal conditions. Fetal nutrient and O_2 restriction induced by occlusion of the umbilical cord for three days reduces lactate output by the fetal hind limbs in

response to a subsequent episode of acute hypoxaemia (Gardner *et al.* 2003). Similarly, glucocorticoid overexposure in utero increases the fetal glycaemic response to acute hypoxaemia 2–6 days after restoration of normal glucocorticoid concentrations (Fletcher *et al.* 2003). These observations suggest that changes in tissue metabolism induced in utero can persist and alter subsequent responses to nutritional challenges later in gestation. This intrauterine programming of metabolic function has several possible explanations.

Systems mechanisms

Development of the placenta

One of the major mechanisms whereby early nutritional or hormonal insults may alter fetal metabolism closer to term is via changes in placental development. Both under- and overnutrition are known to alter placental size, particularly during the period of maximal placenta growth in early gestation. Overexposure to glucocorticoids during this critical period of placental growth has also been shown to alter the size and morphology of the ovine placenta later in gestation (see Dodic *et al.* 2003). During the first 70–80 days of ovine pregnancy, when the placenta is growing most rapidly, moderate undernutrition can increase placental weight and the predominance of fetal tissue in the placentomes late in gestation (McCrabb *et al.* 1991, Kelly 1992, Dandrea *et al.* 2001, Steyn *et al.* 2001, Osgerby *et al.* 2004). Similar compensatory growth of the placenta has been observed in humans undernourished during early pregnancy (Lumey 1998). However, if undernutrition is more severe, placental weight is reduced at term in both sheep and humans (Kelly 1992, Lumey 1998). Maternal undernutrition during mid to late gestation, when the ovine placenta is growing less rapidly, tends to reduce placental weight in late gestation and shift placental morphology towards the everted type of placentome (Ehrhardt and Bell 1995, Osgerby *et al.* 2004). Close to term, maternal undernutrition appears to have little effect on placental weight (Mellor and Murray 1985, Kelly 1992). However, there may be nutritionally induced changes in placental function and ultrastructure that affect nutrient transfer even when placental weight is unaffected. Certainly, when placental growth is impaired in mice by disruption of the placental-specific transcript of the *Igf2* gene, there is reduced

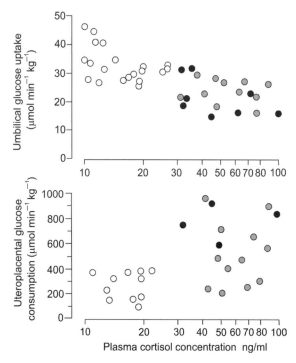

Figure 10.1 The relationship between the plasma cortisol concentration and the rates of umbilical glucose uptake (upper panel) and uteroplacental glucose utilisation (lower panel) in individual sheep fetuses at 127–130 days after 5 days of cortisol (grey circles) or saline infusion (open circles) or at 142–145 days of gestation with high endogenous cortisol concentrations (black circles, term = 145 days). Data from Fowden *et al.* (1998b) and Ward *et al.* (2004).

passive diffusion of hydrophilic molecules and increased amino acid transport per gram of placenta (Fig. 10.2).

Deprivation of nutrients and/or oxygen alters the morphological characteristics of the placenta that influence transplacental diffusion. Maternal undernutrition reduces the surface area and increases the thickness of the exchange barrier, both of which will limit simple diffusion (Roberts *et al.* 2001). Chronic hypoxaemia in pregnant ewes alters gross morphology and increases the branching and volume density of the blood vessels in the placentomes (Krebs *et al.* 1997, Penninga and Longo 1998). In rats and sheep, the abundance of the placental glucose

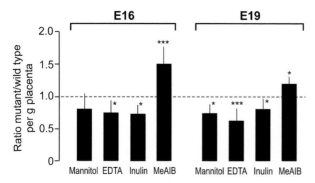

Figure 10.2 Mean (± SD) values of the ratio of mutant to wild-type weight-specific transfer of counts across the placenta for methyl-aminoisobutyric acid (MeAIB), an amino acid analogue transported by the system A transporters, and three hydrophilic molecules of different molecular sizes transported by passive diffusion (mannitol, EDTA and inulin) in pregnant mice on embryonic day 16 (E16) and day 19 (E19). Ratios greater than 1 indicate increased uptake by mutant placentas while ratios less than 1 indicate decreased uptake. * $P < 0.02$; *** $P < 0.01$. Data from Constancia *et al.* (2002) and Sibley *et al.* (2004).

transporters GLUT1 and GLUT3 alters during maternal undernutrition, hypoglycaemia, diabetes and treatment with IGF1 and glucocorticoids (Currie *et al.* 1997, Hahn *et al.* 1999, Das *et al.* 1999, Dandrea *et al.* 2001, Lesage *et al.* 2002). There are also increases in the activity of the system A amino acid transporters in small placentas from growth-retarded human infants (Godfrey *et al.* 1998).

Nutrient consumption by the placenta itself is altered by the prevailing nutritional and hormonal conditions. Short-term undernutrition reduces placental glucose consumption but has little effect on the distribution of uterine glucose uptake between the placental and fetal tissues (Hay *et al.* 1989). However, when maternal hypoglycaemia is prolonged, proportionally more of the uterine glucose uptake is used by the placenta (Carver and Hay 1995). Acute hypoxaemia also increases placental glucose consumption (Jones 1991). In part, these changes may be due to endocrine alterations, as cortisol has been shown to increase placental glucose consumption in parallel with the decline in umbilical glucose uptake

(Fig. 10.1). Similarly, in sheep, the placental production and distribution of lactate alters during hypoxaemia, undernutrition and increased exposure to maternal GH and IGF1 (Liu *et al.* 1994, Hooper *et al.* 1995, Bauer *et al.* 1998). There are also changes in the placental uptake, consumption, handling and transfer of specific amino acids during undernutrition and fetal hormone manipulation (Table 10.2). These alterations in placental nutrient consumption and production affect fetal nutrient delivery but the extent to which they persist after restoration of normal conditions remains unknown.

The placenta also produces and inactivates hormones with metabolic actions. Placental hormones, such as progesterone and placental lactogen, influence maternal metabolism in favour of glucose delivery to the fetus. Changes in these hormone levels will, therefore, affect the partitioning of nutrients between maternal and fetal tissues and alter the availability of substrates for oxidative metabolism and tissue accretion by the fetus. In fetal sheep, the cortisol-induced reduction in the number of placental binucleate cells producing placental lactogen may not only affect placental development and nutrient partitioning before birth but may also compromise mammary development and cause a lactational constraint on nutrition after birth (Ward *et al.* 2002). During undernutrition and glucocorticoid exposure, there are changes in the placental activity of enzymes, such as 11β-hydroxysteroid dehydrogenase and prostaglandin dehydrogenase, that convert biologically active hormones to their inactive metabolites (Yang *et al.* 1997, Clarke *et al.* 2002, Whorwood *et al.* 2001, Challis *et al.* 2002). These changes alter placental hormone exposure and influence the transplacental passage and fetal bioavailability of hormones with metabolic actions.

Development of fetal endocrine glands

Another mechanism that may explain persisting metabolic effects of suboptimal conditions early in gestation is the resetting of endocrine axes involved in metabolic control (Fowden and Forhead 2004). In sheep, periconceptual undernutrition, prolonged maternal hypoglycaemia and cord compression have been shown to alter the subsequent functioning of the hypothalamic–pituitary–adrenal axis and/or the endocrine pancreas of the fetus in late gestation (Hawkins *et al.* 2000, Gardner *et al.* 2001b, Oliver *et al.* 2001, Limesand and Hay 2003). Similarly, there is resetting of the somatotrophic axis in utero by under-nutrition and hormone exposure, which may lead to changes in the relationship between paracrine and endocrine IGF production with adverse seque-lae for both metabolism and growth (Bauer *et al.* 1998, Fowden 2003). Furthermore, alterations in the secretion and function of the orexigenic and anorex-igenic peptides, ghrelin, and leptin, after exposure to suboptimal conditions in utero may cause abnor-malities in energy balance both before and after birth (Forhead *et al.* 2002, Symonds *et al.* 2003). These changes in the set-point and sensitivity of the endocrine axes may lead to permanent changes in basal hormone concentrations and in the endocrine responses to subsequent stimuli (Bertram and Hanson 2001, Fowden and Forhead 2004).

Development of fetal fuel reserves

Early undernutrition and hormone exposure may alter fetal metabolic response later in gestation by altering the fuel reserves of the fetus. Moderate undernutrition during the last 20 days of gestation reduces the body fat content of fetal sheep at term but appears to have little effect on tissue glycogen content (Mellor and Murray 1985, Budge *et al.* 2004). In contrast, acute maternal fasting late in gestation lowers the glycogen content of the fetal liver while undernutrition from earlier in gestation can increase fat deposition in the fetus at mid and late gestation (McCrabb *et al.* 1991, Fowden *et al.* 1998b, Budge *et al.* 2004). Acute deprivation of O_2 depletes fetal glycogen reserves in late gestation, which reduces glucogenesis by the fetus (Jones 1991, Stratford and Hooper 1997). Since the fetus has a limited capacity for lipolysis in utero (Symonds *et al.* 2003), it is the nutritionally induced changes in glycogen deposi-tion and utilisation that are more likely to alter subse-quent metabolic responses to adverse stimuli before

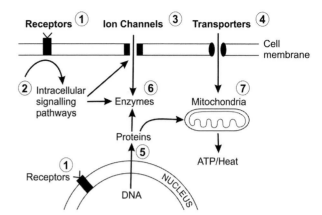

Figure 10.3 A schematic diagram illustrating the cellular processes that may be programmed by intrauterine manipulation of the nutritional or hormonal environment. (1) Hormone receptors; (2) Intracellular signalling pathways; (3) Ion channels; (4) Transporters for nutrients (e.g. glucose or amino acids) or ions; (5) Protein synthesis; (6) Enzyme activities by *de novo* synthesis or phosphorylation through intracellular signalling pathways and/or ion channels; (7) Mitochondrial oxidative phosphorylation and thermogenic activity.

birth (Gardner *et al.* 2003). However, the nutrition-ally induced changes in fat accumulation are likely to have important consequences postnatally, once the constraint on lipolysis is removed at birth.

Cellular mechanisms

At a cellular level, there are several processes that may contribute to the metabolic program-ming of the fetus (Fig. 10.3). These processes affect cell metabolism directly and indirectly and occur at the membrane, cytoplasmic and nuclear levels within the cell. Undernutrition and gluco-corticoid overexposure alter the abundance of mem-brane and nuclear receptors for several hormones with metabolic actions including the glucocorti-coids, catecholamines, GH, IGFs, prolactin and lep-tin (Freemark *et al.* 1992, Hyatt *et al.* 2004, Fowden and Forhead 2004). Changes in receptor density occur in a range of different fetal tissues including the placenta, and, in some instances, can persist to term after a challenge in early to mid gestation (Whorwood *et al.* 2001, Fowden and Forhead 2004). In fetal tissues like the heart and kidneys there are also changes in the expression of transporters and ion channels in the cell membrane after intrauterine nutritional or hormonal manipulation that will alter cellular metabolism and nutrient requirements (Fahmi *et al.* 2004, Nakamura *et al.* 2002, Kamitomo *et al.* 2002).

In the cytoplasm there are changes in intracellular signalling, enzyme activities and mitochondrial oxidative function during undernutrition and/or glucocorticoid exposure in utero. The activities of many enzymes are regulated by nutrient availability and/or hormone manipulation during late gestation (see Fowden and Forhead 2004). Many of these have metabolic functions and may be up- or down-regulated depending on the specific nutrient deficit. For instance, hepatic glucose-6-phosphatase activity is up-regulated by hypoglycaemia and down-regulated by hypoxaemia in fetal sheep (Lemons *et al.* 1986, Stratford and Hooper 1997). Changes in cAMP, gluconeogenic and aminotransferase enzyme activities and in mitochondrial oxidative phosphorylation have been observed in fetal liver in response to restriction of maternal dietary intake or uterine blood flow (Lemons and Snodgrass 1986, Stratford and Hooper 1997, Peterside *et al.* 2003). In fetal rat islets, maternal protein restriction during pregnancy alters enzyme activities in the adenyl cyclase signalling pathway and in the mitochondrial respiratory chain to favour heat over ATP production (Sparre *et al.* 2003). In some tissues, the nutritionally induced changes in enzyme activity and intracellular signalling are due to altered gene expression while, in others, it is the phosphorylation state of existing enzymes and signalling components that is nutritionally regulated (Ozanne *et al.* 1997). Certainly, abnormalities in intracellular signalling are common postnatally in tissues involved in the adult metabolic syndrome associated with impaired intrauterine growth (Ozanne 2001).

At the nuclear level, changes in transcription lead to altered protein synthesis in response to intrauterine undernutrition and hormone exposure. These proteins include the receptors, ion channels, transporters and enzymes known to be regulated by nutrition and hormone exposure in utero. They also include mitochondrial proteins, such as the cytochromes and uncoupling proteins, which alter energy balance and the ability to respond to oxidative stress (Sparre *et al.* 2003, Symonds *et al.* 2003, Bispham *et al.* 2003). There are also changes in the synthesis of binding proteins and cyto-architectural proteins, and in many growth factors (see Fowden 2003, Fowden and Forhead 2004). In particular, the nutritionally induced changes in the synthesis of the IGFs and their binding proteins are likely to have widespread effects on tissue metabolism and growth both before and after birth (Gluckman and Pinal 2002, Fowden 2003). Fetal undernutrition induced by restricting uterine blood flow also reduces DNA synthesis itself in tissues, such as the liver, adrenal and placenta, which have high proliferation rates before birth (McLellan *et al.* 1995, Asano *et al.* 1997).

Molecular mechanisms

At the molecular level, nutritional state and the concomitant endocrine changes affect a number of different aspects of protein synthesis including transcription, mRNA stability, translation and/or the post-translational processing of the protein. Several of the nutritionally regulated genes (e.g. *Igf2*, *GH receptor*, *PEPCK*) have glucocorticoid and thyroid hormone response elements in their promotors to allow transcriptional control of the genes by the hormones that act as nutritional signals. In genes that do not have consensus sequences for the nutritionally sensitive hormones, the effects of nutritional state must be mediated by other transcription factors. Several transcription factors are known to be altered in fetal tissues by manipulation of maternal dietary intake during pregnancy (see Sparre *et al.* 2003). In genes which have multiple mRNA transcripts derived from alternate exon slicing and promotor usage, the effects of nutritional and/or hormone manipulation may be specific to certain leader exons in the genes. Indeed, differential promotor usage has been observed developmentally in the

GH receptor, *Igf1* and *glucocorticoid receptor* genes in fetal ovine liver (see Fowden *et al.* 1998a). Early manipulation of the intrauterine environment may, therefore, initiate use of specific promoters, which, in turn, alters the relative abundance of particular mRNA splice variants with consequences for protein translation and the subsequent metabolism of the fetal tissues.

In genes which are imprinted and expressed from only one parental allele, the effects of adverse intrauterine conditions early in gestation may be mediated through changes in imprint status. Genomic imprinting depends on DNA methylation, an epigenetic modification that confers specificity of allele expression. Since imprinted genes have a key role in placental development (Young 2001), any change in their expression or imprint status is likely to have long-term consequences for nutrient delivery to the fetus (Reik *et al.* 2003). Certainly, disruption of the *H19* gene, which regulates imprinting of the *Igf2* gene, has major consequences for fetoplacental development (Efstratiadis 1998). Methylation of DNA is also important in regulating promotor usage and expression of the *p53* gene, a regulator of apoptosis and growth in many tissues. Hypomethylation of this gene has been shown to occur in fetal kidneys after restriction of uterine blood flow in pregnant rats (Pham *et al.* 2003). Conversely, hypermethylation of DNA has been observed in fetal liver near term during maternal protein deprivation in rats (Rees *et al.* 2000). Epigenetic reprogramming of key imprinted and other genes via changes in methylation may provide the molecular mechanism linking nutrition to gene expression and subsequent fetoplacental metabolism.

Of the nutritionally sensitive genes, it is *Igf* genes that are most likely to have a central role in metabolic programming of the fetus. These genes are expressed in a wide range of tissues throughout gestation and are responsive to both nutritional state and hormone concentrations in utero (see Gluckman and Pinal 2002). They have anabolic effects on fetal metabolism and regulate tissue growth and differentiation from the preimplantation to the late fetal stages of development (Table 10.2). Both *Igf*

genes have multiple mRNA slice variants, which are expressed in a tissue-specific manner and differentially regulated (see Fowden 2003). The *Igf2* gene is also imprinted and sensitive to changes in DNA methylation (Young 2001). It is the actions of the *Igf* genes in the placenta that probably programme the subsequent metabolic phenotype of the fetus, particularly as undernutrition is known to down-regulate expression of these genes in the placenta (Price *et al.* 1992). In mice, deletion of the *Igf2* gene either from all placental cell types (*Igf2* null) or specifically from the labyrinthine trophoblast (P0 null) reduces placental growth from the time in mid gestation when the labyrinthine placenta takes over from the yolk sac as the main source of fetal nutrients (Efstratiadis 1998, Constancia *et al.* 2002). In the P0 mutant placenta, there are also reductions in the surface area and increases in the thickness of the labyrinthine exchange barrier (Sibley *et al.* 2004), which mimic the changes in placental morphology seen during undernutrition (Roberts *et al.* 2001) and limit passive diffusion to a greater extent than predicted by the decrease in placental weight (Figure 10.2). However, there is a compensatory increase in system A transport in the small P0-null placenta (Figure 10.2), which maintains fetal growth until close to term (Constancia *et al.* 2002). Consequently, manipulation of placental *Igf2* gene expression changes both the absolute and relative amounts of specific nutrients supplied to the fetus. Indeed, it may be the composition rather than the magnitude of the nutrient supply that is critical in programming tissue metabolism and growth in utero. Certainly, supplementation of protein-deprived pregnant rats with single amino acids ameliorates the postnatal programming effects of the low-protein diets (Holemans *et al.* 2003).

Conclusions

Deprivation of nutrients and/or O_2 in utero alters fetal metabolism in a manner that changes body growth and the development of individual fetal tissues. When these challenges occur at critical stages of development, there may be permanent changes in fetal metabolism and growth, particularly if the growth and nutrient transfer capacity of the placenta are affected. Interactions between nutrients, hormones and genes early in development may, therefore, alter both the delivery and metabolic fate of nutrients in the fetus closer to term. In particular, prenatal metabolic programming of the liver, skeletal muscle and adipose tissue are likely to have important implications for postnatal energy balance and the aetiology of adult metabolic disease.

REFERENCES

Aldoretta, P. W. and Hay, W. W. (1999). Effect of glucose supply on ovine uteroplacental glucose metabolism. *Am. J. Physiol.*, **277**, R947–58.

Apatu, R. S. K. and Barnes, R. J. (1991). Release of glucose from the liver of fetal and postnatal sheep by portal vein infusion of catecholamines or glucagon. *J. Physiol.*, **436**, 449–68.

Asano, H., Han, V. K., Homan, J. and Richardson, B. S. (1997). Tissue DNA synthesis in the pre-term ovine fetus following 8 hours of sustained hypoxemia. *J. Soc. Gynecol. Investig.*, **4**, 236–40.

Barker, D. J. P. (2001). The malnourished baby and infant. *Br. Med. Bull.*, **60**, 69–88.

Barnes, R. J., Comline, R. S. and Silver, M. (1978). Effect of cortisol on liver glycogen concentrations in hypophysectomized, adrenalectomized and normal fetal lambs during late or prolonged gestation. *J. Physiol.*, **275**, 567–79.

Bassett, J. M. and Hanson, C. (1998). Catecholamines inhibit growth in fetal sheep in the absence of hypoxemia. *Am. J. Physiol.*, **274**, R1536–45.

Bauer, M. K., Bernhard, H. B., Harding, J. E., Veldhuis, J. D. and Gluckman, P. D. (1995). The fetal somatotropic axis during long term maternal undernutrition in sheep: evidence for nutritional regulations in utero. *Endocrinology*, **136**, 1250–7.

Bauer, M. K., Harding, J. E., Bassett, N. S. *et al.* (1998). Fetal growth and placental function. *Mol. Cell. Endocrinol.*, **140**, 115–20.

Bauer, M. K., Harding, J. E., Breier, B. H. and Gluckman, P. D. (2000). Exogenous GH infusion to late-gestational fetal sheep does not alter fetal growth and metabolism. *J. Endocrinol.*, **166**, 591–7.

Bertram, C. E. and Hanson, M. A. (2001). Animal models and programming of metabolic syndrome. *Br. Med. Bull.*, **60**, 103–21.

Bispham, J., Gopalakrishnan, G. C., Dandrea, J. *et al.* (2003). Maternal endocrine adaptation throughout pregnancy to nutrition manipulation: consequences for maternal plasma leptin and cortisol and the programming of fetal adipose tissue development. *Endocrinology*, **144**, 3575–85.

Boyle, D. W., Meschia, G. and Wilkening, R. B. (1992). Metabolism adaptation of fetal hindlimb to severe, nonlethal hypoxia. *Am. J. Physiol.*, **263**, R1130–5.

Budge, H., Edwards, L. J., McMillen, I. C. *et al.* (2004). Nutritional manipulation of fetal adipose tissue deposition and uncoupling protein 1 messenger RNA abundance in the sheep: differential effects of timing and duration. *Biol. Reprod.*, **71**, 359–65.

Carver, T. D. and Hay, W. W. (1995). Uteroplacental carbon substrate metabolism and O_2 consumption after long-term hypoglycemia in pregnant sheep. *Am. J. Physiol.*, **269**, E299–308.

Challis, J. R. G., Sloboda, D., Matthew, S. C. *et al.* (2002). Prostaglandins and the mechanisms of preterm birth. *Reproduction*, **124**, 1–17.

Clarke, K., Ward, J. W., Forhead, A. J., Giussani, D. A. and Fowden, A. L. (2002). Regulation of 11β hydroxysteroid dehydrogenase type 2 (11βHSD2) activity in ovine placenta by fetal cortisol. *J. Endocrinol.*, **172**, 527–34.

Constancia, M., Hemberger, M., Hughes, J. *et al.* (2002). Placental-specific IGF-II is a major modulator of placental and fetal growth. *Nature*, **417**, 945–8.

Currie, M. J., Bassett, N. S. and Gluckman, P. D. (1997). Ovine glucose transporter-1 and -3: cDNA partial sequences and developmental gene expression in the placenta. *Placenta*, **18**, 393–401.

Dalinghaus, M., Rudolph, C. D. and Rudolph, A. M. (1991). Effects of maternal fasting on hepatic glucogenesis and glucose metabolism in fetal lambs. *J. Dev. Physiol.*, **16**, 267–75.

Dandrea, J., Wilson, V., Gopalakrishnan, G. *et al.* (2001). Maternal nutritional manipulation of placental growth and glucose transporter 1 (GLUT-1) abundance in sheep. *Reproduction*, **122**, 793–800.

Das, U. G., Schroeder, R. E., Hay, W. W. and Devaskar, S. U. (1999). Time-dependent and tissue-specific effects of circulating glucose on fetal ovine glucose transporters. *Am. J. Physiol.*, **276**, R809–17.

Devaskar, S. U., Ganguli, S., Styer, D., Devaskar, U. P. and Sperling, M. (1984). Glucagon and glucose dynamics in sheep: evidence for glucagon reistance in the fetus. *Am. J. Physiol.*, **246**, E256–65.

DiGiacomo, J. E. and Hay, W. W. (1990). Fetal glucose metabolism and oxygen consumption during sustained maternal and fetal hypoglycaemia. *Metabolism*, **39**, 139–202.

Dodic, M., Moritz, K. and Wintour, E. M. (2003). Prenatal glu-
cocoticoid exposure and adult disease. *Arch. of Physiol.
Biochem.*, **111**, 61–9.

Efstratiadis, A. (1998). Genetics of mouse growth. *Int. J. Dev. Biol.*,
42, 955–76.

Ehrhardt, R. A. and Bell, A. W. (1975). Growth and metabolism
of the ovine placenta during mid gestation. *Placenta*, **16**,
727–41.

Fahmi, A. I., Forhead, A. J., Fowden, A. L. and Vandenburg, J.
I. (2004). Cortisol influences the ontogeny of both α- and
β-subunits of the cardiac sodium channel in fetal sheep. *J.
Endocrinol.*, **180**, 449–55.

Fletcher, A. J. W., Gardner, D. S., Edwards, C. M. B., Fowden, A.
L. and Giussani, D. A. (2003). Cardiovascular and endocrine
responses to acute hypoxaemia during and following dexamethasone infusion in the ovine fetus. *J. Physiol.*, **549**,
271–87.

Forhead, A. J., Thomas, L., Crabtree, J. *et al.* (2002). Plasma leptin
concentration in fetal sheep during late gestation: ontogeny
and effect of glucocorticoids. *Endocrinology*, **143**, 1166–73.

Forhead, A. J., Ousey, J. C., Allen, W. R. and Fowden, A. L. (2004).
Postnatal insulin secretion and sensitivity after manipu-
lation of fetal growth by embryo transfer in the horse. *J.
Endocrinol.*, **181**, 459–67.

Fowden, A. L. (1995). Endocrine regulation of fetal growth.
Reprod. Fertil. Dev., **7**, 351–63.

(2003). The insulin-like growth factors and feto-placental
growth. *Placenta*, **24**, 803–12.

Fowden, A. L. and Forhead, A. J. (2001). The role of hormones
in intrauterine development. In *Lung Biology in Health &
Disease* (ed. D. J. P. Barker). New York: Dekker, vol. 151, pp.
199–228.

(2004). Endocrine mechanisms of intrauterine programming.
Reproduction. **127**, 515–26.

Fowden, A. L. and Silver, M. (1995). The effects of thyroid hormones on oxygen and glucose metabolism in the sheep
fetus during late gestation. *J. Physiol.*, **482**, 203–13.

Fowden, A. L., Li, J. and Forhead, A. J. (1998a). Glucocorticoids
and the preparation for life after birth: are there long-term
consequences of the life insurance. *Proc. Nutr. Soc.*, **57**, 113–
22.

Fowden, A. L., Mundy, L. and Silver, M. (1998b). Developmental
regulation of glucogenesis in the sheep fetus during late
gestation. *J. Physiol.*, **508**, 937–47.

Freemark, M., Keen, A., Fowlkes, J. *et al.* (1992). The placental lactogen receptor in maternal and fetal sheep liver: regulation
by glucose and role in the pathogenesis of fasting during
pregnancy. *Endocrinology*, **130**, 1063–70.

Gardner, D. S., Fletcher, A. J. W., Fowden, A. L. and Giussani,
D. A. (2001a). A novel method for controlled and reversible

long term compression of the umbilical cord in fetal sheep.
J. Physiol., **535**, 217–29.

(2001b). Adrenocorticotrophin and cortisol during umbilical cord compression and subsequent hypoxaemia in
the late gestation ovine fetus. *Endocrinology*, **142**, 589–
98.

Gardner, D. S., Giussani, D. A. and Fowden, A. L. (2003). Hindlimb
glucose and lactate metabolism during umbilical cord compression and acute hypoxemia in the late-gestation ovine
fetus. *Am. J. Physiol. Regul. Integr. Comp. Physiol.*, **284**,
R954–64.

Gluckman, P. D. and Pinal, C. S. (2002). Maternal–placental–
fetal interactions in the endocrine regulation of fetal growth.
Endocrine, **19**, 81–9.

Godfrey, K. M., Matthews, N., Glazier, J., Jackson, A., Wilman,
C. and Sibley, C. P. (1998). Neutral amino acid uptake by
the microvillous membrane of human placenta is inversely
related to fetal size at birth in normal pregnancy. *J. Clin.
Endocrinol. Metab.*, **83**, 3320–6.

Hahn, T., Barth, S., Graf, R. *et al.* (1999). Placental glucose
transport expression is regulated by glucocorticoids. *J. Clin.
Endorcinol. Metab.*, **84**, 1445–52.

Harding, J. E. and Johnson, B. (1995). Nutrition and fetal growth.
Reprod. Fertil. Dev., **7**, 538–47.

Harding, J. E., Liu, L., Evans, P. C. and Gluckman, P. D. (1994).
Insulin-like growth factor 1 alters feto-placental protein
and carbohydrate metabolism in fetal sheep. *Endocrinology.* **134**, 1509–14.

Harding, J. E., Evans, P. C. and Gluckman, P. D. (1997). Maternal growth hormone treatment increases placental diffusion capacity but not fetal or placental growth in sheep.
Endocrinology, **138**, 5352–8.

Hawkins, P., Steyn, C., McGarrigle, H. H. *et al.* (2000). Cardiovascular and HPA axis development in late gestation fetal
sheep and young lambs following modest maternal nutrient restriction in early gestation. *Reprod. Fertil. Dev.*, **12**,
443–56.

Hay, W. W. (1995). Regulation of placental metabolism by glucose
supply. *Reprod. Fertil. Dev.*, **7**, 365–75.

Hay, W. W., Sparks, J. W., Wilkening, R. B., Battaglia, F. C. and
Meschia, G. (1984). Fetal glucose uptake and utilization as
functions of maternal glucose concentration. *Am. J. Physiol.*, **246**, E237–42.

Hay, W. W., DiGiacomo, J. E., Meznarich, H. K., Hirst, K. and
Zerbe, G. (1989). Effects of glucose and insulin on fetal glucose oxidation and oxygen consumption. *Am. J. Physiol.*,
256, E704–13.

Hendrich, C. E. and Porterfield, S. P. (1996). Ribosomal protein
synthesis in 16 and 19 day gestation fetuses of hypothyroid
mothers. *Proc. Soc. Exp. Biol. Med.*, **213**, 273–80.

Holemans, K, Aerts, L. and Van Assche, F. A. (2003). Fetal growth retardation and consequences for the offspring in animal models. *J. Soc. Gynecol. Investig.*, **10**, 392–9.

Hooper, S. B., Walker, D. W. and Harding, R. (1995). Oxygen, glucose, and lactate uptake by fetus and placenta during prolonged hypoxemia. *Am. J. Physiol.*, **268**, 303–9.

Hyatt, M. A., Walker, D. A., Stephenson, T. and Symonds, M. E. (2004). Ontogeny and nutritional manipulation of the hepatic prolactin–growth hormone–insulin-like growth factor axis in the ovine fetus and in neonate and juvenile sheep. *Proc. Nutr. Soc.*, **63**, 127–35.

Jacobs, R., Owens, J. A., Falconer, J., Webster, M. E. D. and Robinson, J. S. (1988a). Changes in metabolic concentrations in fetal sheep subjected to prolonged hypobaric hypoxia. *J. Dev. Physiol.*, **10**, 113–25.

Jacobs, R., Robinson, J. S., Owens, J. A., Falconer, J. and Webster, M. E. D. (1988b). The effect of prolonged hypobaric hypoxia on growth of fetal sheep. *J. Dev. Physiol.*, **10**, 97–112.

Jenkinson, C. M. C., Min, S. H., Mackenzie, D. D. S., McCutcheon, S. N., Brier, B. H. and Gluckman P. D. (1999). Placental development and fetal growth in growth hormone-treated ewes. *Growth Horm. IGF Res.*, **9**, 11–17.

Jensen, E. C., Harding, J. E., Bauer, M. K. and Gluckman, P. D. (1999). Metabolic effects of IGF-I in the growth retarded fetal sheep. *J. Endocrinol.*, **161**, 485–94.

Jensen, E. C., Gallaher, B. W., Brier, B. H. and Harding, J. E. (2002). The effect of a chronic maternal cortisol infusion on the late-gestation fetal sheep. *J. Endocrinol.*, **174**, 27–36.

Johnson, J. D. and Dunham, T. (1988). Protein turnover in tissues of the fetal rat after prolonged maternal malnutrition. *Pediatr. Res.*, **23**, 534–8.

Jones, C. T. (1991). Control of glucose metabolism in the perinatal period. *J. Dev. Physiol.*, **15**, 81–9.

Kamitomo, M., Onishi, J., Gutierrez, I., Stiffel, V. M. and Gilbert, R. D. (2002). Effects of long-term hypoxia and development on cardiac contractile proteins in fetal and adult sheep. *J. Soc. Gynecol. Investig.*, **9**, 335–41.

Kaneta, M., Liechty, E. A., Moorehead, H. C. and Lemons, J. A. (1991). Ovine fetal and maternal glycogen during fasting. *Biol. Neonate*, **60**, 215–20.

Kelly, R. W. (1992). Nutrition and placental development. *Proc. Nutr. Soc. Aust.*, **17**, 203–11.

Krebs, C., Longo, L. D. and Leiser, R. (1997). Term ovine placental vasculature: comparisons of sea level and high altitude conditions by corrosion. *Placenta*, **18** 43–51.

Lemons, J. A. and Schreiner, R. L. (1983). Amino acid metabolism in the ovine fetus. *Am. J. of Physiol.*, **244**, E459–66.

  (1984). Metabolic balance of the ovine fetus during the fed and fasted states. *Ann. Nutr. Metab.*, **28**, 268–280.

Lemons, J. A. and Snodgrass, P. J. (1986). Effect of maternal fast on the urea cycle enzymes of the ovine fetus. *J. Pediatr. Gastroenterol. Nutr.*, **5**, 138–42.

Lemons, J. A., Moorehead, A. C. and Hage, G. (1986). Effects of fasting on gluconeogenic enzymes in the ovine fetus. *Pediatr. Res.*, **20**, 676–9.

Lesage, J., Hahn, D., Lyonhardt, M., Blondeau, B., Bryant, B. and Dupouy, J. P. (2002). Maternal undernutrition during late gestation-induced intrauterine growth restriction in the rat is associated with impaired placental GLUT3 expression, but does nor correlate with endogenous corticosterone levels. *J. Endocrinol.*, **174**, 37–43.

Leury, B. J., Chandler, K. D., Bird, A. R. and Bell, A. W. (1990). Effects of maternal undernutrition and exercise on glucose kinetics in fetal sheep. *Br. J. Nutr.*, **64**, 463–72.

Levitsky, L., Paton, J. B. and Fisher, D. E. (1988). Precursors to glycogen in ovine fetuses. *Am. J. Physiol.*, **255**, E743–7.

Levitsky, L. L., Stonesweet, B. S., Mink, R. and Zheng, Q. (1993). Glutamine carbon disposal and net glutamine uptake in fetuses of fed and fasted ewes. *Am. J. Physiol.*, **265**, E722–7.

Liechty, E. A. and Lemons, A. J. (1984). Changes in ovine fetal hindlimb amino acid metabolism during maternal fasting. *Am. J. Physiol.*, **246**, E430–5.

Liechty, E. A., Barone, S. and Nutt, M. (1987). Effect of maternal fasting on ovine fetal and maternal branched-chain amino acid transaminase activities. *Biol. Neonate*, **52**, 166–73.

Liechty, E. A., Boyle, D. W., Moorehead, H., Liu, Y. M. and Denne, S. C. (1992). Effect of hyperinsulinemia on ovine fetal leucine kinetics during prolonged maternal fasting. *Am. J. Physiol.*, **263**, E696–702.

Liechty, E. A., Boyle, D. W., Moorehead, H., Lee, W-H., Bowsher, R. R. and Denne, S. C. (1996). Effects of circulating IGF-I on glucose and amino acid kinetics in the ovine fetus. *Am. J. Physiol.*, **271**, E177–85.

Limesand, S. W. and Hay, W. W. (2003). Adaptation of ovine fetal pancreatic insulin secretion to chronic hypoglycaemia and euglycaemic correction. *J. Physiol.*, **547**, 95–105.

Liu, L., Harding, J. E., Evans, P. C. and Gluckman, P. D. (1994). Maternal insulin-like growth factor-I infusion alters feto-placental carbohydrate and protein metabolism in pregnant sheep. *Endocrinology*, **135**, 895–900.

Lorijn, R. H. W., Nelson, J. C. and Longo, L. D. (1980). Induced fetal hyperthyroidism: cardiac output and oxygen consumption. *Am. J. Physiol.*, **239**, H302–7.

Lueder, F. L., Kim, S. B., Buroker, C. A., Bangalore, S. A. and Ogata, E. S. (1995). Chronic maternal hypoxia retards fetal growth and increases glucose utilization of select fetal tissues in the rat. *Metabolism* **44**, 532–7.

Lumey, L. H. (1998). Compensatory placental growth after restricted maternal nutrition in early pregnancy. *Placenta*, **19**, 105–11.

McCrabb, G. J., Egan, A. R. and Hosking, B. J. (1991). Maternal undernutrition during mid-pregnancy in sheep: placental size and its relationship to calcium transfer during late pregnancy. *Br. J. Nutr.*, **65**, 157–68.

McLellan, K. C., Bocking, A. D., White, S. E. and Han, V. K. M. (1995). Placental and fetal hepatic growth are selectively inhibited by prolonged reductions of uterine blood flow in pregnant sheep. *Reprod. Fertil. Dev.*, **7**, 405–10.

Mellor, D. J. and Murray, L. (1985). Effects of maternal nutrition on the availability of energy in the body reserves of fetuses at term and in colostrum from Scottish blackface ewes with twin lambs. *Res. Vet. Sci.*, **3**, 235–40.

Milley, J. R. (1987). Protein synthesis during hypoxia in fetal lambs. *Am. J. Physiol.*, **252**, E519–24.

(1988). Uptake of exogenous substrates during hypoxia in fetal lambs. *Am. J. Physiol.*, **254**, E572–8.

(1994). Effects of insulin on ovine fetal leucine kinetics and protein metabolism. *J. Clin. Investig.*, **93**, 1616–24.

(1995). Effects of increased cortisol concentration on ovine fetal leucine kinetics and protein metabolism. *Am. J. Physiol.*, **268**, E1114–22.

(1996). Fetal substrate uptake during increased ovine fetal cortisol concentration. *Am. J. Physiol.*, **271**, E186–91.

(1997). Ovine fetal metabolism during norepinephrine infusion. *Am. J. Physiol.*, **273**, E336–47.

(1998). Ovine fetal leucine kinetics and protein metabolism during the decreased oxygen availability. *Am. J. Physiol.*, **274**, E618–26.

Nakamura, K., Stokes, J. B. and McCray, P. B. (2002). Endogenous and exogenous glucocorticoid regulation of ENaC mRNA expression in developing kidney and lung. *Am. J. Physiol. Cell Physiol.*, **283**, C762–72.

Oliver, M. H., Hawkins, P., Breier, B. H., Vanzul, P. L., Sargison, S. A. and Harding, J. E. (2001). Maternal undernutrition during the periconceptual period increases plasma taurine levels and insulin response to glucose but not arginine in the late gestation fetal sheep. *Endocrinology*, **142**, 4576–9.

Osgerby, J. C., Wathes, D. C., Howard, D. and Gadd, T. S. (2004). The effect of maternal undernutrition on the placental growth trajectory and the uterine insulin-like growth factor axis in the pregnant ewe. *J. Endocrinol.*, **182**, 89–103.

Ozanne, S. E. (2001). Metabolic programming in animals. *Br. Med. Bull.*, **60**, 143–52.

Ozanne, S. E., Nave, B. T., Wang, C. L., Shepherd, R. P., Prins, J. and Smith, G. D. (1997). Poor fetal nutrition causes long-term changes in expression of insulin signaling components in adipocytes. *Am. J. Physiol.*, **273**, E46–51.

Penninga, L. and Longo, L. D. (1998). Ovine placentome morphology: effect of high altitude, long-term hypoxia. *Placenta*, **19**, 187–93.

Peterside, I. E., Selak, M. A. and Simmons, R. A. (2003). Impaired oxidative phosphorylation in hepatic mitochondria in growth-retarded rats. *Am. J. Physiol. Endocrinol. Metal.*, **285**, E1258–66.

Pham, T. D., MacLennan, N. K., Chiu, C. T., Laksana, G. S., Hsu, J. L. and Lane, R. H. (2003). Uteroplacental insufficiency increases apoptosis and alters p53 gene methylation in the full-term IUGR rat kidney. *Am. J. Physiol. Regul. Integr. Comp. Physiol.*, **285**, R962–70.

Philipps, A. F., Rosenkrantz, T. S., Lemons, J. A., Knox, I., Porte, P. J. and Raye, J. R. (1990). Insulin-induced alterations in amino acid metabolism in the fetal lamb. *J. Dev. Physiol.*, **13**, 251–9.

Price, W. A., Rong, L., Stiles, A. D. and D'Ercole, A. J. (1992). Changes in IGF-I and -II, IGF binding protein, and IGF receptor transcript abundance after uterine artery ligation. *Pediatr. Res.*, **32**, 291–5.

Rae, M. T., Rhind, S. M., Kyle, C. E., Miller, D. W. and Brooks, A. N. (2002). Maternal undernutrition alters triiodothyronine concentration and pituitary response to GnRH in fetal sheep. *J. Endocrinol.*, **173**, 449–55.

Rees, W. D., Hay, S. M., Brown, D. S., Antipatis, C. and Palmer, R. M. (2000). Maternal protein deficiency causes hypermethylation of DNA in the livers of rat fetuses. *J. Nutr.*, **130**, 1821–26.

Reik, W., Constancia, M., Fowden, A. *et al.* (2003). Regulation of supply and demand for maternal nutrients in mammals by imprinted genes. *J. Physiol.*, **547**, 35–44.

Richardson, B. S. and Bocking A. D. (1998). Metabolic and circulatory adaptations to chronic hypoxia in the fetus. *Comp. Biochem. Physiol. A Mol. Integr. Physiol.*, **119**, 717–23.

Roberts, C. T., Sohlstrom, A., Kind, K. L. *et al.* (2001). Maternal food restriction reduces the exchange surface area and increases the barrier thickness of the placenta in the guinea-pig. *Placenta*, **22**, 177–85.

Rosato, R. R., Jahn, G. A. and Gimenez, M. S. (1992). Amelioration of some metabolic effects produced by hyperthyroidism in late pregnant rats and their fetuses: effects on lipids and proteins. *Horm. Metab. Res.*, **24**, 15–20.

Rudolph, C. D., Roman, C. and Rudolph, A. M. (1989). Effect of acute umbilical cord compression on hepatic carbohydrate metabolism in the fetal lamb. *Pediatr. Res.*, **25**, 228–33.

Sibley, C. P., Coan, P. M., Ferguson-Smith, A. C. *et al.* (2004). Placental-specific insulin-like growth factor 2 (Igf2) regulates the diffusional exchange characteristics of the mouse placenta. *Proc. Nat. Acad. Sci. USA*, **101**, 8204–8.

Simmons, M. A., Meschia, G., Makowski, E. L. and Battaglia, F. C. (1974). Fetal metabolic response to maternal starvation. *Pediatr. Res.*, **8**, 830–36.

Sparre, T., Reusens, B., Cherif, H. *et al.* (2003). Intrauterine programming of fetal islet gene expression in rats: effects of maternal protein restriction during gestation revealed by proteome analysis. *Diabetologia*, **46**, 1497–511.

Sperling, M. A., Ganguli, S., Leslie, N. and Landt, K. (1984). Fetal–perinatal catecholamine secretion: role in perinatal glucose homeostasis. *Am. J. Physiol.*, **247**, E69–74.

Steyn, C., Hawkins, P., Saito, T., Noakes, D. E., Kingdom, J. P. C. and Hanson, M. A. (2001). Undernutrition during the first half of gestation increases the predominance of fetal tissue in late-gestation ovine placentomes. *Eur. J. Obstet. Gynecol. Reprod. Biol.*, **98**, 165–70.

Stratford, L. L. and Hooper, S. B. (1997). Effect of hypoxemia on tissue glycogen content and glycolytic enzyme activities in fetal sheep. *Am. J. Physiol.*, **241**, R103–10.

Symonds, M. E., Gopalakrishnan, G., Bispham, J. *et al.* (2003). Maternal nutrient restriction during placental growth, programming of fetal adiposity and juvenile blood pressure control. *Arch. Physiol. Biochem.*, **111**, 45–52.

Teng, C., Battaglia, F. C., Meschia, G., Narkewicz, M. R., and Wilkening, R. B. (2002). Fetal hepatic and umbilical uptakes of glucogenic substrates during a glucagon–somatostatin infusion. *Am. J. Physiol. Endocrinol. Metab.*, **282**, E542–50.

Townsend, S. F., Rudolph, C. D. and Rudolph, A. M. (1991). Cortisol induces perinatal hepatic gluconeogenesis in the lamb. *J. Dev. Physiol.*, **16**, 71–9.

Walker, V., Gentry, A. J., Green, L. R., Hanson, M. A. and Bennet, L. (2000). Effects of hypoxia on plasma amino acids of fetal sheep. *Amino Acids*, **18**, 146–56.

Ward, J. W., Wooding, F. B. P. and Fowden, A. L. (2002). The effects of cortisol on the binucleate cell population in the ovine placenta during late gestation. *Placenta*, **23**, 451–8.

(2004). Ovine feto-placental metabolism. *J. Physiol.*, **554**, 529–41.

Whorwood, C. B., Firth, K. M., Budge, H. and Symonds, M. E. (2001). Maternal undernutrition during early to midgestation programs tissue-specific alterations in the expression of the glucocorticoid receptor, 11β-hydroxysteroid dehydrogenase isoforms, and type1 angiotensin II receptor in neonatal sheep. *Endocrinology*, **142**, 2854–64.

Yang, K., Shearman, K., Asano, H. and Richardson, B. S. (1997). The effects of hypoxemia on 11 beta-hydroxysteroid dehydrogenase types 1 and 2 gene expression in preterm fetal sheep. *J. Soc. Gynecol. Investig.*, **4**, 124–9.

Young, L. E. (2001). Imprinted genes and the Barker hypothesis. *Twins Res.*, **4**, 307–17.

Young, M., Stern, D. R., Horn, J. and Noakes, D. E. (1982). Protein synthetic rate in the sheep placenta in vivo: the influence of insulin. *Placenta*, **3**, 159–64.

11

Lipid metabolism: relevance to developmental origins of health and disease

Graham C. Burdge and Philip C. Calder

University of Southampton

Introduction

Lipids play numerous and diverse roles in the development of the fetus. Fatty acids are required for the synthesis of cell membranes, which are a prerequisite for tissue growth, for the synthesis of second messengers and for generation of energy reserves in adipose tissue. Cholesterol is also required for tissue growth, and for the synthesis of steroid hormones. This chapter discusses how the physiology of the mother adapts to meet the demands of the fetus for fatty acids and cholesterol, the functions of these lipids in the development of specific tissues and the consequences of deficits in lipid accretion for tissue function, with a specific focus on long-chain polyunsaturated fatty acids (PUFAs).

Lipids and fetal development

Fat accumulation and birthweight

In humans, fetal fat accretion into adipose tissues begins between 15 and 20 weeks gestation, but increases exponentially from about 30 g at 30 weeks gestation to 430 g at term (Southgate and Hay 1976). The early phase of adipogenesis is associated with deposition of subcutaneous fat, while visceral fat accumulation occurs during the mid second and third trimesters (Poissonnet et al. 1984). Such deposition may serve to provide insulation during early life, which is important in the absence of body hair (Pawlowski 1998), and it is notable that in non-human primates fat deposition begins after birth (Adolph and Heggeness 1971, Lewis et al. 1983). Prenatal accumulation of adipose tissue may also serve to generate a nutrient reserve to survive infancy (Kuzawa 1998, Correia et al. 2004). Accumulation of adipose tissue accounts for about 50% of weight gain during the third trimester and for approximately 46% of the variation in the weight of human infants at birth (Catalano et al. 1998). A heavier baby is associated with a greater fat mass at any gestational age (Sparks et al. 1980, Sparks 1984). Variations in birthweight are associated with differential risk of a variety of chronic non-communicable diseases (Godfrey and Barker 2001). Since fat accumulation is an important determinant of birthweight, variations in the ability of the mother to supply fatty acids and of the fetus to deposit fatty acids in adipose tissue may either be involved causally in the determination of disease risk or be a marker of underlying pathophysiological process.

In addition to providing an energy reserve for early postnatal life, the rapid increase in fat mass during late gestation may also reflect preferential storage of specific fatty acids. During the last trimester, there is substantial accumulation of the polyunsaturated fatty acid docosahexaenoic fatty acid (22:6n-3, DHA)

Developmental Origins of Health and Disease, ed. Peter Gluckman and Mark Hanson. Published by Cambridge University Press.
© P. D. Gluckman and M. A. Hanson 2006.

into adipose tissue (about 380 mg per week) which is believed to account for about 75% of the total body DHA accumulation (Clandinin *et al.* 1981). This pool is mobilised rapidly after birth (Farquharson *et al.* 1993) and may facilitate supply of DHA to developing tissues during the transition from placental to oral fatty acid supply. Since DHA is important in the development of the brain (Innis 2003), this may explain the positive association between body mass index and head circumference at birth (Correia *et al.* 2004). Although very-low-birthweight infants who are born with lower fat mass may have impaired neurological function in childhood (Hadders-Algra *et al.* 1988, Hack *et al.* 1992), this does not appear to occur in infants born within the normal weight range (Martyn *et al.* 1996). However, this does not exclude the possibility that part of the association between birthweight and later disease may reflect impaired deposition of specific fatty acids during late gestation.

Fatty acids and tissue development

The growth and development of fetal tissues requires a supply of substrates for the synthesis of membrane phospholipids to support cell division. Different cell types maintain unique patterns of fatty acids within membrane phospholipids (Stubbs and Smith 1984). The fatty acid composition of membrane lipids is closely linked to tissue function and primarily reflects the specificity of phospholipid biosynthesis. For example, leukocyte membranes contain large amounts of the eicosanoid precursor arachidonic acid (20:4n-6, AA) (Calder 2001), while the brain and retina contain high concentrations of DHA, which is important for neural function (Innis 2003). Tissue maturation in the fetus is accompanied by selective changes to the composition of membrane phospholipids. Such changes in phospholipid molecular species composition may modify tissue function (Salem and Niebylski 1995). For example, in the developing human, rat and guinea pig lung, there is a progressive increase in the concentration of dipalmitoyl phosphatidylcholine (PC) and a decrease in the amount of *sn*-1-palmitoyl-*sn*-2-oleoyl PC which reflects the maturation of pulmonary surfactant

(Ashton *et al.* 1992). In the developing guinea pig, enrichment in dipalmitoyl PC is due to changes to the specificity of PC biosynthesis (Burdge *et al.* 1993). Similarly, development of the fetal guinea pig brain is associated with a shift in the pattern of incorporation of DHA into membrane phosphatidylethanolamine from *sn*-1-palmitoyl-*sn*-2 docosahexanoyl to *sn*-1-oleoyl or *sn*-1-stearoyl molecular species (Burdge and Postle 1995). This may reflect incorporation of DHA into a more stable membrane pool as the tissue matures (Samborski *et al.* 1990). Overall, developing fetal tissues require the right fatty acid at the appropriate time point. Failure to acquire adequate amounts of the right fatty acids may lead to impaired tissue development and function.

The importance of cholesterol in fetal development

Cholesterol is essential for the normal development of the fetus, and deficit in availability results in developmental abnormalities (Woollett 1993). Cholesterol may be synthesised by fetal tissues. Sterol biosynthesis is greater per gram of liver tissue in the fetus compared to the mother (Dietschy *et al.* 1993). The importance of endogenous cholesterol biosynthesis for fetal development is illustrated by the moderate to severe abnormalities in neurological development and limb deformities in individuals with Smith–Lemli–Opitz syndrome, who are unable to convert 7-dehydrocholesterol to cholesterol (Tint *et al.* 1994). The fetus may also obtain cholesterol from the mother. Human (Wittmaack *et al.* 1995, Grimes *et al.* 1996, Winkler *et al.* 2000) and hamster (Woollett 1996, Wyne and Woollett 1998) placenta express the low-density-lipoprotein (LDL) receptor. This suggests uptake of LDL particles which are rich in cholesterol from the maternal circulation, although the mechanism by which cholesterol is transferred into the fetal circulation is not known. Experimental impairment of the capacity of the fetus to synthesise cholesterol may be offset by increasing the cholesterol concentration in the maternal circulation (Roux *et al.* 2000). This nutritional plasticity highlights the importance of cholesterol in fetal development.

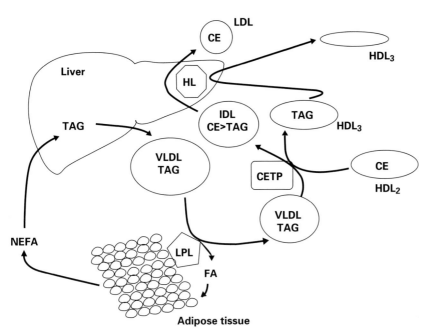

Figure 11.1 Metabolic interrelationships between lipoprotein particles. CE, cholesteryl ester; CETP, cholesteryl ester transfer protein; FA, fatty acid; HDL, high-density lipoprotein; HL, hepatic lipase; IDL, intermediate-density lipoprotein; LDL, low-density lipoprotein; LPL, lipoprotein lipase; NEFA, non-esterified fatty acids; TAG, triacylglycerol; VLDL, very-low-density lipoprotein. A detailed explanation is given in the text.

Maternal lipid metabolism during pregnancy

Importance of the mother as a source of fatty acids for fetal tissues

Although the human fetus does possess some capacity for lipogenesis (Dunlop and Court 1978) it is unlikely to satisfy demands for fatty acids, particularly during the rapid period of fat accretion in late gestation. Thus the developing fetus is essentially dependent upon supply of fatty acids from the mother. This suggests the capacity of the mother to supply fatty acids to the fetus is a potential determinant of fetal fat deposition, and so influences birthweight and the availability of PUFAs for incorporation into fetal tissues.

Interpretation of different circulating lipid pools in mother and fetus

Consideration of the changes to maternal lipid metabolism during pregnancy and the relationship

with the fatty acid composition of the fetal, typically cord, blood requires an understanding of the metabolic origins of different lipid pools. Fatty acids are carried in the circulation either esterified to triacylglycerol (TAG), PC or cholesteryl ester (CE) or, in the case of the non-esterified fatty acid (NEFA) fraction, non-covalently bound to albumin (Fig. 11.1). PC forms the outer coat of lipoproteins, while TAG and CE are present in the core and are distributed differentially between types of lipoprotein particles (Fielding and Frayn 2003). In fasting adults, NEFA are derived primarily by TAG lipolysis in adipose tissue which provides fatty acid and glycerol substrate for uptake by other tissues. Under fasting conditions, TAG is associated primarily with very-low-density lipoprotein (VLDL), while CE is predominantly in LDL and high-density lipoprotein (HDL). PC is present in VLDL, LDL and HDL. Thus fasting plasma TAG and PC fatty acid compositions primarily reflect maternal hepatic fatty acid metabolism, while CE is derived both from maternal liver and

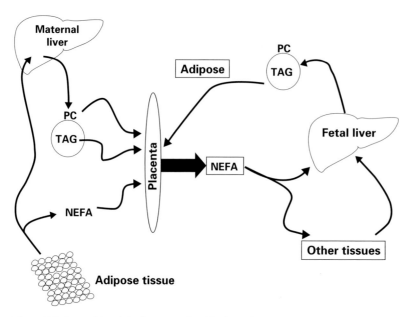

Figure 11.2 Fatty acid pools in the maternal and fetal circulations. NEFA, non-esterified fatty acids; PC, phosphatidylcholine; TAG, triacylglycerol. A detailed explanation is given in the text.

by cholesteryl ester transfer protein (CETP) activity. Unfortunately, many studies simply report total plasma lipid fatty acid compositions or the fatty acid content of a single lipid class, which may mask important data that may identify metabolic adaptations.

Assessment of the fatty acid composition of fetal blood is typically by sampling from the umbilical cord. Since the fetal blood acquires fatty acids as it passes through the placenta, the fatty acid compositions of umbilical vein and artery may differ, although which type of vessel is sampled is often not controlled. In addition, fatty acids enter the fetal circulation bound to α-fetoprotein and represent a NEFA fraction, while PC and TAG in umbilical cord represent fetal hepatic lipid metabolism (Fig. 11.2). Thus the strength of association between the concentrations of fatty acids in the maternal and fetal circulation may be determined in part by the metabolic origin of the lipid class in which they are carried. For example, there is a significant positive relationship between maternal and umbilical cord total TAG concentrations, which suggests a relationship

between maternal and fetal hepatic TAG metabolism (Sherman *et al.* 2001).

Adaptations to maternal lipid metabolism during pregnancy

Maternal hyperphagia during early gestation increases the availability of fatty acids for storage in maternal adipose tissue. The resulting accumulation of fat stores leads to weight gain (Villar *et al.* 1992), although the magnitude is highly dependent upon maternal nutrient intake and is relatively small where maternal nutrition is marginal (Prentice and Goldberg 2000). In relatively poor societies the fetus may account for about 60% of maternal weight gain during pregnancy, but this may be only 25% in well-nourished women (Prentice and Goldberg 2000). In late gestation, maternal adipose stores accumulated earlier in pregnancy are mobilised by increased lypolysis (Williams and Coltart 1978), resulting in an increase in NEFA concentration in the maternal circulation (Benassayag *et al.* 1997). In the rat, this reflects in part increased expression of hormone-sensitive lipase (Martin-Hidalgo *et al.* 1994). The decrease in insulin sensitivity in late gestation (Fraser 1999) may also promote increased lypolysis.

Fatty acids released from maternal adipose tissue in late gestation can be used by the liver for esterification, production of energy or ketone body synthesis. Ketone bodies cross the placenta and may be used either for energy production (Shambaugh 1985) or lipogenesis (Patel *et al.* 1975) by the fetus. In the rat, plasma NEFA concentration rises about twofold, resulting in increased esterification of fatty acids to TAG by the maternal liver and a twofold increase in VLDL TAG secretion (Wasfi *et al.* 1980), leading to an increase in circulating TAG concentration (Smith and Welch 1976). This hyperlipidaemia of pregnancy has also been recognised in women (Williams *et al.* 1976, Darmady and Postle 1982), horses (Jeffcott and Field 1985), sheep (Noble *et al.* 1971), cattle (Vazquez-Anon *et al.* 1994) and nonhuman primates (Schwartz and Kemnitz 1992). This physiological increase in maternal blood lipid concentrations increases supply of fatty acids and cholesterol to the placenta for transfer to the fetus and to the mammary gland for synthesis of milk. In species in which the fetus is born relatively lipid-poor, such as the rat, the primary role of maternal hyperlipidaemia may be to supply fatty acids to the mammary gland rather than the placenta.

In pregnant women, plasma TAG concentration increases threefold to fivefold and is accompanied by a 50% increase in plasma cholesterol level (Darmady and Postle 1982). In addition to an overall increase in VLDL TAG secretion, in pregnant women there are specific changes to the concentrations of individual lipoprotein classes (Sattar *et al.* 1997). The concentrations of $VLDL_1$ and $VLDL_2$ are increased, and this is accompanied by greater transfer of TAG into HDL due to up-regulation of CETP activity. Hepatic lipase activity decreases, resulting in greater concentrations of TAG-rich HDL_2 particles and lower amounts of HDL_3 (Alvarez *et al.* 1996). There is also a shift from LDL_2 to the pro-atherogenic low-density lipoprotein $(LDL)_3$ (Silliman *et al.* 1994, Sattar *et al.* 1997) which may facilitate supply of

cholesterol to the placenta. Maternal hypercholes-terolaemia has been associated with fatty streak formation in human fetal arteries (Palinski and Napoli 2002) and may be associated with increased progression of atherogenesis (Napoli *et al.* 1999). Despite the long recognition of these adaptations to maternal lipid metabolism, the mechanisms which regulate this increase in circulating lipids are not completely understood, although it has been suggested that these adaptations may be due to the action of oestrogen (Knopp 1997). One possibility is that the rise in blood oestrogen concentration due to up-regulation of oestrogen production by the placenta in late gestation drives the increase in hepatic TAG synthesis and secretion. In addition, in women the birthweight of the mother is negatively associated with her plasma TAG concentration in early pregnancy (Dempsey *et al.* 2004). This suggests that patterns of growth of the mother before birth may determine her capacity to supply fatty acids to her offspring during pregnancy.

Since mobilisation of maternal adipose stores is important for supply of fatty acids which are ultimately destined for transfer to the fetus, it may be anticipated that there would be a strong association between maternal fat deposition during early pregnancy and birthweight. Measurement of skinfold thickness in early pregnancy, a marker of maternal fat deposition, failed to show an association with birthweight in some studies (Langhoff-Roos *et al.* 1987) while others have reported a positive relationship (Thorsdottir and Birgisdottir 1998). Pre-pregnancy lean body mass (Allen *et al.* 1994, Langhoff-Roos *et al.* 1987), pre-pregnancy weight (Dougherty and Jones 1982, Langhoff-Roos *et al.* 1987), body mass index (Allen *et al.* 1994) and skinfold thickness during the first and second trimesters (Taggart *et al.* 1967, Pipe *et al.* 1979, Ash *et al.* 1989) have been shown to be positively associated with birthweight. Overall, these studies imply that single measurements of maternal fat mass may be insufficient to describe accurately the dynamic process of fat accumulation and mobilisation in the mother which is central to supply of fatty acids to the fetus. This is supported by the observation that, although skinfold thickness increases

(a)

(b)

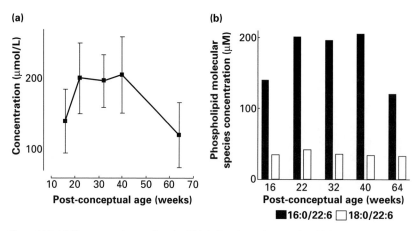

Figure 11.3 (a) Changes to plasma phosphatidylcholine docosahexaenoic acid (22:6n-3) concentration during pregnancy and after delivery in women (Postle *et al.* 1995). (b) The plasma concentrations of *sn*-1-palmitoyl or *sn*-1-stearoyl-*sn*-2-docosahexaenoyl phosphatidylcholine molecular species during pregnancy in women (Postle *et al.* 1995).

during early gestation, there is a decrease associated with the mobilisation of maternal fat stores in late pregnancy (Taggart *et al.* 1967, Pipe *et al.* 1979, Ash *et al.* 1989, Neufeld *et al.* 2004). Thus measurements made in late pregnancy alone will underestimate fat accumulation. In addition, supply of fatty acids to the fetus also depends upon the capacity of the maternal liver to synthesise and mobilise TAG, and of the placenta for uptake and transfer of fatty acids to the fetal circulation. In rhesus monkeys, birthweight of the infants was directly related to that of the mother and to the mother's weight gain in pregnancy (Price and Coe 2000). This suggests a multigenerational influence on birthweight through the maternal line.

There is evidence for adaptations to maternal lipid metabolism that may increase the availability of specific fatty acids for transfer to the fetus. In women (Postle *et al.* 1995, Otto *et al.* 1997), rats and guinea pigs (Burdge *et al.* 1994, Burdge and Postle 1994) pregnancy is associated with a specific physiological increase in the concentrations of AA and DHA in maternal blood which may be important for facilitating the supply of these fatty acids to the fetus, in particular to the central nervous system (Fig. 11.3a). In the rat (Burdge *et al.* 1994a), human (Postle *et al.* 1995, Otto *et al.* 1997) and guinea pig (Burdge and Postle 1994), the increase in plasma

DHA and AA concentrations is specifically due to *sn*-1-palmitoyl, *sn*-2-arachidonoyl or docosahexaenoyl PC species (Fig. 11.3b). This implies that the combination of AA or DHA with palmitic acid is of biological importance. In the rat, the increase in plasma *sn*-1-palmitoyl, *sn*-2-AA or DHA PC is due to a decrease in hepatic conversion of *sn*-1-palmitoyl to *sn*-2-stearoyl PC by the Lands pathway and enrichment of the diacylglycerol substrate pool (Burdge *et al.* 1994). The source of AA and DHA to support this metabolic adaptation is not clear. One possibility is mobilisation of fatty acid stores accumulated before pregnancy or in early gestation (Zeijdner *et al.* 1997). However, since there is no evidence for selective mobilisation of individual fatty acids from adipose tissue during pregnancy this is likely to be the result of specific channelling of DHA and AA into phospholipid precursor pools by the maternal liver. The activity of the rate-limiting enzyme for DHA and AA synthesis is increased in pregnancy (Larque *et al.* 2003a) (Fig.11.4a) and conversion of α-linolenic acid (αLNA) to DHA is greater in women than in men, and is up-regulated by oestrogen (Burdge and Wootton 2002, Burdge 2004) (Fig. 11.4b). Therefore, synthesis of AA and DHA from their precursor essential fatty acids linoleic acid and αLNA, respectively, may be an important source of these fatty acids for incorporation into plasma PC.

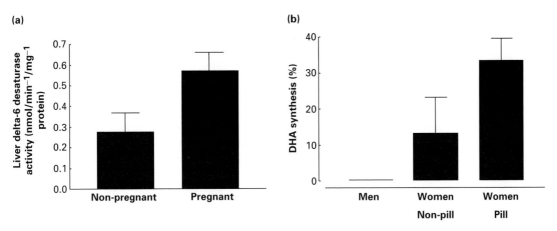

Figure 11.4 (a) Δ6 desaturase activity in livers from non-pregnant and pregnant rats (Larque *et al.* 2003a). (b) Synthesis of docosahexaenoic acid (22:6n-3) from α-linolenic acid in men and women who used or did not use an oral contraceptive pill (Burdge *et al.* 2002, Burdge and Wootton 2002).

Overall, adaptations to maternal hepatic fatty acid metabolism are important for facilitating supply of bulk and specific fatty acids to the fetus. Thus the extent to which fetal and infant demands for individual fatty acids are met by the mother is likely to depend substantially upon her metabolic capacity to mobilise, package and transport fatty acids to the placenta and mammary gland. Although maternal fat consumption is an important determinant of fatty acid supply to the fetus and infant, intakes of other nutrients may markedly alter the supply of fatty acids to the offspring. Feeding pregnant rats a low-protein diet reduced postnatal weight gain in the offspring in a manner dependent on amount of protein in the diet (Langley and Jackson 1994). Since reduced maternal protein intake constrains milk synthesis in the rat (Grigor *et al.* 1987), one explanation for lower weight gain is impaired fat supply in milk. Reduced maternal protein intake during pregnancy also modified the availability of individual fatty acids for transfer to the fetus. Feeding pregnant rats a diet containing 9% (w/w) casein compared to 18% casein (w/w) specifically impaired the pregnancy-associated increase in maternal liver and plasma DHA concentration and resulted in impaired accumulation of DHA into fetal brain phospholipids (Burdge *et al.* 2002). One possible explanation is impaired activity of the rate-limiting enzyme

Δ6-desaturase (De Tomas *et al.* 1983), which is responsible for the first step in the conversion of αLNA to DHA. The deficit in brain DHA content of the offspring was present six days after weaning. This suggests that the effects of impaired maternal DHA status persisted during lactation, although the diet-induced reduction in Δ6-desaturase activity was reversed during this period (De Tomas *et al.* 1983). It is also possible that DHA synthesis in the offspring may have been impaired. This is supported by the lower concentration of DHA in liver and plasma PC (Burdge *et al.* 2003) and lower Δ5-desaturase activity, although Δ6-desaturase activity was not altered (Ozanne *et al.* 1998). Overall, the efficacy of maternal fatty acid supply to the fetus can be constrained by the availability of other nutrients. In addition to poor maternal supply of specific fatty acids, lower synthetic capacity in the offspring may also contribute to the overall deficit in fatty acid accumulation.

Placental fatty acid and cholesterol transport

The placenta provides an interface 4 μm thick and consisting of two membranes between maternal and fetal circulations. This provides the potential for selective nutrient transfer to meet fetal demands. Conversely, impaired function may constrain nutrient transfer, resulting in fetal undernutrition despite apparently normal maternal nutritional status. Understanding of the mechanisms by which lipids are taken up by the placenta, and transferred to the fetus is limited by the difficulties in replicating physiological perfusion in isolated placenta, and by differences between species in placental structure. A detailed review of placental fatty acid metabolism is provided by Haggarty (2002). The lipid pool which represents the primary substrate for placental fatty acid uptake is unclear, although it is possible that different fatty acids may be obtained selectively from different lipid classes in the maternal circulation (G. C. Burdge, unpublished observation, 2004). The placenta is unable to assimilate esterified fatty acids. Placental lipoprotein lipase (pLPL) is able to hydrolyse TAG, and possibly other lipids, thus making the esterified fatty acids available for uptake (Rothwell and Elphick 1982, Shafrir and Barash 1987, Kaminsky et al. 1991, Bonet et al. 1992). The placenta also contains receptors for VLDL, LDL and HDL which may facilitate presentation of esterified fatty acids to pLPL (Cummings et al. 1982, Naoum et al. 1987, Wittmaack et al. 1995). Although free fatty acids can pass passively across cell membranes, uptake across the microvillus surface facing the maternal circulation is mediated by one or more proteins: a fatty acid binding protein which preferentially binds the PUFA AA and DHA (Campbell et al. 1998), and fatty acid transfer proteins. The fatty acid transfer proteins may also be responsible for secretion of fatty acids into the fetal circulation. Within the syncitiotrophoblast layer, fatty acids may be used for energy, transiently esterified into phospholipids or TAG pools, or mobilised directly into the fetal circulation. In perfused human placenta, linoleic acid was secreted into the fetal circulation as free fatty acid while arachidonic acid was secreted esterified to phospholipid (Kuhn and Crawford 1986). However, tracer studies in pregnant women indicate oleic, linoleic and palmitic acids, and DHA are secreted as free fatty acids (Larque et al. 2003b).

The partitioning and uptake of NEFA from the fetal circulation into developing tissues is poorly understood. One determining factor may be the relative blood flow at the ductus venosus between the fetal liver and peripheral circulation. Partitioning of blood flow towards the liver may facilitate incorporation into lipoproteins, which is required for uptake of fatty acids into fetal adipose tissue, by the action of lipoprotein lipase, while shunting towards the peripheral circulation may increase supply of NEFA to other tissues such as the brain, cardiovascular system and skeletal muscle. Although this requires investigation, this suggestion is supported by the observation of preferential blood flow away from the liver and towards the upper body, including the brain, in fetuses with intrauterine growth retardation (Bellotti et al. 2004).

The effects of impaired assimilation of polyunsaturated fatty acids on fetal development

The central nervous system

The brain and retina contain large amounts of DHA, particularly in synaptosomes (in the rat about 30% total fatty acids in phosphatidylethanolamine (PE) and phosphatidylserine) (Breckenridge et al. 1972) and in the outer membrane fraction of rod cells (in the rat 45% of PE total fatty acids) (Sanders et al. 1984). In the brain, DHA is involved in a number of processes associated with neurodevelopment and function, including Na^+/K^+ ATPase activity (Bowen and Clandinin 2002), dopaminergic and serotoninergic receptor activities (Zimmer et al. 2000), GABA receptor A activity (Nabekura et al. 1998), diacylglycerol kinase signalling (Vaidyanathan et al. 1994), gene expression via the activities of peroxisomal proliferator-activated receptors (Rojas et al. 2002) and the retinoid X receptor (De Urquiza et al. 2000), and nerve growth factor secretion (Ikemoto et al. 2000). The DHA content of rod-cell PE in the retina has an important effect on the activity of rhodopsin as it is required for optimal formation of the metarhodopsin–transducin complex (Niu et al. 2001, Mitchell et al. 2003) and for the activation of metarhodopsin 1 to metarhodopsin 2 (Litman *et al.* 2001). These studies also imply that DHA may modulate other receptor/G-protein interactions.

Studies of human infants and of animal models show that the accretion of DHA into neural cell membranes during gestation and early postnatal life is an important determinant of subsequent brain and retinal function. In humans, accumulation of DHA into brain phospholipids occurs principally during the last trimester and during the first two years after birth, which coincides with the major growth phase (Martinez and Mougan 1998). In the rat, DHA accumulation into the brain is largely restricted to the suckling period (Sinclair and Crawford 1972), while in the guinea pig DHA accumulation is essentially complete at birth (Burdge and Postle 1995). Such differences in DHA accumulation are reflected in the level of neurological activity at birth: the newborn rat has poor motor and visual function, while these processes are more advanced in the human infant, but less developed than in the guinea pig, which is able to stand, see and feed soon after birth. Such temporal differences in DHA accretion must be considered in the interpretation of the effects of DHA supply to different species.

The preterm human infant is doubly disadvantaged in terms of DHA accretion. First, placental DHA supply is terminated at birth. Second, the rate of accumulation of DHA into adipose tissue in the human fetus before birth is about 20 times greater than into the brain (Clandinin *et al.* 1981) and this is rapidly mobilised in the early postnatal period, possibly to compensate for the switch in fatty acid supply from the placenta to the mammary gland. Thus infants who are born preterm have smaller DHA reserves that can be mobilised for supply to other tissues. Although the human infant possesses some capacity for conversion of the precursor essential fatty acid αLNA to DHA, this is unlikely to satisfy the demands of developing tissues (Poisson *et al.* 1993, Salem *et al.* 1996). Thus one consequence of preterm birth is reduced accumulation of DHA into the central nervous system, leading to impaired retinal function, in particular reduced visual acu-

ity (Neuringer 2000) and cognitive ability (Carlson *et al.* 1994). Such effects are reversible by feeding milk formula containing preformed DHA (Neuringer 2000). However, supplementation with DHA alone may result in impaired infant growth, which can be corrected by addition of arachidonic acid to the feed (Ryan *et al.* 1999). Unfortunately, there is only limited information on the specific effects of impaired DHA accretion due to preterm birth on long-term neurological function. Infants born preterm and fed milk formula lacking preformed DHA or AA had lower IQ scores at 8 years of age compared with those fed breast milk, which contains about 0.2% DHA and 0.4% AA (Lucas *et al.* 1992), while the persistence of neurological dysfunction in infants born at term was greater in those fed milk formula compared to breast milk (Lanting *et al.* 1994). Although these studies only provide circumstantial evidence for a persistent long-term effect of reduced DHA accretion on neurological function, they are consistent with the observation that consumption of milk formula lacking preformed DHA resulted in lower DHA concentration in brain phospholipids of infants who were born at term but subsequently died of sudden infant death syndrome (Farquharson *et al.* 1992). Furthermore, individuals who suffer from mental illness, including Alzheimer's disease, bipolar disorder and schizophrenia, have lower circulating DHA concentrations, which implies that impaired DHA metabolism may be an important causal factor in these conditions (Horrobin and Bennett 1999, Conquer *et al.* 2000).

The association between fetal growth and subsequent cognitive function is unclear. While lower fetal growth was not associated with impaired cognitive function in adulthood (Martyn *et al.* 1996), individuals with greater head circumference at birth showed a slower decline in memory function in old age (Gale *et al.* 2003). One interpretation of these results may be that there is sufficient neurodevelopmental plasticity to support apparently normal cognitive function in adults despite variations in nutrient accretion in early life, which is consistent with the observation that PUFA status at birth was not related to cognitive function at 7 years of age

(Bakker *et al.* 2003). However, when neural function is in decline, the functional consequences of deficits in DHA become apparent. One possible mechanism is that since DHA protects against neuronal apoptosis (Kim *et al.* 2000), lower DHA status may lead to fewer surviving neurones during development, resulting in a more obvious effect of neurodegeneration on brain function.

The results of studies using animal models of maternal dietary n-3 fatty acid deprivation essentially support the observations in humans and provide important mechanistic insights into the effects of impaired DHA accumulation on neurological function. Typically these studies involve feeding pregnant animals a diet lacking DHA and with reduced αLNA content. Overall, these studies show decreased concentrations of DHA in the brain and retina (Connor and Neuringer 1988, Leat *et al.* 1986). The preferential looking test indicated impaired retinal function in nonhuman primates (Neuringer *et al.* 1984). In rhesus monkeys, postnatal supplementation with DHA reversed the deficit in DHA accumulation into the brain and retina, and decreased the concentration of docospentaenoic acid n-6, indicating plasticity with respect to membrane phospholipid composition (Connor *et al.* 1988, 1990). Maternal dietary n-3 deprivation also decreased cognitive function in the offspring of rats (Catalan *et al.* 2002). Reisbick *et al.* (1990, 1994) assessed the behavioural effects of maternal n-3 PUFA deprivation in offspring at about 3 years of age. These studies showed marked behavioural polydipsia, increased locomotor activity and stereotyped behaviour activity compared to controls. Thus prenatal n-3 fatty acid deprivation results in persistent impairment of brain function in the offspring.

Animal models have provided important insights into the mechanism by which DHA affects neural development and function. In the rat, maternal n-3 fatty acid deprivation during pregnancy results in impaired neurite outgrowth in specific brain regions at 21 days of age (Ahmad *et al.* 2002). For example, the size of neurones was reduced in the CA1, CA3 and CA3/2, but not in the CA2 layers of the hippocampus, and in the dorsomedial, but not ventromedial or arcuate, regions of the hypothalamus. This suggests that the functional effects of impaired DHA accumulation on the brain may be very specific. Impaired DHA incorporation into brain phospholipids is also associated with reduced nerve growth factor secretion, dopaminergic and serotoninergic neurotransmission and reduced Na^+/K^+ ATPase activity (Zimmer *et al.* 2000, Bowen and Clandinin 2002). The importance of the effects of impaired DHA accumulation on behaviour is illustrated by the observation that pigs deprived prenatally of DHA showed reduced maze-learning ability which was partly ameliorated by L-dihydroxyphenylalanine (Ng and Innis 2003). In the retina, substitution of DHA with more saturated fatty acids, such as docosapentaenoic acid n-6, impairs the conformational change in rhodopsin required for activation and the interaction of rhodopsin with transducin (Litman *et al.* 2001, Mitchell *et al.* 2003). The adverse effects of impaired DHA accumulation on retinal function may contribute to reduced performance in tests, such as maze learning, designed to test cognitive function.

Blood pressure

Programming of persistent hypertension in the offspring of rats fed a low-protein diet during pregnancy is a well-established observation (Langley and Jackson 1994), which has been attributed to impaired function of the hypothalamic–pituitary–adrenal (HPA) axis leading to altered corticosteroid action (Langley-Evans *et al.* 1996). Recent studies have demonstrated that n-3 PUFA deprivation during the perinatal period in the rat results in persistent hypertension in the offspring (Weisinger *et al.* 2001, Armitage *et al.* 2003). Since feeding a low-protein diet during pregnancy also compromises DHA accretion in the offspring (Burdge *et al.* 2002, 2003), this may represent one additional mechanism by which maternal dietary restriction may programme hypertension. Interestingly, the n-3-PUFA-deficient diet decreased DHA concentration in the hypothalamus (Armitage *et al.* 2003), and so may influence the regulation of blood pressure via the HPA axis, possible by altering the structural development of the hypothalamus (Ahmad *et al.* 2002).

Immune function

Pregnancy is associated with marked changes in maternal immune function that appear to be required in order to prevent the rejection of the fetus, which bears 'non-self' paternal antigens. Among the most important mechanisms involved is the down-regulation of the T helper 1 (Th1) phenotype of T lymphocytes and the up-regulation of the T helper 2 (Th2) phenotype (Dudley *et al.* 1993, Lin *et al.* 1993, Wegmann *et al.* 1993, Hill *et al.* 1995, Reinhard *et al.* 1998). Although this will most likely result in impairment of maternal defence against intracellular pathogens like bacteria and viruses, the consequence of not undergoing this change can be fetal rejection (Raghupathy 1997, 2001, Reinhard *et al.* 1998). The change in maternal T cell phenotypes has been most frequently reported by sampling maternal peripheral blood (e.g. Reinhard *et al.* 1998), but it has also been observed at the fetomaternal interface (Lin *et al.* 1993) and it seems likely that the immune system of the fetus is also skewed towards the Th 2 phenotype. A number of mechanisms are likely to be involved in the down-regulation of Th1 cells during normal pregnancy. These include a role for progesterone which biases towards the Th2 phenotype (Szerekes-Bartho and Wegmann 1996), a role for upregulation of Fas on some T cells causing their apoptosis (Reinhard *et al.* 1998) and a role for the AA-derived mediator prostaglandin (PG) E_2, which potently down-regulates differentiation to, and activity of, Th1 cells (see Miles *et al.* 2003). Thus there may be a role for an appropriate supply of AA at critical periods of immune change that are required to sustain pregnancy, although this has not been well investigated.

The fetal immune system begins to develop quite early in gestation (reviewed by Whitelaw and Parkin 1988, Kimpton *et al.* 1994). In humans pre-B and pre-T cells arise by eight weeks of gestation, predominantly in the fetal liver. The thymus begins to develop at six weeks gestation, the spleen and lymph nodes later and the gut-associated lymphoid tissue later still. Note however that these organs continue to grow and develop for a substantial period (many years) post-birth (see Prentice *et al.* 1999). Immature B cells express surface immunoglobulin from around 9–12 weeks of gestation and fetal T cells respond to mitogens at around this time. The generation of new immune cells and of lymphoid tissue during pregnancy and after birth will require a suitable supply of fatty acids. Immune cells, at least in adults, are typically rich in PUFA (Calder 2001), and these fatty acids play a role in ensuring appropriate membrane structure and as precursors for eicosanoids involved in regulation of immune development and responses. Thus it seems likely that ensuring an appropriate supply of fatty acids will be important in determining appropriate immune system development, and here there may be competition with other tissues and organs that might have similar demands. The phospholipids of immune cells from human adults contain 15 to 25% of fatty acids as AA and 1.5 to 5% as DHA (Kew *et al.* 2003), although this will depend upon cell type, phospholipid fraction, dietary fatty acid intake, and processes affecting PUFA metabolism and handling. It is known that altering the fatty acid composition of immune cells from adults modifies their function (Calder 2001, 2003), again stressing the importance of ensuring an appropriate supply of fatty acids. The fatty acid composition of human fetal immune cells has been poorly characterised, although one study reported that the proportion of AA in cord mononuclear cells ($11.6 \pm 4.5\%$ of fatty acids) was lower and more variable than that in cells from healthy adults ($15.9 \pm 1.2\%$), and that this was associated with lower production of PGE_2 (Murphy and Reen 1996).

A limited number of studies have investigated the effect of manipulations of the fatty acid composition of the diet in pregnancy on subsequent immune competence. In one study pregnant rats were fed on a diet providing 9% by weight coconut oil plus 1% by weight corn oil, or on a diet providing 10% by weight corn oil. Spleen natural killer-cell activity in the offspring at weaning was lower in the coconut-oil group, even though the dams of both groups had been transferred to standard chow when they gave birth (Calder and Yaqoob 2000). In another study rats were fed on diets providing 10% by weight of either corn oil or fish oil throughout pregnancy and lactation. At the age of 7 days the pups were injected intraperitoneally with live group B *Streptococcus*. Pups from dams fed on the fish-oil diet were more likely to survive (79% survival) than those fed on the corn-oil diet (49% survival), and this was associated with lower lung PGE$_2$ concentrations in the former group (Rayon *et al*. 1997). Human studies in this area are rare. However, one study examined the effect of adding AA and DHA to preterm infant formula on immune cell phenotypes. Preterm infants (gestational age 27–36 weeks) received breast milk, standard preterm formula or formula containing AA and DHA from 14 days after birth for four weeks (Field *et al*. 2000). There were no differences among the groups with respect to the total number of blood lymphocytes or the proportions of lymphocytes, monocytes, granulocytes, T cells or CD8 cells. There were some differences in the proportions of CD4 (helper T) and B cells, but the main finding was a lower proportion of CD45RO$^+$ CD4 cells (memory/mature helper T cells) in the standard-formula group than in the other two groups. The production of the cytokine interleukin-10 decreased in the standard-formula group but not in the breast-milk or formula-plus-PUFA groups. This study suggests that a supply of AA and/or DHA results in better maintenance or maturation of some immune cell phenotypes and responses in preterm infants and may indicate a role for these fatty acids in immune development in the last trimester of normal pregnancy.

Although skewing of the immune response towards the Th2 phenotype appears to be necessary to favour a successful pregnancy, this phenotype is associated with development of atopy and related allergic diseases (Romagnani 2000). Sensitisation to allergens can occur early in life (Jones *et al*. 1996), and one study reported that significant amounts of PGE$_2$ are present in human amniotic fluid at the time at which atopic sensitisation might occur (Jones *et al*. 2001). Thus the presence of excess PGE$_2$ at

certain times during pregnancy may favour allergic sensitisation (via effects on the Th1 and Th2 phenotypes), at least in certain individuals. Some have argued that this situation arises as a result of an absolute or relative excess of n-6 over n-3 fatty acids in the diet (Hodge *et al*. 1994, Black and Sharpe 1997, Kankaanpaa *et al*. 1999), although this is probably a simplistic view. Nevertheless, since it is known from studies in animals and in human adults that consumption of long-chain n-3 PUFAs in the form of fish oil decreases the AA content of immune cells and decreases PGE$_2$ production (Calder 2001, 2003), there has been some interest in the influence of fish oil on the development of allergic diseases (see Prescott and Calder 2004). A limited number of biochemical measurements do suggest an inverse relationship between n-3 PUFA status early in life and atopic disease. For example, the proportions of EPA, docosapentaenoic acid and DHA were higher in umbilical cord serum phospholipids and in breast milk from non-allergic compared with allergic mothers (Yu *et al*. 1996, 1998), while higher n-3 PUFAs in breast milk were associated with decreased likelihood of atopy in the infants (Duchen *et al*. 1998). Intriguingly, there are positive relationships between head circumference at birth and risk of asthma at 16 years of age (Fergusson *et al*. 1997) or likelihood of having an elevated total immunoglobulin E concentration at 50 years of age (Godfrey *et al*. 1994). The mechanism underpinning these associations is not known, but the strong positive relationships between the concentrations of n-6 fatty acids in umbilical cord phospholipids and head circumference at birth (Leaf *et al*. 1992) suggest that there may be subtle relationships between the supply of these fatty acids, brain growth and immune system development.

Despite a biologically plausible mechanism and supportive biochemical data, the key to demonstrating a protective effect of increased n-3 fatty acid consumption towards allergic disease must come from well-designed placebo-controlled intervention studies. Given that atopic sensitisation may occur in utero, such studies need to be performed in pregnant women. The results of one such study have been reported recently (Dunstan *et al.* 2003a, 2003b). In this study women who were proven to be allergic through clinical history and positive skin-prick test results consumed fish oil providing 1.1 g EPA plus 2.2 g DHA per day from 20 weeks gestation until delivery (the placebo group consumed olive oil). There was no effect of fish oil on the numbers or proportions of T cells, helper T cells, suppressor T cells, B cells or natural killer cells in cord blood (Dunstan *et al.* 2003a). Immunoglobuin E and seven cytokines were detectable in only a small minority of cord plasma samples (Dunstan *et al.* 2003a). However, interleukin 13 (IL-13) was detected in 64% of cord plasmas in the placebo group and 45% in the fish-oil group (Dunstan *et al.* 2003a). Overall cord plasma IL-13 concentrations were significantly lower (by 65%) in the fish-oil group; IL-13 production by cord blood T cells may be a useful marker of risk for subsequent atopic disease (Ohshima *et al.* 2002). There was a significant inverse relationship between the proportion of DHA in cord blood erythrocytes and cord plasma IL-13. The authors also studied cord blood lymphocyte responses to ex-vivo stimulation with mitogens and allergens (Dunstan *et al.* 2003b). The cytokine profiles produced by cord blood cells in response to allergens have been reported to be predictive of later atopy (Tang *et al.* 1994, Martinez *et al.* 1995, Smart and Kemp 2001). In general the production of all cytokines investigated (both Th1 and Th2 type) was lower in the fish-oil group, but the differences between groups failed to reach statistical significance in most cases (Dunstan *et al.* 2003b). There were, however, significant negative correlations between the EPA and DHA contents of cord blood erythrocytes and production of some cytokines in response to some allergens (Dunstan *et al.* 2003b). Clinical measurements in the infants at 1 year of age showed lower severity of atopic dermatitis and less skin-prick test positivity, especially to egg allergen, in the fish-oil group (Dunstan *et al.* 2003b). However, the study was not well powered to identify clinical benefits and so the true significance of the cord blood findings is not yet clear.

Conclusions

Fatty acids are involved in a wide range of developmental processes and the demands of different tissues for individual fatty acids change and differ during maturation. There are maternal adaptations during pregnancy that act to ensure appropriate supply of specific fatty acids to the fetus. These adaptations tailor the dietary fatty acid composition to meet fetal demands. Differences between individuals with respect to the magnitude of physiological change during pregnancy may be an important factor in determining differential growth and development of fetal tissues. An inability to meet the fetal demand for specific fatty acids may impair the growth and development of fetal tissues and this may have adverse consequences beyond pregnancy.

REFERENCES

Adolph, E. F. and Heggeness, F. W. (1971). Age changes in body water and fat in fetal and infant mammals. *Growth*, **35**, 55–63.

Ahmad, A., Moriguchi, T. and Salem, N. (2002). Decrease in neuron size in docosahexaenoic acid-deficient brain. *Pediatr. Neurol.*, **26**, 210–18.

Allen, L. H., Lung'aho, M. S., Shaheen, M., Harrison, G. G., Neumann, C. and Kirksey, A. (1994). Maternal body mass index and pregnancy outcome in the Nutrition Collaborative Research Support Program. *Eur. J. Clin. Nutr.*, **48**, (Suppl. 3), S68–76.

Alvarez, J. J., Montelongo, A., Iglesiasm A., Lasuncionm M. A. and Herrera, E. (1996). Longitudinal study on lipoprotein profile, high density lipoprotein subclass, and postheparin lipases during gestation in women. *J. Lipid Res.*, **37**, 299–308.

Armitage, J. A., Pearce, A. D., Sinclair, A. J., Vingrys, A. J., Weisinger, R. S. and Weisinger, H. S. (2003). Increased blood pressure later in life may be associated with perinatal n-3 fatty acid deficiency. *Lipids*, **38**, 459–64.

Ash, S., Fisher, C. C., Truswell, A. S., Allen, J. R. and Irwig, L. (1989). Maternal weight gain, smoking and other factors in pregnancy as predictors of infant birth-weight in Sydney women. *Aust. NZ J. Obstet. Gynaecol.*, **29**, 212–19.

Ashton, M. R., Postle, A. D., Hall, M. A., Smith, S. L., Kelly, F. J. and Normand, I. C. (1992). Phosphatidylcholine composition of endotracheal tube aspirates of neonates and subsequent respiratory disease. *Arch. Dis. Child.*, **67**, 378–82.

Bakker, E. C., Ghys, A. J., Kester, A. D. *et al.* (2003). Long-chain polyunsaturated fatty acids at birth and cognitive function at 7 y of age. *Eur. J. Clin. Nutr.*, **57**, 89–95.

Bellotti, M., Pennati, G., De Gasperi, C., Bozzo, M., Battaglia, F. C. and Ferrazzi, E. (2004). Simultaneous measurements of umbilical venous, fetal hepatic, and ductus venosus blood flow in growth-restricted human fetuses. *Am. J. Obstet. Gynecol.*, **190**, 1347–58.

Benassayag, C., Mignot, T. M., Haouriguim M. *et al.* (1997). High polyunsaturated fatty acid, thromboxane A2, and alpha-fetoprotein concentrations at the human feto-maternal interface. *J. Lipid Res.*, **38**, 276–86.

Black, P. N. and Sharpe, S. (1997). Dietary fat and asthma: is there a connection? *Eur. Respir. J.*, **10**, 6–12.

Bonet, B., Brunzell, J. D., Gown, A. M. and Knopp, R. H. (1992). Metabolism of very-low-density lipoprotein triglyceride by human placental cells: the role of lipoprotein lipase. *Metabolism*, **41**, 596–603.

Bowen, R. A. and Clandinin, M. T. (2002). Dietary low linolenic acid compared with docosahexaenoic acid alter synaptic plasma membrane phospholipid fatty acid composition and sodium-potassium ATPase kinetics in developing rats. *J. Neurochem.*, **83**, 764–74.

Breckenridge, W. C., Gombos, G. and Morgan, I. G. (1972). The lipid composition of adult rat brain synaptosomal plasma membranes. *Biochim. Biophys. Acta*, **266**, 695–707.

Burdge, G. (2004). Alpha-linolenic acid metabolism in men and women: nutritional and biological implications. *Curr. Opin. Clin. Nutr. Metab. Care*, **7**, 137–44.

Burdge, G. C. and Postle, A. D. (1994). Hepatic phospholipid molecular species in the guinea pig: adaptations to pregnancy. *Lipids*, **29**, 259–64.

(1995). Phospholipid molecular species composition of developing fetal guinea pig brain. *Lipids*, **30**, 719–24.

Burdge, G. C. and Wootton, S. A. (2002). Conversion of alpha-linolenic acid to eicosapentaenoic, docosapentaenoic and docosahexaenoic acids in young women. *Br. J. Nutr.*, **88**, 411–20.

Burdge, G. C., Kelly, F. J. and Postle A. D. (1993). Synthesis of phosphatidylcholine in guinea-pig fetal lung involves acyl remodelling and differential turnover of individual molecular species. *Biochim. Biophys. Acta*, **1166**, 251–7.

Burdge, G. C., Hunt, A. N. and Postle, A. D. (1994). Mechanisms of hepatic phosphatidylcholine synthesis in adult rat: effects of pregnancy. *Biochem. J.*, **303**, 941–7.

Burdge, G. C., Dunn, R. L., Wootton, S. A. and Jackson, A. A. (2002). Effect of reduced dietary protein intake on hep-

atic and plasma essential fatty acid concentrations in the adult female rat: effect of pregnancy and consequences for accumulation of arachidonic and docosahexaenoic acids in fetal liver and brain. *Br. J. Nutr.*, **88**, 379–87.

Burdge, G. C., Delange, E., Dubois, L. *et al.* (2003). Effect of reduced maternal protein intake in pregnancy in the rat on the fatty acid composition of brain, liver, plasma, heart and lung phospholipids of the offspring after weaning. *Br. J. Nutr.*, **90**, 345–52.

Calder, P. C. (2001). N-3 polyunsaturated fatty acids, inflammation and immunity: pouring oil on troubled waters or another fishy tale? *Nutr. Res.*, **21**, 309–41.

(2003). N-3 polyunsaturated fatty acids and inflammation: from molecular biology to the clinic. *Lipids*, **38**, 343–52.

Calder, P. C. and Yaqoob, P. (2000). The level of protein and type of fat in the diet of pregnant rats both affect lymphocyte function in the offspring. *Nutr. Res.*, **20**, 995–1005.

Campbell, F. M., Gordon, M. J. and Dutta-Roy, A. K. (1998). Placental membrane fatty acid-binding protein preferentially binds arachidonic and docosahexaenoic acids. *Life Sci.*, **63**, 235–40.

Carlson, S. E., Werkman, S. H., Peeples, J. M. and Wilson, W. M. (1994). Long-chain fatty acids and early visual and cognitive development of preterm infants. *Eur. J. Clin. Nutr.*, **48**, (Suppl. 2), S27–30.

Catalan, J., Moriguchi, T., Slotnick, B., Murthy, M., Greiner, R. S. and Salem, N. (2002). Cognitive deficits in docosahexaenoic acid-deficient rats. *Behav. Neurosci.*, **116**, 1022–31.

Catalano, P. M., Thomas, A. J., Huston, L. P. and Fung, C. M. (1998). Effect of maternal metabolism on fetal growth and body composition. *Diabetes Care*, **21**, (Suppl. 2), B85–90.

Clandinin, M. T., Chappell, J. E., Heim, T., Swyer, P. R. and Chance, G. W. (1981). Fatty acid utilization in perinatal de novo synthesis of tissues. *Early Hum. Dev.*, **5**, 355–66.

Connor, W. E. and Neuringer, M. (1988). The effects of n-3 fatty acid deficiency and repletion upon the fatty acid composition and function of the brain and retina. *Prog. Clin. Biol. Res.*, **282**, 275–94.

Connor, W. E., Neuringer, M. and Lin, D. S. (1990). Dietary effects on brain fatty acid composition: the reversibility of n-3 fatty acid deficiency and turnover of docosahexaenoic acid in the brain, erythrocytes, and plasma of rhesus monkeys. *J. Lipid Res.*, **31**, 237–47.

Conquer, J. A., Tierney, M. C., Zecevic, J., Bettger, W. J. and Fisher, R. H. (2000). Fatty acid analysis of blood plasma of patients with Alzheimer's disease, other types of dementia, and cognitive impairment. *Lipids*, **35**, 1305–12.

Correia, H. R., Balseiro, S. C., Correia, E. R., Mota, P. G. and de Areia, M. L. (2004). Why are human newborns so fat?

Relationship between fatness and brain size at birth. *Am. J. Hum. Biol.*, **16**, 24–30.

Cummings, S. W., Hatley, W., Simpson, E. R. and Ohashi, M. (1982). The binding of high and low density lipoproteins to human placental membrane fractions. *J. Clin. Endocrinol. Metab.*, **54**, 903–8.

Darmady, J. M. and Postle, A. D. (1982). Lipid metabolism in pregnancy. *Br. J. Obstet. Gynaecol.*, **89**, 211–15.

De Tomas, M. E., Mercuri, O. and Serres, C. (1983). Effect of cross-fostering rats at birth on the normal supply of essential fatty acids during protein deficiency. *J. Nutr.*, **113**, 314–19.

de Urquiza, A. M., Liu, S., Sjoberg, M. *et al.* (2000). Docosahexaenoic acid, a ligand for the retinoid X receptor in mouse brain. *Science*, **290**, 2140–4.

Dempsey, J. C., Williams, M. A., Leisenring, W. M., Shy K. and Luthy, D. A. (2004). Maternal birth weight in relation to plasma lipid concentrations in early pregnancy. *Am. J. Obstet. Gynecol.*, **190**, 1359–68.

Dietschy, J. M,, Turley, S. D. and Spady, D. K. (1993). Role of liver in the maintenance of cholesterol and low density lipoprotein homeostasis in different animal species, including humans. *Jo. Lipid Res.*, **34**, 1637–59.

Dougherty, C. R. and Jones, A. D. (1982). The determinants of birth weight. *Am. J. Obstet. Gynecol.*, **144**, 190–200.

Duchen, K., Yu, G. and Bjorksten, B. (1998). Atopic sensitization during the first year of life in relation to long chain polyunsaturated fatty acid levels in human milk. *Pediatr. Res.*, **44**, 478–84.

Dudley, D. J., Chen, C. L., Mitchell, M. D., Daynes, R. A. and Araneo, B. A. (1993).Adaptive immune responses during murine pregnancy: pregnancy-induced regulation of lymphokine production by activated T lymphocytes. *Am. J. Obstet. Gynecol.*, **168**, 1155–63.

Dunlop, M. and Court, J. M. (1978). Lipogenesis in developing human adipose tissue. *Early Hum. Dev.*, **2**, 123–30.

Dunstan, J. A., Mori, T. A., Barden, A. *et al.* (2003a). Maternal fish oil supplementation in pregnancy reduces interleukin-13 levels in cord blood of infants at high risk of atopy. *Clin. Exp. Allergy*, **33**, 442–8.

(2003b). Fish oil supplementation in pregnancy modifies neonatal allergen-specific immune responses and clinical outcomes in infants at high risk of atopy: a randomized, controlled trial. *J. Allergy Clin. Immunol.*, **112**, 1178–84.

Farquharson, J., Cockburn, F., Patrick, W. A., Jamieson, E. C. and Logan, R. W. (1992). Infant cerebral cortex phospholipid fatty-acid composition and diet. *Lancet*, **340**, 810–13.

(1993). Effect of diet on infant subcutaneous tissue triglyceride fatty acids. *Arch. Dis. Child.*, **69**, 589–93.

Fergusson, D. M., Crane, J., Beasley, R. and Horwood, L. J. (1997). Perinatal factors and atopic diseases in childhood. *Clin. Exp. Allergy*, **27**, 1394–401.

Field, C. J., Thomson, C. A., Van Aerde, J. E. *et al.* (2000). Lower proportion of CD45R0+ cells and deficient interleukin-10 production by formula-fed infants, compared with human-fed, is corrected with supplementation of long-chain polyunsaturated fatty acids. *J. Pediatr. Gastroenterol. Nutr.*, **31**, 291–9.

Fielding, B. A. and Frayn, K. N. (2003). Lipid metabolism. *Curr. Opin. Lipidol.*, **14**, 389–91.

Fraser, R. (1999) Insulin resistance in pregnancy. *Med. Biochem.*, **1**, 155–66.

Gale, C. R., Walton, S. and Martyn, C. N. (2003). Foetal and postnatal head growth and risk of cognitive decline in old age. *Brain*, **126**, 2273–8

Godfrey, K. M. and Barker, D. J. P. (2001). Fetal programming and adult health. *Public Health Nutr.*, **4**, 611–24.

Godfrey, K. M., Barker, D. J. P. and Osmond, C. (1994). Disproportionate fetal growth and raised IgE concentration in adult life. *Clin. Exp. Allergy*, **24**, 641–8.

Grigor, M. R., Allan, J. E., Carrington, J. M. *et al.* (1987). Effect of dietary protein and food restriction on milk production and composition, maternal tissues and enzymes in lactating rats. *J. Nutr.*, **117**, 1247–58.

Grimes, R. W., Pepe, G. J. and Albrecht, E. D. (1996). Regulation of human placental trophoblast low-density lipoprotein uptake in vitro by estrogen. *J. Clin. Endocrinol. Metab.*, **81**, 2675–9.

Hack, M., Breslau, N., Aram, D., Weissman, B., Klein, N. and Borawski-Clark, E. (1992). The effect of very low birth weight and social risk on neurocognitive abilities at school age. *J. Dev. Behav. Pediatr.*, **13**, 412–20.

Hadders-Algra, M., Huisjes, H. J. and Touwen, B. C. (1988). Preterm or small-for-gestational-age infants: neurological and behavioural development at the age of 6 years. *Eur. J. Pediatr.*, **147**, 460–7.

Haggarty, P. (2002). Placental regulation of fatty acid delivery and its effect on fetal growth: a review. *Placenta.* **23**, (Suppl. A), S28–38.

Hill, J. A., Polgar, K. and Anderson, D. J. (1995). T-helper 1-type immunity to trophoblast in women with recurrent spontaneous abortion. *JAMA*, **273**, 1933–6.

Hodge, L., Peat, J. K. and Salome, C. (1994). Increased consumption of polyunsaturated oils may be a cause of increased prevalence of childhood asthma. *Aust. NZ J. Med.*, **24**, 727.

Horrobin, D. F. and Bennett, C. N. (1999). Depression and bipolar disorder: relationships to impaired fatty acid and phospholipid metabolism and to diabetes, cardiovascular disease,

immunological abnormalities, cancer, ageing and osteoporosis. Possible candidate genes. *Prostaglandins Leukot.
Essent. Fatty Acids*, **60**, 217–34.

Ikemoto, A., Nitta, A., Furukawa, S. *et al.* (2000). Dietary n-3 fatty
acid deficiency decreases nerve growth factor content in rat
hippocampus. *Neurosci. Lett.*, **285**, 99–102.

Innis, S. M. (2003). Perinatal biochemistry and physiology of
long-chain polyunsaturated fatty acids. *J. Pediatr.*, **143**
(Suppl. 4), S1–8.

Jeffcott, L. B. and Field, J. R. (1985). Current concepts of hyper-
lipaemia in horses and ponies. *Vet. Rec.*, **116**, 461–6.

Jones, A., Miles, E., Warner, J., Colwell, B., Bryant, T. and Warner,
J. (1996). Fetal peripheral blood mononuclear cell proliferative responses to mitogenic and allergenic stimuli during
gestation. *Pediatr. Allergy Immunol.*, **7**, 109–16.

Jones, C. A., Vance, G. H. S., Power, L. L., Pender, S. L. F., MacDon-
ald, T. T. and Warner, J. O. (2001). Costimulatory molecules
in the developing human gastrointestinal tract: a pathway
for fetal allergen priming. *J. Allergy Clin. Immunol.*, **108**,
235–41.

Kaminsky, S., D'Souza, S. W., Massey, R. F., Smart, J. L. and Sibley,
C. P. (1991). Effects of maternal undernutrition and uterine
artery ligation on placental lipase activities in the rat. *Biol.
Neonate*, **60**, 201–6.

Kankaanpaa, P., Sutas, Y., Salminen, S., Lichtenstein, A. and Iso-
lauri, E. (1999). Dietary fatty acids and allergy. *Ann. Med.*,
31, 282–7.

Kew, S., Banerjee, T., Minihane, A. M., Finnegan, Y. E., Williams,
C. M. and Calder, P. C. (2003). Relation between the fatty
acid composition of peripheral blood mononuclear cells
and measures of immune cell function in healthy, free-
living subjects aged 25–72 y. *Am. J. Clin. Nutr.*, **77**, 1278–86.

Kim, H. Y., Akbar. M., Lau, A. and Edsall, L. (2000). Inhibition
of neuronal apoptosis by docosahexaenoic acid (22:6n-3):
role of phosphatidylserine in antiapoptotic effect. *J. Biol.
Chem.*, **275**, 35215–23.

Kimpton, W. G., Washington, E. A. and Cahill, R. N. P. (1994). The
development of the immune system in the fetus. In: *Textbook of Fetal Physiology* (ed. G. D. Thorburn and R. Harding,
R). Oxford: Oxford University Press, pp. 245–55.

Knopp, R. H. (1997). Hormone-mediated changes in nutrient
metabolism in pregnancy: a physiological basis for normal
fetal development. *Ann. NY Acad. Sci.*, **817**, 251–71.

Kuhn, D. C. and Crawford, M. (1986). Placental essential fatty
acid transport and prostaglandin synthesis. *Prog. Lipid Res.*,
25, 345–53.

Kuzawa, C. W. (1998). Adipose tissue in human infancy and
childhood: an evolutionary perspective. *Am. J. Phys. Anthropol.*, **27**, (Suppl.), 177–209.

Langhoff-Roos, J., Lindmark, G. and Gebre-Medhin, M. (1987).
Maternal fat stores and fat accretion during pregnancy in
relation to infant birthweight. *Br. J. Obstet. Gynaecol.*, **94**,
1170–7.

Langley, S. C. and Jackson, A. A. (1994). Increased systolic blood
pressure in adult rats induced by fetal exposure to maternal
low protein diets. *Clin. Sci.*, **86**, 217–22.

Langley-Evans, S. C., Gardner, D. S. and Jackson, A. A. (1996).
Maternal protein restriction influences the programming
of the rat hypothalamic–pituitary–adrenal axis. *J. Nutr.*, **126**,
1578–85.

Lanting, C. I., Fidler, V., Huisman, M., Touwen, B. C. and
Boersma, E. R. (1994). Neurological differences between
9-year-old children fed breast-milk or formula-milk as
babies. *Lancet*, **344**, 1319–22.

Larque, E., Garcia-Ruiz, P. A., Perez-Llamas, F., Zamora, S. and
Gil, A. (2003a). Dietary trans fatty acids alter the compositions of microsomes and mitochondria and the activities of microsome delta6-fatty acid desaturase and glucose-
6-phosphatase in livers of pregnant rats. *J. Nutr.*, **133**,
2526–31.

Larque, E., Demmelmair, H., Berger, B., Hasbargen, U. and Koletzko, B. (2003b). In vivo investigation of the placental transfer of [^{13}C]-labeled fatty acids in humans. *J. Lipid Res.*, **44**,
49–55.

Leaf, A. A., Leighfield, M. J., Costeloe, K. L. and Crawford, M. A.
(1992). Long chain polyunsaturated fatty acids and fetal
growth. *Early Hum. Dev.*, **30**, 183–91.

Leat, W. M., Curtis, R., Millichamp, N. J. and Cox, R. W. (1986).
Retinal function in rats and guinea-pigs reared on diets low
in essential fatty acids and supplemented with linoleic or
linolenic acids. *Ann. Nutr. Metab.*, **30**, 166–74.

Lewis, D. S., Bertrand, H. A., Masoro, E. J., McGill, H. C., Carey,
K. D. and McMahan, C. A. (1983). Preweaning nutrition and
fat development in baboons. *J. Nutr.*, **113**, 2253–9.

Lin, H., Mosmann, T. R., Guilbert, L., Tuntipopipat, S. and Wegmann, T. G. (1993). Synthesis of T helper 2-type cytokines
at the maternal–fetal interface. *J. Immunol.*, **151**, 4562–73.

Litman, B. J., Niu, S. L., Polozova, A. and Mitchell, D. C. (2001).
The role of docosahexaenoic acid containing phospholipids in modulating G protein-coupled signaling pathways:
visual transduction. *J. Mol. Neurosci.*, **16**, 237–42

Lucas, A., Morley, R., Cole, T. J., Lister, G. and Leeson-Payne, C.
(1992). Breast milk and subsequent intelligence quotient in
children born preterm. *Lancet*, **339**, 261–4.

Martin-Hidalgo, A., Holm, C., Belfrage, P., Schotz, M. C. and Herrera, E. (1994). Lipoprotein lipase and hormone-sensitive
lipase activity and mRNA in rat adipose tissue during pregnancy. *Am. J. Physiol.*, **266**, E930–5.

Martinez, M. and Mougan, I. (1998). Fatty acid composition of human brain phospholipids during normal development. *J. Neurochem.*, **71**, 2528–33.

Martinez, F., Stern, D., Wright, A., Holberg, C., Taussig, L. and Halonen, M. (1995). Association of interleukin-2 and interferon-γ production by blood mononuclear cells in infancy with parental allergy skin tests and with subsequent development of atopy. *J. Allergy Clin. Immunol.*, **96**, 652–660.

Martyn, C. N., Gale, C. R., Sayer, A. A. and Fall, C. (1996). Growth *in utero* and cognitive function in adult life: follow up study of people born between 1920 and 1943. *BMJ*, **312**, 1393–6.

Miles, E. A., Aston, L. and Calder, P. C. (2003). In vitro effects of eicosanoids derived from different 20-carbon fatty acids on T helper type 1 and T helper type 2 cytokine production in human whole-blood cultures. *Clin. Exp. Allergy*, **33**, 624–32.

Mitchell, D. C., Niu, S. L. and Litman, B. J. (2003). Enhancement of G protein-coupled signaling by DHA phospholipids. *Lipids*, **38**, 437–43.

Murphy, F. J. and Reen, D. J. (1996). Diminished production of prostaglandin E2 by monocytes of newborns is due to altered fatty acid membrane content and reduced cyclooxygenase activity. *J. Immunol.*, **157**, 3116–21.

Nabekura, J., Noguchi, K., Witt, M. R., Nielsen, M. and Akaike, N. (1998). Functional modulation of human recombinant gamma-aminobutyric acid type A receptor by docosahexaenoic acid. *J. Biol. Chem.*, **273**, 11056–61.

Naoum, H. G., De Chazal, R. C., Eaton, B. M. and Contractor, S. F. (1987). Characterization and specificity of lipoprotein binding to term human placental membranes. *Biochim. Biophys. Acta*, **902**, 193–9.

Napoli, C., Glass, C. K., Witztum, J. L., Deutsch, R., D'Armiento, F. P. and Palinski, W. (1999). Influence of maternal hypercholesterolaemia during pregnancy on progression of early atherosclerotic lesions in childhood: Fate of Early Lesions in Children (FELIC) study. *Lancet*, **354**, 1234–41.

Neufeld, L. M., Haas, J. D., Grajeda, R. and Martorell, R. (2004). Changes in maternal weight from the first to second trimester of pregnancy are associated with fetal growth and infant length at birth. *Am. J. Clin. Nutr.*, **79**, 646–52.

Neuringer, M. (2000). Infant vision and retinal function in studies of dietary long-chain polyunsaturated fatty acids: methods, results, and implications. *Am. J. Clin. Nutr.*, **71**, (Suppl.1), 256–67S.

Neuringer, M., Connor, W. E., Van Petten, C. and Barstad, L. (1984). Dietary omega-3 fatty acid deficiency and visual loss in infant rhesus monkeys. *J. Clini. Investig.*, **73**, 272–6.

Ng, K. F. and Innis, S. M. (2003). Behavioral responses are altered in piglets with decreased frontal cortex docosahexaenoic acid. *J. Nutr.*, **133**, 3222–7.

Niu, S. L., Mitchell, D. C. and Litman, B. J. (2001). Optimization of receptor-G protein coupling by bilayer lipid composition II: formation of metarhodopsin II-transducin complex. *J. Biol. Chem.*, **276**, 42807–11.

Noble, R. C., Steele, W. and Moore, J. H. (1971). The plasma lipids of the ewe during pregnancy and lactation. *Res. Vet. Sci.*, **12**, 47–53.

Ohshima, Y., Yasutomi, M., Omata, N. *et al.* (2002). Dysregulation of IL-13 production by cord blood CD4$^+$ T cells is associated with the subsequent development of atopic disease in infants. *Pediatr. Res.*, **51**, 195–200.

Otto, S. J., Houwelingen, A. C., Antal, M. *et al.* (1997). Maternal and neonatal essential fatty acid status in phospholipids: an international comparative study. *Eur. J. Clin. Nutr.*, **51**, 232–42.

Ozanne, S. E., Martensz, N. D., Petry, C. J., Loizou, C. L. and Hales, C. N. (1998). Maternal low protein diet in rats programmes fatty acid desaturase activities in the offspring. *Diabetologia*, **41**, 1337–42.

Palinski, W. and Napoli, C. (2002). The fetal origins of atherosclerosis: maternal hypercholesterolemia, and cholesterol-lowering or antioxidant treatment during pregnancy influence in utero programming and postnatal susceptibility to atherogenesis. *FASEB J.*, **16**, 1348–60.

Patel, M. S., Johnson, C. A., Rajan, R. and Owen, O. E. (1975). The metabolism of ketone bodies in developing human brain: development of ketone-body-utilizing enzymes and ketone bodies as precursors for lipid synthesis. *J. Neurochem.*, **25**, 905–8.

Pawlowski, B. (1998). Why are human newborns so big and fat? *Hum. Evol.*, **13**, 65–72.

Pipe, N. G., Smith, T., Halliday, D., Edmonds, C. J., Williams, C. and Coltart, T. M. (1979). Changes in fat, fat-free mass and body water in human normal pregnancy. *Br. J. Obstet. Gynaecol.*, **86**, 929–40.

Poisson, J. P., Dupuy, R. P., Sarda, P. *et al.* (1993). Evidence that liver microsomes of human neonates desaturate essential fatty acids. *Biochim. Biophy. Acta*, **1167**, 109–13.

Poissonnet, C. M., Burdi, A. R. and Garn, S. M. (1984). The chronology of adipose tissue appearance and distribution in the human fetus. *Early Hum. Dev.*, **10**, 1–11.

Postle, A. D., Al, M. D., Burdge, G. C. and Hornstra, G. (1995). The composition of individual molecular species of plasma phosphatidylcholine in human pregnancy. *Early Hum. Dev.*, **43**, 47–58.

Prentice, A. M. and Goldberg, G. R. (2000). Energy adaptations in human pregnancy: limits and long-term consequences. *Am. J. Clin. Nutr.*, **71**, (Suppl. 5), 1226–32S.

Prentice, A. M., Cole, T. J., Moore, S. E. and Collinson, A. C. (1999). Programming the adult immune system. In *Fetal Programming: Influences on Development and Disease in Later Life* (ed. P. M. S. O'Brien, T. Wheeler and D. J. P. Barker). London: Royal College of Gynaecology Press, pp. 399–413.

Prescott, S. L. and Calder, P. C. (2004). N-3 polyunsaturated fatty acids and allergic disease. *Curr. Opin. Clin. Nutr. Metab. Care*, **7**, 123–9.

Price, K. C. and Coe, C. L. (2000). Maternal constraint on fetal growth patterns in the rhesus monkey (*Macaca mulatta*): the intergenerational link between mothers and daughters. *Hum. Reprod.*, **15**, 452–7.

Raghupathy, R. (1997). Th1-type immunity is incompatible with successful pregnancy. *Immunol. Today*, **18**, 478–82.

    (2001). Pregnancy: success and failure within the Th1/Th2/Th3 paradigm. *Semin. Immunol.*, **13**, 219–27.

Rayon, J. I., Carver, J. D., Wyble, L. E. *et al.* (1997). The fatty acid composition of maternal diet affects lung prostaglandin E2 levels and survival from group B streptococcal sepsis in neonatal rat pups. *J. Nutr.*, **127**, 1989–92.

Reinhard, G., Noll, A., Schlebusch, H., Mallmann, P. and Ruecker, A. V. (1998). Shifts in the TH1/TH2 balance during human pregnancy correlate with apoptotic changes. *Biochem. Biophys. Res. Comm.*, **245**, 933–8.

Reisbick, S., Neuringer, M., Hasnain, R. and Connor, W. E. (1990). Polydipsia in rhesus monkeys deficient in omega-3 fatty acids. *Physiol. Behav.*, **47**, 315–23.

    (1994). Home cage behaviour of rhesus monkeys with long-term deficiency of omega-3 fatty acids. *Physiol. Behav.*, **55**, 231–9.

Rojas, C. V., Greiner, R. S., Fuenzalida, L. C., Martinez, J. I., Salem, N. and Uauy, R. (2002). Long-term n-3 FA deficiency modifies peroxisome proliferator-activated receptor beta mRNA abundance in rat ocular tissues. *Lipids*, **37**, 367–74.

Romagnani, S. (2000). The role of lymphocytes in allergic disease. *J. Allergy Clin. Immunol.*, **105**, 399–408.

Rothwell, J. E. and Elphick, M. C. (1982). Lipoprotein lipase activity in human and guinea-pig placenta. *J. Dev. Physiol.*, **4**, 153–9.

Roux, C., Wolf, C., Mulliezm N. *et al.* (2000). Role of cholesterol in embryonic development. *Am. J. Clin. Nutr.*, **71** (Suppl. 5), 1270–9S.

Ryan, A. S., Montalto, M. B., Groh-Wargo, S. *et al.* (1999). Effect of DHA-containing formula on growth of preterm infants to 59 weeks postmenstrual age. *Am. J. Hum. Biol.*, **11**, 457–67.

Salem, N. and Niebylski, C. D. (1995). The nervous system has an absolute molecular species requirement for proper function. *Mol. Membr. Biol.*, **12**, 131–4.

Salem, N., Wegher, B., Mena, P. and Uauy, R. (1996). Arachidonic and docosahexaenoic acids are biosynthesized from their 18-carbon precursors in human infants. *Proc. Natl. Acad. Sci. USA*, **93**, 49–54.

Samborski, R. W., Ridgway, N. D. and Vance, D. E. (1990). Evidence that only newly made phosphatidylethanolamine is methylated to phosphatidylcholine and that phosphatidylethanolamine is not significantly deacylated-reacylated in rat hepatocytes. *J. Biol. Chem.*, **265**, 18322–9.

Sanders, T. A., Mistry, M. and Naismith, D. J. (1984). The influence of a maternal diet rich in linoleic acid on brain and retinal docosahexaenoic acid in the rat. *Br. J. Nutr.*, **51**, 57–66.

Sattar, N., Greer, I. A., Louden, J. *et al.* (1997). Lipoprotein subfraction changes in normal pregnancy: threshold effect of plasma triglyceride on appearance of small, dense low density lipoprotein. *J. Clin. Endocrinol. Metab.*, **82**, 2483–91.

Schwartz, S. M. and Kemnitz, J. W. (1992). Age- and gender-related changes in body size, adiposity, and endocrine and metabolic parameters in free-ranging rhesus macaques. *Am. J. Phys. Anthropol.*, **89**, 109–21.

Shafrir, E. and Barash, V. (1987). Placental function in maternal–fetal fat transport in diabetes. *Biol. Neonate*, **51**, 102–12.

Shambaugh, G. E. (1985). Ketone body metabolism in the mother and fetus. *Fed. Proc.*, **44**, 2347–51.

Sherman, R. C., Burdge, G. C., Ali, Z., Singh, K. L., Wootton, S. A. and Jackson, A. A. (2001). Effect of pregnancy on plasma lipid concentration in Trinidadian women: result of a pilot study. *West Indian Med. J.*, **50**, 282–7.

Silliman, K, Shore, V. and Forte, T. M. (1994). Hypertriglyceridemia during late pregnancy is associated with the formation of small dense low-density lipoproteins and the presence of large buoyant high-density lipoproteins, *Metabolism*, **43**, 1035–41.

Sinclair, A. J. and Crawford, M. A. (1972). The accumulation of arachidonate and docosahexaenoate in the developing rat brain. *J. Neurochem.*, **19**, 1753–8.

Smart, J. M. and Kemp, A. S. (2001). Ontogeny of T-helper 1 and T-helper 2 cytokine production in childhood. *Pediatr. Allergy Immunol.*, **12**, 181–7.

Smith, R. W. and Welch, V. A. (1976). Effect of pregnancy and lactation on triglycerides of very-low-density lipoproteins of rat plasma. *J. Dairy Sci.*, **59**, 876–9.

Southgate, D. A. T. and Hay, E. N. (1975). Chemical and biochemical development of the fetus. In *The Biology of Fetal Growth* (ed. D. F. Roberts and A. M. Thomson). Symposia of the Society for the Study of Human Biology, vol. 15, pp. 195–209.

Sparks, J. W. (1984). Human intrauterine growth and nutrient accretion. *Semin. Perinatol.*, **8**, 74–93.

Sparks, J. W., Girard, J. R. and Battaglia, F. C. (1980). An estimate of the caloric requirements of the human fetus. *Biol. Neonate*, **38**, 113–19.

Stubbs, C. D. and Smith, A. D. (1984). The modification of mammalian membrane polyunsaturated fatty acid composition to membrane fluidity and function. *Biochim. Biophys. Acta*, **779**, 89–137.

Szerekes-Bartho, J. and Wegmann, T. G. (1996). A progesterone-dependent immunomodulatory protein alters the Th1/Th2 balance. *J. Reprod. Immunol.*, **31**, 81–95.

Taggart, N. R., Holliday, R. M., Billewicz, W. Z., Hytten, F. E. and Thomson, A. M. (1967). Changes in skinfolds during pregnancy, *Br. J. Nutr.*, **21**, 439–51.

Tang, M. L. K., Kemp, A. S., Thorburn, J. and Hill, D. (1994). Reduced interferon gamma secretion in neonates and subsequent atopy. *Lancet*, **344**, 983–5.

Thorsdottir, I. and Birgisdottir, B. E. (1998). Different weight gain in women of normal weight before pregnancy: postpartum weight and birth weight. *Obstet. Gynecol.*, **92**, 377–83.

Tint, G. S., Irons, M., Elias, E. R. *et al.* (1994). Defective cholesterol biosynthesis associated with the Smith–Lemli–Opitz syndrome. *N. Engl. J. Med.*, **330**, 107–13.

Vaidyanathan, V. V., Rao, K. V. and Sastry, P. S. (1994). Regulation of diacylglycerol kinase in rat brain membranes by docosahexaenoic acid. *Neurosci. Lett.*, **179**, 171–4.

Vazquez-Anon, M., Bertics, S., Luck, M., Grummer, R. R. and Pinheiro, J. (1994). Peripartum liver triglyceride and plasma metabolites in dairy cows. *J. Dairy Sci.*, **77**, 1521–8.

Villar, J., Cogswell, M., Kestler, E., Castillo, P., Menendez, R. and Repke, J. T. (1992). Effect of fat and fat-free mass deposition during pregnancy on birth weight. *Am. J. Obstet. Gynecol.*, **167**, 1344–52.

Wasfi, I., Weinstein, I. and Heimberg, M. (1980). Increased formation of triglyceride from oleate in perfused livers from pregnant rats. *Endocrinology*, **107**, 584–90.

Wegmann, T. G., Lin, H., Guilbert, L. and Mosmann, T. R. (1993). Bidirectional cytokine interactions in the maternal–fetal relationship: is successful pregnancy a TH2 phenomenon? *Immunol. Today*, **14**, 353–6.

Weisinger, H. S., Armitage, J. A., Sinclair, A. J., Vingrys, A. J., Burns, P. L. and Weisinger, R. S. (2001). Perinatal omega-3 fatty acid deficiency affects blood pressure later in life. *Nat. Med.*, **7**, 258–9.

Whitelaw, A. and Parkin, J. (1988). Development of immunity. *Br. Med. Bull.*, **44**, 1037–51.

Williams, C. and Coltart, T. M. (1978). Adipose tissue metabolism in pregnancy: the lipolytic effect of human placental lactogen. *Br. J. Obstet. Gynaecol.*, **85**, 43–6.

Williams, P. F., Simons, L. A. and Turtle, J. R. (1976). Plasma lipoproteins in pregnancy. *Horm. Res.*, **7**, 83–90.

Winkler, K., Wetzka, B., Hoffmann, M. M. *et al.* (2000). Low density lipoprotein (LDL) subfractions during pregnancy: accumulation of buoyant LDL with advancing gestation. *J. Clin. Endocrinol. Metab.*, **85**, 4543–50.

Wittmaack, F. M., Gafvels, M. E., Bronnerm M. *et al.* (1995). Localization and regulation of the human very low density lipoprotein/apolipoprotein-E receptor: trophoblast expression predicts a role for the receptor in placental lipid transport. *Endocrinology*, **136**, 340–8.

Woollett, L. A. (1993). The origins and roles of cholesterol and fatty acids in the fetus. *Curr. Opin. Lipidol.*, **12**, 305–12.

Woollett, L. A. (1996). Origin of cholesterol in the fetal golden Syrian hamster: contribution of de novo sterol synthesis and maternal-derived lipoprotein cholesterol. *J. Lipid Res.*, **37**, 1246–57.

Wyne, K. L. and Woollett, L. A. (1998). Transport of maternal LDL and HDL to the fetal membranes and placenta of the golden Syrian hamster is mediated by receptor-dependent and receptor-independent processes. *J. Lipid Res.*, **39**, 518–30.

Yu, G., Kjellman, N. I. and Bjorksten, B. (1996). Phospholipid fatty acids in cord blood: family history and development of allergy. *Acta Paediatr.*, **85**, 679–83.

Yu, G., Duchen, K. and Bjorksten, B. (1998). Fatty acid composition in colostrum and mature milk from non-atopic and atopic mothers during the first 6 months of lactation. *Acta Paediatr.*, **87**, 729–36.

Zeijdner, E. E., van Houwelingen, A. C., Kester, A. D. and Hornstra. G. (1997). Essential fatty acid status in plasma phospholipids of mother and neonate after multiple pregnancy. *Prostaglandins Leukot. Essent. Fatty Acids,*. **56**, 395–401.

Zimmer, L., Delpal, S., Guilloteau, D., Aioun, J., Durand, G. and Chalon, S. (2000). Chronic n-3 polyunsaturated fatty acid deficiency alters dopamine vesicle density in the rat frontal cortex. *Neurosci. Lett.*, **284**, 25–8.

12

Prenatal hypoxia: relevance to developmental origins of health and disease

Dino A. Giussani

University of Cambridge

Introduction

The compelling evidence linking small size at birth with later cardiovascular disease, obtained from epidemiological studies of human populations from more than a dozen countries (Barker 1998), has clearly renewed and amplified a clinical and scientific interest in the determinants of fetal growth, birthweight and the development of cardiovascular function before and after birth. As early as the 1950s Penrose highlighted that an important determinant of birthweight was the quality of the intrauterine environment, being twice as great a determinant of the rate of fetal growth as the maternal or fetal genotype. Studies of birthweights of relatives (Penrose 1954), together with strong evidence from animal crossbreeding experiments (Walton and Hammond 1938, Giussani *et al.* 2003), have clearly supported this contention. One of the important modifiers of the fetal environment is maternal nutritional status during pregnancy. The reciprocal association between low birthweight and increased risk of high blood pressure in adulthood, as described by Barker (1998), has exploded into a new field of research investigating the effects of maternofetal nutrition on fetal growth, birthweight and subsequent cardiovascular disease. However, the fetus nourishes itself also with oxygen, and in contrast to the international effort which is assessing the effects of maternofetal undernutrition on early development, the

effects of maternofetal under-oxygenation on fetal growth, birthweight and subsequent increased risk of disease have been little addressed. Moreover, the physiological mechanisms linking intrauterine growth retardation, as a result of either fetal undernutrition or under-oxygenation or both, to abnormalities in physiological function before and after birth also remain unknown.

Interestingly, a growing number of clinical and experimental studies have now shown that the association between impaired growth in utero and cardiovascular dysfunction in postnatal life is also coupled to altered regulation of the stress system. This system coordinates the adaptive responses of the organism to stressors or stimuli that threaten homeostasis of any kind (Chrousos 1998). Its main central components are the locus coeruleus–noradrenaline autonomic complex (LC/NA) and the corticotrophin-releasing hormone (CRH) neurones. The peripheral effectors of the stress system are the sympathoadrenomedullary and the pituitary–adrenocortical axes, respectively (Chrousos 1998). Repeated or sustained activation of these components of the stress system during times of increased brain plasticity, such as the prenatal period, can clearly have profound effects on the function of its peripheral effectors throughout life, increasing the risk of pathology. However, it remains unresolved whether altered activities of both peripheral components of the stress system provide a

Developmental Origins of Health and Disease, ed. Peter Gluckman and Mark Hanson. Published by Cambridge University Press.
© P. D. Gluckman and M. A. Hanson 2006.

final common mechanistic pathway underlying the association between impaired fetal growth and increased risk of developing disease in adulthood, or whether altered activities of the sympatho-adrenomedullary system and the HPA axis and in the control of blood pressure and growth in the fetus simply reflect parallel tracking of programmed changes in these systems by adverse intrauterine conditions. Nevertheless, in this chapter, evidence is provided to show that altered regulation of the sympathoadrenomedullary system and the pituitary–adrenocortical axis are also hallmarks associated with slow growth in the fetus and cardiovascular dysfunction in adulthood as a result of intrauterine under-oxygenation, independent of the nutritional status of the mother and of the unborn child. This strongly supports the concept that fetal hypoxia alone may provide a candidate prenatal stimulus contributing to the developmental origins of health and disease.

Prenatal hypoxia and the fetal cardiovascular defence

Fetal hypoxia is one of the major challenges that the fetus may face during gestation, and it may occur by insufficiency of either uterine blood flow or umbilical blood flow, or by a decrease in maternal arterial oxygen content (Parer 1988). Other mechanisms such as fetal anaemia or increased fetal oxygen consumption (e.g. in pyrexia) are relatively rare in clinical practice (see Thakor and Giussani 2005). Risk factors which predispose to the development of fetal hypoxia can be classified into maternal (e.g. diabetes, pregnancy-induced or chronic hypertension, Rh sensitisation, maternal infection, sickle cell anaemia, chronic substance abuse, asthma, seizure disorders, smoking), intrapartum (e.g. multiple pregnancy, premature or post-term birth, prolonged labour, placental abruption, placenta praevia, prolapsed umbilical cord, abnormal presentation of the fetus) or iatrogenic (e.g. epidural anaesthesia; for details see Thakor and Giussani 2005).

Acute hypoxia

The strategy of the fetal cardiovascular defence to hypoxia will clearly depend not only on the magnitude but also on the duration of the challenge. In simple terms, the fetal cardiovascular defence to an acute, short-term episode of hypoxia (lasting minutes to an hour) is represented via three changes: changes in heart rate, changes in arterial blood pressure and changes in the distribution of the fetal cardiac output to the various organs. The pattern and magnitude of the fetal heart, blood-pressure and circulatory defence responses to acute hypoxia are dependent on the stage of gestation at which the challenge occurs and, consequently, the maturity of the mechanisms which mediate them. In the late-gestation sheep fetus (>120 days; term ~150 days), the cardiovascular defence to an hour-long episode of acute hypoxia involves a transient fall in heart rate, a progressive increase in arterial blood pressure, a fall in carotid vascular resistance and an increase in femoral vascular resistance (Giussani *et al.* 1993). The carotid vasodilatation and femoral vasoconstriction are good continuous indices of the redistribution of the fetal cardiac output away from the peripheral circulations towards the brain (Cohn *et al.* 1974). The fetal bradycardic and peripheral constrictor responses to episodes of reduced oxygenation have also been shown in fetuses of other species such as the rhesus monkey (Jackson *et al.* 1987), cat, guinea pig, rabbit (Rosen and Kjellmer, 1975), llama (Llanos *et al.* 2002), dog (Monheit *et al.* 1988), seal (Liggins *et al.* 1980), and even in embryonic chicks (Mulder *et al.* 1998) and alligators (Warburton *et al.* 1995) in late incubation. In human obstetric practice, fetal hypoxia secondary to uterine contractions during the actual processes of labour and delivery is also associated with fetal heart decelerations (Beard and Rivers 1979) and Doppler velocimetric evidence of redistribution in the fetal arterial circulation. The latter results in the 'brain sparing' effect, represented by falls in indices of resistance and an increase in the blood velocity in the common carotid and middle cerebral arteries, and reductions in blood velocities to the umbilical artery and descending aorta

(a) Acute hypoxia

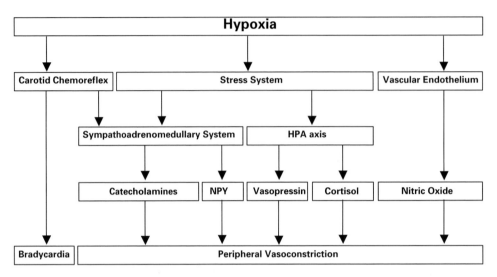

Figure 12.1 Mechanisms controlling the fetal cardiovascular responses to (a) acute hypoxia and (b) chronic hypoxia. Fetal exposure to chronic hypoxia leads to combined up-regulation of the sympathoadrenomedullary system coupled with down-regulation of NO-dependent dilator mechanisms in the fetal peripheral vascular endothelium (bold symbols). Persistent redistribution of blood flow towards central, and away from peripheral, circulations aids the maintenance of oxygen delivery to hypoxia-sensitive organs in the face of chronic reductions in fetal blood oxygen content. The biological trade-offs are increased cardiac afterload, ventricular and aortic hypertrophy, and asymmetric intrauterine growth retardation (IUGR), providing a link between hypoxia and the developmental origin of cardiovascular disease.

resulting from increases in resistance in those circulations (Akalin-Sel and Campbell 1992). Therefore, typically in obstetric medicine, an increase in the ratio of the resistance indices in central (ascending aorta, carotid artery or middle cerebral artery) relative to peripheral (descending aorta, umbilical, internal iliac or femoral arteries) circulations is representative of redistribution of the fetal combined ventricular output (CVO) in favour of the brain at the expense of the fetal trunk (Akalin-Sel and Campbell 1992).

The physiological mechanisms controlling the fetal cardiovascular responses to acute hypoxia involve at least four components (Fig. 12.1a). First, there is a rapid reflex component that is initiated selectively by the carotid chemoreceptors (Giussani et al. 1993). During hypoxia, the increased frequency discharge of chemosensory fibres arriving at the nucleus of the solitari tract (NTS) alters the balance of autonomic efferent output from the cardiac and vasomotor centres of the fetal brainstem to trigger bradycardia and to initiate vasoconstriction in peripheral circulations. Bradycardia occurs as a result of efferent vagal dominance, and peripheral vasoconstriction as a result of increased sympathetic outflow (Giussani et al. 1993). The neurogenic vasoconstriction is mediated via both α_1-adrenoreceptors and neuropeptide Y (NPY) Y_1 receptors (Giussani et al. 1993, Fletcher et al. 2000). Second, hypoxia stimulates the fetal stress system, activating the sympathoadrenomedullary system and the HPA axis (Chrousos 1998). This leads to an increase in the circulating concentrations of catecholamines, vasopressin and cortisol in the fetal blood (Gardner et al. 2002). Neuronal spillover from sympathetic terminals may also elevate the circulating concentrations of noradrenaline and NPY (Fletcher et al. 2000, Gardner et al. 2002).

(b) Chronic hypoxia

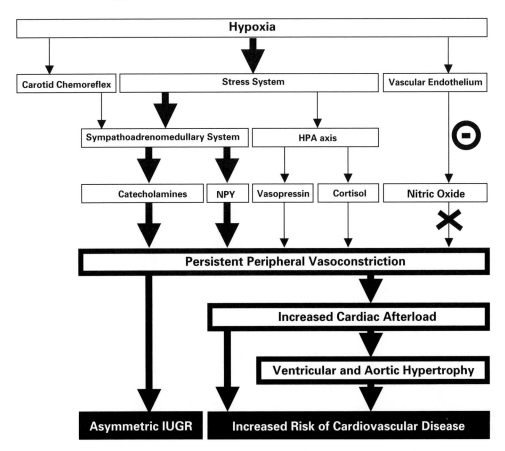

Figure 12.1 (*cont.*)

During hypoxia, the increased levels of fetal plasma catecholamines oppose vagal tone and return fetal heart rate to baseline, and, together with elevations in vasopressin and NPY, maintain the peripheral vasoconstriction (Fletcher *et al.* 2000, Gardner *et al.* 2002). Elevations in plasma cortisol sensitise the constrictor actions on the peripheral vasculature of the sympathetic nervous system and of sympathomimetic agents (Yang and Zhang 2004). The third component determining the pattern and magnitude of the fetal cardiovascular defence to oxygen deprivation is due to the direct effects of hypoxia on the fetal vascular endothelium. In the fetus, as in the adult, the vascular endothelium

acts as a hypoxic sensor and effector system that releases vasoactive agents, such as nitric oxide (NO; see Morrison *et al.* 2003). It is well accepted that enhanced NO synthesis in the cerebral, myocardial and adrenal vascular beds will promote vasodilation in these essential vascular beds (see Morrison *et al.* 2003). However, only comparatively recently has it become appreciated that the peripheral vasoconstrictor response to acute hypoxaemia actually represents the balance between neural and endocrine vasoconstrictor influences and local vasodilator actions of NO in the peripheral vascular beds. Hence, treatment of the sheep fetus with the NO clamp, a technique that permits blockade of

NO synthesis whilst maintaining basal cardiovascular function (Gardner *et al.* 2001a), revealed that hypoxia-induced NO production in the fetus acts to offset or fine-tune the extent of neural and endocrine constrictor influences on the fetal peripheral vascular beds (Morrison *et al.* 2003). Finally, if fetal hypoxia results from maternal hypoxia, as during pregnancy at high altitude, the placenta may also release vasodilator agents into the fetal circulation. These include prostaglandin E_2, adenosine, oestrogen, corticotrophin-releasing hormone and adrenomedullin. They may act to modify the fetal cardiovascular responses to acute hypoxia by NO-dependent and NO-independent mechanisms (see Di Iorio *et al.* 1998).

Chronic hypoxia

Less information is available regarding the fetal cardiovascular defence to sustained periods of hypoxaemia, lasting hours to days to months, owing to the technical difficulty in producing sustained, controlled, reproducible reductions in oxygen delivery to the fetus. Experimental approaches in pregnant sheep have included the surgical removal of endometrial caruncles prior to conception (carunclectomy; Robinson *et al.* 1979), the induction of maternal hypobaric (Ducsay 1998) or isobaric (Kitanaka *et al.* 1989) hypoxia, the embolisation of the uteroplacental (Creasy *et al.* 1972) or umbilical (Gagnon *et al.* 1996) circulations with microspheres, and the sustained partial compression of the uterine artery (Bocking *et al.* 1989) or of the umbilical cord (Gardner *et al.* 2001b). An alternative approach has been to study the fetal cardiovascular physiology of the llama, a species adapted to the chronic hypobaric hypoxia of life at high altitude for generational times (Llanos *et al.* 2002). Most recently, sustained isobaric (Mulder *et al.* 1998) or hypobaric (Salinas *et al.* 2003a) hypoxia has also been induced in the chick embryo for most of the incubation period. Combined, the available information obtained from experiments in fetal sheep, chick embryos and fetal llamas suggests that the fetal cardiovascular defence strategy to sustained periods of hypoxaemia focuses on the main-

tenance of the redistribution of the CVO, away from peripheral circulations towards the brain, the heart and the adrenal glands. Data from chronically instrumented fetal sheep preparations show that partial compression of uterine artery for 48 hours leads to maintained increases in cerebral, myocardial and adrenal blood flow (Bocking *et al.* 1989). Partial compression of the ovine umbilical cord for three days via automated servo-controlled inflation of an occluder cuff elevated fetal femoral vascular resistance for the duration of the reduction in umbilical blood flow (Gardner *et al.* 2001b). Measurement of the distribution of cardiac output via microspheres in the chick embryo revealed less blood flow apportioned to the peripheral circulations in embryos exposed to chronic hypoxia throughout the incubation period, relative to normoxic controls (Mulder *et al.* 1998). Data obtained from the chronically instrumented llama preparation show that fetal basal peripheral vascular resistance and the femoral vasoconstrictor response to acute hypoxia in this species are both much greater than those calculated for fetal sheep at equivalent gestational ages (Giussani *et al.* 1996).

Intuitively, persistent peripheral vasoconstriction in response to chronic hypoxia in the fetus should result from differential alteration of constrictor and dilator component mechanisms mediating the fetal peripheral vascular response to oxygen deprivation. Accumulating evidence supports this thesis and shows that fetal exposure to chronic hypoxia leads to combined up-regulation of the sympathoadrenomedullary system coupled with down-regulation of NO-dependent dilator mechanisms in the fetal peripheral vascular endothelium (Fig. 12.1b). Chronically hypoxaemic fetal sheep (Gardner *et al.* 2002) and fetal llamas (Llanos *et al.* 2003) have higher resting plasma concentrations of noradrenaline than normoxic fetal sheep at equivalent stages of gestation. Studies in the chick embryo have shown that incubation at high altitude of fertilised eggs laid by hens native to sea level elevates the adrenal catecholamine content in the chick embryo at the end of the incubation period (unpublished data). Elegant studies by Ruijtenbeek and colleagues (2000) have reported that incubation of chick embryos under chronic isobaric hypoxia from 0.3 to 0.9 of the incubation leads to elevation in the noradrenaline content of the femoral but not the carotid vessels. In the femoral vasculature of hypoxic embryos the density of catecholamine-containing perivascular nerves and cocaine-sensitive neuronal uptake of noradrenaline were also elevated. The same group of investigators have later shown that femoral arterial segments of embryos chronically exposed to hypoxia were significantly less sensitive to acetylcholine, but not to sodium nitroprusside, when compared with femoral arteries isolated from normoxic control embryos or, interestingly, from undernourished embryos (Ruijtenbeek et al. 2003). Combined, these findings strongly suggest that chronic hypoxia, but not undernutrition, down-regulates the capacity of the vascular endothelium in the peripheral vasculature to synthesise NO, but that it does not affect the capacity of the smooth muscle cells to relax in response to NO.

Prenatal hypoxia and fetal growth

Persistent redistribution of blood flow towards central circulations, secondary to sustained elevations in peripheral vascular tone, may offer a physiological advantage to the fetus that aids the maintenance of oxygen delivery to hypoxia-sensitive organs in the face of chronic reductions in fetal blood oxygen content. However, this homeostatic vascular response in the fetus comes with important biological trade-offs. Not only does hypoxia reduce the overall rate of growth in the whole fetus (Malaspina et al. 1971), but the sustained reduction in nutrient delivery to the periphery worsens the problem in these circulations, leading to pronounced asymmetric growth retardation. Although several studies in animals have shown that chronic hypoxia during pregnancy can lead to slow, disproportionate fetal growth (Chang et al. 1984, De Grauw et al. 1986), whether the effects are due to sustained under-oxygenation or partial undernutrition is uncertain, as chronic hypoxia also reduces maternal food intake (De Grauw et al. 1986). In human populations, maternofetal hypoxia occurs

most commonly during the hypobaric hypoxia of pregnancy at high altitude. In support of data gathered from animal experiments, several investigators have also reported reduced birthweight and asymmetric growth retardation in human babies with increasing altitude (Gonzales and Guerra Gracia 1993, Zamudio et al. 1993, Giussani et al. 2001). However, because most high-altitude populations are also impoverished, the extent to which this reduction in fetal growth is governed by maternal nutritional status or the hypoxia of high altitude again remains uncertain. To assess the partial contributions of fetal under-oxygenation and undernutrition in the control of fetal growth, we have recently adopted a two-pronged approach, addressing questions in a specific human population and in a specific experimental animal model.

Epidemiological studies of human populations were carried out in Bolivia, as this country is geographically and socioeconomically unique. Bolivia lies in the heart of South America and it is split by the Andean cordillera into areas of very high altitude (4000 m) to the west of the country and sea-level areas as the east of the country spans into the Brazilian Amazon. Facilitating the study design, the two largest cities, and therefore the most populated with approximately two million inhabitants each, are La Paz (4000 m) and Santa Cruz (400 m). Bolivia is also socioeconomically unique as both La Paz and Santa Cruz are made up of striking economically divergent populations (Mapa de Pobreza 1995). In developing countries, and especially in Bolivia, there is an unsurprising strong relationship between socioeconomic status and nutritional status (Post et al. 1994). Joining strengths with Barker, a recent study investigated whether the intrauterine growth retardation observed in the high-altitude regions of Bolivia was primarily due to intrauterine hypoxia or due to the maternal socioeconomic nutritional status (Giussani et al. 2001). Birthweight records were obtained from term pregnancies in La Paz and Santa Cruz, especially from obstetric hospitals selectively attended by wealthy or impoverished mothers. Plots of the cumulative frequency distribution across all birthweights gathered revealed a pronounced shift to the left in the curve of babies from

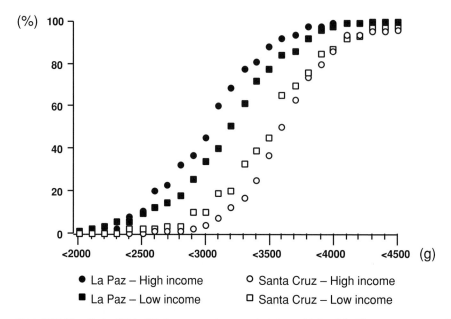

Figure 12.2 The effects of high altitude versus socioeconomic status on birthweight. The curves represent the cumulative frequency distribution across all birthweights in term babies born from mothers of opposing economic status in La Paz (4000 m) and in Santa Cruz (400 m), Bolivia. Modified with permission from Giussani *et al.* (2001).

high altitude versus those from low altitude, despite similarly high maternal economic status (Fig. 12.2). Interestingly, when lowland babies born from mothers with high and low economic status were compared, a shift to the left in birthweight occurred in low- versus high-income groups; however, this shift was not as pronounced as the effect on birthweight of high-altitude hypoxia alone. Additional data also showed that highland babies from poor families did not have the greatest leftward shift of the relationship, as one would have expected. Rather, these babies were actually heavier than highland babies born from families with a high socioeconomic status. The apparent conundrum is easily explained by assessing the ancestry of the families. In our study, the low socioeconomic group of La Paz contained a high percentage (92%) of women of Amerindian origin with Aymara Indian paternal and maternal surnames (Giussani *et al.* 2001). In contrast, the high-socioeconomic group of La Paz contained a high European admixture. These findings are reminiscent of the observations of Haas *et al.* (1980) and

Moore (1990), who suggested that fetal growth retardation at altitude is correlated with the duration of high-altitude residence, independent of maternal nutrition, the longest-resident population experiencing the least decline and the shortest-residence groups demonstrating the most reduction in birthweight. Accordingly, reductions in birthweight at elevations greater than 3000 m above sea level are greatest in Colorado, intermediate in Andeans and least in Tibetans (Moore 1990). Thus, women from high-altitude-residence ancestry like the Tibetans (Moore 1990) and the Aymaras (Haas *et al.* 1980) give birth to heavier babies than women from low-altitude-residence ancestry like Han women in China and women from European or mestizo ancestry in South America.

The second prong of our approach exploited the chick embryo as an animal model. In contrast to all mammals, in avian species the effects of hypoxia on the fetus can be assessed directly, without additional effects of hypoxia on the mother and the placenta, and without confounding problems associated with reductions in maternal food intake. The study reasoned that if oxygen alone has a real role in the direct control of fetal growth, then fertilised eggs from hens native to sea level should show growth restriction when incubated at high altitude, and fertilised eggs from hens native to high altitude, which usually show growth restriction, should at least recover their growth when incubated at sea level (Salinas *et al.* 2003a). Again, the study was done in Bolivia, in the cities of La Paz and Santa Cruz. The data show that incubation of sea-level embryos at high altitude led to a 50% growth restriction, but incubation at high altitude of embryos from hens native to high altitude only led to 30% growth restriction. The embryonic growth restriction of incubations at high altitude was asymmetric, as brain weight was preserved at the expense of body length. Furthermore, incubation at sea level of embryos from hens native to high altitude not only restored their symmetric growth, but these embryos were larger than sea-level control embryos incubated at sea level (Salinas *et al.* 2003a).

Combined, our observation in human babies and our experiments in the chick embryo not only strongly support the hypothesis that fetal oxygen, independent of genetic and maternal nutritional factors, regulates fetal growth but they also highlight that in both human and avian species prolonged high-altitude-residence ancestry can develop a protection against unwanted biological trade-offs. The mechanism of this protection is clearly of paramount scientific interest and has important clinical applications.

Prenatal hypoxia, other models of adverse intrauterine conditions and the HPA axis

It is well established that fetal exposure to elevated glucocorticoid concentrations can reduce the rate of fetal growth (Fowden 1995) and promote an increase in fetal peripheral vascular resistance and arterial blood pressure (Derks *et al.* 1997). Because a large number of clinical and experimental studies have shown that the relationship between impaired growth in utero and hypertension in postnatal life is also coupled to altered regulation of the HPA axis, sustained fetal exposure to elevated glucocorticoid concentrations during gestation has been proposed as a final common mechanistic pathway underlying the association (Newnham *et al.* 2002). For example, human adults whose birthweight was low show elevated basal circulating concentrations of cortisol (Phillips *et al.* 2001) and enhanced adrenocortical responsiveness to ACTH (Reynolds *et al.* 2001). In addition, the offspring of pregnant ewes which were undernourished in early gestation showed enhanced pituitary and adrenal responsiveness to exogenous and endogenous stimuli in the fetal and postnatal periods (Hoet and Hanson 1999, Edwards and McMillen 2002). In some of these studies, the augmented pituitary–adrenal responsiveness was associated with a higher resting arterial blood pressure in lambs (see Hoet and Hanson 1999). Numerous other studies have shown that exposure of the human (Kari *et al.* 1994), sheep (Dodic *et al.* 1999), rat (Benediktsson *et al.* 1993) or guinea pig (Dean and Matthews 1999) fetus to increased glucocorticoid concentration, either by exogenous treatment or by elevating endogenous steroid bioactivity secondary to inactivation of placental 11β-hydroxysteroid dehydrogenase, can be associated with impaired fetal growth and postnatal hypertension.

Opposing this thesis, an accumulating number of studies show that persistent elevations in circulating fetal glucocorticoid concentrations are not an absolute prerequisite for growth-restriction and cardiovascular dysfunction in either the fetal or adult period. For example, in a study which used between-breed embryo transfer in the horse, thoroughbred embryos transferred into pony mares yielded growth-restricted foals with appropriate basal blood pressure and adrenocortical function. In contrast, pony embryos transferred into thoroughbred mares produced very large foals with significantly elevated basal blood pressure and enhanced adrenocortical responsiveness to ACTH (Giussani *et al.* 2003). Thus, the data obtained from equine breeds showed that growth-enhanced, rather than growth-restricted, foals had the increased adrenocortical responsiveness to ACTH. In addition, fetal growth restriction secondary to chronic hypoxia is mostly, if not exclusively, associated with diminished, rather than enhanced, basal adrenocortical function. Clearly, the fetal pituitary–adrenocortical responses to hypoxia will depend on the duration of the oxygen deprivation. In ovine pregnancies in late gestation, it is well established that the fetus responds to 1-hour episodes of hypoxia with elevations in plasma ACTH and cortisol (Gardner *et al.* 2002). If the fetal exposure to hypoxia lasts from hours to days, dissociation in the plasma ACTH and cortisol responses occurs, such that cortisol is maintained high despite plasma ACTH concentrations returning to basal levels (Gardner *et al.* 2001c). If the fetal exposure to hypoxia is more prolonged, lasting months, plasma cortisol concentrations return to basal levels (Ducsay 1998). In fact, incubation at high altitude of fertilised eggs from sea-level hens from day 0 to day 20 of the incubation period produced severely-growth-restricted embryos with basal plasma corticosterone concentrations even lower than sea-level control embryos (Giussani *et al.* 2004).

In addition to basal changes in adrenocortical function, the responsiveness of the fetal HPA axis to a challenge following chronic hypoxia is variable. Harvey *et al.* (1993) showed that sheep undergoing pregnancy at high altitude had markedly attenuated fetal cortisol responses to an ACTH challenge when compared with sea-level control fetuses, supporting diminished adrenocortical responsiveness. However, the same group of investigators reported enhanced adrenocortical responsiveness to acute hypotension or acute occlusion of the umbilical cord (see Imamura *et al.* 2004) in fetal sheep following long-term exposure to high-altitude hypoxia for most of gestation. Conversely, a recent study in the newborn period showed that high-altitude lambs had normal plasma ACTH, but markedly diminished plasma cortisol, responses to acute hypoxia relative to sea-level lambs (Riquelme *et al.* 2004).

Despite inconsistencies in the perinatal responsiveness to a challenge of the HPA axis following development under long-term hypoxia, most studies agree that basal adrenocortical function is suppressed following fetal exposure to chronic hypoxia.

Blunting of fetal basal adrenocortical sensitivity to ACTH may be an appropriate homeostatic response to prolonged periods of hypoxia, such as those associated with high-altitude pregnancy, to protect sensitive tissues from sustained elevations in plasma cortisol levels during fetal development. The biological trade-off may yield newborns with adrenocortical suppression, which if proven in human babies may support the global use of antenatal glucocorticoid therapy in human pregnancy at high altitude, irrespective of threatened preterm labour. Interestingly, a few studies have reported that adrenarche and menarche are delayed in highland boys and girls relative to lowland children (Goñez *et al.* 1993, Gonzales and Villena 1996), supporting basal suppression of the hypothalamic–pituitary–adrenal and gonadal axes following development under long-term exposure to hypoxia in the human.

Taken together, evidence to date therefore suggests that enhanced activity of the HPA axis cannot be the final common mechanism linking fetal growth restriction with cardiovascular dysfunction following development under adverse intrauterine conditions, as a number of studies show clear dissociation between growth restriction and enhanced glucocorticoid concentrations. Rather, the evidence suggests that alterations in HPA axis function, above and below the normal basal status, are associated with alterations in growth and cardiovascular function during development.

Summary and perspectives

In response to acute hypoxia, the fetus redistributes its cardiac output via vasoconstriction in peripheral vascular beds and vasodilatation in essential vascular beds (Cohn *et al.* 1974, Giussani *et al.* 1993). Peripheral vasoconstriction represents the balance between constrictor influences triggered by a carotid chemoreflex and from activation of the sympatho-adrenomedullary system, and dilator influences resulting from the direct effects of hypoxia on NO synthesis in the vascular endothelium (Morrison *et al.* 2003). In this chapter, it is proposed that in response to chronic hypoxia the fetal homeostatic response becomes exaggerated, by up-regulation of the sympathoadrenomedullary axis and down-regulation of NO activity in the peripheral vascular endothelium, thereby promoting persistent peripheral vasoconstriction. Whether this exaggerated homeostatic response in the fetus becomes a mal-adaptation, akin to the erythrocytotic (Monge *et al.* 1992) or the pulmonary vasoconstrictor (Maggiorini and León-Velarde 2003) responses to hypoxia in highland neonates and adults which are beneficial if transient, but if persistent lead to pathology, is unclear at present. However, it is proposed that plausible biological trade-offs of fetal persistent peripheral vasoconstriction are asymmetric growth retardation and increased cardiac afterload, suggesting that the classical phenotypic association between intrauterine growth retardation and cardiovascular dysfunction in adult life may originate from the same developmental stimulus – fetal hypoxia.

An increasing number of experimental studies in animal models are beginning to support this argument. Studies in fetal sheep have shown that chronic hypoxia, secondary to pregnancy at high altitude, sustained anaemia or chronic fetal placental embolisation, led to suppressed cardiac function and contractility, increased myocardial lactate dehydrogenase and citrate synthase and resulted in cardiac hypertrophy (see Bae *et al.* 2003). Studies in chick and rat embryos have shown that exposure to sustained hypoxia during development, which leads to asymmetrical growth retardation, can be accompanied by ventricular and aortic hypertrophy (Bae *et al.* 2003, Salinas *et al.* 2003b). Three elegant studies have now shown that fetal hypoxia alone may have persisting consequences for cardiac and vascular health in the offspring at adulthood. Li *et al.* (2003) reported that exposure of pregnant rats to hypoxia from day 15 to 21 of gestation produced offspring with increased cardiac susceptibility to ischaemic-reperfusion injury at 6 months of age. Williams *et al.* (2004) reported that exposure of pregnant rats to hypoxia from day 15 to 21 of gestation produced offspring with impaired NO-dependent vasodilatation in the mesenteric circulation at 4 months of age.

Ruijtenbeek *et al.* (2003) reported that exposure of chick embryos to hypoxia from day 6 to 19 of the incubation period produced offspring with exaggerated responses to peri-arterial sympathetic nerve stimulation and down-regulated NO-dependent dilator function in the femoral vascular endothelium at 15–16 weeks of adulthood.

Conclusion

In humans, it remains to be elucidated whether hypoxia-induced reductions in birthweight, as a result of placental insufficiency or of pregnancy at high altitude, are clearly associated with increased health risks after birth. Clearly, it is close to impossible to isolate the partial effects of fetal hypoxia and fetal undernutrition in promoting intrauterine growth retardation in human pregnancies complicated with placental insufficiency. In contrast, investigation of the contribution of fetal hypoxia alone in promoting effects on fetal growth and programming health risks before and after birth can be achieved in human pregnancy at high altitude, carefully controlled for maternal nutritional status, making this a powerful model. Preliminary data (Giussani 2003) suggest that the rates of infant mortality, within the first year of newborn life, are positively correlated with altitude, increasing at a rate of *c.* 8 deaths per 1000 live births per 1000 m increase in altitude, and that this relationship is independent of the maternal socioeconomic and nutritional status. However, the negligible number of studies in which basal arterial blood pressure was measured in residents rather than climbers at high altitude report conflicting results suggesting either a higher incidence of hypertension in the inhabitants of high-altitude regions of Saudi Arabia (Khalid *et al.* 1994) or lower resting blood pressure in Peruvian highlanders (Ruiz and Peñaloza 1977). These inconsistencies may be related to the high-altitude-residence ancestry of the individuals being studied. Thus, while hypoxia during development may increase the risk of hypertension at adulthood in people who originated from sea-level regions, highland natives may have developed a protection, masking the effect. This final point re-emphasises the clear need for future epidemiological studies of human populations at altitude to relate the effects of prenatal hypoxia to postnatal cardiovascular function in lowland and highland natives separately. It is also likely that the deleterious programming effects of prenatal hypoxia on cardiovascular function in later life may express themselves not during basal conditions but only once the cardiovascular system is stressed. In this context, it is extremely interesting to highlight one study in India reporting a much higher incidence of ischaemic stroke in 20–50-year-old men resident at high altitude (Jha *et al.* 2002).

REFERENCES

Akalin-Sel, T. and Campbell, S. (1992). Understanding the pathophysiology of intra-uterine growth retardation: the role of the 'lower limb reflex' in redistribution of blood flow. *Eur. J. Obstet. Gynaecol. Reprod. Biol.*, **46**, 79–86.

Bae, S., Xiao, Y., Li, G., Casiano, C. A. and Zhang, L. (2003). Effect of maternal chronic hypoxic exposure during gestation on apoptosis in fetal rat heart. *Am. J. Physiol. Heart Circ. Physiol.*, **285**, H983–90.

Barker, D. J. P. (1998). *Mothers, Babies, and Disease in Later Life.* Edinburgh: Churchill Livingstone.

Beard, R. W. and Rivers, R. P. (1979). Fetal asphyxia in labour. *Lancet*, **2**, 1117–19.

Benediktsson, R., Lindsay, R. S., Noble, J., Seckl, J. R. and Edwards, C. R. (1993). Glucocorticoid exposure in utero: new model for adult hypertension. *Lancet*, **341**, 339–41.

Bocking, A. D., White, S. E., Gagnon, R. and Hansford, H. (1989). Effect of prolonged hypoxaemia on fetal heart rate accelerations and decelerations in sheep. *Am. J. Obstet. Gynecol.*, **159**, 1418–24.

Chang, J. H.T, Rutledge, J. C., Stoops, D. and Abbe, R. (1984). Hypobaric hypoxia-induced intrauterine growth retardation. *Biol. Neonate*, **46**, 10–13.

Chrousos, G. P. (1998). Stressors, stress, and neuroendocrine integration of the adaptive response: the 1997 Hans Selye Memorial Lecture. *Ann. NY Acad. Sci.*, **30**, 311–35.

Cohn, H. E., Sacks, E. J., Heymann, M. A. and Rudolph, A. M. (1974). Cardiovascular responses to hypoxemia and acidemia in fetal lambs. *Am. J. Obstet. Gynecol.*, **120**, 817–24.

Creasy, R. K., Barrett, C. T., de Swiet M., Kahanpaa, K. V. and Rudolph, A. M. (1972). Experimental intrauterine growth retardation in the sheep. *Am. J. Obstet. Gynecol.*, **112**, 566–73.

Dean, F. and Matthews, S. G. (1999). Maternal dexamethasone treatment in late gestation alters glucocorticoid and mineralocorticoid receptor m RNA in the fetal guinea pig brain. *Brain Res.*, **6**, 253–9.

De Grauw, T. J., Myers, R. and Scott, W. J. (1986). Fetal growth in rats from different levels of hypoxia. *Biol. Neonate*, **49**, 85–9.

Derks, J. B., Giussani, D. A., Jenkins, S. L. *et al.* (1997). A comparative study of the cardiovascular, endocrine and behavioural effects of betamethasone and dexamethasone administration to fetal sheep. *J. Physiol.*, **499**, 217–26.

Di Iorio, R., Marinoni, E. and Cosmi, E. V. (1998). New peptides, hormones and parturition. *Gynecol. Endocrinol.*, **12**, 429–34.

Dodic, M., Peers, A., Coghlan, J. P. and Wintour, M. (1999). Can excess glucocorticoid, in utero, predispose to cardiovascular and metabolic disease in middle age? *Trends Endocrinol. Metab.*, **10**, 86–91.

Ducsay, C. A. (1998). Fetal and maternal adaptations to chronic hypoxia: prevention of premature labor in response to chronic stress. *Comp. Biochem. Physiol. A Mol. Integr. Physiol.*, **119**, 675–81.

Edwards, L. J. and McMillen, I. C. (2002). Impact of maternal undernutrition during the periconceptional period, fetal number, and fetal sex on the development of the hypothalamo-pituitary adrenal axis in sheep during late gestation. *Biol. Reprod.*, **66**, 1562–69.

Fletcher, A. J. W., Edwards, C. M. B., Gardner, D. S., Fowden, A. L. and Giussani, D. A. (2000). Neuropeptide Y in the sheep fetus: effects of acute hypoxemia and dexamethasone during late gestation. *Endocrinology*, **141**, 3976–82.

Fowden, A. L. (1995). Endocrine regulation of fetal growth. *Reprod. Fertil. Dev.*, **7**, 351–63.

Gagnon, R., Johnston, I. and Murotsuki, J. (1996). Fetal–placental embolization in the late-gestation ovine fetus: alterations in umbilical blood flow and fetal heart rate patterns. *Am. J. Obstet. Gynecol.*, **175**, 63–72.

Gardner, D. S., Powlson, A. S. and Giussani, D. A. (2001a). An in vivo nitric oxide clamp to investigate the influence of nitric oxide on continuous umbilical blood flow during acute hypoxaemia in the sheep fetus. *J. Physiol.*, **537**, 587–96.

Gardner, D. S., Fletcher, A. J. W., Swann, M., Fowden, A. L. and Giussani, D. A. (2001b). A novel method for controlled, long term compression of the umbilical cord in fetal sheep. *J. Physiol.*, **535**, 217–29.

Gardner, D. S., Fletcher, A. J., Fowden, A. L. and Giussani D. A. (2001c). Plasma adrenocorticotropin and cortisol concentrations during acute hypoxemia after a reversible period of adverse intrauterine conditions in the ovine fetus during late gestation. *Endocrinology*, **142**, 589–98.

Gardner, D. S., Fletcher, A. J. W., Bloomfield, M. R., Fowden, A. L. and Giussani, D. A. (2002). Effects of prevailing hypoxaemia, acidaemia or hypoglycaemia upon the cardiovascular, endocrine and metabolic responses to acute hypoxaemia in the ovine fetus. *J. Physiol.*, **540**, 351–66.

Giussani, D. A. (2003). High altitude and infant mortality: a study of 99 provinces in Bolivia. *J. Soc. Gynecol. Investig.*, **10** (Suppl.), 308A.

Giussani, D. A., Spencer, J. A. D., Moore, P. J., Bennet, L. and Hanson, M. A. (1993). Afferent and efferent components of the cardiovascular reflex responses to acute hypoxia in term fetal sheep. *J. Physiol.*, **461**, 431–49.

Giussani, D. A., Riquelme, R. A., Moraga, F. A. *et al.* (1996). Chemoreflex and endocrine components of the cardiovascular response to acute hypoxaemia in the llama fetus. *Am. J. Physiol.*, **271**, R73–83.

Giussani, D. A., Phillips, P. S., Anstee, S. and Barker, D. J. P. (2001). Effects of altitude vs. economic status on birth weight and body shape at birth. *Pediatr. Res.*, **49**, 490–4.

Giussani, D. A., Forhead, A. J., Gardner, D. S., Fletcher, A. J. W., Allen, W. R. and Fowden, A. L. (2003). Postnatal cardiovascular function after manipulation of fetal growth by embryo transfer in the horse. *J. Physiol.*, **547**, 67–76.

Giussani, D. A., Salinas, C. E., Villena, M. and Blanco, C. E. (2004). Reversible adrenocortical suppression in chick embryos during incubation at high and low altitude. *J. Soc. Gynecol. Investig.*, **10** (Suppl.), 306A.

Goñez, C., Villena, A. and Gonzales, G. F. (1993). Serum levels of adrenal androgens up to adrenarche in Peruvian children living at sea level and at high altitude. *J. Endocrinol.*, **136**, 517–23.

Gonzales, G. F. and Guerra-Gracia, R. (1993). Características hormonales y antropométricas del embarazo y del recien nacido en la altura. In *Reproducción humana en la Altura*, (ed. G. F. Gonzales). Lima: Consejo Nacional de Ciencia y Tecnología, pp. 125–41.

Gonzales, G. F. and Villena A. (1996). Body mass index and age at menarche in Peruvian children living at high altitude and at sea level. *Hum. Biol.*, **68**, 265–75.

Haas, J. D., Frongillo, E. F., Stepcik, C., Beard, J. and Hurtado, L. (1980). Altitude, ethnic and sex differences in birthweight and length in Bolivia. *Hum. Biol.*, **52**, 459–77.

Harvey, L. M., Gilbert, R. D., Longo, L. D. and Ducsay, C. A. (1993). Changes in ovine fetal adrenocortical responsiveness after long-term hypoxia. *Am. J. Physiol.*, **264**, E741–9.

Hoet, J. J. and Hanson, M. A. (1999). Intrauterine nutrition: its importance during critical periods for cardiovascular and endocrine development. *J. Physiol.*, **514**, 617–27.

Imamura, T., Umezaki, H., Kaushal, K. M. and Ducsay, C. A. (2004). Long-term hypoxia alters endocrine and physiologic responses to umbilical cord occlusion in the ovine fetus. *J. Soc. Gynecol. Investig.*, **11**, 131–40.

Jackson, B. T., Piasecki, G. J. and Novy, M. J. (1987). Fetal responses to altered maternal oxygenation in rhesus monkey. *Am. J. Physiol.*, **252**, R94–101.

Jha, S. K., Anand, A. C., Sharma, V., Kumar, N. and Adya, C. M. (2002). Stroke at high altitude: Indian experience. *High Alt. Med. Biol.*, **3**, 21–7.

Kari, M. A., Hallman, M., Eronen, M. *et al.* (1994). Prenatal dexamethasone treatment in conjunction with rescue therapy of human surfactant: a randomized placebo-controlled multicenter study. *Pediatrics*, **93**, 730–6.

Khalid, M. E., Ali, M. E., Ahmed, E. K. and Elkarib, A. O. (1994). Pattern of blood pressures among high and low altitude residents of southern Saudi Arabia. *J. Hum. Hypertens.*, **8**, 765–9.

Kitanaka, T., Alonso, J. G., Gilbert, R. D., Siu, B. L., Clemons, G. K. and Longo, L. D. (1989). Fetal responses to longterm hypoxemia. *Am. J. Physiol.*, **256**, R1348–54.

Li, G., Xiao, Y., Estrella, J. L., Ducsay, C. A., Gilbert, R. D. and Zhang, L. (2003). Effect of fetal hypoxia on heart susceptibility to ischemia and reperfusion injury in the adult rat. *J. Soc. Gynecol. Investig.*, **10**, 265–74.

Liggins, G. C., Qvist, J., Hochachka, P. W. *et al.* (1980). Fetal cardiovascular and metabolic responses to simulated diving in the Weddell seal. *J. Appl. Physiol.*, **49**, 424–30.

Llanos, A. J., Riquelme, R. A., Sanhueza, E. M., Cabello, G., Giussani, D. A. and Parer, J. T. (2002). Regional brain blood flow and cerebral hemispheric oxygen consumption during acute hypoxaemia in the llama fetus. *J. Physiol.*, **538**, 975–83.

Llanos, A. J., Riquelme, R. A., Sanhueza, E. M. *et al.* (2003). The fetal llama versus the fetal sheep: different strategies to withstand hypoxia. *High Alt. Med. Biol.*, **4**, 193–202.

Maggiorini, M. and León-Velarde, F. (2003). High-altitude pulmonary hypertension: a pathophysiological entity to different diseases. *Eur. Respir. J.*, **22**, 1019–25.

Malaspina, L., Quilici, J. C. and Ergueta Collao, J. (1971). Modificaciones de las condiciones del cultivo celular en la altura. *Annales del Instituto Boliviano de Biología de la Altura*, **2**, 3–5.

Mapa de Pobreza (1995): *Una guía para la acción social*, 2nd edn. La Paz: Ministerio de Desarrollo Humano, República de Bolivia.

Monge, C. C., Arregui, A. and León-Velarde, F. (1992). Pathophysiology and epidemiology of chronic mountain sickness. *Int. J. Sports Med.*, **13** (Suppl. 1), S79–81.

Monheit, A. G., Stone, M. L. and Abitbol, M. M. (1988). Fetal heart rate and transcutaneous monitoring during experimentally induced hypoxia in the fetal dog. *Pediatr. Res.*, **23**, 548–52.

Moore, L. G. (1990). Maternal O_2 transport and fetal growth in Colorado, Peru and Tibet high-altitude residents. *Am. J. Hum. Biol.*, **2**, 627–37.

Morrison, S., Fletcher, A. J. W., Gardner, D. S. and Giussani, D. A. (2003). Enhanced nitric oxide activity offsets peripheral vasoconstriction during acute hypoxaemia via chemoreflex and adrenomedullary actions. *J. Physiol.*, **547**, 283–91.

Mulder, A. L., van Golde, J. C., Prinzen, F. W. and Blanco, C. E. (1998). Cardiac output distribution in response to hypoxia in the chick embryo in the second half of the incubation time. *J. Physiol.*, **508**, 281–7.

Newnham, J. P., Moss, T. J., Nitsos, I., Sloboda, D. M. and Challis, J. R. (2002). Nutrition and the early origins of adult disease. *Asia Pac. J. Clin. Nutr.*, **11** (Suppl. 3), S537–42.

Parer, J. T. (1988). Measurement of fetal heart rate: techniques and significance. In *Research in Perinatal Medicine*. VII. *Fetal and Neonatal Development* (ed. C. T. Jones). Ithaca, NY: Perinatology Press, pp. 511–20.

Penrose, L. S. (1954). Some recent trends in human genetics. *Cardiologia*, **6** (Suppl.), 521–9.

Phillips, D. I., Walker, B. R., Reynolds, R. M. *et al.* (2001). Low birthweight predicts elevated plasma cortisol concentrations in adults in 3 populations. *Hypertension*, **35**, 1301–6.

Post, G. B., Lujan, C., San-Miguel, J. L. and Kemper, H. C. (1994). The nutritional intake of Bolivian boys: the relation between altitude and socioeconomic status. *Int. J. Sports Med.*, **15** (Suppl. 2), S100–5.

Reynolds, R. M., Walker, B. R., Syddall, H. E. *et al.* (2001). Altered control of cortisol secretion in adult men with low birthweight and cardiovascular risk factors. *J. Clin. Endocrinol. Metab.*, **86**, 245–50.

Riquelme, R. A., Herrera, E. A., Sanhueza, E. M. *et al.* (2004). Lambs born at high altitude have a blunted pituitary–adrenal axis response to acute hypoxia. *J. Soc. Gynecol. Investig.*, **11** (Suppl.), 212A.

Robinson, J. S., Kingston, E. J., Jones, C. T. and Thorburn, G. D. (1979). Studies on experimental growth retardation in sheep: the effect of removal of endometrial caruncles on fetal size and metabolism. *J. Dev. Physiol.*, **1**, 379–98.

Rosen, K. G. and Kjellmer, I. (1975). Changes in the fetal heart rate and ECG during hypoxia. *Acta Physiol. Scand.*, **93**, 59–66.

Ruijtenbeek, K., Le Noble, F. A., Janssen, G. M. *et al.* (2000). Chronic hypoxia stimulates periarterial sympathetic nerve development in chicken embryo. *Circulation*, **102**, 2892–7.

Ruijtenbeek, K., Kessels, C. G., Janssen, B. J. *et al.* (2003). Chronic moderate hypoxia during in ovo development alters arterial reactivity in chickens. *Pflugers Arch.*, **447**, 158–67.

Ruiz, L. and Peñaloza, D. (1977). Altitude and hypertension. *Mayo Clin. Proc.*, **52**, 442–5.

Salinas, C. E., Villena, M., Blanco, C. E. and Giussani, D. A. (2003a). The role of oxygen in fetal growth. *J. Soc. Gynecol. Investig.*, **10** (Suppl.), 305A.

 (2003b). Protection against hypoxia-induced cardiomegaly in chick embryos from hens native to high altitude. *J. Soc. Gynecol. Investig.*, **10** (Suppl.), 108A.

Thakor, A. S. and Giussani, D. A. (2005). Calcitonin gene-related peptide contributes to the umbilical haemodynamic defence response to acute hypoxaemia. *J. Physiol.*, **563**, 309–17.

Walton, A. and Hammond, J. (1938). The maternal effects on growth and conformation in Shire horse–Shetland pony crosses. *Proc. R. Soc. Lond. B Biol. Sci.*, **125**, 311–35.

Warburton, S. J., Hastings, D. and Wang, T. (1995). Responses to chronic hypoxia in embryonic alligators. *J. Exp. Zool.*, **273**, 44–50.

Williams, S. J., Hemmings, D. G., McMillen, I. C. and Davidge, S. T. (2004). Maternal hypoxia during late gestation in rats impairs endothelium-dependent relaxation in mesenteric arteries from four month old male offspring. *J. Soc. Gynecol. Investig.*, **10** (Suppl.), 184A.

Yang, S. and Zhang, L. (2004). Glucocorticoids and vascular reactivity. *Curr. Vasc. Pharmacol.*, **2**, 1–12.

Zamudio, S., Droma, T., Norkyel, K. Y. *et al.* (1993). Protection from intrauterine growth retardation in Tibetans at high altitude. *Am. J. Phys. Anthropol.*, **91**, 215–24.

13

The fetal hypothalamic–pituitary–adrenal axis: relevance to developmental origins of health and disease

Deborah M. Sloboda,[1] John P. Newnham,[1] Timothy J. M. Moss[1]
and John R. G. Challis[2]

[1]University of Western Australia
[2]University of Toronto

Introduction

A clear relationship exists between intrauterine development and predisposition to postnatal disease. It is now understood that pre- and periconceptional nutritional status, glucocorticoid exposure and immediate postnatal development including catch-up growth may all contribute to these influences of early development on later-life disease. Barker and colleagues have described in detail the potential influence that an adverse intrauterine environment could play in the risk of developing particular diseases later in life (Barker 1994a, 1994b, 1995). It has been proposed that resetting of endocrine axes controlling growth and development could be one pathway for the developmental programming of later health and wellbeing. The fetal hypothalamic–pituitary–adrenal (HPA) axis in particular is highly vulnerable to changes in the intrauterine environment. Fetal HPA axis activity increases with gestation in most species and contributes to increased fetal levels of circulating glucocorticoids (Fowden *et al.* 1998). Even subtle changes in the intrauterine environment can disrupt the delicate balance of fetal HPA development and glucocorticoid production and can therefore alter long-term HPA activity and function. HPA hyperactivity has been demonstrated in animals after prenatal undernutrition (Lingas *et al.* 1999), prenatal stress (Takahashi and Kalin 1991) and maternal syn-

thetic glucocorticoid administration (Uno *et al.* 1990, Sloboda *et al.* 2000).

Programming of the fetal HPA axis during development appears to play a central role in the link between fetal growth and long-term disease in adulthood. Prenatal programming of HPA axis function may increase the risk of developing cardiovascular and metabolic diseases. Cognitive and behavioural modifications have also been associated with fetal programming and linked to alterations in HPA axis activity and prenatal glucocorticoid exposure (Welberg and Seckl 2001, Phillips 2001, French *et al.* 2004). Indeed, stress has been associated with changes in memory and behaviour, and with disorders such as depression, anxiety, chronic fatigue syndrome and schizophrenia (Kofman 2002). This chapter will outline normal HPA axis development, and will review current literature regarding the mechanisms programming HPA axis function and how HPA programming contributes to later disease.

The developing hypothalamic–pituitary–adrenal axis

A functional HPA axis is made up of the hippocampus, the hypothalamus and the pituitary and adrenal glands. In most species, normal fetal HPA axis function is essential for growth, development and for the onset of birth (Liggins 1994). Glucocorticoids

Developmental Origins of Health and Disease, ed. Peter Gluckman and Mark Hanson. Published by Cambridge University Press.
© P. D. Gluckman and M. A. Hanson 2006.

promote tissue and organ maturation and are responsible for the maturational changes in a variety of organ systems which prepare the fetus for extrauterine life (Liggins 1994, Fowden *et al.* 1998). In most species, there is an increase in fetal circulating glucocorticoid concentrations towards term, although the timing and the magnitude of this increase depends largely upon brain development (Fowden *et al.* 1998). In species that give birth to mature offspring (primates, sheep, guinea pigs) most brain and HPA development occurs in utero, whereas in species that give birth to immature offspring (rodents) most brain development occurs in the early postnatal days (Dobbing and Sands 1979). Therefore, as a result, the impact of prenatal versus postnatal manipulations on HPA axis programming is species-specific.

The hippocampus

The hippocampal formation is made up of four cortical regions that include the dentate gyrus, the hippocampus proper (CA1–CA4), the subicular complex and the entorhinal cortex (Amaral and Witter 1989), and it plays a major role in learning, memory and the regulation of HPA activity. The hippocampus exerts an inhibitory influence on basal, circadian and stress-induced HPA activity primarily by mediating glucocorticoid feedback (Jacobson and Sapolsky 1991). In rats, removal of the dorsal hippocampus has been shown to result in elevated basal and stress-induced adrenocortical responses (Feldman and Conforti 1980). Conversely, stimulation of the hippocampus results in decreased basal plasma corticosteroid levels (Mandell *et al.* 1963, Rubin *et al.* 1966). Central corticosteroid receptors in the hippocampus play a critical role in the regulation of HPA activity (De Kloet *et al.* 1998). Two corticosteroid receptors are present in the hippocampus: type 1, mineralocorticoid receptor (MR), identical to the kidney MR; and type 2, the classic glucocorticoid receptor (GR). MR bind glucocorticoids with an affinity that is 10 times greater ($Kd \sim 0.5$ nM) than that of GR ($Kd \sim 5.0$ nM) (Bamberger *et al.* 1996, De Kloet *et al.* 1998). In most species, the hippocampus

exhibits the highest levels of corticosteroid receptors of any brain region (Reul and De Kloet 1985, Jacobson and Sapolsky 1991, De Kloet *et al.* 1998) and is one of the few regions to express both MR and GR (Reul and De Kloet 1985). The hippocampus therefore represents a negative feedback site over a wide range of corticosteroid concentrations (Jacobson and Sapolsky 1991). Due to their high affinity, MR have been shown to be $\sim$90% occupied by endogenous corticosteroids under most circumstances and are thought to regulate basal or circadian trough levels of ACTH and cortisol (Reul and De Kloet 1985). GR occupancy varies from a minimum of 10% at basal and circadian trough corticosteroid levels to a maximum of $\sim$75% with stress or administration of synthetic corticosteroids (Reul and De Kloet 1985), and is proposed to mediate the effects of circadian peak or stress-induced increases in HPA activity (Reul and De Kloet 1985, Jacobson and Sapolsky 1991). Alterations in hippocampal MR and GR expression levels therefore could influence basal and stress-induced increases in HPA activity.

In the rat, the period of rapid brain growth occurs after birth, unlike that of the human, sheep or guinea pig (Dobbing and Sands 1979). In this species, hippocampal corticosteroid receptors increase gradually after birth, MR expression reaching adult levels by the second week of life and GR expression increasing somewhat later (Meaney *et al.* 1985). In species that give birth to mature offspring, GR mRNA is present at all levels of the axis (hippocampus, hypothalamus, pituitary, adrenal) during fetal life and increases gradually with gestation (Owen and Matthews 2003). Matthews and colleagues (2004) have recently shown in the fetal guinea pig hippocampus that steroid receptor signalling also changes with gestation, perhaps contributing to the normal increase in fetal HPA activity and glucocorticoids output observed at term (Setiawan *et al.* 2004).

The hypothalamus

The hypothalamus is divided into several nuclei including the paraventricular (PVN) and supraoptic nuclei (SON). The PVN is a highly differentiated nucleus containing discrete regions of neurons (Kupfermann 1991). It is within this nucleus that corticotrophin-releasing hormone (CRH) and arginine vasopressin (AVP) neurons are primarily localised in discrete areas. AVP is also localised in the SON (Page 1988). CRH-containing neurons are localised primarily to the parvocellular neuroendocrine cells of the PVN. AVP-containing neurons are localized to both parvocellular and magnocellular neuroendocrine cells of the PVN as well as magnocellular neurons of the SON (Page 1988). The axons of the parvocellular neurons project through the external lamina of the median eminence, where neuropeptides are secreted into the hypophyseal portal vessels to reach ultimately the anterior pituitary (pars distalis) and influence the synthesis and secretion of adrenocorticotrophin (ACTH), which then drives adrenal glucocorticoid secretion (Swanson and Sawchenko 1983, Levidiotis *et al.* 1987). The axons of the magnocellular neurons of both the PVN and the SON project through the internal lamina of the median eminence to nerve terminals in the posterior pituitary (pars nervosa) (Swanson and Sawchenko 1983). Therefore the parvocellular neurons of the PVN are thought to modulate pars distalis function, and magnocellular neurons subserve pars nervosa function and systemic AVP and oxytocin (OT) levels (Swanson and Simmons 1989).

The pituitary gland

The pituitary gland (hypophysis) is a small endocrine gland situated within the sella turcica at the base of the brain. It is composed of two morphologically discrete regions. The posterior lobe or pars nervosa is of neural origin, and represents a collection of axons whose cell bodies lie in the hypothalamus (see above). Peptide hormones that are synthesised in these neurons travel down their axons and are stored in the nerve terminals within the pars nervosa. The anterior lobe (pars distalis), the intermediate lobe (pars intermedia) and the stalk (pars tuberalis) represent the remainder of the pituitary gland. The pars distalis of the pituitary contains at least five

different types of secretory cells, 3–10% of which are estimated to be corticotroph cells (Page 1988). It is these cells that synthesise and process the polypeptide precursor pro-opiomelanocortin (POMC) into ACTH. ACTH then drives the release of glucocorticoids from the adrenal cortex.

The histological maturation of fetal pituitary corticotrophs has been well documented in the fetal sheep. Immunoreactive (ir) ACTH levels increase with advancing gestation both in fetal plasma and in the pars distalis (Perry *et al.* 1985). Corticotroph maturation is regulated by the fetal hypothalamus and adrenal (McDonald *et al.* 1992). The pars intermedia contains secretory cells (melanotrophs) that are cytologically different from the pars distalis (Perry *et al.* 1982). Secretory cells of the pars intermedia synthesise and secrete primarily α-melanocyte-stimulating hormone (αMSH), made up of amino acids 1–13 of the ACTH peptide (Lunblad and Roberts 1988). This reflects an altered pattern of POMC processing and prevalence of prohormone convertase (PC) 2 in the pars intermedia. The pars intermedia is well developed in the fetus, but diminishes in size with advancing gestation and is absent in the human adult. In lower mammals the pars intermedia remains distinctive (Mulchahey *et al.* 1987). It is well established that CRH and AVP are potent stimulators of ACTH synthesis and secretion. CRH stimulates ACTH secretion from fetal corticotrophs in vivo (Brooks and Challis 1989) and *in vitro* (Lu and Challis, 1994). Ir-ACTH has been detected in plasma from fetal sheep from 59 days of gestation (term is 150 days) and concentrations gradually increase over the last 25 days of gestation to reach peak levels at term (Norman *et al.* 1985).

The adrenal cortex

For most of gestation the primate fetal adrenal cortex is divided into three morphologically distinct zones: from outermost to innermost, the definitive or adult zone, the transitional zone and the fetal zone. Rapid growth of the adrenal begins at about 10 weeks of gestation and continues to term. Growth is almost entirely due to the development of the fetal zone of the gland. The primate adrenal, unlike that of fetal sheep, primarily secretes androgens, specifically dehydroepiandrostendione (DHEA), due to the low expression of the steroidogenic enzyme 3β-hydroxysteroid dehydrogenase (3β-HSD) in the fetal zone.

In fetal sheep, the adrenal gland is present very early in gestation (Wintour *et al.* 1975) and two distinct zones within the cortex are observed by day 60 (Webb 1980). Maturation of these zones begins later in gestation and, although the outer zone resembles a mature zona glomerulosa and the inner zone resembles the zona fasciculata, the zona reticularis does not develop until postnatal life (Webb 1980). The size and weight of the fetal sheep adrenal increases progressively throughout gestation from day 53 to day 130 and then further increases dramatically over the last 15–20 days of gestation (Boshier and Holloway 1989). This increase in growth late in gestation has been shown to be mainly due to an increase in the zona fasciculata (Boshier and Holloway 1991), which develops in three phases: the first phase at 53–100 days, the second phase from day 100 to day 130, and a third phase between 130 days of gestation and 2 days postpartum (Boshier and Holloway 1989). It has been shown in vivo that ACTH is a potent stimulus for the growth of the adrenal cortex (Liggins 1969) and fetal pituitary ablation results in adrenal cortical hypoplasia (Liggins and Kennedy 1968). These observations demonstrate the importance of ACTH in adrenal growth and maturation.

Fetal adrenal responsiveness to ACTH changes over the course of gestation (Glickman and Challis 1980). Fetal sheep adrenal cells respond to exogenous ACTH with elevated cortisol output early in gestation (50–60 days), followed by a loss in responsiveness at mid gestation (90–125 days) and a re-emergence of responsiveness at term (150 days) (Wintour *et al.* 1975, Glickman and Challis 1980). Increased adrenal responsiveness in late gestation has been attributed to an increase in ACTH receptor number (Durand *et al.* 1980), enhanced sensitivity to ACTH via increased adenylyl cyclase activity, increased cAMP levels (Durand *et al.* 1981) or enhanced steroidogenic enzyme expression

and activity (Challis *et al.* 1986). Among the five melanocortin receptors (MC1-R to MC5-R), MC2-R is known as the classical ACTH receptor (ACTH-R) of the adrenal cortex (Liakos *et al.* 1998). Once bound to its receptor, ACTH stimulates adenylate cyclase activity via G_s proteins, resulting in an accumulation in cAMP, stimulation of cAMP-dependent kinases and enhanced steroidogenesis (Reperant and Durand 1997). In fetal sheep, both ACTH-R mRNA levels and receptor number increase significantly in the last 20–25 days of gestation (Fraser *et al.* 2001a). This increase in receptor number is correlated directly with an increase in circulating cortisol levels (Durand 1979, Wang *et al.* 2004). Most evidence suggests that the up-regulation of ACTH-R number and activity, as well as increases in steroidogenic enzyme activity, by ACTH or cortisol in the fetal sheep are important events late in gestation, increasing adrenal responsiveness at the time of labour.

Premature fetal HPA axis activation: prenatal stress, undernutrition and synthetic glucocorticoids

There are several lines of evidence linking HPA axis maturation with fetal programming and the predisposition to adult disease (Challis *et al.* 2001, Bertram and Hanson 2002). Studies in humans have shown that cord blood levels of ACTH and cortisol are increased in association with reduced fetal growth (Goland *et al.* 1993). Glucocorticoids increase blood pressure in adults (Tonolo *et al.* 1988) and cortisol infusion into the fetal sheep results in elevated fetal blood pressure (Dodic and Wintour 1994). Low birthweight has been associated with increased urinary concentrations of glucocorticoid metabolites in children 9 years of age (Clark *et al.* 1996) and with significant changes in sympathetoadrenomedullary system activity and behaviour in school-aged children (Fernald and Grantham-McGregor 2002). Low birthweight correlates with increased adult cortisol levels as well as with insulin resistance and elevated blood pressure (Levitt *et al.* 2000, Reynolds *et al.* 2001a, 2001b). Given these relationships, it is essential to ascertain the role of fetal HPA activation in programming. Possible mechanisms for the programming of HPA hyperactivity have been proposed, although none has been fully defined.

Prenatal stress

Prenatal stress has a profound effect on neuroendocrine development and function. Stress during pregnancy in the rat results in basal and stimulated HPA hyperactivity (Takahashi and Kalin 1991, Weinstock 1996) and altered anxiety behaviour in offspring (Weinstock et al. 1992). Prenatal stress also results in abnormal corticosterone circadian rhythm in adult rats (Koehl et al. 1997), which is further modified by postnatal manipulations. Prenatal stress modifies the HPA axis in other species. A recent report has demonstrated that lambs born to prenatally stressed ewes exhibited altered behaviour and elevated basal cortisol concentrations (Roussel et al. 2004). Prenatal stress significantly elevated basal and stimulated ACTH and basal cortisol concentrations in rhesus monkeys (Clarke et al. 1994). The effects of maternal stress on HPA axis function in offspring is sex-dependent. Female offspring of prenatally stressed pregnant rats demonstrate elevated basal ACTH but not corticosterone and elevated pituitary–adrenal responses to stress, whereas male offspring demonstrate no change in basal HPA activity and have reduced stress responsiveness (McCormick et al. 1995). Little is known regarding the pathways regulating these gender-specific responses in HPA function, although it is evident that male and female neuroendocrine pathways are differently affected by prenatal stress.

Exposure of the fetus to elevated glucocorticoids appears to be the central link between prenatal stress and modification in the HPA axis development and function. Maternal stress in rats results in elevated maternal and fetal plasma corticosterone (Takahashi 1998). Administration of ACTH to pregnant sows (thereby partially mimicking the effects of maternal stress) resulted in a hyperactive HPA axis response to stress in offspring in the first 10 days of postnatal life. This was accompanied by elevated ACTH-R mRNA in the adrenal, increased adrenal cortex to medulla ratio and an increase in the number of ACTH-positive corticotrophs in the pituitary. Most of these changes persisted to 60 days of postnatal age (Haussmann et al. 2000). Prenatal hypoxic stress is associated with fetal HPA hyperactivity, which resulted in elevations in fetal ACTH and cortisol levels and increased fetal pituitary and hypothalamic neuropeptide expression levels (Matthews and Challis 1995). Maternal stress alters fetal hippocampal, hypothalamic and/or pituitary glucocorticoid receptors, and resulted in alterations in negative feedback (Lemaire et al. 2000).

Stress and anxiety during pregnancy in humans are associated with alterations in fetal growth and neonatal behaviour, although reports are somewhat conflicting (Austin and Leader 2000, Field et al. 2003). There is evidence, however, that antenatal stress/anxiety has a programming effect on the fetus which lasts at least until middle childhood and results in higher rates of behavioural and emotional problems (O'Connor et al. 2003). Recently, Van den Bergh and colleagues have reported that high maternal anxiety between 12 and 22 weeks of gestation is associated with the development of attention deficit hyperactivity disorder (ADHD) symptoms, externalising problems and anxiety during childhood (Van den Bergh and Marcoen 2004). Anxiety during pregnancy may significantly influence neuronal migration and synaptic contacts in the developing brain. Asymmetry in the brain has been identified in a number of regions in the cerebral cortex, and similar asymmetries have been identified in the fetal brain (Habib and Galaburda 1986). Functional asymmetries such as handedness and hemispheric dominance for language are most likely dependent upon neuronal migration and a consequence of synaptic competition in different cortical areas of the brain, regulating neuronal growth and death (Habib and Galaburda 1986). Recently, Glover et al. (2004) have demonstrated that elevated anxiety at 18 weeks of gestation was associated with a 20% increase in mixed-handedness in children at 3.5 years of age. This observation may further implicate the fetal endocrine environment in the mechanisms regulating postnatal brain activity and function.

Behavioural modifications have been demonstrated in animal models as well as in humans. In rodents, prenatal stress has been reported to result in offspring that exhibit elevated anxiety and alterations in behaviour (Weinstock *et al.* 1992, Vallee *et al.* 1996, Vazquez *et al.* 1996, Lemaire *et al.* 2000, Welberg *et al.* 2000). Alterations in HPA axis function, behaviour and cognition as a result of prenatal stress have been related to changes in brain corticosteroid receptor populations and alterations in hippocampal and hypothalamic neuronal development (Vazquez *et al.* 1996, Lemaire *et al.* 2000, Welberg and Seckl 2001).

Prenatal undernutrition

HPA regulation can be programmed by nutrient restriction. Studies in animals have shown that nutrient restriction in the rat results in blunted diurnal patterns of ACTH at 4 weeks of postnatal age (Holmes *et al.* 1997), alterations in basal plasma corticosterone in adulthood (Jacobson *et al.* 1997), and altered basal HPA axis activity in offspring (Sebaai *et al.* 2004). Maternal nutrient restriction in the sheep results in reductions in pituitary and adrenal responsiveness to endogenous and exogenous stimulation (Hawkins *et al.* 1999, 2000) and in significant alterations in fetal adrenal P450$_{C17}$ and 3β-HSD steroidogenic enzymes (Fraser *et al.* 2001b).

Many of these alterations in HPA axis function in the offspring have been attributed to changes in corticosteroid receptor populations in higher brain centres (hippocampus and hypothalamus) (Langley-Evans *et al.* 1996a). Recently Sebaai *et al.* (2004) demonstrated that rats exposed to prenatal nutrient restriction exhibited reduced body weight, increased hippocampal MR : GR mRNA ratio and increased POMC and GR mRNA in the pituitary. These changes were accompanied by an increase in basal corticosterone levels. In the sheep, a modest 15% reduction in maternal nutrition early in pregnancy resulted in a decrease in CRH mRNA in the hypothalamic PVN of near-term fetuses (Hawkins

et al. 2001). In the guinea pig, 48 hours of maternal nutrient deprivation resulted in a significant reduction in GR mRNA levels in the regions of the hypothalamic PVN and hippocampal CA1–2 in females and hippocampal CA1–2 in male fetuses at 52 days of gestation. Furthermore, maternal and fetal cortisol levels were increased significantly after maternal nutrient restriction, but these increases in cortisol concentrations were associated with elevated ACTH levels only in the maternal circulation. This study demonstrated that nutrient deprivation increased maternal HPA activity and resulted in an increase in placental transfer of maternal glucocorticoids to the fetal circulation (Lingas *et al.* 1999). Alterations in maternal nutrition have been linked to changes in offspring endocrine function in humans as well. Herrick *et al.* (2003) reported that an unbalanced high-meat/fish, low-green-vegetable diet during pregnancy may present a metabolic stress to the mother and programme the HPA axis of offspring, leading to hypercortisolaemia.

The presence of the enzyme 11β-hydroxysteroid dehydrogenase type 2 (11β-HSD2) in the placental syncytiotrophoblasts protects the fetus from maternally derived glucocorticoids (Edwards *et al.* 1993). Maternal glucocorticoid levels are much higher than fetal levels for most of pregnancy, so a relative deficiency in placental 11β-HSD2 would put the fetus at great risk of glucocorticoid exposure (Edwards *et al.* 1993, Fowden and Forhead 2004). In some studies a strong positive correlation exists between placental 11β-HSD2 activity and fetal weight at term (Benediktsson *et al.* 1993, Stewart *et al.* 1995), and birthweights in preterm infants (Kajantie *et al.* 2003). Maternal protein restriction in rats is associated with elevations in systolic blood pressure in adult offspring and attenuated placental 11β-HSD2 activity (Langley-Evans *et al.* 1996a, 1996b). In sheep, nutrient restriction results in a significant decrease in 11β-HSD2 activity in association with growth restriction (McMullen *et al.* 2004). In early studies, Lindsay *et al.* (1996) demonstrated that treatment of pregnant rats with carbenoxolone, a potent inhibitor of placental 11β-HSD2, resulted in significant reductions in birth weight, and in elevated basal concentrations of corticosterone and hypothalamic neuropeptides responsible for HPA axis regulation. These offspring also exhibited metabolic dysfunction and glucose intolerance. These effects were abolished by maternal adrenalectomy; therefore the effects must have been mediated via fetal exposure to maternally derived glucocorticoids (Lindsay *et al.* 1996). Strong evidence therefore exists to suggest that a deficiency in placental 11β-HSD2, resulting in the increased exposure of the fetus to maternally derived glucocorticoids, can programme the HPA axis and influence postnatal endocrine dysfunction.

Elevated HPA axis activity in the fetus not only has important implications for long-term endocrine regulation and health, but could also contribute to the process and timing of parturition. Recently, Bloomfield and colleagues (2003) have demonstrated that modest periconceptional undernutrition in pregnant sheep resulted in precocious prepartum fetal cortisol output and preterm birth. The authors suggest that modest changes in nutrition at around the time of conception resulted in accelerated HPA axis maturation late in gestation, subsequently initiating a cascade of molecular events leading to preterm labour. These data therefore suggest that the programming of HPA axis function may contribute to the initiation of preterm labour (and possibly preterm delivery) as well as sustained effects into adulthood by way of disease onset.

Synthetic glucocorticoids

In the rat, maternal dexamethasone administration ($100\ \mu g\ kg^{-1}\ day^{-1}$) over the last few days of pregnancy resulted in a reduction in birthweight, and the offspring had significantly elevated basal levels of corticosterone and blood pressure and a significant decrease in GR and MR mRNA levels in specific hippocampal subfields (Levitt *et al.* 1996). Maternal administration of dexamethasone to the rhesus monkey at 132 and 133 days of gestation (term is 165 days) resulted in significant alterations in the cytoarchitectural development of hippocampal neurons at 135 days of gestation (Uno *et al.* 1990) and at 10 months of postnatal age. Dexamethasone-treated

offspring also demonstrated higher basal cortisol levels and higher plasma cortisol levels following stress (Uno *et al.* 1994). Maternal dexamethasone treatment in the guinea pig resulted in significant changes in fetal basal cortisol and alterations in MR and GR mRNA in the hippocampus (Dean and Matthews 1999). Negative feedback at the level of the hippocampus results in an inhibition of HPA activity; therefore reduced glucocorticoid feedback through alterations in receptor number would elevate HPA activity (Jacobson and Sapolsky 1991).

Since fetal glucocorticoid exposure can alter the expression of GR, synthetic glucocorticoids can potentially impact at every level of the HPA axis. In the fetal sheep, maternal administration of dexamethasone early in gestation (40–41 days) resulted in significant elevations in basal ACTH and cortisol levels in fetuses at 131 days of gestation, in addition to elevated ACTH responses to an exogenous CRH challenge (Cox *et al.* 1999). Benediktsson *et al.* (1993) demonstrated that dexamethasone treatment of pregnant rats resulted in offspring with a significant reduction in birthweight and elevations in systolic blood pressure. Bakker *et al.* (1995) showed that maternal administration of dexamethasone on day 17 and 19 of pregnancy in the rat significantly decreased birthweight, did not alter basal HPA function, but significantly decreased the ratio of CRH to AVP in the hypothalamus of offspring at 20 days postnatal age (Bakker *et al.* 1995). This may reflect subtle long-term effects on HPA regulation at the level of the hypothalamus. We have shown that maternal betamethasone administration in sheep resulted in HPA hyperactivity before birth (Sloboda *et al.* 2000) without associated changes in fetal hypothalamic and pituitary neuropeptide expression. We have also demonstrated that offspring of pregnant sheep treated with maternal betamethasone exhibited HPA hyperactivity in early adulthood (Sloboda *et al.* 2002), but later in life the adrenal became incapable of sustaining cortisol output and relative adrenal insufficiency developed (Sloboda *et al.* 2003). In these animals there is a dose-dependent increase in basal ACTH levels in adulthood, associated with significant reductions in basal cortisol levels. These alterations in HPA function were most pronounced in offspring that were exposed to multiple doses (Sloboda *et al.* 2003).

Glucocorticoids are critical for normal brain development, exerting effects on neuronal growth, cell-to-cell interactions and neuronal reorganisation (for review see Matthews 2001). Exposure of the developing brain to inappropriate levels of glucocorticoids during critical periods can modify both the structure and function of neurons. In sheep, fetal exposure to repeated doses of maternal betamethasone results in significant reductions in fetal brain growth (Newnham *et al.* 1999, Huang *et al.* 1999), and brain weight is reduced in adulthood (Moss *et al.* 2005). Fetal betamethasone exposure also resulted in reduced myelination of the optic nerve and corpus callosum of fetal sheep (Dunlop *et al.* 1997, Huang *et al.* 1999, Quinlivan *et al.* 1999), and decreased neuronal cytoskeletal microtubule-associated proteins (MAPs) and synapse-associated protein (synaptophysin) in the frontal cortex of fetal baboons (Antonow-Schlorke *et al.* 2003).

Programming of neuroendocrine development and HPA axis function may also be regulated through the serotonergic system. Nuclei within the hypothalamus that secrete CRH receive input from the forebrain through serotonergic inputs that are regulated by serotonin receptors 5-HT$_{1A}$ and 5-HT$_{2A}$ (for review see Dinan 1996). Alterations in serotonin receptors and transporters have been linked to hippocampal glucocorticoid receptor programming (Muneoka *et al.* 1997, Laplante *et al.* 2002). Andrews *et al.* (2004) have demonstrated in guinea pigs that prenatal dexamethasone treatment results in sex- and dose-dependent changes in serotonin receptor 5-HT$_{1A}$ expression in the fetal hippocampus. Whether these changes persist postnatally is unknown, although alterations in 5-HT$_{1A}$ have been associated with modified postnatal behaviour. Knockout mice lacking 5-HT$_{1A}$ receptors exhibit increased anxiety-like behaviour (Toth 2003). The link between HPA axis activity (and circulating glucocorticoids), serotonin receptor populations and behaviour is unclear, although current proposals suggest that glucocorticoids modulate/regulate neuroendocrine development through glucocorticoid receptor populations and significantly impact on serotonin receptor levels.

Fetal exposure to inappropriate levels of glucocorticoids has direct clinical relevance. Synthetic glucocorticoids are administered to women threatened with preterm delivery to enhance fetal maturation and reduce morbidity and mortality (Crowley 2003). In these cases, the fetus is exposed to high levels of potent synthetic glucocorticoids at a time in gestation when endogenous fetal cortisol levels may be quite low. Over 30 years ago, Liggins demonstrated that lambs delivered prematurely after fetal infusions of ACTH, cortisol or synthetic glucocorticoids have improved maturation in lung tissue (Liggins, 1969). Subsequently, Liggins and Howie, (1972) were the first to demonstrate that administration of synthetic glucocorticoids to women at risk of preterm delivery significantly reduced neonatal morbidity and mortality from respiratory distress. Since this first report a number of clinical trials have reported a decrease in the number of cases of RDS and mortality among infants whose mothers were treated with antenatal corticosteroids (Kari *et al.* 1994, Ballard and Ballard 1996, Anyaegbunam and Adetona, 1997). The National Institutes of Health Consensus Developmental Conference on the Effects of Corticosteroid for Fetal Maturation (NIH 1995) suggested that corticosteroids should be administered to women at risk of preterm birth between 24 and 34 weeks of gestation and in a treatment window of 24 hours to 7 days prior to delivery in order to reduce mortality, respiratory distress syndrome and intraventricular haemorrhage in preterm infants. As a result, the administration of synthetic glucocorticoids to women threatened with preterm delivery became routine practice. Until recently, because of the difficulty in diagnosing preterm labour and a reduction in the efficacy of the drug after seven days, multiple courses were administered.

In humans, neonatal head circumference decreases with increasing numbers of antenatal glucocorticoid courses (French *et al.* 1999). Repeated courses of glucocorticoids before birth were associated with a reduction in risk of cerebral palsy but with an increased risk of subsequent disorder in aggressive–destructive behaviour, hyperactivity and distractibility (Fig. 13.1; French *et al.* 2004). Reduced head-circumference at birth and head-circumference growth velocity during the first year of life have been strongly associated with learning difficulties and cognition in school-aged children (Stathis *et al.* 1999). Infants exposed to 3–11 courses of prenatal glucocorticoids exhibited lower whole-brain cortex convolution indices and a smaller surface area (Modi *et al.* 2001). It is likely that brain function and HPA axis regulation could be related to brain growth and exposure to glucocorticoids during development. Gale *et al.* (2003) demonstrated that individuals who had larger head circumference as adults gained significantly higher scores on intelligence tests and were less likely to show a decline in memory performance with age.

Due to the overwhelming amount of data that has emerged from animal and human studies investigating the effects of this practice, a recent NIH Consensus Statement (2001) has recommended that repeated courses of maternal synthetic glucocorticoid should not be administered to women threatened with preterm delivery, except for those enrolled in randomised controlled trials. In spite of this recommendation, however, a recent report has demonstrated that 40% of obstetricians surveyed in the Royal Australian and New Zealand College of Obstetricians and Gynaecologists still prescribe repeated doses of antenatal corticosteroids to their pregnant patients (McLaughlin and Crowther 2003).

HPA axis programming and long-term outcomes

Adverse behaviour, cognition disorders and mood disorders such as anxiety and depression may involve pathways that include intrauterine exposure to cortisol and programming of the fetal HPA axis. The first reports describing the fetal and obstetric determinants of 'mental deficiency' and 'mental

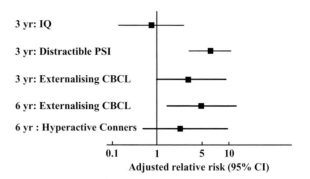

Figure 13.1 Relative risks and 95% confidence intervals at 3 and 6 years of age for children who had received three or more doses of antenatal glucocorticoids. All data were adjusted for maternal smoking, socioeconomic score, and gestational age at birth, sex and IQ. CBCL, Child Behaviour Check List; IQ, intelligence quotient; PSI, Parenting Stress Index (French *et al.* 2004).

disease' were published over 50 years ago (Pasamanick and Lilienfeld 1955, Barker 1966, Leon 2001). Subtle fetal adaptations to changes in the intrauterine environment may not display gross abnormalities (such as growth restriction) but still exhibit changes in function later in life. Richards *et al.* (2001) demonstrated that birthweight was associated with cognitive ability at age 8 in the general population within the normal birthweight range. Furthermore, a recent study demonstrates that DNA methylation can be modified in rats through behavioural programming and may be reversible (Weaver *et al.* 2004), suggesting that a new era of potential mechanisms has emerged in the fetal programming arena.

In an ideal intrauterine environment, fetal endocrine development would progress along a trajectory that permits optimal growth and appropriate timing of maturation of organ systems that contribute to long-term health. However, in circumstances where this environment changes, or in some cases becomes overtly adverse, the fetus has the capacity to adapt in a way that facilitates survival. In extreme cases the fetus may even initiate its own delivery from this environment through the process of premature birth. The fetal endocrine environment plays a central role in these adaptive processes.

Perinatal growth and development and long-term health are associated with fetal endocrine status, and HPA axis programming appears to play a central role. Premature exposure of the fetus to cortisol may thus prepare the fetus for a world perceived by the maternal endocrine system to be hostile and stressful, resulting in changes in long-term stress responsiveness, behaviour and cognition. Although this field of research has expanded dramatically in the last decade, further studies are required to elucidate the exact mechanism linking prenatal adaptive processes, HPA axis development and long-term postnatal modifications.

REFERENCES

Amaral, D. G. and Witter, M. P. (1989). The three dimensional organization of the hippocampal formation: a review of anatomical data. *Neuroscience*, **31**, 571–91.

Andrews, M. H., Kostaki, A., Setiawan, E. *et al.* (2004). Developmental regulation of 5-HT7 receptor and NGFI-A in the fetal limbic system: influence of glucocorticoid. *J. Physiol.*, **555**, 659–70.

Antonow-Schlorke, I., Schwab, M., Li, C. and Nathanielsz, P. W. (2003). Glucocorticoid exposure at the dose used clinically alters cytoskeletal proteins and presynaptic terminals in the fetal baboon brain. *J. Physiol.*, **547**, 117–23.

Anyaegbunam, W. I. and Adetona, A. B. (1997). Use of antenatal corticosteroids for fetal maturation in preterm infants. *Am. Fam. Physician*, **56**, 1093–6.

Austin, M. P. and Leader, L. (2000). Maternal stress and obstetric and infant outcomes: epidemiological findings and neuroendocrine mechanisms. *Aust. NZ J. Obstet. Gynaecol.*, **40**, 331–7.

Bakker, J. M., Schmidt, E. D., Kroes, H. *et al.* (1995). Effects of short-term dexamethasone treatment during pregnancy on the development of the immune system and the hypothalamo-pituitary adrenal axis in the rat. *J. Neuroimmunol.*, **63**, 183–91.

Ballard, R. A. and Ballard, P. L. (1996). Antenatal hormone therapy for improving the outcome of the preterm infant. *J. Perinatol.*, **16**, 390–6.

Bamberger, C. M., Schulte, H. M. and Chrousos, G. P. (1996). Molecular determinants of glucocorticoid receptor function and tissue sensitivity to glucocorticoids. *Endocr. Rev.*, **17**, 245–60.

Barker, D. J. P. (1966). Low intelligence: its relation to length of gestation and rate of foetal growth. *Br. J. Prev. Soc. Med.*, **20**, 58–66.

(1994a). The fetal origins of adult disease. *Fetal Matern. Med. Rev.*, **6**, 71–80.

(1994b). *Mothers, Babies and Disease in Later Life.*, London: BMJ Publishing Group.

(1995). The fetal and infant origins of disease. *Eur. J. Clini. Investiga.*, **25**, 457–63.

Benediktsson, R., Lindsay, R. S., Noble, J. M., Seckl, J. R. and Edwards, C. R. W. (1993). Glucocorticoid exposure in utero: new model for adult hypertension. *Lancet*, **341**, 339–41.

Bertram, C. E. and Hanson, M. A. (2002). Prenatal programming of postnatal endocrine responses by glucocorticoids. *Reproduction*, **124**, 459–67.

Bloomfield, F. H., Oliver, M. H., Hawkins, P. *et al.* (2003). A periconceptional nutritional origin for noninfectious preterm birth. *Science*, **300**, 606.

Boshier, D. P. and Holloway, H. (1989). Morphometric analyses of adrenal gland growth in fetal and neonatal sheep. I. The adrenal cortex. *J. Anat.*, **167**, 1–14.

(1991). Morphometric analyses of adrenal gland growth in fetal and neonatal sheep. III. Volumes of the major organelles within the zona fasciculata steroidogenic cells. *J. Anat.*, **178**, 175–87.

Brooks, A. N. and Challis, J. R. G. (1989). Effects of CRF, AVP and opioid peptides on pituitary–adrenal responses in sheep. *Peptides*, **10**, 1291–3.

Challis, J. R. G., Lye, S. J. and Welsh, J. (1986). Ovine fetal adrenal maturation at term and during fetal ACTH administration: evidence that the modulating effect of cortisol may involve cAMP. *Can. J. Physiol. Pharmacol.*, **64**, 1085–90.

Challis, J. R. G., Sloboda, D., Matthews, S. G. *et al.* (2001). The fetal placental hypothalamic–pituitary–adrenal (HPA) axis, parturition and post natal health. *Mol. Cell. Endocrinol.*, **185**, 135–44.

Clark, P. M. S., Hindmarsh, P. C., Shiell, A. W., Law, C. M., Honour, J. W. and Barker, D. J. P. (1996). Size at birth and adrenocortical function in childhood. *Clin. Endocrinol.*, **45**, 721–6.

Clarke, A. S., Wittwer, D. J., Abbott, D. H. and Schneider, M. L. (1994). Long-term effects of prenatal stress on HPA axis activity in juvenile rhesus monkeys. *Dev. Psychobiol.*, **27**, 257–69.

Cox, D. B., Brubaker, P., Fraser, M., Whittle, W. and Challis, J. R. G. (1999). The effect of maternal dexamethasone during early pregnancy on fetal growth, HPA development and the control of glucose homeostasis. *J. Soc. Gynecol. Investig.*, **6**, 110A.

Crowley, P. (2003). Antenatal corticosteroids: current thinking. *BJOG*, **110** (Suppl. 20), 77–8.

Dean, F. and Matthews, S. G. (1999). Maternal dexamethasone treatment in late gestation alters glucocorticoid and mineralocorticoid receptor mRNA in the fetal guinea pig brain. *Brain Res.*, **846**, 253–9.

De Kloet, E. R., Vreugdenhil, E., Oitzl, M. S. and Joels, M. (1998). Brain corticosteroids receptor balance in health and disease. *Endocr. Rev.*, **19**, 269–301.

Dinan, T. G. (1996). Serotonin and the regulation of hypothalamic–pituitary–adrenal axis function. *Life Sci.*, **58**, 1683–94.

Dobbing, J. and Sands, J. (1979). Comparative aspects of the brain growth spurt. *Early Hum. Dev.*, **3**, 79–83.

Dodic, M. and Wintour, E. M. (1994). Effects of prolonged (48 h) infusion of cortisol on blood pressure, renal function and fetal fluids in the immature ovine foetus. *Clin. Exp. Pharmacol. Physiol.*, **21**, 971–80.

Dunlop, S. A., Archer, M. A., Quinlivan, J. A., Beazley, L. D. and Newnham, J. P. (1997). Repeated prenatal corticosteroids delay myelination in the ovine central nervous system. *J. Matern. Fetal Med.*, **6**, 309–13.

Durand, P. (1979). ACTH receptor levels in lamb adrenals at late gestation and early neonatal stages. *Biol. Reprod.*, **20**, 837–45.

Durand, P., Bosc, M. J. and Locatelli, A. (1980). Adrenal maturation of the sheep fetus during late pregnancy. *Reprod. Nutr. Dev.*, **20**, 339–47.

Durand, P., Locatelli, A., Cathiard, A. M., Dazord, A. and Saez, J. M. (1981). ACTH induction of the maturation of ACTH-sensitive adenylate cyclase system in the ovine fetal adrenal. *J. Steroid Biochem.*, **15**, 445–8.

Edwards, C. R. W., Benediktsson, R., Lindsay, R. S. and Seckl, J. R. (1993). Dysfunction of placental glucocorticoid barrier: link between fetal environment and adult hypertension? *Lancet*, **341**, 355–7.

Feldman, S. and Conforti, N. (1980). Participation of the dorsal hippocampus in the glucocorticoid feedback effect on adrenocortical activity. *Neuroendocrinology*, **30**, 52–5.

Fernald, L. C. and Grantham-McGregor, S. M. (2002). Growth retardation is associated with changes in the stress response system and behavior in school-aged Jamaican children. *J. Nutr.*, **132**, 3674–9.

Field, T., Diego, M., Hernandez-Reif, M. *et al.* (2003). Pregnancy anxiety and comorbid depression and anger: effects on the fetus and neonate. *Depress. Anxiety*, **17**, 140–51.

Fowden, A. L. and Forhead, A. J. (2004). Endocrine mechanisms of intrauterine programming. *Reproduction*, **127**, 515–26.

Fowden, A. L., Li, J. and Forhead, A. J. (1998). Glucocorticoids and the preparation for life after birth: are there long-term consequences of the life insurance? *Proc. Nutr. Soc.*, **57**, 113–22.

Fraser, M., Braems, G. and Challis, J. R. G. (2001a). Developmental regulation of corticotrophin receptor gene expression in the adrenal gland of the ovine fetus and newborn lamb: effects of hypoxia during late pregnancy. *J. Endocrinol.*, **169**, 1–10.

Fraser, M., Oliver, M. H., Harding, J. E., Gluckman, P. D. and Challis, J. R. G. (2001b). Alterations in ovine fetal adrenal corticotropin receptor and steroidogenic enzyme mRNA expresssion following maternal undernutrition in late pregnancy. *J. Soc. Gynecol. Investig.*, **6**, 116A.

French, N. P., Evans, S. F., Godfrey, K. M. and Newnham, J. P. (1999). Repeated antenatal corticosteroids: size at birth and subsequent development. *Am. J. Obstet. Gynecol.*, **180**, 114–21.

French, N. P., Hagan, R., Evans, S. F., Mullan, A. and Newnham, J. P. (2004). Repeated antenatal corticosteroids: effects on cerebral palsy and childhood behaviour. *Am. J. Obstet. Gynecol.*, **190**, 588–95.

Gale, C. R., Walton, S. and Martyn, C. N. (2003). Foetal and postnatal head growth and risk of cognitive decline in old age. *Brain*, **126**, 2273–8.

Glickman, J. A. and Challis, J. R. G. (1980). The changing response pattern of sheep fetal adrenal cells throughout the course of gestation. *Endocrinology*, **106**, 1371–6.

Glover, V., O'Connor, T. G., Heron, J. and Golding, J. (2004). Antenatal maternal anxiety is linked with atypical handedness in the child. *Early Hum. Dev.*, **79**, 107–18.

Goland, R. S., Jozak, S., Warren, W. B., Conwell, I. M., Stark, R. I. and Tropper, P. J. (1993). Elevated levels of umbilical cord plasma corticotropin-releasing hormone in growth retarded fetuses. *J. Clin. Endocrinol. Metab.*, **77**, 1174–9.

Habib, M. and Galaburda, A. M. (1986). [Biological determinants of cerebral dominance]. *Rev. Neurol. (Paris)*, **142**, 869–94.

Haussmann, M. F., Carroll, J. A., Weesner, G. D., Daniels, M. J., Matteri, R. L. and Lay, D. C. Jr. (2000). Administration of ACTH to restrained, pregnant sows alters their pigs' hypothalamic–pituitary–adrenal (HPA) axis. *J. Anim. Sci.*, **78**, 2399–411.

Hawkins, P., Steyn, C., McGarrigle, H. H. G. *et al.* (1999). Effect of maternal nutrient restriction in early gestation on development of the hypothalamic pituitary adrenal axis in fetal sheep at 0.8–0.9 of gestation. *J. Endocrinol.*, **163**, 553–61.

(2000). Effect of maternal nutrient restriction in early gestation on hypothalamic pituitary adrenal axis responses during acute hypoxemia in late gesation fetal sheep. *Exp. Physiol.*, **85**, 85–96.

Hawkins, P., Hanson, M. A. and Matthews, S. G. (2001). Maternal undernutrition in early gestation alters molecular regulation of the hypothalamic–pituitary–adrenal axis in the ovine fetus. *J. Neuroendocrinol.*, **13**, 855–61.

Herrick, K., Phillips, D. I., Haselden, S., Shiell, A. W., Campbell-Brown, M. and Godfrey, K. M. (2003). Maternal consumption of a high-meat, low-carbohydrate diet in late pregnancy: relation to adult cortisol concentrations in the offspring. *J. Clin. Endocrinol. Metab.*, **88**, 3554–60.

Holmes, M. C., French, K. L. and Seckl, J. R. (1997). Dysregulation of diurnal rhythms of serotonin 5-HT$_{2C}$ and corticosteroid receptor gene expression in the hippocampus with food restriction and glucocorticoids. *J. Neurosci.*, **17**, 4056–65.

Huang, W. L., Beazley, L. D., Quinlivan, J. A., Evans, S., Newnham, J. and Dunlop, S. A. (1999). Effect of corticosteroids on brain growth in fetal sheep *Obstet. Gynecol.*, **94**, 213–18.

Jacobson, L. and Sapolsky, R. M. (1991). The role of the hippocampus in feedback regulation of the hypothalamic–pituitary–adrenocortical axis. *Endocr. Rev.*, **12**, 118–34.

Jacobson, L., Zurakowski, D. and Majzoub, J. A. (1997). Protein malnutrition increases plasma adrenocorticotropin and anterior pituitary proopiomelanocortin messenger ribonucleic acid in the rat. *Endocrinology*, **138**, 1048–57.

Kajantie, E., Dunkel, L., Turpeinen, U. *et al.* (2003). Placental 11β-hydroxysteroid dehydrogenase-2 and fetal cortisol/cortisone shuttle in small preterm infants. *J. Clin. Endocrinol. Metab.*, **88**, 493–500.

Kari, M. A., Hallman, M., Eronen, M. *et al.* (1994). Prenatal dexamethasone treatment in conjunction with rescue therapy of human surfactant: a randomized placebo-controlled multicenter study. *Pediatrics*, **93**, 730–6.

Koehl, M., Barbazanges, A., Le Moal, M. and Maccari, S. (1997). Prenatal stress induces a phase advance of circadian corticosterone rhythm in adult rats which is prevented by postnatal stress. *Brain Res.*, **759**, 317–20.

Kofman, O. (2002). The role of prenatal stress in the etiology of developmental behavioural disorders. *Neurosci. Biobehav. Rev.*, **26**, 457–70.

Kupfermann, I. (1991). Hypothalamus and limbic system: peptidergic neurons, homeostasis, and emotional behavior. In *Principles of Neural Science* (ed. E. R. Kandel, J. H. Schwartz and T. M. Jessell). New York, NY: Elsevier, pp. 735–49.

Langley-Evans, S. C., Gardner, D. S. and Jackson, A. A. (1996a). Maternal protein restriction influences the programming of the rat hypothalamic–pituitary–adrenal axis. *J. Nutr.*, **126**, 1578–85.

Langley-Evans, S. C., Phillips, G. J., Benediktsson, R. *et al.* (1996b). Protein intake in pregnancy, placental glucocorticoid metabolism and the programming of hypertension in the rat. *Placenta*, **17**, 169–72.

Laplante, P., Diorio, J. and Meaney, M. J. (2002). Serotonin regulates hippocampal glucocorticoid receptor expression via a 5-HT7 receptor. *Brain Res. Dev. Brain Res.*, **139**, 199–203.

Lemaire, V., Koehl, M., LeMoal, M. and Abrous, D. N. (2000). Prenatal stress produces learning deficits associated with an inhibition of neurogenesis in the hippocampus. *Proc. Natl. Acad. Sci. USA*, **97**, 11032–7.

Leon, D. A. (2001). Commentary. Getting to grips with fetal programming: aspects of a rapidly evolving agenda. *Int. J. Epidemiol.*, **30**, 96–8.

Levidiotis, M. L., Oldfield, B. J. and Wintour, E. M. (1987). Corticotropin-releasing factor and arginine vasopressin fibre projections to the median eminence of fetal sheep. *Neuroendocrinology*, **46**, 453–6.

Levitt, N. S., Lindsay, R. S., Holmes, M. C. and Seckl, J. R. (1996). Dexamethasone in the last week of pregnancy attenuates hippocampal glucocorticoid receptor gene expression and elevates blood pressure in the adult offspring in the rat. *Neuroendocrinology*, **64**, 412–19.

Levitt, N. S., Lambert, E. V., Woods, D., Hales, C. N., Andrew, R. and Seckl, J. R. (2000). Impaired glucose tolerance and elevated blood pressure in low birth weight, nonobese, young south african adults: early programming of cortisol axis. *J. Clin. Endocrinol. Metab.*, **85**, 4611–18.

Liakos, P., Chambaz, E. M., Feige, J. J. and Defaye, G. (1998). Expression of ACTH receptors (MC2-R and MC5-R) in the glomerulosa and the fasciculata-reticularis zones of bovine adrenal cortex. *Endocr. Res.*, **24**, 427–32.

Liggins, G. C. (1969). Premature delivery of fetal lambs infused with glucocorticoids. *J. Endocrinol.*, **45**, 515–23.

  (1994). The role of cortisol in preparing the fetus for birth. *Reprod., Fertil. Dev.*, **6**, 141–50.

Liggins, G. C. and Howie, R. N. (1972). A controlled trial of antepartum glucocorticoid treatment for prevention of the respiratory distress syndrome in premature infants. *Pediatrics*, **50**, 515–25.

Liggins, G. C. and Kennedy, P. C. (1968). Effects of electrocoagulation of the fetal lamb hypophysis on growth and development. *J. Endocrinol.*, **40**, 371–81.

Lindsay, R. S., Lindsay, R. M., Waddell, B. J. and Seckl, J. R. (1996). Prenatal glucocorticoid exposure leads to offspring hyperglycaemia in the rat: studies with the 11β-hydroxysteroid dehydrogenase inhibitor carbenoxolone. *Diabetologia*, **39**, 1299–305.

Lingas, R., Dean, F. and Matthews, S. G. (1999). Maternal nutient restriction (48h) modifies brain corticosteorid receptor expression and endocrine function in the fetal guinea pig. *Brain Res.*, **846**, 236–42.

Lu, F. and Challis, J. R. G. (1994). Regulation of ovine fetal pituitary function by corticotrophin-releasing hormone, arginine vasopressin and cortisol in vitro. *J. Endocrinol.*, **143**, 199–208.

Lunblad, J. R. and Roberts, J. L. (1988). Regulation of proopiomelanocortin gene expression in pituitary. *Endocr. Rev.*, **9**, 135–58.

Mandell, A. J., Chapman, L. F., Rand, R. W. and Walter, R. D. (1963). Plasma corticosteroids: changes in concentration after stimulation of hippocampus and amygdala. *Science*, **139**, 1212.

Matthews, S. G. (2001). Antenatal glucocorticoids and the developing brain: mechanisms of action. *Semin. Neonatol.*, **6**, 309–17.

Matthews, S. G. and Challis, J. R. G. (1995). Levels of proopiomelanocortin and prolactin mRNA in the fetal sheep pituitary following hypoxemia and glucocorticoid treatment in late gestation. *J. Endocrinol.*, **147**, 139–46.

Matthews, S. G., Owen, D., Kalabis, G. *et al.* (2004). Fetal glucocorticoid exposure and hypothalamo–pituitary–adrenal (HPA) function after brith.. *Endocr. res.*, **30**, 827–36.

McCormick, C. M., Smythe, J. W., Sharma, S. and Meaney, M. (1995). Sex specific effects of prenatal stress on hypothalamic-pituitary adrenal responses to stress and brain glucocorticoid receptors density in rats. *Dev. Brain Res.*, **84**, 55–61.

McDonald, T. J., Hoffman, G. E. and Nathaneilsz, P. W. (1992). Hypothalamic paraventricular nuclear lesions delay corticotroph maturation in the fetal sheep anterior pituitary. *Endocrinology*, **131**, 1101–6.

McLaughlin, K. J. and Crowther, C. A. (2003). Repeat prenatal corticosteroids: who still recommends their use and why? *Aust. NZ J. Obstet. Gynaecol.*, **43**, 199–202.

McMullen, S., Osgerby, J. C., Thurston, L. M. *et al.* (2004). Alterations in placental 11 beta-hydroxysteroid dehydrogenase (11 betaHSD) activities and fetal cortisol: cortisone ratios induced by nutritional restriction prior to conception and at defined stages of gestation in ewes. *Reproduction*, **127**, 717–25.

Meaney, M., Sapolsky, R. M. and McEwen, B. S. (1985). The development of the glucocorticoid receptor system in the rat limbic brain. I. Ontogeny and autoregulation. *Dev. Brain Res.*, **18**, 159–164.

Modi, N., Lewis, H., Al-Naqeeb, N., Ajayi-Obe, M., Dore, C. J. and Rutherford, M. (2001). The effects of repeated antenatal glucocorticoid therapy on the developing brain. *Pediatr. Res.*, **50**, 581–5.

Moss, T. J. M., Doherty, D., Nitsos, I., Sloboda, D. M., Harding, R. and Newnham, J. P. (2005). Effects into adulthood of single or repeated antenatal corticosteroids in sheep. *Am. J. Obstet. Gynecol.*, **192**, 146–52.

Mulchahey, J. J., DiBlasio, A. M., Martin, M. C., Blumenfeld, Z. and Jaffe, R. B. (1987). Hormone production and peptide regulation of the human fetal pituitary gland. *Endocr. Rev.*, **8**, 406–425.

Muneoka, K., Mikuni, M., Ogawa, T. *et al.* (1997). Prenatal dexamethasone exposure alters brain monoamine metabolism and adrenocortical response in rat offspring. *Am. J. Physiol.*, **273**, R1669–75.

Newnham, J. P., Evans, S. F., Godfrey, M., Huang, W., Ikegami, M. and Jobe, A. (1999). Maternal, but not fetal, administration of corticosteroids restricts fetal growth. *J. Matern. Fetal Med.*, **8**, 81–7.

NIH (1995). Effect of corticosteroids for fetal maturation on perinatal outcomes, NIH Consensus Development Panel on the Effect of Corticosteroids for Fetal Maturation on Perinatal Outcomes. *JAMA*, **273**, 413–18.

(2001). Antenatal corticosteroids revisited: repeat courses. National Institutes of Health Consensus Development Conference Statement, August 17–18, 2000. *Obstet. Gynecol.*, **98**, 144–50.

Norman, L. J., Lye, S. J., Wlodek, M. E. and Challis, J. R. G. (1985). Changes in pituitary responses to synthetic ovine corticotrophin releasing factor in fetal sheep. *Can. J. Physiol. Pharmacol.*, **63**, 1398–403.

O'Connor, T. G., Heron, J., Golding, J. and Glover, V. (2003). Maternal antenatal anxiety and behavioural/emotional problems in children: a test of a programming hypothesis. *J. Child Psychol. and Psychiatry.*, **44**, 1025–36.

Owen, D. and Matthews, S. G. (2003). Glucocorticoids and sex-dependent development of brain glucocorticoid and mineralocorticoid receptors. *Endocrinology*, **144**, 2775–84.

Page, R. B. (1988). The anatomy of the hypothalamo-hypophyseal complex. In *The Physiology of Reproduction* (ed. E. Knobil and J. D. Neill). New York, NY: Raven Press pp. 1161–233.

Pasamanick, B. and Lilienfeld, A. M. (1955). Association of maternal and fetal factors with development of mental deficiency. 1. Abnormalities in the prenatal and paranatal periods. *J Am Med Assoc*, **159**, 155–60.

Perry, R. A., Robinson, P. M. and Ryan, G. B. (1982). Ultrastructure of the pars intermedia of the developing sheep hypophysis *Cell Tissue Res.*, **224**, 369–81.

Perry, R. A., Mulvogue, H. M., McMillen, I. C. and Robinson, P. M. (1985). Immunohistochemical localization of ACTH in the adult and fetal sheep pituitary. *J. Dev. Physiol.*, **7**, 397–404.

Phillips, D. I. (2001). Fetal growth and programming of the hypothalamic–pituitary–adrenal axis. *Clin. Exp. Pharmacol. Physiol.*, **28**, 967–70.

Quinlivan, J. A., Dunlop, S. A., Newnham, J., Evans, S. F. and Beazley, L. D. (1999). Repeated, but not single, maternal administration of corticosteroids delays myelination in the brain of fetal sheep. *Prenat. Neonatal Med.*, **4**, 47–55.

Reperant, E. N. and Durand, P. (1997). The development of the ovine fetal adrenal gland and its regulation. *Reprod. Nutr. Dev.* **37**, 81–95.

Reul, J. M. H. M. and De Kloet, E. R. (1985). Two receptor systems for corticosterone in rat brain: microdistribution and differential occupation. *Endocrinology*, **117**, 2505–11.

Reynolds, R. M., Walker, B. R., Syddall, H. E. *et al.* (2001a). Altered control of cortisol secretion in adult men with low birth weight and cardiovascular risk factors. *J. Clin. Endocrinol. Metab.*, **86**, 245–50.

(2001b). Elevated plasma cortisol in glucose-intolerant men: differences in responses to glucose and habituation to venepuncture. *J. Clin. Endocrinol. Metab.*, **86**, 1149–53.

Richards, M., Hardy, R., Kuh, D. and Wadsworth, M. E. J. (2001). Birth weight and cognitive function in the British 1946 birth cohort: longitudinal population based study. *BMJ*, **322**, 199–203.

Roussel, S., Hemsworth, P. H., Boissy, A. and Duvaux-Ponter, C. (2004). Effects of repeated stress during pregnancy in ewes on the behavioural and physiological responses to stressful events and birth weight of their offspring. *Appl. Anim. Behav. Sci.*, **85**, 259–76.

Rubin, R. T., Mandell, A. J. and Crandall, P. H. (1966). Corticosteroid responses to limbic stimulation in man: localization of stimulus site. *Science*, **153**, 767–8.

Sebaai, N., Lesage, J., Breton, C., Vieau, D. and Deloof, S. (2004). Perinatal food deprivation induces marked alterations of the hypothalamo–pituitary–adrenal axis in 8-month-old male rats both under basal conditions and after a dehydration period. *Neuroendocrinology*, **79**, 163–73.

Setiawan, E., Owen, D., McCabe, L., Kostaki, A., Andrews, M. H. and Matthews, S. G. (2004). Glucocorticoids do not alter developmental expression of hippocampal or pituitary steroid receptor coactivator-1 and -2 in the late gestation fetal guinea pig. *Endocrinology*, **145**, 3796–803.

Sloboda, D. M., Newnham, J. and Challis, J. R. G. (2000). Effects of repeated maternal betamethasone administration on growth and hypothalamic–pituitary–adrenal function of the ovine fetus at term. *J. Endocrinol.*, **165**, 79–91.

Sloboda, D. M., Moss, T. J., Gurrin, L. C., Newnham, J. and Challis, J. R. G. (2002). The effect of prenatal betamethasone administration on postnatal ovine hypothalamic–pituitary–adrenal function. *J. Endocrinol.*, **172**, 71–81.

Sloboda, D. M., Moss, T., Nitsos, I., Doherty, D. A., Challis, J. R. G. and Newnham, J. P. (2003). Antenatal glucocorticoid treatment in sheep results in adrenal suppression in adulthood. *J. Soc. Gynecol. Investig.*, **10**, 233A.

Stathis, S. L., O'Callaghan, M., Harvey, J. and Rogers, Y. (1999). Head circumference in ELBW babies is associated with learning difficulties and cognition but not ADHD in the school-aged child. *Dev. Med. Child Neurol.*, **41**, 375–80.

Stewart, P. M., Rogerson, F. M. and Mason, J. I. (1995). Type 2 11β hydroxysteroid dehydrogenase messenger ribonucleic acid and activity in human placenta and fetal membranes: its relationship to birth weight and putative role in fetal adrenal steroidogenesis. *J. Clin. Endocrinol. Metab.*, **80**, 885–90.

Swanson, L. W. and Sawchenko, P. E. (1983). Hypothalamic integration: organization of the paraventricular and supraoptic nuclei. *Ann. Rev. Neurosci.*, **6**, 269–324.

Swanson, L. W. and Simmons, D. M. (1989). Differential steroid hormone and neural influences on peptide mRNA levels in CRH cells of the paraventricular nucleus: a hybridization histochemical study in the rat. *J. Comp. Neurol.*, **285**, 413–35.

Takahashi, L. K. (1998). Prenatal stress: consequences of glucocorticoids on hippocampal development and function. *Internat. J. Neurosci.*, **16**, 199–207.

Takahashi, L. K. and Kalin, N. H. (1991). Early developmental and temporal characteristics of stress-induced secretion of pituitary adrenal hormones in prenatally stressed rat pups. *Brain Res.*, **558**, 75–8.

Tonolo, G., Fraser, G., Connell, J. M. and Kenyon, C. J. (1988). Chronic low dose infusions of dexamethasone in rats: effects on blood pressure, body weight and plasma atrial natriuretic peptide. *J. Hypertens.*, **6**, 25–31.

Toth, M. (2003). 5-HT1A receptor knockout mouse as a genetic model of anxiety. *Eur. J. Pharmacol.*, **463**, 177–84.

Uno, H., Lohmiller, L., Thieme, C. *et al.* (1990). Brain damage induced by prenatal exposure to dexamethasone in fetal rhesus macaques. I. Hippocampus. *Dev. Brain Res.*, **53**, 157–67.

Uno, H., Eisele, S., Sakai, A. *et al.* (1994). Neurotoxicity of glucocorticoids in the primate brain. *Horm. Behav.*, **28**, 336–48.

Vallee, M., Mayo, W., Maccari, S., Le Moal, M. and Simon, H. (1996). Long-term effects of prenatal stress and handling on metabolic parameters: relationship to corticosterone secretion response. *Brain Res.*, **712**, 287–92.

Van den Bergh, B. R. and Marcoen, A. (2004). High antenatal maternal anxiety is related to ADHD symptoms, externalizing problems, and anxiety in 8- and 9-year-olds *Child Dev.*, **75**, 1085–97.

Vazquez, D. M., Van Oers, H., Levine, S. and Akil, H. (1996). Regulation of glucocorticoid and mineralocorticoid receptor mRNAs in the hippocampus of the maternally deprived infant rat. *Brain Res.*, **761**, 79–90.

Wang, J. J., Valego, N. K., Su, Y., Smith, J. and Rose, J. C. (2004). Developmental aspects of ovine adrenal adrenocorticotropic hormone receptor expression. *J. Soc. Gynecol. Investig.*, **11**, 27–35.

Weaver, I. C., Cervoni, N., Champagne, F. A. *et al.* (2004). Epigenetic programming by maternal behavior. *Nat. Neurosci.*, **7**, 847–54.

Webb, P. D. (1980). Development of the adrenal cortex in the fetal sheep: an ultrastructural study. *J. Dev. Physiol.*, **2**, 161–81.

Weinstock, M. (1996). Does prenatal stress impair coping and regulation of hypothalamic–pituitary–adrenal axis? *Neurosci. Biobehav. Rev.*, **21**, 1–10.

Weinstock, M., Matlina, E., Maor, G. I., Rosen, H. and McEwen, B. S. (1992). Prenatal stress selectively alters the reactivity of the hypothalamic–pituitary–adrenal system in the female rat *Brain Res.*, **595**, 195–200.

Welberg, L. A. M. and Seckl, J. R. (2001). Prenatal stress, glucocorticoids and the programming of the brain. *J. Neuroendocrinol.*, **13**, 113–28.

Welberg, L. A. M., Seckl, J. R. and Holmes, M. C. (2000). Inhibition of 11β-hydroxysteroid dehydrogenase, the fetal–placental barrier to maternal glucocorticoids, permanenetly programs amygdala GRmRNA expression and anxiety-like behaviour in the offspring. *Eur. J. Neurosci.*, **12**, 1047–54.

Wintour, E. M., Brown, E. H., Denton, D. A. *et al.* (1975). The ontogeny and regulation of corticosteroid secretion by the ovine foetal adrenal. *Acta Endocrinol.*, **79**, 301–16.

14

Perinatal influences on the endocrine and metabolic axes during childhood

W. S. Cutfield, C. A. Jefferies and P. L. Hofman

University of Auckland

Introduction

Over the past 15 to 20 years, David Barker and colleagues at the Southampton Epidemiology Unit have made a sequence of landmark epidemiological observations linking reduction in birthweight with increasing risk of diseases in late adult life that included type 2 diabetes mellitus, syndrome X, hypertension, cerebrovascular disease, coronary artery disease and chronic bronchitis (Barker *et al.* 1989a, 1989b, 1993, Hales *et al.* 1991, Hales and Baker 1992, Robinson *et al.* 1992, Martyn *et al.* 1996). These observations were possible due to the meticulous neonatal and infancy records kept across several places in England, including Hertfordshire and Preston from 1911 onwards. These initial studies led Barker to propose the fetal origins of adult disease hypothesis (also known as the Barker hypothesis). This hypothesis proposes that the origins of adult disease begin in utero. The observations made by the Southampton Epidemiology Unit linking reduction in birthweight with disordered glucose metabolism in adult life have been confirmed by other research groups across ethnicities and countries including the Netherlands, USA, Sweden and India (Valdez *et al.* 1994, Curhan *et al.* 1996, Lithell *et al.* 1996, McCance *et al.* 1996, Ravelli *et al.* 1998). Arguably, the most important of these studies was conducted on adult survivors of the Second World War Dutch famine, in whom 2-hour plasma glucose values following

an oral glucose tolerance test were higher than in those born before or conceived after the famine (Ravelli *et al.* 1998). Furthermore, late-gestation famine exposure was associated with the highest 2-hours plasma glucose values. This was the first study in humans to link fetal undernutrition to long-term abnormalities in glucose regulation.

These epidemiological associations at the extremes of life relating birth size and diseases in late adult life do not establish a causative relationship. However, the relationship can be further strengthened if similar pathophysiological relationships are found between birth and childhood. In this chapter three groups of children will be examined: (1) those born small for gestational age (SGA, arbitrarily defined as a birthweight <10th percentile for gestational age); (2) those born prematurely and of very low birthweight (VLBW, arbitrarily defined as born at $\leq$32 weeks gestation); and (3) twins. Hales and Barker (1992) have shown that the relationship between a reduction in birthweight and either glucose intolerance or syndrome X in adult males is nonlinear. In those with a birthweight of <2.5 kg (<10th percentile, which equates to the definition of SGA), there is a marked increased risk of both disorders. In Barker's original cohorts from Preston and Hertfordshire, those of low birthweight did not include adults born prematurely. It is only in the past 20 years or so that those born VLBW have survived without major handicap. The Dutch

Developmental Origins of Health and Disease, ed. Peter Gluckman and Mark Hanson. Published by Cambridge University Press.
© P. D. Gluckman and M. A. Hanson 2006.

famine study data suggest that poor nutrition during the last trimester of pregnancy is associated with disordered glucose regulation and risk of diabetes mellitus (Ravelli *et al.* 1998). Consequently, it would seem reasonable to hypothesise that under- or malnutrition in the equivalent of the last trimester, whether in utero (as with SGA fetuses) or in a neonatal unit (as with VLBW infants) could lead to disordered glucose regulation. Twins are more likely to be born both SGA and premature, thus theoretically enhancing the risk of later metabolic abnormalities.

Small-for-gestational-age children

Auxological characteristics

The most commonly studied long-term sequelae of SGA infants are poor postnatal growth and short stature (Fitzhardinge and Steven 1972, Westwood *et al.* 1983, Tenovuo *et al.* 1987, Sung *et al.* 1993, Boguszewski *et al.* 1995, Karlberg and Albertsson-Wikland 1995). Most SGA children display growth acceleration to achieve a length in the normal range by 6 months of age, with a small portion exhibiting delayed growth acceleration during childhood. Despite differences in SGA definition, 80% of SGA children achieve a length within the normal range by 6 months of age, and this is only increased to 86% by 12 months of age (Tenovuo *et al.* 1987, Karlberg and Albertsson-Wikland 1995). Of those that are short at 12 months of age, 50% remained short at final adult height (Karlberg and Albertsson-Wikland 1995). Overall, 8–14% of SGA infants become short adults (Albertsson-Wikland and Karlberg 1994, Karlberg and Albertsson-Wikland 1995, Lundgren *et al.* 2003). There is a greater risk of short adult stature in those with a birth length rather than birthweight standard deviation score (SDS) of ≤ -2. Interestingly, the SGA group represents a large proportion of all short adults: 22% when SGA was defined as birth length ≤ -2 SD from the mean and 14% when defined as birthweight ≤ -2 SD (Karlberg and Albertsson-Wikland 1995). Although puberty has been reported

to occur earlier in some SGA children, in most of these children pubertal onset is delayed (Vincens-Calvert *et al.* 2002). When corrected for the age of onset of puberty, the size of the pubertal growth spurt of short SGA children of both sexes is normal (Fitzhardinge and Steven 1972, Ledger *et al.* 1997).

The influence of parental heights on the height of SGA children has been overlooked in most studies. When adjustment is made for parents' heights, SGA subjects of both sexes achieve an adult height that is 4 cm below mid-parental height (Ledger *et al.* 1997). In the first two years of life, shorter birth length is the major influence on SGA catch-up growth into the normal height range, whereas throughout the rest of childhood, parents' heights had the greatest influence on catch-up growth, with SGA children who had tall parents showing the most impressive catch-up growth of all (Luo *et al.* 1998).

The endocrine axis

In late gestation and at birth the changes to the insulin-substrate and growth-hormone–IGF axes can be largely attributed to poor nutrition, with the majority of studies demonstrating elevated serum GH, low IGF1, IGF2 and IGFBP3, together with low insulin and increased IGFBP1 levels, as summarised in Table 14.1 (De Zegher *et al.* 1990, Lassarre *et al.* 1991, Giudice *et al.* 1995, Leger *et al.* 1996). These changes are in sharp contrast to the changes seen in these axes during childhood when nutritional constraint is removed.

Postnatally, there are major changes to the GH-IGF-binding protein axis as the uteroplacental constraint is removed. In the first few days of life, spontaneous pulsatile GH hypersecretion occurs (De Zegher *et al.* 1993). Moreover, exogenous GH-releasing hormone elicits an exaggerated GH response in SGA neonates during the early phase of catch-up growth (Deiber *et al.* 1989). Three days after birth, exaggerated GH secretion in SGA neonates was associated with increased levels of circulating IGF1, suggesting that nutritional inhibition of IGF1 secretion is removed before GH hypersecretion is inhibited (Deiber *et al.* 1989). The transient GH

Table 14.1 Comparison of circulating hormone levels from the growth and nutrition axes from fetal life to childhood in the SGA subject. Note that the short SGA childhood values are compared to short normal children to highlight the characteristics unique to being SGA.

	SGA fetus	SGA child
GH	↑	←→?
IGF1	↓	↑
IGF2	↓	↑
IGFBP3	↓	↑
IGFBP1	↑	↓
Insulin	↓	↑
Leptin	↓	↑
Adiponectin	↓	↓

hypersecretion in SGA neonates may drive the early growth acceleration that occurs to some degree in virtually all SGA infants. The mechanisms orchestrating neonatal catch-up growth in SGA infants remain enigmatic. Clearly genetic growth potential has a role, as earlier discussed, but there are no auxological, recognised biochemical or endocrine markers that reliably and accurately predict catch-up growth into the normal range in SGA infants.

There have been conflicting reports regarding the characteristics of the GH–IGF axis in SGA children, often attributable to the lack of matching or adjustment of key variables such as age, height or BMI. Both diminished and elevated spontaneous GH secretion in short SGA children have been reported; however, on closer scrutiny of the data these findings are rather unconvincing (Stanhope *et al.* 1989, Boguszewski *et al.* 1995, Woods *et al.* 2002). GH secretion rates increase with age in SGA children (Boguszewski *et al.* 1995). The reported changes in spontaneous GH secretion may be due simply to differences in the ages of the SGA and appropriate-for-gestational-age (AGA) cohorts studied (Boguszewski *et al.* 1989, Woods *et al.* 2002). Stanhope and colleagues (1989) found a reduction in the number of overnight GH pulses in short SGA children, but these occurred almost exclusively in children with Russell–Silver syndrome. No differences in stimulated GH levels

were found between short children born SGA or AGA (Boguszewski *et al.* 1989, De Waal *et al.* 1994).

Initial published studies found either lower or similar serum IGF1 and IGF2 levels and comparable IGFBP3 levels in SGA when compared to normal children of normal height. Low IGF1 values have been interpreted to be due to either GH deficiency or GH resistance, raising the possibility of partial GH deficiency or resistance (Boguszewski *et al.* 1989, De Waal *et al.* 1994, Leger *et al.* 1996). Unfortunately, height and weight were not matched between the SGA and control groups in these studies. Unlike normal-statured children, short SGA children are usually thin. Age, height and nutritional status (as measured by body mass index) have all been shown to positively influence IGFBP3 and IGF1 levels in normal and SGA children (Boguszewski *et al.* 1989, Stanhope *et al.* 1989).

We have shown that when short prepubertal SGA children are matched to normal prepubertal children for these three variables SGA children display higher serum IGF1, IGF2 and IGFBP3 values (Cutfield *et al.* 2002). The SGA children also had fasting hyperinsulinaemia that was directly and highly correlated with fasting plasma IGF1 levels, as shown in Fig. 14.1. We have demonstrated that these children have reduced insulin sensitivity (see below) and it is likely that the compensatory hyperinsulinaemia

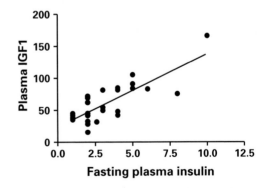

Figure 14.1 Correlation between fasting plasma insulin (mU L^{-1}) and IGF1 (µg m^{-1}) in 27 short prepubertal children born either SGA or of normal birthweight ($r^2 = -0.65$, $p < 0.0001$).

required to maintain euglycaemia was responsible for the elevated IGF1 and IGFBP3 levels observed. Insulin is thought to regulate circulating IGF1 levels by facilitating GH binding to the GH receptor in the liver and by stimulating IGF1 mRNA production in cultured hepatocytes (Boni-Schnetzler *et al.* 1991, O'Brien and Granner 1991, Bereket *et al.* 1995). Insulin may increase circulating IGFBP3 levels by reducing IGFBP3 degradation through reduction in serine protease activity (Baxter and Martin 1986, Yeoh and Baxter 1988).

The metabolic axis

The studies performed by the Southampton Epidemiology Unit linking reduction in birthweight and type 2 diabetes mellitus or syndrome X led Hales to propose the thrifty phenotype hypothesis, a refinement of the Barker hypothesis (Hales and Barker 1992). According to this hypothesis, insulin resistance and deficiency (due to β-cell hypoplasia) are the outcome of the undernourished fetus having to be nutritionally thrifty. For as long as an individual remains undernourished during postnatal life, glucose regulation remains normal. However, a sudden move to overnutrition, as occurs in energy-rich modern diets, exposes the deficiencies in insulin sensitivity and insulin secretory capacity, enhancing the risk of type 2 diabetes mellitus.

If adverse prenatal events lead to programmed alterations in insulin action and sensitivity that ultimately result in the development of type 2 diabetes mellitus in adult life, these changes should be present from birth. Reduced insulin sensitivity (i.e. insulin resistance) has been demonstrated in 20-year-old SGA subjects during an oral glucose tolerance test when compared to age-matched controls (Ledger *et al.* 1997). Insulin resistance was confirmed in a similar age group of young adults with the euglycaemic hyperinsulinaemic clamp, which identified a reduction in peripheral glucose uptake (Jaquet *et al.* 2000). It appears that reduced insulin sensitivity is the only overt feature of syndrome X present in young adults with SGA, although subtle differences in lipid parameters and adiposity have been documented

(Ledger *et al.* 1997, Jaquet *et al.* 2000). We have further extended the observation of reduced insulin sensitivity into the prepubertal years in SGA subjects. From our validated modification of Bergman's minimal model we found that prepubertal short children born at term and SGA were markedly insulin-resistant compared to an age-, height- and weight-matched group of normal children born at term (Cutfield *et al.* 1990, Hofman *et al.* 1997). The plasma glucose and insulin profiles during the frequently sampled IV glucose test in the two groups are shown in Fig. 14.2. To maintain euglycaemia an appropriate degree of compensatory hyperinsulinemia was observed in the SGA children, which indicates that these children do not have appreciable β-cell hypoplasia as proposed by Barker and Hales (Hales *et al.* 1991, Barker *et al.* 1993, Hofman *et al.* 1997, Ledger *et al.* 1997). The relationship between reduction in birthweight and insulin resistance was strengthened by the correlation between reduction in birthweight and progressive insulin resistance (Hofman *et al.* 1997). Subsequent studies have indirectly observed insulin resistance in SGA children as young as 12 months of age, adding further weight to the view that the defect in insulin sensitivity occurs prior to birth (Soto *et al.* 2003).

We proposed the fetal salvage hypothesis to explain the adaptive physiological changes of insulin resistance seen in those born with SGA (Hofman *et al.* 1997). The malnourished fetus receives inadequate nutrition for optimal growth. To ensure that adequate amounts of glucose are delivered to essential organs such as the brain, peripheral insulin resistance occurs, which allows for a redistribution of nutrient supply within the fetus. In this critical phase of development, inadequate nutrition leads to a permanent reduction in insulin-responsive skeletal muscle glucose transporter number or function. Support for such a hypothesis comes from intrauterine growth retardation studies in rats, in which there is a reduction in the glucose transporter GLUT1 in skeletal muscle but not the brain of affected fetuses.

The long-term consequences and associations of insulin resistance include not only the obvious potential risk of type 2 diabetes mellitus, but also

(a)

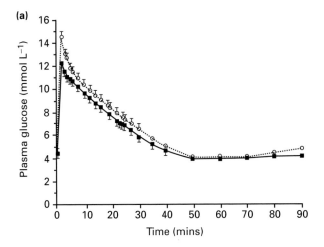

(b)

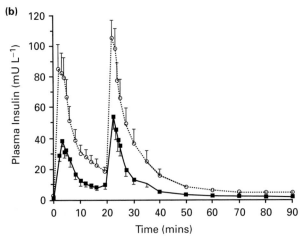

Figure 14.2 The glucose (a) and insulin (b) profiles during frequently sampled IV glucose tolerance testing in short prepubertal children born at full term and either SGA (open circles) or of normal birthweight (closed circles). From Hofman *et al.* (1997).

a diverse range of age-related diseases that include hypertension, coronary artery disease, cerebrovascular accident and cancer (Reaven *et al.* 1996, Facchini *et al.* 2001). Martin *et al.* (1992) showed that an isolated reduction in insulin sensitivity in those at risk of type 2 diabetes mellitus, such as a first-degree relative of a type 2 diabetic, was associated with a 40% cumulative incidence of type 2 diabetes over

25 years, whereas the relatives with a normal insulin sensitivity had a <5% risk of diabetes over the same interval.

Most insulin-resistant individuals will not develop type 2 diabetes mellitus. The two most likely explanations for this are:

(1) unless severe, insulin resistance may not lead to β-cell exhaustion and ultimately β-cell failure. A second inherent defect in glucose regulation may not be present. A triad of factors are responsible for normal glucose regulation: insulin-mediated glucose uptake (insulin sensitivity), glucose uptake independent of insulin (glucose effectiveness) and insulin secretory capacity (Bergman 1989). Insulin sensitivity has an inverse hyperbolic relationship with insulin secretion (Kahn *et al.* 1993). In other words, with increasing insulin resistance, a compensatory increase in insulin secretion must occur to maintain normal plasma glucose. The relationship between increasing insulin resistance and insulin secretion is not linear, and individuals shift their positioning on this relationship with changes in dietary and activity patterns. There are changes in both insulin, secretion and sensitivity, as shown in Fig. 14.3 which shows the relationship between insulin sensitivity and the acute insulin response (which is an indicator of insulin secretory capacity) in 120 prepubertal children born SGA, twin, prematurely or of normal birthweight and gestation. Major defects in at least two of these three parameters are needed before type 2 diabetes mellitus develops (Bergman 1989). An isolated defect in insulin sensitivity was seen in SGA children (Hofman *et al.* 1997).

(2) Active lifestyle changes that include exercise, reduction in food intake (particularly fat), increasing fibre intake and avoidance of smoking and other drugs that exacerbate insulin resistance can markedly improve insulin sensitivity. Generally, however, insulin resistance tracks through life, as too few individuals actively change their lifestyles to improve physiological wellbeing (Martin *et al.* 1992). Current data suggest that SGA subjects have a high risk of

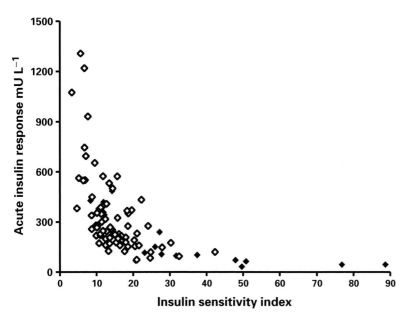

Figure 14.3 The hyperbolic relationship between insulin sensitivity and insulin response in prepubertal twin, SGA and prematurely born children (open diamonds), and normal prepubertal children (closed diamonds). Insulin sensitivity index expressed as 10^{-4} min^{-1} per $\mu U/ml$.

developing type 2 diabetes mellitus in late adult life, as seen in first-degree relatives of those with type 2 diabetes mellitus. These risks likely increase into adulthood as insulin resistance increases with the cumulative effect of puberty, sedentary lifestyle and obesity. There is evidence to suggest that children born SGA have an increased risk of adult obesity, and this may be the added metabolic burden that eventually leads to β-cell failure and type 2 diabetes mellitus (Byberg *et al.* 2000, Roseboom *et al.* 2001, Ong and Dunger 2002). In addition, genetic polymorphisms have been shown to exacerbate insulin resistance that include polymorphisms of IGF1, angiotensin-converting enzyme 1, the β-3 adrenoreceptor and PPARγ (Cambien *et al.* 1998, Arends *et al.* 2002, Jaquet and Czernichow 2003).

Adiponectin is an adipokine secreted from adipose tissue and has important roles in enhancing insulin sensitivity and in preventing atherosclerosis and inflammation. Plasma adiponectin levels are lower in SGA than in appropriate-for-gestational-age neonates (Kamoda *et al.* 2004). In addition, during childhood, plasma adiponectin levels are lower in normal or obese children and lowest of all in SGA children that exhibit catch-up growth (Cianfarani *et al.* 2004). The adiponectin levels were lower than expected in SGA neonates and children when correcting for fat mass, suggesting that hypoadiponectinaemia may reflect insulin resistance present in fetal life and during childhood (Cianfarani *et al.* 2004, Kamoda *et al.* 2004). It is also conceivable that the lower adiponectin levels seen in SGA children will enhance the risk of future atherosclerosis, given the potent anti-atherosclerotic and anti-inflammatory role that adiponectin displays (Goldstein and Scalia 2004).

Leptin is produced primarily in adipose tissue and reflects body fat mass. Leptin signals the amount of energy stores to the brain and has a role in appetite and energy metabolism. SGA newborns have lower leptin levels than AGA infants, probably reflecting the lower fat mass of the poorly nourished SGA fetus (Stoll-Becker *et al.* 2003). During childhood and adolescence short slim SGA children exhibit lower leptin levels than AGA children of normal weight (Pulzer *et al.* 2001, Doyle *et al.* 2004). However, we have found higher leptin levels in SGA prepubertal children compared to controls when correcting for DEXA-determined fat mass, again underpinning the importance of ensuring an appropriate control group (unpublished data). Thus it is conceivable that SGA children are in fact leptin-resistant. Interestingly, an exponential relationship was seen between increasing insulin resistance and increasing plasma leptin levels. Predictably, SGA children that exhibit acceleration in height and weight velocity during childhood have higher leptin levels than those that remain short and slim, indicating an increase in fat mass of those with height and weight acceleration (Doyle *et al.* 2004).

The reproductive/adrenal axis

Abnormalities in the reproductive and adrenal axes of SGA children and adolescents have recently been described. Precocious pubarche was initially reported in a cohort of north Spanish female adolescents born low-birthweight (Ibáñez *et al.* 1998). Compared to a control group of normal birthweight adolescents, this group demonstrated elevated dehydroepiandrosterone (DHEA) levels and a much higher risk of ovarian hyperandrogenism and developing polycystic ovarian syndrome (PCOS). This group was shown to be insulin-resistant, with the hyperandrogenism and menstrual abnormalities improved with insulin sensitisers (Ibáñez *et al.* 2002a). As insulin resistance is a recognised association with both SGA and PCOS it is not surprising the two have been linked. Indeed, insulin resistance is believed to be a prime early factor in the pathogenesis of PCOS (Dunaif 1997). Premature pubarche due to premature adrenache has also long been recognised as associated with PCOS. Thus these observations in SGA children are not unexpected. The risk of developing premature pubarche appears related not only to being SGA but also to postnatal growth rates, with children showing greatest postnatal weight gain

between 0 and 3 years having the highest DHEA levels (Ong *et al.* 2004).

Other reproductive abnormalities have been documented in female SGA adolescents, including smaller uterine volumes, reduced ovarian response to FSH (as determined by follicle number generation) and hypergonadotrophinaemia (Ibáñez *et al.* 2003). In infant SGA girls and boys elevated FSH levels have been observed, with normal inhibin B and LH levels (Ibáñez *et al.* 2002b). The later consequences of these metabolic abnormalities on reproductive function remain unclear, and follow-up of these subjects into adulthood is necessary.

Very-low-birthweight premature children

Over the past 20–25 years there have been considerable improvements in neonatal care leading to improved survival of VLBW (defined as birthweight < 1500 g) and extremely low-birthweight infants (ELBW, defined as birthweight < 1000 g). Analysis of outcome data from National Women's Hospital in Auckland, New Zealand, demonstrates that survival of infants with a birthweight between 1000 and 1500 g has improved by 12%, and of infants with a birthweight < 1000 g by 60%, from 1980 to 2000. Currently in New Zealand 7% of all live births are born premature (defined as < 37 weeks gestation) and 1.2% of live births are < 32 weeks gestation (approximating the formal VLBW infant definition of a birthweight < 1500 g). In addition, the number of VLBW and ELBW infants born between 1980 and 2000 has approximately doubled. Predictably, there are greater numbers of these children surviving into childhood with fewer major handicaps such as neurological, cognitive or visual impairment and chronic lung disease. While the major focus of long-term outcome data in these children has been the major handicaps outlined, scant attention has been paid to the endocrine and metabolic axes.

Auxological characteristics

The early pattern of growth of VLBW and ELBW infants is very similar to that seen in term children born small for gestational age (SGA). A rapid increase in height velocity results in a height within the normal range in more than 80% of children within the first six months of life in both of these groups. A small proportion of ELBW children have delayed height acceleration that may not become obvious until approximately 5 years of age (Doyle *et al.* 2004). Early studies that examined the growth pattern of prematurely born children through childhood found that these children achieved a height within the normal range (Sann *et al.* 1985, Elliman *et al.* 1992). However, most of these infants were not very premature at 34 to 36 weeks gestation. Recently the heights of young adults born VLBW and ELBW during the late 1970s and early 1980s have been reported. Final height data from these studies and others performed in adolescence reveal conflicting results. Hack *et al.* (2003) assessed 195 young adults of VLBW and compared them to 208 young adults born of normal birthweight. VLBW adult males were approximately 0.5 SD (standard deviations) shorter than control males, whereas there was no difference in the heights of the female VLBW and normal-birthweight groups. Conversely, Cooke (2004) found that low-birthweight young adult females were 8 cm shorter than those of normal birthweight, with only 4 cm difference in height between the low-birthweight and normal-birthweight young adult males. Doyle *et al.* (2004) presented longitudinal auxological data on 40 ELBW subjects to 20 years of age with assessments through childhood. At 2 years of age the height SD score approximated that at 20 years of age. Several other studies of adolescents born ELBW consistently show that these children are −0.5 to −0.7 SD shorter than adolescents born of normal birthweight (Hirata and Bosque 1998, Peralta-Carcelen *et al.* 2000, Siagal *et al.* 2001). As growth patterns usually stabilise in early childhood in this population these SD values are likely to reflect adult-height SD values. Remarkably few auxological studies of children born VLBW or ELBW have attempted to determine whether these children approximate genetic height potential. Although Doyle *et al.* (2004) found that young adults born ELBW were short, their parents were similarly short, with matching final height and

mid-parental height SD score. This is in contrast to our finding that in mid to late childhood, VLBW children were approximately 0.7 SD shorter than their parents right across the height range (Cutfield *et al.* 2004).

There are several possible explanations for the apparent conflicting height data in late childhood and at final height in those born VLBW and ELBW. First, none of these studies have attempted to determine just what proportion of the children evaluated exhibited short stature. Second, although considered a homogenous group as defined by birthweight, these children display considerable heterogeneity in the prenatal events that lead to premature birth and even greater heterogeneity in the way in which they are managed and the illnesses suffered during the critical first two months of life. Remarkably few studies have attempted to define whether either prenatal or neonatal events have a long-term influence on growth. Dexamethasone therapy has a dramatic short-term effect on growth in VLBW infants, with no lower-leg growth occurring during dexamathasone treatment (Gibson *et al.* 1993) Neonatal dexamethasone treatment adversely affects growth throughout childhood. In a randomised study of early dexamethasone therapy, the dexamethasone-treated children, assessed at 7 to 10 years of age, were shorter than untreated children (Yeh *et al.* 2004). This is the first study to identify a single perinatal characteristic in VLBW infants that led to adverse long-term consequences. The presence of SGA has been found to increase the risk of short adult stature in VLBW young adults, as has duration of neonatal hospital stay (Hack *et al.* 2003). Dissecting out specific prenatal and neonatal events in VLBW and ELBW infants that constrain long-term growth offers a more focused approach to better identify and characterise those at risk of short stature.

Neonatal intensive care continues to evolve decade by decade. Pre- and neonatal management strategies will continue to change; hence any long-term programmed auxological, endocrine, or metabolic sequelae may also change. Therefore it may not be valid to assume that the programmed sequelae encountered in young adults born with VLBW will occur in infants born today.

Table 14.2 Comparison of IGFs during mid childhood in prepubertal children between premature (< 33 weeks gestation) and short SGA, short normal and normal children.

	Premature		Term		Normal stature AGA controls
	AGA	SGA	AGA	SGA	
Height SDS	-0.8 ± 0.3	-1.9 ± 0.3	-2.6 ± 0.1	-2.4 ± 0.2	$0.1 \pm 0.3^*$
Weight-for-length index %	97 ± 9	80 ± 11	85 ± 10	84 ± 12	103 ± 8
IGF1 (μg L^{-1})	$57.5 \pm 5.6^*$	$53.4 \pm 7.0^*$	$36.8 \pm 3.6^*$	$82.7 \pm 8.3^*$	$117 \pm 9.1^*$
IGF2 (μg L^{-1})	582 ± 32	538 ± 65	$297 \pm 21^*$	$379 \pm 15^*$	–
IGFBP3 (μg L^{-1})	$1101 \pm 61^*$	$1065 \pm 101^*$	$1683 \pm 83^*$	$2107 \pm 134^*$	$2340 \pm 220^*$

$^*p < 0.001$

ELBW young adults tend to be heavy, which does not appear to occur in VLBW young adults. From the age of 5 years there is a progressive increase in weight velocity in those born ELBW, who ultimately become short, relatively heavy young adults with 30% being overweight (Doyle *et al.* 2004).

The endocrine axis

Although there are similarities between the growth patterns of children born SGA and VLBW, there are major differences in the circulating indicies of the growth-hormone–IGF1 axis. VLBW children display elevated growth-hormone levels during early infancy. Infants born at 24–34 weeks of gestation have elevated 6–12 hour spontaneous serum growth-hormone levels during the neonatal period when compared with term or SGA infants or older normal children (Miller *et al.* 1992, Wright *et al.* 1992). This increased GH secretion was the result of increased GH production rates with higher GH secretory burst amplitudes (Wright *et al.* 1992). VLBW infants have 24-hour urinary growth-hormone levels that are 7- to 72-fold higher in early infancy when compared with those of either preterm children of 34–37 weeks gestation or full-term infants (Quattrin *et al.* 1990, Fuse *et al.* 1993).

In complete contrast to SGA children, VLBW children exhibited low plasma IGF1 and IGFBP3 levels compared with term children of the same age, height and nutritional status, as shown in Table 14.2 (Cutfield *et al.* 2004). All three of these factors have been shown to have a major influence on plasma IGF1 and IGFBP3, hence the need for several control groups (Juul *et al.* 1995, Ong *et al.* 2002). Comparison of short, thin, term SGA children to short, thin, preterm SGA children enabled us to examine the effect of prematurity alone on the IGF–IGF-binding-protein axis (Cutfield *et al.* 2004). Similarly, comparison of the premature AGA to the normal-statured AGA control group enabled comparison of two groups of children of normal heights and weights, with prematurity the only difference between them. Interestingly, the combination of prematurity and SGA did not have any further influence on serum IGF1 or IGFBP3 levels than did prematurity alone (Cutfield *et al.* 2004). This suggests that there may be a threshold effect such that being born prematurely results in metabolic perturbations that are not further influenced by other adverse antenatal events such as being born SGA. The combination of elevated circulating growth-hormone levels in infancy and low plasma IGF1 and IGFBP3 levels in mid childhood raises the possibility that growth of VLBW infants is constrained by partial growth-hormone resistance. More formal assessment of growth-hormone sensitivity is required to test this hypothesis.

Elevated plasma IGF2 levels were seen in the term SGA children we studied. However, even higher values were seen in the preterm SGA and AGA children, as shown in Table 14.2. The reason for the elevated IGF2 levels is unclear. IGF2 levels have been shown to be associated with fat mass in normal children, with higher levels seen in obese children (Juul *et al.* 1995, Ong *et al.* 2002). However, there was no difference in IGF2 levels between the lean premature SGA group and the normally nourished premature AGA group. In one of the few follow-up studies of young adults born prematurely, those infants born AGA were heavier than those born at term of normal birth weight (Irving *et al.* 2002). Therefore, it is conceivable that the elevated plasma IGF2 levels we observed in premature children play a role in the development of later obesity during adult life.

The metabolic axis

The majority of studies evaluating the impact of perinatal events on glucose regulation after birth have focused on reduced birthweight, including SGA, in children and adults born at term. If metabolic abnormalities observed in later life reflect programming from an early adverse environment, then groups other than those born of reduced birthweight at term may also be at risk. Prematurely born children also suffer from an adverse early environment. The postnatal environment occurs during the equivalent of the third trimester of pregnancy and is similar to the adverse late in-utero environment seen in those born SGA. VLBW infants are physiologically immature and have a range of problems from nutrient access and growth to respiratory, CNS and immunological immaturity.

The few studies published to date support the hypothesis that prematurity may also result in metabolic programming. Irving *et al.* (2002) found that young adults born weighing < 2000 g and at 34 weeks gestation had an elevated BMI and systolic blood pressure compared to the controls. Baseline fasting insulin, an indirect marker of insulin resistance, was also significantly raised in the premature group. Fewtrell and colleagues (2000) recently studied 200 premature 12-year-olds using a 30-minute glucose and insulin following a standard oral glucose load. They found an association with birthweight and glucose level but not insulin when adjusted for current weight. However, this study had the major flaw of the subjects being at various stages of puberty, which markedly alters insulin resistance. Nonethe-

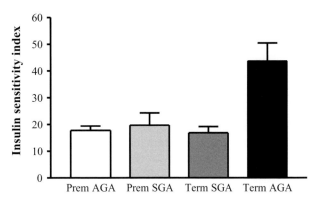

Figure 14.4 Insulin sensitivity values in premature and term children, subdivided into appropriate-for-gestational-age (AGA) and small-for-gestational-age (SGA) groups. Values expressed as mean ± SEM. Premature AGA and SGA compared to term AGA $p < 0.001$. Insulin sensitivity index expressed as 10^{-4} min^{-1} per μU/ml. Data from Hofman *et al.* (2004).

less, these studies both suggested a possible effect of prematurity on insulin sensitivity.

We have recently found (Hofman *et al.* 2004) that 50 prepubertal children born VLBW (24–32 weeks gestation) had an approximately 50% reduction in insulin sensitivity when compared to 22 term, normal birthweight control subjects, as shown in Fig. 14.4. The reduction in insulin sensitivity in the premature SGA and AGA groups is similar to that observed in term SGA subjects. Unlike term SGA children, the prematurely born children also had a reduction in glucose effectiveness, which reflects glucose's ability to increase its own uptake and suppress its own production. It has been demonstrated that defects in both insulin sensitivity and glucose effectiveness are additive and greatly increase the risk of later metabolic complications such as type 2 diabetes mellitus (Bergman 1989). There was no association between insulin sensitivity and either birthweight or degree of prematurity. We also did not see any difference in any metabolic parameters between premature AGA and premature SGA subjects. The effect of prematurity alone seemed to predominate, suggesting that the postnatal environment was more important in metabolic programming in prematurely born subjects. VLBW infants with a gestation < 32 weeks exhibit metabolic abnormalities, similar to those observed in term SGA subjects. However, unlike the SGA group, the timing of the insult to the post-natal period in VLBW infants suggests there may well be an accessible window in which therapeutic interventions could be implemented to ameliorate these metabolic sequelae. To identify the possible aetiology of insulin resistance in VLBW infants we have subsequently assessed a number of potentially important early postnatal events that could impact on glucose regulation. For example, infection stim-ulates cytokine production such as TNFα and IL6, both of which are known to reduce insulin sensitivity (Rosen and Spiegelman 1999). The fetus is exposed to potent synthetic glucocorticoids to inhibit labour. In addition, prolonged courses of high-dose dexamethasone, commenced in the first two weeks of life, are commonly administered to prevent chronic lung disease. Glucocorticoids have been shown to lead to marked insulin resistance (Paguano *et al.* 1983, Delaunay *et al.* 1997). Furthermore, premature neonates receiving glucocorticoids have higher fasting insulin values (Leipala *et al.* 2002). In our cohort we found no significant associations in any of these variables with the observed reduction in insulin sensitivity. However, it was clear that all the premature children were protein-malnourished, with none receiving the recommended adequate protein intake in the first month and the major-ity receiving less than the recommended amount over the following two months (Hofman *et al.* 2004). In addition, a disproportionately high quan-tity of fat was consumed in this first month of life. Rodent models of maternal protein malnu-trition result in a metabolic syndrome phenotype in the offspring, raising the interesting possibil-ity that the metabolic changes we have observed may be in part related to disordered macronu-trient intake (Woodall *et al.* 1996). Thus we pro-pose that low protein intake during the critical first month of life may lead to a programmed irreversible reduction in insulin sensitivity. This is in contrast to the conclusion of Singhal *et al.* (2003) that a nutrient-enriched diet in the first two to four weeks of life in premature children was associated with

reduced insulin sensitivity when assessed at 13 to 16 years of age. These authors compared 106 infants fed an enriched preterm formula with 110 infants who received standard term formula, either with or without expressed breast milk, until a weight of 2000 g was achieved. Higher levels of 32–33 split proinsulin, a very indirect marker of insulin sensi-tivity, were observed in the preterm formula group, which led the authors to conclude that relative undernutrition early in life in preterm children may have beneficial effects on insulin resistance. The authors appear to have over-interpreted their data. Fasting plasma insulin, a less indirect marker of insulin sensitivity, was the same in both groups, invalidating the claim that there was indeed any real difference in insulin sensitivity with the two dif-ferent early nutritional regimens. The recommen-dation that nutrition should be restricted in early infancy in those born prematurely to avoid later insulin resistance (Singhal *et al.* 2003) is inappro-priate when the data are more closely scrutinised. Clearly, further research is needed to evaluate more precisely the impact of early nutrition on glucose regulation across the gestational range of preterm children.

Twins

The metabolic axis

There are conflicting results from studies that have examined the relationship between birthweight and reduced insulin sensitivity or overt type 2 diabetes mellitus in adults. Poulsen and colleagues (2002) examined insulin sensitivity with the euglycaemic clamp in monozygotic and dizygotic twins in two age groups (25–34 and 57–66 years). Interestingly, in the younger group, monozygotic twins were found to be more insulin-sensitive than younger dizygotic twins. Conversely, in the older group the monozygotic twins were more insulin-resistant than the dizygotic twins. In contrast to the fetal-origins hypothesis, birth-weight was not found to be associated with insulin secretion or action in the younger adult twins. How-ever, there appeared to be an association between low birthweight and reduced insulin sensitivity and low insulin secretion in elderly monozygotic twins. These authors postulated that ageing could unmask the influence of an adverse intrauterine environment that leads to insulin resistance and low insulin secretion in twins. Vaag *et al.* (1995) found no difference in insulin sensitivity as assessed by the area under the insulin curve from glucose tolerance testing in adult monozygotic twins discordant for type 2 diabetes mellitus. Not surprisingly, β-cell function was reduced in the diabetic twin, consistent with the progressive nature of β-cell decline in the development of type 2 diabetes mellitus (Vaag *et al.* 1995, Gerich 1998, Kahn 2001).

Lifestyle influences such as obesity, activity levels, smoking, sex hormone use etc. were not usually considered in these adult twin studies, and may have served to increase variability in the assessment of insulin sensitivity. We examined insulin sensitivity in prepubertal twin children to minimise many of these lifestyle effects. We found there there was no difference in insulin sensitivity or insulin secretion between monozygotic and dizygotic twins ($p = 0.7$) (Jefferies *et al.* 2004). This observation argues against a genetic influence on insulin sensitivity during the prepubertal years in twins. There was concordance for insulin sensitivity within twin pairs, that was predictably higher in the genetically identical monozygotic twins, ($r^2 = 0.84$, $p = 0.004$) than within dizygotic twin pairs, ($r^2 = 0.32$, $p = 0.03$).

However, the prepubertal twins we studied had considerably lower insulin sensitivity values than control subjects matched for age and body mass index ($p < 0.01$). There was a slightly greater reduction in insulin sensitivity in twins than seen during childhood in those born either SGA or VLBW, as shown in Fig. 14.5. To compensate for insulin resistance the twins displayed compensatory hyperinsulinism when compared to control subjects, indicating an isolated defect in insulin sensitivity. The insulin resistance in twins compared to singletons was independent of gestational age, birthweight, zygosity, age, sex, and body mass index ($p < 0.001$). In twins insulin sensitivity was only weakly associated with birthweight SD score ($p = 0.14$) and gestation ($p = 0.09$). Most impor-

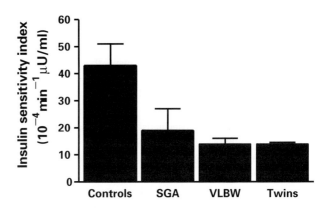

Figure 14.5 Comparison of insulin sensitivity values in prepubertal twin, very-low-birthweight, small-for-gestational-age and control children. Data from Hofman *et al.* (1997, 2004), Jefferies *et al.* (2004).

tantly, there was no difference in insulin sensitivity when the heavier-born twins were compared to the lighter-born twins in either monozygotic or dizygotic pairs ($p = 0.6$); therefore all twins regardless of birthweight had lower insulin sensitivity indexes than control subjects.

Glucose regulation appears to be fundamentally different in twins regardless of birthweight, suggesting that fetal undernutrition is unlikely to be a major factor in the development of insulin resistance in twins, as has been proposed for SGA children (Hofman *et al.* 1997). Other potential candidates that lead to insulin resistance in twins include placental factors or genetic polymorphisms that enhance twin survival. As twins, irrespective of birth size, are insulin-resistant they can no longer be considered a valid group to test the fetal-origins hypothesis linking birth size and later adult disease.

Summary

Prepubertal children born SGA, premature VLBW and twin all exhibit marked insulin resistance. There are similarities between SGA and VLBW children in that both are exposed to suboptimal environments that probably include undernutrition or malnutrition during the equivalent of the last trimester of pregnancy. Conversely, twins irrespective of birth size are insulin-resistant, suggesting that mechanisms other than undernutrition – such as placental factors or genetic polymorphisms that may improve twin survival – may cause insulin resistance in this group. Although both SGA and VLBW groups do not reach genetic height potential, and SGA and VLBW are recognised causes of short stature in childhood, there are differences between the groups in the growth-hormone and IGF1 axis. SGA children have elevated IGF1 levels, possibly due to either hyperinsulinaemia or partial IGF1 resistance, whereas VLBW children have low IGF1 and IGFBP3 levels suggestive of GH resistance. Thus the nature and timing of the early insult may lead to discordant changes to the metabolic and endocrine axes. The evolving programmed manifestations of adverse perinatal events in humans have become quite detailed; however, the specific insults and pathways that lead to these changes remain an enigma and will inevitably be the focus of future research in this fascinating and important field.

REFERENCES

Albertsson-Wikland, K. and Karlberg, J. (1994). Natural growth in children born small for gestational age with and without catch-up growth. *Acta Paediatr. Scand.*, **399** (Suppl.), 64–70.

Arends, N., Johnston, L., Hokken-Koelega, A. *et al.* (2002). Polymorphism in the IGF-I gene: clinical relevance for short children born small for gestational age (SGA). *J. Clin. Endocrinol. Metab.*, **87**, 2720.

Barker, D. J. P., Osmond, C. and Law, C. M. (1989a). The intrauterine and early postnatal origins of cardiovascular disease and chronic bronchitis. *J. Epidemiol. Community Health*, **43**, 237–40.

Barker, D. J. P., Osmond, C., Dolding, J., Kuh, D. and Wadsworth, M. E. J. (1989b). Growth in utero, blood pressure in childhood and adult life, and mortality from cardiovascular disease. *BMJ*, **298**, 564–7.

Barker, D. J. P., Hales, C. N., Fall, C. H. D., Osmond, C., Phipps, K. and Clark, P. M. S. (1993). Type 2 (non-insulin-dependent) diabetes mellitus, hypertension and hyperlipidaemia (syndrome X): relation to reduced foetal growth. *Diabetologia*, **36**, 62–7.

Baxter, R. C. and Martin, J. L. (1986). Radioimmunoassay of growth hormone-dependent insulin like growth factor binding protein in human plasma. *J. Clin. Invest.*, **78**, 1504–12.

Bereket, A., Lang, C. H., Fan, J., Frost, R. A. and Wilson, T. A. (1995). Insulin-like growth factor binding protein (IGFBP)-3 proteolysis in children with insulin dependent diabetes mellitus: a possible role for insulin in the regulation of IGFBP-3 protease activity. *J. Clin. Endocrinol. Metab.*, **80**, 2282–8.

Bergman, R. N. (1989). Lilly lecture 1989. Toward physiological understanding of glucose tolerance: minimal-model approach. *Diabetes*, **38**, 1512–27.

Boguszewski, M., Rosberg, S. and Albertsson-Wikland, K. (1995). Spontaneous 24-hour growth hormone profiles in prepubertal small for gestational age children. *J. Clin. Endocrinol. Metab.*, **80**, 2599–606.

Boni-Schnetzler, M., Schmid, C., Meier, P. J. and Froesch, E. R. (1991). Insulin regulates insulin like growth factor-1 mRNA in rat hepatocytes. *Am. J. Physiol.*, **260**, E846–51.

Byberg, L., McKeigue, P. M., Zethelius, B. and Lithell, H. O. (2000). Birth weight and the insulin resistance syndrome: association of low birth weight with truncal obesity and raised plasminogen activator inhibitor-1 but not with abdominal obesity or plasma lipid disturbances. *Diabetologia*, **43**, 54–60.

Cambien, F., Leger, J., Mallet, C., Levy-Marchal, C., Collin, D. and Czernichow, P. (1998). Angiotensin I-converting enzyme gene polymorphism modulates the consequences of *in utero* growth retardation on plasma insulin in young adults. *Diabetes*, **47**, 470–5.

Cianfarani, S., Martinez, C., Maiorana, A., Scire, G., Spadoni, G. L. and Boemi, S. (2004). Adiponectin levels are reduced in children born small for gestational age and are inversely related to postnatal catch-up growth. *J. Clin. Endocrinol. Metab.*, **89**, 1346–51.

Cooke, R. W. I. (2004). Health, lifestyle and quality of life for young adults born very preterm. *Arch. Dis. Child.*, **89**, 201–6.

Curhan, G. C., Willet, W. C., Rimm, E. B. and Stampfer, M. J. (1996). Birth weight and adult hypertension and diabetes mellitus in US men. *Am. J. Hypertens.*, **9**, 11A.

Cutfield, W. S., Bergman, R. N., Menon, R. K. and Sperling, M. A. (1990). The modified minimal model: a novel tool to measure insulin sensitivity in children. *J. Clin. Endocrinol. Metab.*, **70**, 1644–50.

Cutfield, W. S., Hofman, P. L., Vickers, M., Breier, B., Blum, W. E. and Robinson, E. M. (2002). Insulin-like growth factors and binding proteins in short children with intrauterine growth retardation. *J. Clin. Endocrinol. Metab.*, **87**, 235–9.

Cutfield, W. S., Regan, F. A., Jackson, W. E. *et al.* (2004). The endocrine consequences for very low birth weight premature infants. *Growth Horm. IGF Res.*, **14** (Suppl. A), S130–5.

Deiber, M., Chatelain, P., Naville, D., Putet, G. and Salle, B. (1989). Functional hypersomatotropism in small for gestational age (SGA) newborn infants. *J. Clin. Endocrinol. Metab.*, **68**, 232–4.

Delaunay, F., Khan, A., Cintra, A. *et al.* (1997). Pancreatic beta cells are important targets for the diabetogenic effects of glucocorticoids. *J. Clin. Invest.*, **100**, 2094–8.

De Waal, W. J., Hokken-Koelega, A. C., Stijen, T., de Muinck Keizer-Schrama, S. M. and Drop, S. L. (1994). Endogenous and stimulated GH secretion, urinary GH excretion, and plasma IGF-I and IGF-II levels in prepubertal children with short stature after intrauterine growth retardation. The Dutch Working Group on Growth Hormone. *Clin. Endocrinol.*, **41**, 621–30.

De Zegher, F., Kimpen, J., Raus, J. and Vanderschueren-Lodeweyckx, M. (1990). Hypersomatotropism in the dysmature infant at term and preterm birth. *Biol. Neonate*, **58**, 188–91.

De Zegher, F., Devlieger, H. and Veldhuis, J. D. (1993). Properties of growth hormone and prolactin hypersecretion by the human newborn on the day of birth. *J. Clin. Endocrinol. Metab.*, **76**, 1177–81.

Doyle, L. W., Faber, B., Callanan, C., Ford, G. W. and Davis, N. M. (2004). Extremely low birth weight and body size in early adulthood. *Arch. Dis. Child.*, **89**, 347–50.

Dunaif, A. (1997). Insulin resistance and the polycystic ovary syndrome: mechanism and implications for pathogenesis. *Endocr. Rev.* **18**, 774–800.

Elliman, A., Bryan, E., Walker, J. and Harvey, D. (1992). The growth of low-birth-weight children. *Acta Paediatr. Scand.*, **81**, 311–14.

Facchini, F. S., Hua, N., Abbasi, F. and Reaven, G. M. (2001). Insulin resistance as a predictor age related disease. *J. Clin. Endocrinol. Metab.*, **86**, 3574–9.

Fewtrell, M. S., Doherty, C., Cole, T. J., Stafford, M., Hales, C. N. and Lucas, A. (2000). Effects of size at birth, gestational age and early growth in preterm infants on glucose and insulin concentrations at 9–12 years. *Diabetologia*, **43**, 714–17.

Fitzhardinge, P. and Steven, E. (1972). The small-for-date-infant I. Later growth patterns. *Pediatrics*, **46**, 671–81.

Fuse, Y., Nemoto, Y., Wakae, E., Tada, H., Miyachi, Y. and Irie, M. (1993). Maturational changes of urinary growth hormone excretion in the premature infant. *J. Clin. Endocrinol. Metab.*, **76**, 1511–15.

Gerich, J. E. (1998). The genetic basis of type 2 diabetes mellitus: impaired insulin secretion versus impaired insulin sensitivity. *Endocr. Rev.*, **19**, 491–503.

Gibson, A. T., Pearse, R. G. and Wales, J. K. (1993). Growth retardation after dexamethasone administration: assessment by knemometry. *Arch. Dis. Child.*, **69**, 505–9.

Giudice, L. C., DeZegher, F., Gargosky, S. E. *et al.* (1995). Insulin-like growth factors and their binding proteins in the term and preterm human fetus and neonate with normal and extremes of intrauterine growth. *J. Clin. Endocrinol. Metab.*, **80**, 1548–55.

Goldstein, B. J. and Scalia, R. (2004). Adiponectin: a novel adipokine linking adipocytes and vascular function. *J. Clin. Endocrinol. Metab.*, **89**, 2563–8.

Hack, M., Schluchter, M., Cartar, L., Rahman, M., Cuttler, L. and Borawski, E. (2003). Growth of very low birth weight infants to 20 years. *Pediatrics*, **112**, e30–8.

Hales, C. N. and Barker, D. J. P. (1992). Type 2 (non-insulin-dependent) diabetes mellitus: the thrifty phenotype hypothesis. *Diabetologia*, **35**, 595–601.

Hales, C. N., Barker, D. J. P., Clark, P. M. S. *et al.* (1991). Fetal and infant growth and impaired glucose tolerance at age 64. *BMJ*, **303**, 1019–22.

Hirata, T. and Bosque, E. (1998). When they grow up: the growth of extremely low birth weight ($\leq$ 1,000 gm) infants at adolescence. *J. Paediatr.*, **132**, 1033–5.

Hofman, P. L., Cutfield, W. S., Robinson, E. M. *et al.* (1997). Insulin resistance in short children with intrauterine growth retardation. *J. Clin. Endocrinol. Metab.*, **82**, 402–6.

Hofman, P. L., Regan, F., Jackson, W. E. *et al.* (2004). Premature birth and later insulin resistance. *N. Engl. J. Med.*, **18**, 2179–86.

Ibáñez, L., Potau, N., Francois, I. *et al.* (1998). Precocious pubarche, hyperinsulinism, and ovarian hyperandrogenism in girls: relation to reduced fetal growth. *J. Clin. Endocrinol. Metab.*, **83**, 3558–62.

Ibáñez, L., Potau, N., Ferrer, A. *et al.* (2002a). Anovulation in eumenorrheic, nonobese adolescent girls born small for gestational age: insulin sensitization induces ovulation, increases lean body mass, and reduces abdominal fat excess, dyslipidemia, and subclinical hyperandrogenism. *J. Clin. Endocrinol. Metab.*, **87**, 5702–5.

Ibáñez, L., Valls, C., Cols, M. *et al.* (2002b). Hypersecretion of FSH in infant boys and girls born small for gestational age. *J. Clin. Endocrinol. Metab.*, **87**, 1986–8.

Ibáñez, L., Potau, N., Enriquez, G. *et al.* (2003). Hypergonadotrophinaemia with reduced uterine and ovarian size in women born small-for-gestational-age. *Hum. Reprod.*, **18**, 1565–9.

Irving, R. J., Belton, N. R., Elton, R. A. and Walker, B. R. (2002). Adult cardiovascular risk factors in premature babies. *Lancet*, **355**, 2135–6.

Jaquet, D. and Czernichow, P. (2003). Born small for gestational age: increased risk of type 2 diabetes, hypertension and hyperlipidaemia in adulthood. *Horm. Res.*, **59**, 131–7.

Jaquet, D., Gaboriau, A., Czernichow, P. and Levy-Marchal, C. (2000). Insulin resistance early in adulthood in subjects born with intrauterine growth retardation. *J. Clin. Endocrinol. Metab.*, **85**, 1401–6.

Jefferies, C. A., Hofman, P. L., Knoblauch, H., Luft, F. C., Robinson, E. M. and Cutfield, W. S. (2004). Insulin resistance in healthy prepubertal twins. *J. Pediatr.*, **144**, 608–13.

Juul, A., Dalgard, P., Blum, W. F. *et al.* (1995). Serum levels of insulin-like growth factor binding protein-3 in healthy infants, children and adolescents: the relation to IGF-I, IGF-II, IGFBP-1, IGFBP-2, age, sex, body mass index, and pubertal maturation. *J. Clin. Endocrinol. Metab.*, **80**, 2534–42.

Kahn, S. E. (2001). The importance of β-cell failure in the development and progression of type 2 diabetes. *J. Clin. Endocrinol. Metab.*, **86**, 4047–58.

Kahn, S. E., Prigeon, R. L., McCulloch, D. K. *et al.* (1993). Quantification of the relationship between insulin sensitivity and beta-cell function in human subjects. *Diabetes*, **42**, 1663–72.

Kamoda, T., Saitoh, H., Saito, M., Sugiura, M. and Matsui, A. (2004). Serum adiponectin concentrations in newborn infants in early postnatal life. *Pediatr. Res.*, **56**, 690–3.

Karlberg, J. and Albertsson-Wikland, K. (1995). Growth in full-term small for gestational age infants: from birth to final height. *Pediatr. Res.*, **38**, 733–9.

Lassarre, C., Hardoiun, S., Daffos, F., Forestier, F., Frankenne, F. and Binoux, M. (1991). Serum insulin-like growth factors and insulin-like growth factor binding proteins in the human fetus: relationships with growth in normal subjects and in subjects with intrauterine growth retardation. *Pediatr. Res.*, **29**, 219–25.

Ledger, J., Levy-Marchal, C., Bloch, J. *et al.* (1997). Reduced final height and indications for insulin resistance in 20 year olds born small for gestational age: regional cohort study. *BMJ*, **315**, 341–7.

Leger, J., Oury, J. F. and Noel, M. (1996). Growth factors and intrauterine growth retardation. I. Serum growth hormone, insulin-like growth factor (IGF)-I, IGF-II, and IGF binding protein 3 levels in normally grown and growth retarded human fetuses during the second half of gestation. *Pediatr. Res.*, **40**, 94–100.

Leipala, J., Raivio, K., Sarnesto, A. *et al.* (2002). Intrauterine growth restriction and postnatal steroid treatment effects on insulin sensitivity in preterm neonates. *J. Pediatr.*, **141**, 472–6.

Lithell, H. O., McKeigue, P. M., Berglund, L., Mohsen, R., Lithell, U. B. and Leon, D. A. (1996). Relation of size at birth to non-insulin dependent diabetes and insulin concentrations in men aged 50–60 years. *BMJ*, **312**, 406–10.

Lundgren, E. M., Cnattingius, S., Jonsson, B. and Tuvemo, T. (2003). Prediction of adult height and risk of overweight in females born small-for-gestational-age. *Paediatr. Perinat. Epidemiol.*, **17**, 156–63.

Luo, Z. C., Albertsson-Wikland, K. and Karlberg, J. (1998). Length and body mass index at birth and target height influences on patterns of postnatal growth in children born small for gestational age. *Pediatrics*, **102**, 72–82.

Martin, B. C., Warram, J. H., Krolewski, A. S., Bergman, R. N., Soeldner, J. S. and Kahn, C. R. (1992). Role of glucose and insulin resistance in development of type 2 diabetes mellitus; results of a 25-year follow-up study. *Lancet*, **340**, 925–9.

Martyn, C. N., Barker, D. J. P. and Osmond, C. (1996). Mother's pelvic size, fetal growth, and death from stroke and coronary heart disease in men in the UK. *Lancet*, **348**, 1264–8.

McCance, D. R., Pettitt, D. J., Hanson, R. L., Jacobsson, L. T. H., Knowler, W. C. and Bennett, P. H. (1996). Birth weight and non-insulin dependent diabetes: thrifty genotype, thrifty phenotype or surviving small baby genotype? *BMJ*, **308**, 942–5.

Miller, J. D., Wright, N. M., Esparza, A. *et al.* (1992). Spontaneous pulsatile growth hormone release in male and female premature infants. *J. Clin. Endocrinol. Metab.*, **75**, 1508–13.

O'Brien, R. M. and Granner, D. K. (1991). Regulation of gene expression by insulin. *Biochem J.*, **278**, 609–19.

Ong, K., Kratzsch, J., Keiss, W. and Dunger, D. (ALSPAC Study Team) (2002). Circulating IGF-I levels in childhood are related to both current body composition and early postnatal growth rate. *J. Clin. Endocrinol. Metab.*, **87**, 1041–4.

Ong, K. K. and Dunger, D. B. (2002). Perinatal growth failure: the road to obesity, insulin resistance and cardiovascular disease in adults. *Best Pract. Res. Clin. Endocrinol. Metab.*, **16**, 191–207.

Ong, K. K., Potau, N., Petry, C. J. *et al.* (Avon Longitudinal Study of Parents and Children Study Team) (2004). Opposing influences of prenatal and postnatal weight gain on adrenarche in normal boys and girls. *J. Clin. Endocrinol. Metab.*, **89**, 2647–51.

Paguano, G., Cavallo-Perin, P., Cassander, M. *et al.* (1983). An in vivo and in vitro study of the mechanism of prednisone-induced insulin resistance in healthy subjects. *J. Clin. Invest.*, **72**, 1814–20.

Peralta-Carcelen, M., Jackson, D. S., Goran, M. I. *et al.* (2000). Growth of adolescents who were born at extremely low birth weight without major disability. *J. Paediatr.*, **136**, 633–40.

Poulsen, P., Levin, K., Beck-Nielsen, H. and Vaag, A. (2002). Age-dependent impact of zygosity and birth weight on insulin secretion and insulin action in twins. *Diabetologia*, **45**, 1649–57.

Pulzer, F., Haase, U., Knupfer, M. *et al.* (2001). Serum leptin in formerly small-for-gestational-age children during adolescence: relationship to gender, puberty, body composition, insulin sensitivity, creatinine, and serum uric acid. *Metabolism*, **50**, 1141–6.

Quattrin, T., Albini, C. H., Mills, B. J. and Macgillivray, M. H. (1990). Comparison of urinary growth hormone and IGF-I excretion in small- and appropriate-for-gestational-age infants and healthy children. *Pediatr. Res.*, **28**, 209–12.

Ravelli, A. C. J., van der Meulen, J. H. P., Michels, R. P. J. *et al.* (1998). Glucose tolerance in adults after prenatal exposure to the Dutch famine. *Lancet*, **351**, 173–7.

Reaven, G. M., Lithell, H. and Landsberg, L. (1996). Hypertension and associated metabolic abnormalities: the role of insulin resistance and the sympathoadrenal system. *N. Engl. J. Med.*, **334**, 374–81.

Robinson, S., Walton, R. J., Clark, P. M., Barker, D. J. P., Hales, C. N. and Osmond, C. (1992). The relation of fetal growth to insulin secretion in young men. *Diabetologia*, **35**, 444–6.

Roseboom, T. J., van der Meulen, J. H., Ravelli, A. C., Osmond, C., Barker, D. J. P. and Bleker, O. P. (2001). Effects of prenatal exposure to the Dutch famine on adult disease in later life: an overview. *Mol. Cell. Endocrinol.*, **185**, 93–8.

Rosen, E. D. and Spiegelman, B. M. (1999). Tumour necrosis factor alpha as a mediator of the insulin resistance of obesity. *Curr. Opin. Endocrinol. Diabetes*, **6**, 170–6.

Sann, L., Darre, E., Lasne, Y. *et al.* (1985). Effects of prematurity and dysmaturity on growth at age 5 years. *J. Pediatr.*, **109**, 681–6.

Siagal, S., Stoskopf, B. L., Streiner, D. L. *et al.* (2001). Physical growth and current health status of infants who were of extremely low birth weight and controls at adolescence. *Pediatrics*, **108**, 407–15.

Singhal, A., Fewtrell, M., Cole, T. J. and Lucas, A. (2003). Low nutrient intake and early growth for later insulin resistance in adolescents born preterm. *Lancet*, **361**, 1089–97.

Soto, N., Bazaes, R. A., Pena, V. *et al.* (2003). Insulin sensitivity and secretion are related to catch up growth in small-for-gestational age infants at age 1 year: results from a prospective cohort. *J. Clin. Endocrinol. Metab.*, **88**, 3645–50.

Stanhope, R., Ackland, F., Hamill, G., Clayton, J., Jones, J. and Preece, M. A. (1989). Physiological growth hormone secretion and response to growth hormone treatment in children with short stature and intrauterine growth retardation. *Acta Paediatr. Scand.*, **349** (Suppl.), 47–52.

Stoll-Becker, S., Kreuder, J., Reiss, I., Etspuler, J., Blum, W. F. and Gortner, L. (2003). Influence of gestational age and intrauterine growth on leptin concentrations in venous cord blood of human newborns. *Klin. Padiatr.*, **215**, 2–8.

Sung, I., Vohr, B. and Zoh, W. (1993). Growth and neurodevelopmental outcome of very low birth weight infants with intrauterine growth retardation: comparison with control subjects matched by birthweight and gestational age. *J. Pediatr.*, **123**, 618–24.

Tenovuo, A., Kero, P., Piekkala, P., Korvenranta, H., Sillanpaa, M. and Erkkola, R. (1987). Growth of 519 small for gestational age infants during the first two years of life. *Acta Paediatr. Scand.*, **76**, 636–46.

Vaag, A., Henriksen, J. E., Madsbad, S., Holm, N. and Beck-Nielsen, H. (1995). Insulin secretion, insulin action, and hepatic glucose production in identical twins discordant for non insulin dependent diabetes mellitus. *J. Clin. Invest.*, **95**, 690–8.

Valdez, R., Athens, M. A., Thompson, G. H., Bradshaw, B. S. and Stern, M. P. (1994). Birthweight and adult health outcomes in a biethnic population in the USA. *Diabetologia*, **37**, 624–31.

Vincens-Calvert, E., Espadero, R. M. and Carrascosa, A. (2002). Longitudinal study of the pubertal growth spurt in children born small for gestational age without postnatal catch-up growth. *J. Pediatr. Endocrinol. Metab.*, **15**, 381–8.

Westwood, M., Kramer, M., Munz, D., Lovett, J. and Watters, G. (1983). Growth and development of full-term, nonasphyxiated small-for-gestational-age newborns; followup through adolescence. *Pediatrics*, **71**, 376–82.

Woodall, S. M., Breier, B. H., Johnson, B. M. and Gluckman, P. D. (1996). A model of intrauterine growth retardation caused by chronic maternal undernutrition in the rat: effects on the somatotropic axis and postnatal growth. *J. Endocrinol.*, **150**, 231–42.

Woods, K. A., Van Helvoirt, M., Ong, K. K. L. *et al.* (2002). The somatotropic axis in short children born small for gestational age: relation to insulin resistance. *Pediatr. Res.*, **51**, 76–80.

Wright, N. M., Northington, F. J., Miller, J. D., Veldhuis, J. D. and Rogol, A. D. (1992). Elevated growth hormone secretory rate in premature infants: deconvolution analysis of pulsatile growth hormone secretion in the neonate. *Pediatr. Res.*, **32**, 286–90.

Yeh, T. F., Lin, Y. F., Lin, H. C. *et al.* (2004). Outcomes at school age after postnatal dexamethasone therapy for lung disease of prematurity. *N. Engl. J. Med.*, **350**, 1304–13.

Yeoh, S. I. and Baxter, R. C. (1988). Metabolic regulation of the growth hormone independent insulin-like growth factor binding protein in human plasma. *Acta Endocrinol.*, **119**, 465–73.

15

Patterns of growth: relevance to developmental origins of health and disease

Johan G. Eriksson

National Public Health Institute, Finland

Introduction

Epidemiological studies have contributed enormously to our understanding of the natural history of many non-communicable diseases like coronary heart disease (CHD) and type 2 diabetes. Although clinical manifestations of these conditions normally become evident in adult life, early signs are recognisable already in children (Holman *et al*. 1958, Strong and McGill 1962, Berenson *et al*. 1979). A greater understanding of the evolution of many chronic diseases and their risk factors early in life is important for their primary prevention as well as in order to get a better understanding of the disease pathogenesis. The discovery that people who develop CHD and many of its risk factors in adult life grow differently during early life has led to the recognition of new developmental models for the disease and its risk factors. In this chapter, patterns of growth will be focused upon primarily in relation to CHD and type 2 diabetes as disease outcomes.

Prenatal growth

David Barker proposed that the epidemic of CHD in Western countries might have its origin in fetal life. He observed that areas in the UK with the highest rates of neonatal mortality in the 1910s and 1920s had the highest rates of CHD in the 1970s and 1980s. Based on these observations he postulated that impaired fetal growth predisposes to heart disease in adult life; studies in Hertfordshire, UK, proved the hypothesis to be correct (Osmond *et al*. 1993). Similar relationships had been put forward earlier by Forsdahl (1977) in Norway, although he never aimed at proving his theories scientifically.

The associations between small birth size and later cardiovascular morbidity and mortality have since been widely replicated in studies in Asia, Europe and the USA (Frankel *et al*. 1996, Stein *et al*. 1996, Rich-Edwards *et al*. 1997, Eriksson *et al*. 1999, 2001). In other words, findings point towards the importance of events during critical periods of growth and development in the pathogenesis of many non-communicable diseases like CHD, hypertension, stroke, type 2 diabetes and osteoporosis. It is now well established that the development of a fetus in a non-optimal intrauterine environment implies structural and functional adaptations with long-lasting consequences later in life – mediated by biological programming. Although a small birth size, due to restricted growth rather than preterm delivery, has originally been associated with unfavourable long-term health outcomes, the effect of programming does not necessarily affect birth size. Findings from the Dutch 'hunger winter' show that programming or induction of a risk factor or disease can occur without growth failure (Roseboom *et al*. 2000). Furthermore, it has been shown that both

Developmental Origins of Health and Disease, ed. Peter Gluckman and Mark Hanson. Published by Cambridge University Press.

extremes of the birthweight spectrum can be associated with an increased risk for type 2 diabetes, implying the importance of programming instead of absolute size attained (McCance *et al.* 1994, Eriksson *et al.* 2003a, Wei *et al.* 2003). One has to keep in mind that birth size is a surrogate for summing the interaction between environmental and genetic influences. Consequently, although birth size is a convenient marker in epidemiological research it gives an inadequate description of the phenotypic characteristics of a baby with regard to long-term health outcomes. Several paths of fetal growth can achieve the same birth size. Therefore for clinical purposes no cutoff points – associated with a higher disease risk – can be set.

Infant growth and adult health outcomes

In several aspects infant growth can be seen as a continuation of fetal growth, and consequently a strong relationship between birthweight and weight at 1 year exists. Among men born in Hertfordshire, UK, death rates from CHD doubled across the range of weight at 1 year from 11.8 kg to 8.2 kg (Barker *et al.* 1989). Among 4630 Finnish men, a similar relation with weight at age 1 was observed. Hazard ratios for CHD doubled between men who weighed ≥ 12 kg and those who weighed <9 kg (Eriksson *et al.* 2001). Low weight gain during infancy increased the risk of CHD independently of birthweight. Similar trends were observed with height and body mass index at 1 year. Table 15.1 shows the hazard ratios for coronary heart disease according to birthweight and weight at 1 year (Eriksson *et al.* 2001).

It has been argued that most published data on the relationship between infant growth and adult health outcomes are observational and retrospective, making interpretations difficult and therefore providing an insecure basis for clinical practice. It has even been proposed that a high-nutrient diet in infancy adversely programmes the principal components of the metabolic syndrome – thereby suggesting that slower infant growth and relative undernutrition benefit later cardiovascular disease and its risk fac-

Table 15.1 Hazard ratios for coronary heart disease in adult life among Finnish men according to birthweight and weight at 12 months.

Birthweight (g)	Hazard ratio
≤ 2500	3.63
$- 3000$	1.83
$- 3500$	1.99
$- 4000$	2.08
> 4000	1.00
p value for trend	0.006

Weight at 12 months (kg)	Hazard ratio
≤ 9	1.82
$- 10$	1.17
$- 11$	1.12
$- 12$	0.94
> 12	1.00
p value for trend	<0.0001

Data from Eriksson *et al.* (2001).

tors (Singhal *et al.* 2004, Singhal and Lucas 2004). This argument gets support from the fact that in some species accelerated early growth has short-term benefits but adverse long-term consequences (Metcalfe and Monaghan 2001). However, these arguments and interpretations have largely been based upon studies performed in preterm individuals followed up and studied at age 8–12 years (Singhal *et al.* 2003, 2004, Singhal and Lucas 2004). Therefore, these conclusions cannot be generalised to full-term infants, or to adult health outcomes. Various proxies for adult health outcomes have been used, and a critical re-evaluation of the results in relation to early growth and, for example, insulin resistance would not support the conclusions drawn by the authors (Singhal *et al.* 2003). A Dutch study assessing beta-cell capacity and insulin sensitivity in a contemporary group of children using highly validated methods for the assessment of insulin sensitivity (hyperinsulinaemic euglycaemic clamp) found no association between change in body mass index between birth and 2 years and later insulin resistance in children born small for gestational age (Veening *et al.* 2003). An increase in

BMI in the first two years of life was not related to decreased insulin sensitivity. Children who gained weight after the second year of life were at higher risk of developing type 2 diabetes later in life. Therefore the authors speculate that high-energy intake during infancy would be desirable for low-birthweight children. In the ALSPAC birth cohort study (Ong *et al.* 2004) insulin resistance in children at 8 years of age was associated with small birth size and rapid weight gain during the early postnatal years. Lower insulin sensitivity was predicted by greater weight gain between birth and 3 years of age.

By far the vast majority of the published human studies support the view that promoting infant growth seems to have long-term beneficial health effects. Another important issue causing difficulties in interpretation of human studies is to distinguish between the effects of fetal and early postnatal growth restriction. It will be of great importance to try to determine which changes in postnatal growth are caused by antenatal programming and which are caused primarily by postnatal factors.

Childhood growth and CHD

Is the increased risk for CHD and type 2 diabetes associated with a small body size at birth and at infancy, modified by growth during childhood? The Finnish birth cohort studies have largely contributed to our present knowledge in this field by having the possibility of simultaneously assessing size at birth, childhood growth and adult health outcomes (Eriksson and Forsen 2002). Deaths from CHD are associated with a small body size at birth, impaired growth during infancy and an average body mass index during childhood. Measures of childhood growth often interact with birth measurements in the prediction of adult disease. This is illustrated in Fig. 15.1, showing that an increase in body size from birth to 11 years of age was associated with an increased risk of CHD in adult life primarily in those who were small or thin at birth. In contrast, boys who were not small at birth did not seem to be at an increased CHD risk despite their higher child-

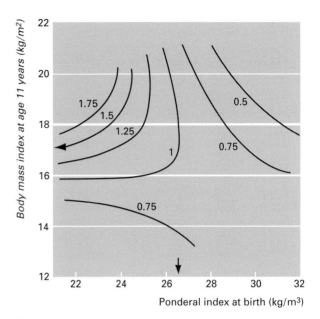

Figure 15.1   Hazard ratios for CHD according to birth size (ponderal index) and body mass index at 11 years of age. The average values are marked with arrows. Lines join points with the same hazard ratios. From Eriksson *et al.* (2001); reproduced with permission.

hood BMI (Eriksson *et al.* 2001). Therefore the consequences of achieved childhood body size are conditioned by growth in utero and infancy and do not depend only on the absolute level of weight attained. Furthermore, adult obesity adds to and interacts with the effects of low birthweight. An adverse CHD risk profile is quite consistently found in individuals who were small at birth but became obese as adults.

Early and childhood growth of men who developed CHD are shown in Fig. 15.2. In the figure the *z* score for the whole cohort is set at zero and so an individual maintaining a steady position as large or small in relation to other subjects would follow a horizontal path on the figure. Those who later developed CHD had been small at birth and during infancy, then experienced accelerated gain in weight and body mass index thereafter, but their heights remained below average – this is consistent with the known association between CHD and short adult stature (Eriksson *et al.* 2001). These findings also support

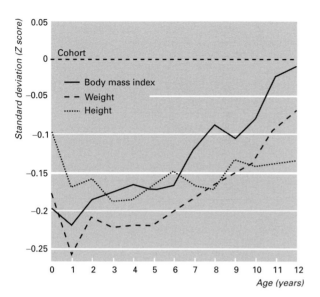

Figure 15.2 Patterns of growth associated with CHD in adult life among Finnish men born 1934–44. From Eriksson *et al.* (2001); reproduced with permission.

the view that there is a reduced incidence of CHD in those whose weight and/or body mass index increase during infancy.

The associations between early growth and CHD in adult life are strong and graded. A theoretical calculation based upon data from the Helsinki Birth Cohort Study shows that men who had a ponderal index at birth $>26 \text{ kg m}^{-3}$ and whose height and body mass index at 1 year were above the average for the cohort (76.2 cm and 17.7 kg m^{-2}) had half the risk of CHD occurring before age 65 years. It is obvious that these calculations are made from a historical cohort but they give a picture of the magnitude of risk associated with various patterns of growth.

Women are known to have lower rates of CHD than men. There are also fewer studies focusing on the relationship between early growth and CHD among women. However, the findings in women usually follow those in men, and CHD among women seems to be associated with small size at birth (Osmond *et al.* 1993, Rich-Edwards *et al.* 1997, Forsen *et al.* 1999, 2004). However, the paths of fetal growth among women and men seem to differ. Whilst boys tended

to be thin, the girls tended to be short at birth. The effects of fetal growth retardation on the risk of CHD were increased by accelerated childhood growth but it was unrelated to body size at 1 year. These findings in relation to patterns of growth need to be interpreted carefully due to the small number of CHD cases among the women studied (Forsen *et al.* 2004).

The patterns of growth that predispose to adult diseases are complex, and the importance of distinguishing between earlier and later 'catch-up' in growth needs to be stressed (Eriksson 2001). Early 'catch-up' growth, during infancy, seems to be beneficial, while crossing of centiles in later childhood is associated with an increased disease risk. There is no evidence in the current literature that supports the view that accelerated growth during infancy in low-birthweight babies would be harmful. This is important, because promoting weight gain in infancy is standard practice. In contrast, there is considerable evidence of the deleterious effects of childhood overweight and obesity, so treatment and prevention of childhood obesity should be high health priorities, especially in high-risk individuals.

Adiposity rebound and later disease risk

Type 2 diabetes and hypertension are associated with similar patterns of growth to those associated with CHD. In general the risk for these disorders falls with increasing birthweight and rises with increasing childhood BMI. A link between small body size at birth and later type 2 diabetes has been repeatedly documented, but less is known about the associations between the disease and growth during childhood (Hales *et al.* 1991, Lithell *et al.* 1996, Rich-Edwards *et al.* 1999, Forsen *et al.* 2000, Eriksson *et al.* 2002a, Barker *et al.* 2002, 2003).

The growth of children who later developed type 2 diabetes in the Helsinki Birth Cohort Study showed several similarities with the growth of those who developed CHD. Children who later developed type 2 diabetes had small body size at birth and at 1 year, after which their weights and BMIs rose progressively

Table 15.2 Age at adiposity rebound in relation to BMI and weight at 1 year of age, BMI at 12 years of age and cumulative incidence of type 2 diabetes in adult life.

Age at adiposity rebound (years)	BMI at 1 year ($kg\,m^{-2}$)	Weight at 1 year (kg)	BMI at 12 years ($kg\,m^{-2}$)	Prevalence of type 2 diabetes (%)
≤4	16.9	9.7	20.1	8.6
5	16.9	9.6	17.9	4.4
6	17.7	10.3	17.2	3.2
7	18.2	10.4	17.1	2.2
≥8	18.4	10.5	16.9	1.8
p value for trend	<0.001	<0.001	<0.001	<0.001

Data from Eriksson *et al.* (2003b).

to exceed the average. Their heights rose more slowly and reached the average (Eriksson *et al.* 2003b).

Type 2 diabetes is strongly associated with obesity and therefore its association with the tempo of growth in childhood is of great interest. After the age of 2 years the degree of obesity of young children as measured by BMI decreases to a minimum around 6 years of age before increasing again, i.e. the so-called adiposity rebound (Rolland-Cachera *et al.* 1984, 1987). Figure 15.3 shows the changes in BMI between birth and 12 years according to the age at adiposity rebound. Children who had an adiposity rebound at the earliest ages had the highest BMI in later childhood and the highest prevalence of type 2 diabetes in adult life. The prevalence of type 2 diabetes decreased from 8.6% in those in whom the adiposity rebound occurred before the age of 5 years to 1.8% in those in whom it occurred after the age of 7 years. The figure also shows that an early adiposity rebound was associated with low weight gain between birth and 1 year and thinness up to 3 years of age.

Table 15.2 shows the relation between age at adiposity rebound and BMI and weight at 1 year, BMI at 12 years of age and the cumulative incidence of type 2 diabetes. In contrast to its association with later high BMI, early adiposity rebound is preceded by thinness at birth, low BMI and weight at 1 year of age, and high rates of type 2 diabetes in adult life.

Early age at adiposity rebound has previously been related to an increased risk for obesity (Rolland-

Cachera *et al.* 1984, 1987, Whitaker *et al.* 1998). While an early adiposity rebound is associated with the development of both obesity and type 2 diabetes, the patterns of growth that lead to these two disorders differ. People who become obese tend to be big at birth, whereas people who develop type 2 diabetes tend to have low birthweight and to be small or thin at birth (Forsen *et al.* 2000, Eriksson *et al.* 2003b, 2003c).

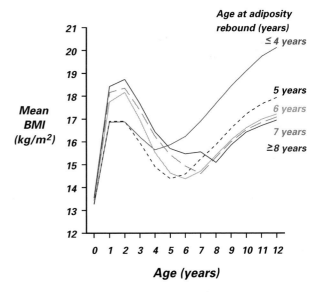

Figure 15.3 Mean body mass index during childhood according to age of adiposity rebound. From Eriksson *et al.* (2003b); reproduced with permission.

The findings described above have been replicated in a unique population-based longitudinal study of children born in Delhi, India, about 30 years ago. Those individuals who developed impairment in their glucose metabolism had a low body mass index up to 2 years of age, followed by an early adiposity rebound and accelerated increase in body mass index until adult life (Barghava *et al.* 2004).

The processes that link low weight gain in infancy and thinness at 1 year with an early adiposity rebound are not known. It could reflect a post-weaning infant diet that is low in fat but high in protein, followed by a childhood diet that is high in fat. Another possible explanation for the association between small body size at birth, early adiposity rebound and later type 2 diabetes is that there are persisting alterations in body composition. An early adiposity rebound could be associated with lifelong setting of hormones and growth factors that facilitate the deposition of fat, thereby predisposing to obesity and type 2 diabetes

Different patterns of growth, same disease outcome

Various patterns of growth can lead to the same disease; this has been shown for both CHD and type 2 diabetes. Two separate patterns of growth leading to type 2 diabetes will be discussed. In the Helsinki Birth Cohort Study both low birthweight and low weight at age 1 year were associated with an increased risk of type 2 diabetes in adult life. The disease was also associated with higher body mass index in later childhood. A highly significant interaction between childhood BMI and birthweight suggests that there may be two separate patterns of growth leading to type 2 diabetes – one among children with below-average birthweights and another among children who had above-average birth size (Eriksson *et al.* 2003a).

In the Finnish study about two thirds of the type 2 diabetes cases were observed among subjects with birthweights <3500 g. Rate of infant growth was unrelated to type 2 diabetes in this group. Among those with birthweights >3500 g slow growth in length between birth and 3 months of age predicted later disease. Growth in length was inversely related to the cumulative incidence of type 2 diabetes in adult life. Accelerated gain in body mass index after the age of 2 years increased the risk of later disease in both groups, the effect being greatest among children who had slow growth in length between birth and 3 months (Eriksson *et al.* 2003a).

The two patterns of growth associated with type 2 diabetes are shown in Fig. 15.4. Changes in heights, weights and BMIs between birth and 12 years are shown as z scores, with the z score for the cohort as a whole being set at zero. In general, the group with birthweights <3500 g tended to regress towards the zero line in height, weight and BMI. Those who later developed type 2 diabetes had lower birthweights, and they also regressed towards the mean, but their heights, weights and BMIs remained below those of the other children until the age of 5–7 years. After age 7 they became larger than the other children and the difference, especially in weight and BMI, progressively increased.

Among children with birthweights >3500 g the z scores for heights, weights, and BMIs tended to regress towards zero. Mean birthweight of those who later developed type 2 diabetes was similar to that of the other children in this group. Their heights and weights also regressed towards the average, but fell more steeply than those of the other children. After the age of 2 years a steep rise in weight and BMI began, and after the age of 4 years they were larger in weight and BMI than the other children. This difference progressively increased.

Type 2 diabetes has previously been reported in babies of above-average birthweight among the Pima Indians and among schoolchildren in Taiwan (McCance *et al.* 1994, Wei *et al.* 2003). In both studies the association between the disease and birthweight was U-shaped. Among the Pima Indians the findings were largely explained by a high incidence of gestational diabetes. Among the schoolchildren in Taiwan those with higher birthweight who developed type 2 diabetes were more likely to have a higher BMI and a family history of type 2 diabetes compared

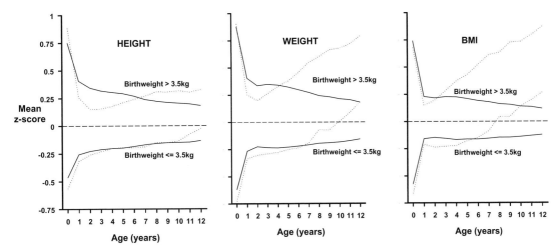

Figure 15.4 Growth of 8760 children in two birthweight groups: above or below 3.5 kg. The solid lines represent the growth in height, weight and BMI of all children in the two birthweight groups. The dotted lines represent the growth in height, weight and BMI of the 290 children who later developed type 2 diabetes, divided into two groups according to birthweight. The z scores for the entire cohort are set at zero, represented by the dashed line. From Eriksson *et al.* (2003a); reproduced with permission.

to those with a low birthweight and later type 2 diabetes.

The diabetes epidemic in India is more common and severe among urban than rural Indians, despite the higher birthweights of urban babies. This certainly suggests that postnatal factors must contribute highly to the pathogenesis and the increase in diabetes in India (Yajnik 2004). The existence of two separate pathways of growth that lead to the same disease may explain some of the heterogeneity in its manifestations which are encountered in clinical practice.

Gene–environment interactions early in life

The reported association between altered early growth and CHD and type 2 diabetes in adult life has led to the suggestion that these diseases might originate through a phenomenon called developmental plasticity. This is a phenomenon whereby one genotype gives rise to a range of different physiological states in response to various environmental conditions during development. There is some

evidence of gene–early-environment interactions in the genesis of insulin resistance, type 2 diabetes and dyslipidaemia (Eriksson *et al.* 2002b, 2003d, 2003e).

There is a well-established association between the *PPARγ2* gene and type 2 diabetes, while the *Pro12Ala* genotype seems to offer some protection against type 2 diabetes. However, the effects of the *Pro12Ala* polymorphism of the *PPARγ2* gene on insulin sensitivity and type 2 diabetes in adult life are modified by size at birth. The well-known association between small birth size and insulin resistance and type 2 diabetes was observed among elderly Finns only in individuals with the high-risk *Pro12Pro* genotype. In those who had low birthweight, the *Pro12Pro* polymorphism of the PPARγ2 gene was associated with increased insulin resistance and elevated insulin concentrations (Eriksson *et al.* 2002b). Table 15.3 shows the interactions between the *PPARγ2* gene polymorphism and birth length in relation to type 2 diabetes. The *Pro12Pro* genotype was weakly associated with a higher incidence of type 2 diabetes, but this was confined to people with a shorter birth length. In the group with

Table 15.3 Cumulative incidence of type 2 diabetes according to birth size (length) and PPAR $\gamma 2$ gene polymorphism in 476 elderly subjects.

	Genotype		
	Pro12Pro	*Pro12Ala*	*p* value
Birth length (cm)			
≤49	24.5	14.3	0.02
>49	19.6	17.9	0.54
p value	0.02	0.94	0.08

Data from Eriksson *et al.* (2003e).

the *Pro12Pro* genotype and short length at birth the prevalence of type 2 diabetes was 24.5%, while it was 14.3% in the group with the *Pro12Ala* genotype and short length at birth (Eriksson *et al.* 2003e). Interestingly, the *PPARγ 2* gene polymorphism *Pro12Ala* has been shown to beneficially influence insulin resistance and its tracking from childhood to adulthood in the Bogalusa Heart Study (Li *et al.* 2003). To study the impact of this polymorphism in longitudinal birth cohort settings would certainly be of great interest.

Conclusion

Slow growth during fetal life and infancy is often followed by accelerated weight gain in childhood. These patterns of growth seem to precede the development of CHD and type 2 diabetes in adult life. We are beginning to see that adult degenerative diseases are associated with different patterns of infant and childhood growth. Furthermore, the same disease may even originate through more than one pathway. Unfortunately it is not clear what optimal growth is and how it can be achieved; obviously this is also related to the measured health outcome. Most data suggest that the development of many non-communicable diseases involve a number of interactions including genetic ones. Therefore these diseases can best be focused upon from a lifecycle perspective. From a preventive point of view one must keep in mind that in most cases adult diseases are not programmed per

se, although the tendency towards the disease seems to be programmed. In other words it is important to consider impaired early growth as a major risk factor for adult disease, not as a causative factor. The early risk factors are to a large degree modified by various factors during childhood and adult life (Eriksson *et al.* 2004).

REFERENCES

Barghava, S. K., Sachdev, H. S., Fall, C. H. D. *et al.* (2004). Relation of serial changes in childhood body-mass index to impaired glucose tolerance in young adulthood. *N. Engl. J. Med.*, **350**, 865–75.

Barker, D. J. P., Osmond, C., Winter, P. D., Margetts, B. and Simmonds, S. J. (1989). Weight in infancy and death from ischaemic heart disease. *Lancet*, **2**, 577–80.

Barker, D. J. P., Forsen, T., Eriksson, J. G. and Osmond, C. (2002). Growth and living conditions in childhood and hypertension in adult life: a longitudinal study. *J. Hypertens.*, **20**, 1951–6.

Barker, D. J. P., Hales, C. N., Fall, C. H. D., Osmond, C., Phipps, K. and Clark, P. M. S. (1993). Type 2 (non-insulin-dependent) diabetes mellitus, hypertension and hyperlipidaemia (syndrome X): relation to reduced fetal growth. *Diabetologia*, **36**, 62–7.

Berenson, G. S., Blonde, C. V., Farris, R. P. *et al.* (1979). Cardiovascular disease risk factor variables during the first year of life. *Am. J. Dis. Child.*, **133**, 1049–57.

Eriksson, J. G. (2001). Commentary: early 'catch-up' growth is good for later health. *Int. J. Epidemiol.*, **30**, 1330–1.

Eriksson, J. G. and Forsen, T. J. (2002). Childhood growth and coronary heart disease in later life. *Ann. Med.*, **34**, 157–61.

Eriksson, J. G., Forsen, T., Tuomilehto, J., Winter, P. D., Osmond, C. and Barker, D. J. P. (1999). Catch-up growth in childhood and death from coronary heart disease: longitudinal study. *BMJ*, **318**, 427–31.

Eriksson, J. G., Forsen, T., Tuomilehto, J., Osmond, C. and Barker, D. J. P. (2001). Early growth and coronary heart disease in later life: longitudinal study. *BMJ*, **322**, 949–53.

Eriksson, J. G., Forsen, T., Tuomilehto, J., Jaddoe, V. W. V., Osmond, C. and Barker, D. J. P. (2002a). Effects of size at birth and childhood growth on the insulin resistance syndrome in elderly individuals. *Diabetologia*, **45**, 342–7.

Eriksson, J. G., Lindi, V., Uusitupa, M. *et al.* (2002b). The effects of the Pro12Ala polymorphism of the peroxisome proliferator-activated receptor-gamma2 gene on insulin sensitivity and insulin metabolism interact with size at birth. *Diabetes*, **51**, 2321–4.

Eriksson, J. G., Forsen, T. J., Osmond, C. and Barker, D. J. P. (2003a). Pathways of infant and childhood growth that lead to type 2 diabetes. *Diabetes Care*, **26**, 3006–10.

Eriksson, J. G., Forsén, T., Tuomilehto, J., Osmond, C. and Barker, D. J. P. (2003b). Early adiposity rebound in childhood and risk of type 2 diabetes in adult life. *Diabetologia*, **46**, 190–4.

Eriksson, J. G., Forsen, T., Osmond, C. and Barker, D. (2003c). Obesity from cradle to grave. *Int. J. Obes. Relat. Metab. Disord.*, **27**, 722–7.

Eriksson, J. G., Lindi, V., Uusitupa, M. *et al.* (2003d). The effects of the Pro12Ala polymorphism of the PPARgamma-2 gene on lipid metabolism interact with body size at birth. *Clin. Genet.*, **64**, 366–70.

Eriksson, J. G., Osmond, C., Lindi, V. *et al.* (2003e). Interactions between peroxisome proliferator-activated receptor gene polymorphism and birth length influence risk for type 2 diabetes. *Diabetes Care*, **26**, 2476–7.

Eriksson, J. G., Ylihärsilä, H., Forsén, T., Osmond, C. and Barker, D. J. P. (2004). Exercise protects against type 2 diabetes in persons with a small body size at birth. *Prev. Med.*, **39**, 164–7.

Forsdahl, A. (1977). Are poor living conditions in childhood and adolescence an important risk factor for arteriosclerotic heart disease? *Br. J. Prev. Soc. Med.*, **31**, 91–5.

Forsen, T., Eriksson, J. G., Tuomilehto, J., Osmond, C. and Barker, D. J. P. (1999). Growth in utero and during childhood among women who develop coronary heart disease: longitudinal study. *BMJ*, **319**, 1403–7.

Forsen, T., Eriksson, J., Tuomilehto, J., Reunanen, A., Osmond, C. and Barker, D. (2000). The fetal and childhood growth of persons who develop type 2 diabetes. *Ann. Intern. Med.*, **133**, 176–82.

Forsen, T., Osmond, C., Eriksson, J. G. and Barker, D. J. P. (2004). Growth of girls who later develop coronary heart disease. *Heart*, **90**, 20–4.

Frankel, S., Elwood, P., Sweetnam, P., Yarnell, J. and Davey Smith, G. (1996). Birthweight, adult risk factors and incident coronary heart disease: the Caerphilly study. *Public Health*, **110**, 139–43.

Hales, C. N., Barker, D. J. P., Clark, P. M. S. *et al.* (1991). Fetal and infant growth and impaired glucose tolerance at age 64. *BMJ*, **303**, 1019–22.

Holman, R. L., McGill, H. C. Jr., Strong, J. P. and Geer, J. C. (1958). The natural history of atherosclerosis: the early aortic lesions as seen in New Orleans in the middle of the 20th century. *Am. J. Pathol.*, **34**, 209–35.

Li, S., When, W., Srinivasan, S. R., Boerwinkle, E. and Berenson, G. S. (2003). The peroxisome proliferator-activated receptor-gamma2 gene polymorphism (Pro12Ala) beneficially influences insulin resistance and its tracking from childhood to adulthood. The Bogalusa Heart Study. *Diabetes*, **52**, 1265–9.

Lithell, H. O., McKeigue, P. M., Berglund, L., Mohsen, R., Lithell, U. B. and Leon, D. A. (1996). Relation of size at birth to non-insulin dependent diabetes and insulin concentrations in men aged 50–60 years. *BMJ*, **312**, 406–10.

McCance, D. R., Pettitt, D. J., Hanson, R. L., Jacobsson, L. T. H., Knowler, W. C. and Bennett, P. H. (1994). Birth weight and non-insulin dependent diabetes: thrifty genotype, thrifty phenotype, or surviving small baby genotype? *BMJ*, **308**, 942–5.

Metcalfe, N. B. and Monaghan, P. (2001). Compensation for a bad start: grow now, pay later? *Trends Ecol. Evol.*, **16**, 254–60.

Ong, K. K., Petry, C. J., Emmett, P. M. *et al.* (2004). Insulin sensitivity and secretion in normal children related to size at birth, postnatal growth, and plasma insulin-like growth factor-I levels. *Diabetologia*, **47**, 1064–70.

Osmond, C, Barker, D. J. P., Winter, P. D., Fall, C. H. D. and Simmonds, S. J. (1993). Early growth and death from cardiovascular disease in women. *BMJ*, **307**, 1519–24.

Rich-Edwards, J. W., Stampfer, M. J., Manson, J. E. *et al.* (1997). Birth weight and risk of cardiovascular disease in a cohort of women followed up since 1976. *BMJ*, **315**, 396–400.

Rich-Edwards, J. W., Colditz, G. A., Stampfer, M. J. *et al.* (1999). Birthweight and the risk for type 2 diabetes mellitus in adult women. *Ann. Intern. Med.*, **130**, 278–84.

Rolland-Cachera, M. F., Deheeger, M., Bellisle, F., Sempe, M., Guilloud-Bataille, M. and Patois, E. (1984). Adiposity rebound in children: a simple indicator for predicting obesity. *Am. J. Clin. Nutr.*, **39**, 129–35.

Rolland-Cachera, M. F., Deheeger, M., Guilloud-Bataille, M., Avons, P., Patois, E. and Sempe, M. (1987). Tracking the development of adiposity from one month of age to adulthood. *Ann. Hum. Biol.*, **14**, 219–29.

Roseboom, T. J., van der Meulen, J. H., Osmond, C. *et al.* (2000). Coronary heart disease after prenatal exposure to the Dutch famine, 1944–45. *Heart*, **84**, 595–8.

Singhal, A. and Lucas, A. (2004). Early origins of cardiovascular disease: is there a unifying hypothesis? *Lancet*, **363**, 1642–5.

Singhal, A., Fewtrell, M., Cole, T. J. and Lucas, A. (2003). Low nutrient intake and early growth for later insulin resistance in adolescents born preterm. *Lancet*, **361**, 1089–97.

Singhal, A., Cole, T. J., Fewtrell, M., Deanfield, J. and Lucas, A. (2004). Is slower early growth beneficial for long-term cardiovascular health. *Circulation*, **109**, 1108–13.

Stein, C. E., Fall, C. H. D., Kumaran, K., Osmond, C., Cox, V. and Barker, D. J. P. (1996). Fetal growth and coronary heart disease in South India. *Lancet*, **348**, 1269–73.

Strong, J. P. and McGill, H. C. Jr. (1962). The natural history of coronary atherosclerosis. *Am. J. Pathol.*, **40**, 37–49.

Veening, M. A., Weissenbruch, M. M., Heine, R. J. and Dellemarre-van de Waal, H. A. (2003). β-cell capacity and insulin sensitivity in prepubertal children born small for gestational age: influence of body size during childhood. *Diabetes*, **52**, 1756–60.

Wei, J. N., Sung, F. C., Li, C. Y. *et al.* (2003). Low birth weight and high birth weight infants are both at an increased risk to have type 2 diabetes among schoolchildren in Taiwan. *Diabetes Care*, **26**, 343–8.

Whitaker, R. C., Pepe, M. S., Wright, J. A., Seidel, K. D. and Dietz, W. H. (1998). Early adiposity rebound and the risk of adult obesity. *Pediatrics*, **101**, 1–6.

Yajnik, C. S. (2004). Early life origins of insulin resistance and type 2 diabetes in India and other Asian countries. *J. Nutr.*, **134**, 205–10.

16

The developmental environment and the endocrine pancreas

Brigitte Reusens, Luise Kalbe and Claude Remacle

Université Catholique de Louvain

Introduction

The intrauterine environment is the first to which the conceptus is exposed and it is strongly influenced by the mother's health. In this chapter we will focus on the development of the endocrine pancreas. A disturbed intrauterine metabolic milieu would contribute to inappropriate β-cell ontogeny, resulting in a population of β cells that does not adequately cope with metabolic or oxidative stress later in life. This hypothesis obviously cannot be verified in humans; therefore various animal models have been established.

Development of the endocrine pancreas in the rodent

The development of the pancreas in rodents shows similarities to that in humans. However, while fetal β cells are functioning as true endocrine cells at the end of the first trimester in humans (Piper *et al.* 2004), this occurs only during the last third of gestation in the rat. The development of the pancreas is a fascinating event, starting from a pool of common progenitor cells (multipotent endodermal progenitors) which will be committed into the endocrine or exocrine cell lineages or become duct cells. Then, within the endocrine compartment, the cells will

have to further differentiate into α, β, δ or PP cells producing glucagon, insulin, somatostatin or the pancreatic polypeptide respectively. This is regulated by the expression of distinct genes, under the control of a hierarchy of various specific networks of transcription factors. It is thus obvious that any disturbance in the environment of the future endocrine cell may alter the relative participation of factors involved in this network and then drive the β-cell mass into a corner, contributing to β-cell failure and diabetes later in life.

Endocrine cells are organised in highly vascularised and innervated micro-organs distributed throughout the exocrine tissue. They represent 2–4% of the total pancreatic tissue at birth, decreasing to 1% in adulthood, with 60–80% of the islet cell population being β cells. Figure 16.1 illustrates the different steps of pancreatic development. In response to signals coming from the mesodermal tissues, pancreatic morphogenesis begins with the evagination of foregut endoderm to form a dorsal, and then a ventral pancreatic bud. The region which will become the pancreas receives signals from the notochord and dorsal aorta, leading to the expression of essential pancreatic transcription factor genes such as pancreatic–duodenal homeobox genes (*Pdx1/Ppf1*) (Hebrok *et al.* 1998, Lammert *et al.* 2001). One of the important components of the early specification of the pancreatic programme within the region of the gut endoderm involves the exclusion of the

Developmental Origins of Health and Disease, ed. Peter Gluckman and Mark Hanson. Published by Cambridge University Press.
© P. D. Gluckman and M. A. Hanson 2006.

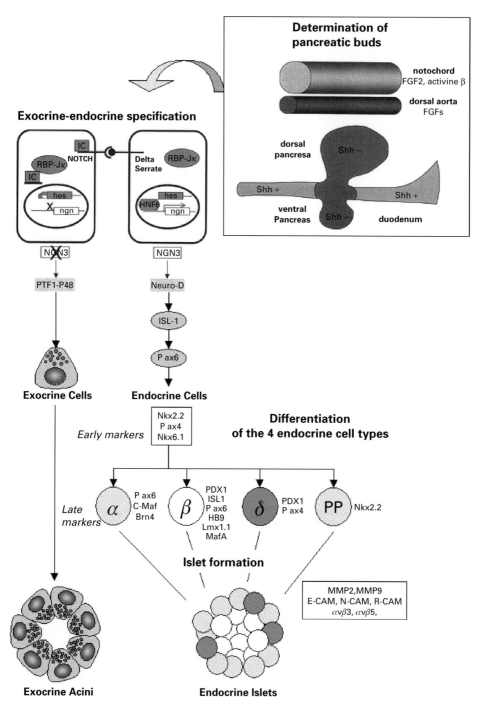

Figure 16.1 Schematic representation of the different steps of the development of the pancreas. Adapted from Grapin-Botton *et al.* (2001) and Wilson *et al.* (2003).

expression of the hedgehog gene family (*Shh* and *Ihh*) that is expressed elsewhere in the primitive gut (Hebrok *et al.* 1998). Early morphogenetic signalling may depend on the interplay between peptide growth factors and tissue transcription factors. The activin β (a member of the transforming growth factor family, TGF) and fibroblast growth factor 2 (FGF2) are notochord factors that can repress endodermal *Shh*, permitting expression of pancreas genes including *Pdx1* and *insulin* (Hebrok *et al.* 1998). The dorsal and ventral buds fuse at E16.5 in the rat. A branched structure is distinguishable at E14.5 in which endocrine cells can be identified by E15.5. The endocrine tissue is derived from epithelial duct cells. After divisions, the cells will form small clusters budding out from the pancreatic ducts. The vascularisation begins to invade these immature endocrine cell clusters that coexpress several pancreatic hormones and neuropeptides and will become 'islets of Langerhans' (Reusens *et al.* 2000).

The classical way of specifying a particular cell fate within a field of initially equivalent cells is the lateral specification mediated by the Notch–Delta-serrate pathway. In the pancreas, blocking the activation of the Notch receptor results in high neurogenin 3 gene (*ngn3*) expression, and promotes the endocrine fate. In contrast, cells with active Notch signalling adopt the exocrine fate and/or remain as undifferentiated progenitor cells (Edlund 2001).

The final fate of the individual endocrine cells is determined by the expression of a series of transcription factors specific for each type of endocrine cell. Some of them are early markers such as Pax4, Nk2.2 and Nk6.1 coexpressed with neurogenin 3, others are late markers such as Pax6, Isl1, Hb9 and Pdx1 for the β cells. The transcription factor network is very complicated because several factors involved are expressed more than once during the differentiation process and play more than one role. As mentioned above, one of the key players is the homeodomain transcription factor Pdx1, which is not only important in the regulation of insulin gene expression, but is also required for the differentiation of the mature pancreas (Hebrok *et al.* 1998).

Other growth factors such PDGF, VEGF, FGF7, which are expressed within the pancreatic stroma adjacent to the ductal epithelium, may also intervene. The ongoing proliferation and developmental differentiation of β cells, once formed, are highly dependent on the expression of the IGFs within the islets.

Beta-cell function and insulin action

In adults, β cells synthesise and store insulin as well as C-peptide within their granules. After enhanced glucose uptake via the low-affinity glucose transporter GLUT2, glucose enters the cell, is phosphorylated by glucokinase and metabolised, leading to a rise in the ATP/ADP ratio. This increase induces a blockage of the K^+ ATP-dependent channels, which in turn will lead to membrane depolarisation and subsequently to the activation of the voltage-dependent Ca^{++} channels. Ca^{++} will enter into the β cell and stimulate the release of insulin by exocytosis. Amino acids have been shown to stimulate insulin release in the absence of glucose. In the fetus, insulin secretion is more sensitive to amino acids than to glucose (de Gasparo *et al.* 1978), its full response to glucose beginning after birth. In humans as well as in rats, fetal β cells show an immature or poor response to nutrient, especially to glucose. In contrast to adult pancreas, fetal β cells never display a biphasic pattern of insulin secretion (Hughes 1994).

Early malnutrition programmes the endocrine pancreas and its β cells

In the rat fetus, the β-cell mass increases rapidly at the end of gestation due to replication and recruitment of undifferentiated β-cell precursors in the pancreatic duct (neogenesis). Following birth, the growth rate of each islet cell population, including β cells, declines within 3–4 days. A wave of apoptosis occurs in the neonatal rat islets between 2 and 3 weeks of age (Scaglia *et al.* 1997), the loss of the β cells being compensated by replication and neogenesis. Although insulin-producing β cells in the adult pancreas were thought to derive from pancreatic stem cells, it seems now that they arise abundantly from pre-existing β cells themselves (Dor *et al.* 2004). The early development of the β-cell mass thus determines the islet mass in adulthood. Therefore, any deficiency occurring in utero or soon after birth is unlikely to be completely compensated for later in life. Alterations of the β-cell mass by maternal malnutrition were demonstrated in humans four decades ago (Winick and Noble 1966), but the mechanisms involved in these alterations were only deciphered when animal models were developed.

In our rat model of protein restriction, animals receive either a diet containing 20% protein or an isocaloric protein-restricted diet containing only 8% protein throughout gestation or gestation and lactation. Maternal low-protein (LP) diet modifies the β-cell expansion, with ensuing depletion of the β-cell mass at birth and after weaning in the offspring. Islet size and pancreatic insulin content are reduced and islet cell replication is decreased by almost 50% preferentially in the β cells, due to a lengthening of their cell cycle (Snoeck *et al.* 1990, Petrik *et al.* 1999).

The modulation of the β-cell mass during development also involves β-cell death. Although the timing of the neonatal apoptotic wave described previously was not affected by the maternal diet, the rate of islet cell apoptosis was increased in protein-restricted offspring at every age analysed. This suggests that the event is quantitatively dependent upon, but qualitatively independent of, the diet. A simultaneous reduction of IGF2 (insulin-like growth factor 2) expression (Petrik *et al.* 1999), which acts as a growth factor as well as a survival factor to prevent apoptosis in β cells (Petrik *et al.* 1998), suggests a link to the increased apoptosis and the reduced β-cell proliferation seen in islets of LP offspring.

The deleterious effect of fetal malnutrition on the development of the β-cell mass is also apparent in other animal models of fetal malnutrition. Fetuses from mothers subjected to 50% calorie restriction during the last week of gestation were growth-retarded. They were also born with a significantly altered development of their endocrine pancreas, including a lower β-cell mass. Different mechanisms from those observed in the case of protein deprivation were involved, since in this model the reduction in β-cell mass appears to be due to reduced neogenesis rather than alteration of the islet cell proliferation or apoptotic rate (Garofano *et al.* 1997). *Pdx1* expression was diminished in these fetal pancreatic buds and islets which was not the case in low protein islets (L. Kalbe, unpublished data).

The endocrine pancreas is a richly vascularised tissue. Blood vessels provide metabolic sustenance and inductive signals for the endocrine pancreas development. Pancreatic and vascular development cooperate during embryogenesis. Pancreatic buds develop precisely where endoderm previously contacted the endothelium of the dorsal aorta and the vitelline veins (Lammert *et al.* 2001; Fig. 16.1). Islet blood vessel development is very sensitive to the specific lack of protein availability in utero, since both the volume occupied by blood-vessels and the blood vessel number were lower in protein-restricted fetal islets (Snoeck *et al.* 1990, Boujendar *et al.* 2003). This was associated with an altered expression of a major factor of endothelium–endocrine cell interactions, i.e. vascular endothelial cell growth factor (VEGF) and its receptor Flk1 in fetal low-protein islets and/or duct cells (Boujendar *et al.* 2003). Interestingly, the islet vascularisation was not affected in calorie-restricted fetal islets (L. Kalbe, unpublished data).

What are the nutrients that may be responsible for the dramatic effects on the endocrine pancreas observed at birth in the offspring of a protein-restricted mother? Although the development of fetal islet cell is dependent on the availability of glucose, amino acids appear to be more potent than glucose in stimulating β-cell differentiation and proliferation (de Gasparo *et al.* 1978). Amino acids, but not glucose, potentiate the release of immunoreactive IGF2 from isolated fetal rat islets (Hogg *et al.* 1993). As mentioned above, less IGF2 was observed in the pancreas of the fetus which grew in an intrauterine milieu poor in amino acids. In protein-restricted animals, plasma glucose levels were normal, but the amino acid profile was perturbed in the fetomaternal unit (Reusens *et al.* 1995), several amino acids being significantly decreased. Taurine, which does not participate in protein synthesis, but which is important during development for several tissues (Sturman 1993), was the most affected. Supplementation of the drinking water of the protein-restricted pregnant rats with taurine prevented the reduction of the β-cell mass by enhancing β-cell proliferation and decreasing islet cell apoptosis. This was achieved, in part, by the normalisation of the number of islet cells expressing IGF2 (Boujendar *et al.* 2002). The islet blood vessels are also sensitive to the depletion of taurine that occurs in LP fetuses, since addition of this amino acid to the protein-restricted diet of the dams was sufficient to restore a well-vascularised endocrine pancreas in the progeny and restore the expression of VEGF and its receptor in islets (Boujendar *et al.* 2003). It is unclear, however, if the primary effect of taurine is on the endothelial or the endocrine cells of the pancreas.

In a study comparing the effect of maternal isocaloric low-protein, low-calorie and low-protein/low-calorie diets, Bertin *et al.* (2002) demonstrated that, although the three approaches to inducing fetal malnutrition all induced 50% reduction of the fetal β-cell mass, plasma taurine was only depleted in the fetuses that were protein-deprived. Taurine can thus not be involved in the reduction of β-cell mass observed in calorie-restricted fetuses. Other factors have been suggested. During development, a negative role of glucocorticoids on the fetal β cell has been demonstrated (Blondeau *et al.* 2001). Maternal food restriction increased maternal and fetal corticosterone levels (Lesage *et al.* 2001). A normalisation of the glucocorticoid levels in the IUGR calorie-restricted fetus restored a normal β-cell mass that was associated with the correction of the decreased β-cell neogenesis (Blondeau *et al.* 2001).

Maternal diabetes affects also fetal tissue development. In the rat, diabetes may be induced experimentally by streptozotocin, which selectively destroys β cells. Mild or severe diabetic states ensue, depending on the dose used. The progeny of mildly diabetic mothers were macrosomic. The development of the endocrine pancreas was enhanced. Hypertrophy and hyperplasia of fetal islets were already observed at two days before birth (Aerts *et al.* 1990). At birth, islet cell proliferation was enhanced by 42% (Reusens-Billen *et al.* 1984), leading to increased β-cell mass. Islet vascularisation was increased by 36% (Reusens and Remacle 2001a). By contrast, the pancreatic insulin content and insulin secretion were also raised in these fetuses (Kervran *et al.* 1978). The fetuses of severely diabetic mothers were small for gestational age. Due to an overstimulation by the excessive glucose concentration, their β cells were almost degranulated, leading to lower pancreatic insulin content and plasma secretion (Kervran *et al.* 1978).

In conclusion, these three experimental conditions in dams – low-protein and low-calorie diet as well as streptozotocin-induced diabetes – demonstrate that early nutritional events in utero impinge upon the development of β-cell mass, its vascularisation and its secretory function.

To address the key issue of the fetal programming of the endocrine pancreas, we used two approaches. In the first, we highlighted the short-term programming of fetal β cells by culturing islets that were taken from the disturbed metabolic maternal environment. Long-term consequences were revealed by a second approach, i.e. a feeding the offspring with a normal diet after birth or after weaning and analysing the adult progeny. This long-term programming will be addressed in the section below.

In the first approach, pancreatic cells were cultured for seven days. They proliferated and differentiated into pseudo-islets rich in β cells. Although cultured in the same medium as the control islets and free of the poor maternal milieu, low-protein islet cells retained the lower proliferation rate (Cherif *et al.* 2001) and the higher apoptotic rate (Merezak *et al.* 2001) that were observed in vivo. In addition, insulin secretion in response to glucose and various amino acids was dramatically altered in islets of the LP fetus, depending on the secretagogues used. This reduction of insulin release was more pronounced when the islets were challenged with amino acids than with glucose (Cherif *et al.* 2001). Although a reduction of cAMP concentration was detected in these islets, and might explain in part the reduced insulin release, we demonstrated that the main defect in insulin secretion was at the level of exocytosis (Cherif *et al.* 2001). The persisting reduction of the insulin secretion and replication, as well as the increased apoptotic rate of fetal β cells in LP offspring, even when they have been withdrawn from the maternal environment and cultured for one week, demonstrates that protein restriction during pregnancy induces lasting impairments.

Early malnutrition programmes glucose metabolism and insulin action: type 2 diabetes

Type 2 diabetes is characterised by hyperglycaemia, resulting from insulin resistance, β-cell dysfunction, or both. β-cell dysfunction occurs because of an inability to synthesise and secrete active insulin in sufficient amount to meet the increased demand for insulin (Kahn 1998). Type 2 diabetic patients often show a reduced β-cell number compared to weight-matched non-diabetic patients. This suggests that these patients had fewer cells prior to the onset of diabetes, or that they failed to enhance their β-cell mass in response to the demand (Clark *et al.* 1988). However, Guiot *et al.* (2001) were unable to demonstrate a decreased β-cell mass in type 2 diabetes after morphometric analysis. Individuals with type 2 diabetes are not at increased risk for autoimmune diseases. Nevertheless, a recent study showed that one-third of patients aged 15–34 with clinical type 2 diabetes had objectively type 1 diabetes based on the evolution of their anti-islet antibodies (Borg *et al.* 2003).

The underdevelopment of the endocrine pancreas as a response to malnutrition may be a survival advantage in early life, but may be a risk factor for the appearance of diabetes later on. In rat, early protein restriction leads in adulthood to a blunted insulin secretion in response to the oral

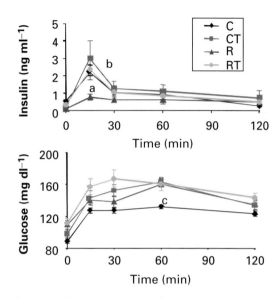

Figure 16.2 Glucose tolerance and plasma insulin response of adult (11 weeks) female rats to an oral glucose challenge $(0.7\,\mathrm{g\,kg^{-1}})$. These animals were born from mothers fed, during gestation and lactation: R, a low-protein (LP) diet; C, a control diet; RT, a LP diet with taurine (2.5%) in the drinking water or; CT, a control diet with taurine. Values are means $\pm$ SE of 7–8 animals per group. a: $p < 0.05$ vs. C; b: $p < 0.05$ vs. R; c: $p < 0.05$ vs CT. From Merezak *et al.* (2004).

glucose challenge despite a normal diet after birth or weaning (Dahri *et al.* 1991, Reusens and Remacle 2001b). This suggests that the early low-protein diet causes fundamental changes in the programming of the β-cell phenotype with critical periods both in fetal and neonatal life. Indeed, when taurine was added to the maternal low-protein diet during those periods, the adult offspring had adequate basal and glucose-stimulated insulin secretion (Merezak *et al.* 2004, Fig. 16.2).

Changes in such programming of the β cells were also observed following fetal (last week of gestation) and early postnatal calorie restriction. The β-cell mass that was depressed by 66% at weaning remained reduced by 35% at 3 months (Garofano *et al.* 1998). When the calorie restriction was more severe (30% of the *ad libitum* available food) and was applied from the first day of gestation until birth, 4-month-old male offspring developed obesity, hyperinsulinaemia and hyperlipidaemia, which was even amplified by hypercaloric nutrition postnatally (Vickers *et al.* 2000).

The limited capacity of the β cells to regenerate following poor development of the endocrine pancreas after early malnutrition leaves the offspring with a suboptimal complement of functional units in the pancreas. This will not be a real handicap as long as the individual is young, thin and does not face ageing, overfeeding or pregnancy. Should such events occur, long-term consequences of early malnutrition, such as insulin resistance proceeding to glucose intolerance and diabetes, would appear in the adult offspring (see Chapter 17).

Fetal malnutrition as a consequence of utero-placental insufficiency occurring over the last three days of gestation in the rat also programmes the development of the endocrine pancreas and glucose metabolism later in life. Although no difference in the β-cell mass was detected at 1 and 7 weeks, a reduction of the β-cell proliferation was reported at 14 days, associated with a dramatic reduction of Pdx1 expression (Boloker *et al.* 2002, Stoffers *et al.* 2003). The malnourished offspring developed marked fasting hyperglycaemia and hyperinsulinaemia at 10 weeks. It deteriorated into glucose intolerance and insulin resistance at 15 weeks, which evolved to a severe lack of insulin secretion at 26 weeks of age.

Intrauterine exposure to diabetes conveys risks for type 2 diabetes and obesity as in the Pima Indian population, where diabetes has the highest prevalence (Dabelea *et al.* 2000). Indeed, the risk for diabetes was higher in siblings born from a diabetic mother than in those born before the mother became diabetic. The effect of maternal diabetes can be thought of as a vicious cycle with consequences for the offspring extending well beyond the neonatal period.

Adult offspring of severely diabetic rats kept a lower body weight. They had a normal endocrine pancreas and a normal plasma glucose concentration under basal conditions (Aerts *et al.* 1990). As in protein restriction, they maintained glucose levels within the control range, but at the expense of high insulin levels after three hours of glucose infusion. After euglycaemic hyperinsulinaemic clamp, offspring were resistant to insulin at the hepatic and peripheral levels (Holemans *et al.* 1991).

In summary, the endocrine pancreas is altered at birth in the various experimental animal models: low-protein and low-calorie diets, as well as streptozotocin-induced diabetes. As a consequence, insulin secretion is abnormal at adulthood despite the withdrawal of the early metabolic insult. Later, with age or with overweight, glucose intolerance may ensue, rendering the progeny prone to developing diabetes.

Transgenerational programming of the endocrine pancreas

The impact of the early events is not limited to the first generation but seems to persist in the second, because the altered endocrine pancreas of the mother is unable to adapt correctly to the challenging situation which is the pregnancy. Pregnancy is associated with peripheral insulin resistance and increased insulin secretion in association with normoglycaemia or slight hypoglycaemia (Freinkel 1980). This leads to a state of increased functional load on the endocrine pancreas. Mechanisms of adaptation include growth of the islets and a decreased threshold for glucose-induced insulin secretion. Beta-cell mass doubles by the end of gestation in rat (Bone and Taylor 1976, Sorenson and Brelje 1997). An altered β-cell mass is of course a limiting factor for this adaptation.

When female offspring from malnourished (protein- or calorie-restriction) mothers became pregnant, adaptation of their endocrine pancreas could not be fully achieved. Low-protein pregnant offspring showed a lower pancreatic insulin content and a reduced insulin secretion after an oral glucose tolerance test (OGTT) (Reusens and Remacle 2001b) while offspring of calorie-restriction mothers exhibited inability to increase their β-cell mass (Blondeau *et al.* 1999). This abnormal intrauterine milieu impacted upon the next generation. Just before birth, the pups whose grandmothers were protein- or calorie-restricted during pregnancy also clearly exhibited lower plasma insulin levels and pancreatic insulin content, as a consequence of their reduced β-cell-mass development (Reusens and Remacle 2001b, Blondeau *et al.* 2002).

Female offspring from streptozotocin-diabetic rats developed diabetes when they became pregnant. Their fetuses were macrosomic, displaying islet hyperplasia, β-cell degranulation and hyperinsulinaemia resulting from the maternal hyperglycaemia. (Aerts *et al.* 1990).

In the model of placental insufficiency, female offspring exhibited a clear insulin resistance and glucose intolerance when pregnant, and consequences were apparent when the second generation was examined. Pups were born slightly heavier and remained so throughout life. They were insulin-resistant very early in life and they featured progressive glucose intolerance. At 26 weeks the β-cell mass was dramatically reduced (Boloker *et al.* 2002). Thus, the endocrine pancreas of the second generation is clearly damaged, but the pathways responsible for this are far from defined.

Early malnutrition and susceptibility to type 1 diabetes

In type 1 diabetes β cells are selectively destroyed by apoptosis because of the invasion of the islets by immune cells (insulitis) releasing free radicals and cytokines, and also because they have poor defence mechanisms. It has always been known as a disease of childhood and adolescence, but more recent epidemiological studies have indicated that the incidence is comparable in adults and that some patients diagnosed with type 2 diabetes actually have type 1 diabetes (Turner *et al.* 1997). The traditional view of type 1 diabetes postulates that environmental agents trigger the onset of disease in genetically susceptible individuals. However, recent observations from humans and in animals support a more complex model wherein the penetration and expression of heritable immune aberrations

(immune dysfunction), in combination with inherent target-organ defects, are part of the lifelong influence of multiple environmental factors such as infectious agents, diet factors and environmental toxins (Atkinson and Eisenbarth 2001).

Among the limited epidemiological evidence available, only viral infections such as coxsackie B4 appear to support the idea of early programming of type 1 diabetes in humans (Hyöty and Taylor 2002). In spontaneously diabetic animals it has been hypothesised that insulitis is induced by an exaggerated wave of apoptosis just after birth, and this has been proposed as a pathway to the early programming of type 1 diabetes (Trudeau *et al.* 2000).

Islet apoptotic rate was increased in the pancreas at fetal and neonatal stages in the offspring of mothers fed a low-protein diet. We therefore asked about the possible increased susceptibility of the β cell to the effects of agents known to be involved in type 1 diabetes, and we demonstrated that it was the case. When β cells from fetuses of protein-deprived mothers were challenged in culture with a NO donor or IL1β, they exhibited a higher apototic rate than the control fetal β cells (Merezak *et al.* 2001). Moreover, the increased susceptibility was maintained throughout life despite adequate feeding after weaning, since adult islets were also more vulnerable in presence of cytokines (Merezak *et al.* 2004, Fig. 16.3). The lack of protein during development thus generated a β-cell population that is more sensitive to cytokines, perhaps because of a low level of IGF2 (Petrik *et al.* 1999) or altered defence mechanisms. The low level of taurine present during development may also be involved, since supplementation of the low-protein diet with taurine, which restored a normal β-cell mass with adequate numbers of cells positive for IGF2, a normal vascularisation and a normal insulin secretion at birth, prevented the hypersensitivity of the fetal and adult islets to cytokines (Merezak *et al.* 2001, 2004; Fig. 16.3). An adequate level of taurine during fetal and early life thus seems critical to achieving normal development and function of the endocrine pancreas. Should that not be present, β-cell vulnerability will ensue and remain throughout life.

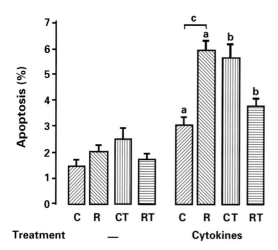

Figure 16.3 Effect of low-protein diet and taurine on the sensitivity of adult islets to cytokines. Control diet (C group) or low-protein diet (R group) was given during gestation and lactation. To test the effect of taurine, 2.5% of taurine was added to the drinking water during gestation and lactation (CT and RT groups). At 12 weeks of age, islets were isolated and cultivated without (−) or with cytokines (IL1β, TNFα and IFNγ) for 24 hours. Apoptosis was measured by the TUNEL method. Values are means ± SE of 3–4 separate experiments providing >4.5 × 10⁴ of islet cells per group. a: $p < 0.01$ vs. no cytokine treatment, b: $p < 0.01$ vs. cytokine treatment without taurine supplementation, c: $p < 0.01$ C vs. R. From Merezak *et al.* (2004).

Conclusions

Epidemiological observations identify the phenomenon of fetal programming without explaining the underlying mechanisms that establish causation. Animal models have been established and have demonstrated that alteration in the availability of nutrients during fetal development programmes the endocrine pancreas and the insulin-sensitive tissues. Independently of the type of fetal malnutrition, i.e. whether it involves dietary calorie or protein restriction or placental deficiency, or too much glucose, pups are born with a defect in their β-cell mass that will never completely recover. Insulin-sensitive tissues will be definitively altered. Despite the similar defects arising from different approaches,

different mechanisms seem to operate. A lack of taurine in the case of protein restriction and high levels of glucocorticoids in case of the calorie-restriction model have been the focus of much interest. Addition of taurine to maternal low-protein diet, or the normalisation of the maternal plasma glucocorticoid level in the calorie-restricted mother, prevents the alterations of the endocrine pancreas observed with these interventions.

ACKNOWLEDGMENTS

The authors are grateful to the Parthenon Trust for financial support.

REFERENCES

Aerts, L., Holemans, K. and Van Assche, F. A. (1990). Maternal diabetes during pregnancy: consequences for the offspring. *Diabetes Metab. Rev.*, **16**, 147–67.

Atkinson, M. A. and Eisenbarth, G. S. (2001). Type 1 diabetes: new perspectives on disease pathogenesis and treatment. *Lancet*, **358**, 221–9.

Bertin, E., Gangnerau, M. N., Bellon, G., Bailbe, D., Arbelot de Vacqueur, A. and Portha, B. (2002). Development of β-cell mass in fetuses of rats deprived of protein and/or energy in last trimester of pregnancy. *Am. J. Physiol. Regul. Integr. Comp. Physiol.*, **283**, R623–30.

Blondeau, B., Garofano, A., Czernichow, P. and Bréant, B. (1999). Age-dependant inability of the endocrine pancreas to adapt to pregnancy: a long term consequence of perinatal malnutrition in the rat. *Endocrinology*, **40**, 4208–13.

Blondeau, B., Lesage, J., Czernichow, P., Dupouy, J. P. and Bréant, B. (2001). Glucocorticoids impair fetal β-cell development in rat. *Am. J. Physiol. Endocrinol. Metab.*, **281**, E592–9.

Blondeau, B., Avril, I., Duchene, B. and Bréant, B. (2002). Endocrine pancreas development is altered in fetuses from rats previously showing intra-uterine growth retardation in response to malnutrition. *Diabetologia*, **45**, 394–401.

Boloker, J., Shira, J. G. and Simmons, R. (2002). Gestational diabetes leads to the development of diabetes in adulthood in the rat. *Diabetes*, **51**, 1499–506.

Bone, A. and Taylor, K. (1976). Metabolic adaptation to pregnancy shown by increased biosynthesis of insulin islets of Langerhans isolated from pregnant rats. *Nature*, **262**, 501–2.

Borg, H., Arnqvit, H. J., Bjork, E. *et al.* (2003). Evaluation of the new ADA and WHO criteria for classification of diabetes mellitus in young adult people (15–34 yrs) in the Diabetes Incidence Study in Sweden (DISS). *Diabetologia*, **46**, 173–81.

Boujendar, S., Reusens, B., Merezak, S. *et al.* (2002). Taurine supplementation to a low protein diet during fetal and early postnatal life restores a normal proliferation and apoptosis of rat pancreatic islets. *Diabetologia*, **45**, 856–66.

Boujendar, S., Arany, E., Hill, D., Remacle, C. and Reusens, B. (2003). Taurine supplementation of a low protein diet fed to rat dams normalized the vascularization of the fetal endocrine pancreas. *J. Nutr.*, **133**, 2820–5.

Cherif, H., Reusens, B., Dahri, S. and Remacle, C. (2001). A protein-restricted diet during pregnancy alters in vitro insulin secretion from islets of fetal Wistar rat. *J. Nutr.*, **131**, 1555–9.

Clark, A., Wells, C. A., Buley, I. D. *et al.* (1988). Islet amyloid, increased A-cells, reduced B-cell and exocrine fibrosis: quantitative changes in the pancreas in type 2 diabetes. *Diabetes Res.*, **9**, 151–9.

Dabelea, D., Knowler, W. C. and Pettitt, D. J. (2000). Effect of diabetes in pregnancy on offspring: follow-up research in the Pima Indians. *J. Matern. Fetal. Med.*, **9**, 83–8.

Dahri, S., Snoeck, A., Reusens, B., Remacle, C. and Hoet, J. J. (1991). Islet function in offspring of mothers on low-protein diet during gestation. *Diabetes*, **40**, 115–20.

de Gasparo, M., Milner, G. R., Norris, P. D. and Milner, R. D. G. (1978). Effect of glucose and amino acids on fetal rat pancreatic growth and insulin secretion *in vitro*. *J. Endocrinol.*, **77**, 241–8.

Dor, Y., Brown, J., Martinez, O. and Melton, D. (2004). Adult pancreatic beta cells are formed by self-duplication rather than stem-cell differentiation. *Nature*, **429**, 41–6.

Edlund, H. (2001). Factors controlling pancreatic cell differentiation and function. *Diabetologia*, **44**, 1071–9.

Freinkel, N. (1980). Banting Lecture 1980. Of pregnancy and progeny. *Diabetes*, **29**, 1023–35.

Garofano, A., Czernichow, P. and Bréant, B. (1997). In utero undernutrition impairs rat β-cell development. *Diabetologia*, **40**, 1231–4.

(1998). Beta-cell mass and proliferation following late fetal and early postnatal malnutrition in the rat. *Diabetologia*, **34**, 373–84.

Grapin-Botton, A., Majithia, A. R. and Melton, D. A. (2001). Key events of pancreas formation are triggered in gut endoderm by ectopic expression of pancreatic regulatory genes. *Genes Dev.*, **15**, 44–54.

Guiot, Y., Sempoux, C., Moulin, P. and Rahier, J. (2001). No decrease of the beta-cell mass in type 2 diabetic patients. *Diabetes*, **50** (Suppl. 1), S188.

Hebrok, M., Kim, S. G. and Douglas, A. M. (1998). Notochord repression of endodermal Sonic hedgehog permits pancreas development. *Genes Dev.*, **12**, 1705–13.

Hogg, J., Han, V. K. M., Clemmons, D. and Hill, D. J. (1993). Interactions of glucose, insulin like growth factors (IGFs) and IGF binding proteins in the regulation of DNA synthesis by isolated fetal rat islets of Langerhans. *J. Endocrinol.*, **138**, 401–12.

Holemans, K., Aerts, L. and Van Assche, F. A. (1991). Evidence for an insulin resistance in the adult offspring of pregnant streptozotocin-diabetic rats. *Diabetologia*, **34**, 81–5.

Hughes, S. J. (1994). The role of reduced glucose transporter content and glucose metabolism in the immature secretory responses of fetal rat pancreatic islets. *Diabetologia*, **37**, 134–40.

Hyöty, H. and Taylor, K. W. (2002). The role of viruses in human diabetes. *Diabetologia* **45**, 1353–61.

Kahn, B. B. (1998). Type 2 diabetes: when insulin secretion fails to compensate for insulin resistance. *Cell*, **92**, 593–6.

Kervran, A., Guillaume, M. and Jost, A. (1978). The endocrine pancreas of the fetus from diabetic pregnant rat. *Diabetologia*, **15**, 387–93.

Lammert, E., Cleaver, O. and Melton, D. (2001). Induction of pancreatic differentiation by signals from blood vessels. *Science*, **294**, 564–7.

Lesage, J., Blondeau, B., Grino, M., Bréant, B. and Dupouy, J. P. (2001). Maternal undernutrition during late gestation induces fetal overexposure to glucocorticoids and intrauterine growth retardation, and disturbs the hypothalamo-pituitary adrenal axis in the newborn rat. *Endocrinology*, **142**, 1692–702.

Merezak, S., Hardikar, A., Yajnick, C. S., Remacle, C. and Reusens, B. (2001). Intraurerine low protein diet increases fetal β cell sensitivity to NO and IL-1-β: the protective role of taurine. *J. Endocrinol.*, **171**, 299–308.

Merezak, S., Reusens, B., Ahn, M. T. and Remacle, C. (2004). Effect of maternal low protein diet and taurine on the vulnerability of Wistar rat islets to cytokines. *Diabetologia*, **7**, 669–75.

Petrik, J., Arany, E., McDonald, T. J. and Hill, D. J. (1998). Apoptosis in the pancreatic islet cells of the neonatal rat is associated with a reduced expression of insulin-like growth factor II that may act as a survival factor. *Endocrinology*, **139**, 2994–3004.

Petrik, J., Reusens, B., Arany, E. *et al.* (1999). A low protein diet alters the balance of islet cell replication and apoptosis in the fetal and neonatal rat and is associated with a reduced pancreatic expression of insulin like growth factor II. *Endocrinology*, **140**, 4861–73.

Piper, K., Brickwood, S., Turnpenny, L. W. *et al.* (2004). Beta cell differentiation during human pancreas development *J. Endocrinol.*, **181**, 11–23.

Reusens, B. and Remacle, C. (2001a). Intergenerational effects of adverse intrauterine environment on perturbation of glucose metabolism. *Twin Res.*, **4**, 406–11.

(2001b). Effects of maternal nutrition and metabolism on the developing endocrine pancreas. In *Fetal Origins of Cardiovascular and Lung Disease* (ed. D. Barker). New York, NY: Marcel Dekker, pp. 339–58.

Reusens, B., Dahri, S., Snoeck, A., Bennis-Taleb, N., Remacle, C. and Hoet, J. J. (1995). Long-term consequences of diabetes and its complications may have a fetal origin: experimental evidence. In *Diabetes* (ed. R. M. Cowett). New York, NY: Raven Press, pp. 187–98.

Reusens, B., Hoet, J. J. and Remacle, C. (2000). Anatomy, developmental biology and pathology of the pancreatic islets. In *Endocrinology* (ed. L. J. De Groot *et al.*). Philadelphia, PA: Saunders, pp. 5024–35.

Reusens-Billen, B., Remacle, C., Daniline, J. and Hoet, J. J. (1984). Cell proliferation in pancreatic islets of rat fetus and neonates from normal and diabetic mothers: an in vitro and in vivo study. *Horm. Metab. Res.*, **16,** 565–71.

Scaglia, L., Cahill, C. J., Finegood, D. T. and Bonner-Weir, S. (1997). Apoptosis participates in the remodelling of the endocrine pancreas in the neonatal rat. *Endocrinology*, **138**, 1736–41.

Snoeck, A., Remacle, C., Reusens, B. and Hoet, J. J. (1990). Effect of a low protein diet during pregnancy on the fetal rat endocrine pancreas. *Biol. Neonate*, **57**, 107–18.

Sorenson, R. L. and Brelje, T. C. (1997). Adaptation of islets of Langerhans to pregnancy: beta-cell growth, enhanced insulin secretion and the role of lactogenic hormones. *Horm. Metab. Res.*, **29**, 301–7.

Stoffers, D. A., Desai, B. M., DeLeon, D. D. and Simmons, R. (2003). Neonatal Exendin-4 prevents the development of diabetes in the intrauterine growth retarded rat. *Diabetes*, **52**, 734–40.

Sturman, G. A. (1993). Taurine in development. *Physiol. Rev.*, **73**, 119–47.

Trudeau, J., Dutz, J. P., Arany, E., Hill, D., Fieldus, W. and Finegood, D. (2000). Perspectives in diabetes. Neonatal β-cell apoptosis: a trigger for autoimmune diabetes. *Diabetes*, **49**, 1–7.

Turner, R., Stratton, I., Horton, V. *et al.* (1997). UKPDS 25: autoantibodies to islet cell cytoplasm and glutamic acid decarboxylase for prediction of insulin requirement in type 2 diabetes. *Lancet*, **350**, 1288–93.

Vickers, M. H., Breier, B. H., Cutfield, W. S., Hofman, P. L. and Gluckman, P. D. (2000). Fetal origin of hyperphagia, obesity and hypertension and its postnatal amplification by hypercaloric nutrition. *Am. J. Physiol. Endocrinol. Metab.*, **279**, E83–7.

Wilson, M. E., Scheel, D. and German, M. S. (2003). Gene expression cascades in pancreas development. *Mech. Dev.*, **120**, 65–80.

Winick, M. and Noble, A. (1966). Cellular response in rats during malnutrition at various ages. *J. Nutr.*, **89**, 300–6.

17

The developmental environment and insulin resistance

Noel H. Smith and Susan E. Ozanne

University of Cambridge

Introduction

The detrimental effects of an insult during a critical period of development have been recognised for many years. In the past 15 years there have been a number of epidemiological studies which have shown that there is a relationship between early growth restriction and the subsequent development of adult degenerative diseases such as ischaemic heart disease, hypertension, type 2 diabetes and the metabolic syndrome. The mechanistic basis and the relative roles of genetic and environmental factors are unclear. However, there is growing evidence that the fetal and early environment play an important role in this relationship.

A number of different factors can result in intrauterine growth restriction (IUGR). Maternal malnutrition during pregnancy is one cause of IUGR, because of inadequate nutrient delivery to the fetus. Growth restriction in offspring can be induced by the reduction of all nutrients in the mother's diet (global food restriction) or by the reduction of specific dietary nutrients such as protein and iron. Maternal stress can lead to IUGR, and this is thought at least in part to be mediated by overexposure to glucocorticoids. Overexposure of the fetus to glucocorticoids is known to lead to reductions in birthweight. In the Western world placental insufficiency is one of the most common causes of IUGR. It is not known if all modes of growth restriction result in

the same phenotypic outcomes. To investigate these forms of growth restriction, animal models mimicking each of these causes of IUGR have been developed. This chapter will review the current evidence gained from these animal models and how we can take these findings into human studies.

Maternal calorie restriction

Undernourishment in the developing world is known to be a major cause of famine and disease. It is well known that with maternal food restriction comes a decreased nutrient supply to the fetus, due to the decreased availability of nutrients and decreased placental blood flow to the fetus (Rosso and Kava 1980), leading to IUGR. Animal models have been used to investigate the effects of maternal food restriction on the growth and development of the offspring. Both mild (50% of normal food intake) and severe (30% of normal food intake) food restriction regimens have been used in rats. Mild reductions in nutrient supply have been shown to lead to growth restriction in the fetus and also a failure to stimulate the development of the fetal endocrine pancreas (Holemans et $al.$ 1996). Prolonged mild maternal food restriction during pregnancy and lactation maintains the growth restriction and reduction in β-cell mass compared to controls (Garofano et $al.$ 1997). When the offspring of food-restricted mothers

Developmental Origins of Health and Disease, ed. Peter Gluckman and Mark Hanson. Published by Cambridge University Press.
© P. D. Gluckman and M. A. Hanson 2006.

are nursed by mothers on a normal food intake their body weight normalises by weaning. In adulthood, offspring of mothers fed a severely restricted diet (to only 30% of *ad libitum* intake) during pregnancy and lactation have elevated systolic blood pressures and increased fasting plasma insulin concentrations (Vickers *et al.* 2000). These offspring remain smaller even when weaned onto a control diet, and they show a more sedentary behaviour and an increased food intake compared to control offspring (Vickers *et al.* 2000, 2003). This hyperphagia increases with age and can be amplified by hypercaloric nutrition (Vickers *et al.* 2003). Hyperphagia has also been suggested in humans, where early growth restriction is thought to be associated with adult central obesity (Law *et al.* 1992). Less severe food restriction in rats (50% of *ad libitum* intake) from day 15 of pregnancy to weaning has been shown to result in insulinopaenia and an age-dependent loss of glucose tolerance which is apparent at 12 months of age (Garofano *et al.* 1999).

Maternal low protein

Along with global food restriction, specific nutrients in the diet have also been shown to cause IUGR. Reduced protein intake during late pregnancy has been shown to suppress the growth of the fetus (Godfrey *et al.* 1996). The maternal-low-protein model has been widely used to study growth restriction in the past 15 years. The low-protein rat model involves feeding rats an 8% protein diet during pregnancy, which leads to fetal growth restriction (Desai *et al.* 1996). If the protein restriction is maintained into the lactation period, permanent growth restriction occurs even if the offspring themselves are weaned onto a normal 20% protein diet (Desai *et al.* 1996). During early life these offspring (termed LP offspring) seem to show a significantly better glucose tolerance than controls (Shepherd *et al.* 1997, Holness and Sugden 1999). However, they undergo a greater age-dependent loss of glucose tolerance such that by 15 months of age their glucose tolerance is significantly worse than that of

controls (Hales *et al.* 1996), which is also associated with insulin resistance, and by 17 months of age they have frank diabetes (Petry *et al.* 2001). Maternal protein restriction has also been shown to be associated with hypertension (Langley-Evans *et al.* 1999), which is thought to be related not only to changes in kidney structure but also to the activity of the renin–angiotensin system (Langley-Evans *et al.* 1999). It has also been shown that when maternal low protein is combined with obesity they have an independent and additive effect on blood pressure (Petry *et al.* 1997). Many of these complications in the maternal-low-protein rats are also seen in individuals with type 2 diabetes and/or the metabolic syndrome. Both maternal-low-protein rats and humans with the metabolic syndrome are born small and have a short stature, and go on to develop diabetes, insulin resistance and hypertension.

The growth restriction caused by low-protein feeding during pregnancy can be rescued by cross-fostering to control mothers fed a normal 20% control diet during lactation. These recuperated offspring rapidly gain weight such that by weaning (21 days of age) they are of similar weight to controls. The catch-up growth of these animals, however, appears to have a detrimental effect on their longevity. Recuperated offspring die prematurely, which is thought to be due to the accelerated loss of kidney telomeric DNA (Jennings *et al.* 1999). The detrimental effects of catch-up growth have also been demonstrated in human populations. Studies in Sweden have shown that men who were born small but then grew to above average height have raised blood pressure (Leon *et al.* 1996). It has also been shown that catch-up growth in a Finnish cohort is associated with increased risk of both diabetes and cardiovascular disease (Eriksson *et al.* 2000). Recent studies have shown that male mice that have been growth-restricted by maternal protein restriction during pregnancy undergo catch-up growth during lactation and have a significantly shorter life expectancy than controls. This effect is exaggerated if the animals are weaned onto an obesity-inducing cafeteria-style diet. In contrast, control offspring that are

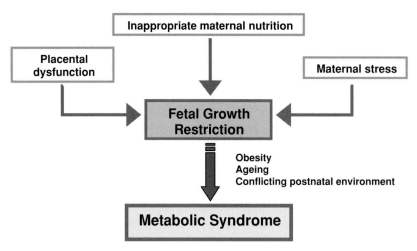

Figure 17.1 Fetal origins of adult disease.

cross-fostered to protein-restricted mothers during lactation live significantly longer than controls that are not so fostered (Hales and Ozanne 2004). The mechanisms responsible for this are unknown. These studies suggest that minor nutritional interventions during critical periods of development can significantly increase lifespan.

Many studies have also investigated the long-term effects of maternal protein restriction on the structure and function of major organs. A large number of these studies have concentrated on the effects of maternal protein restriction on the endocrine pancreas. Rat fetuses of protein-restricted mothers have been shown to have smaller islets and reduced β-cell proliferation compared to controls (Snoeck *et al.* 1990). There is also evidence of reduced islet vascularisation (Snoeck *et al.* 1990) and increased β-cell apoptosis (Petrik *et al.* 1999) in these fetuses. Impaired insulin secretion in vitro has also been reported in fetuses of low-protein mothers, caused by a defect in the exocytosis step of the secretion cascade and no reduction in the insulin pool of the β cell (Cherif *et al.* 2001). Decreases in expression of IGF2 may contribute to the reduced proliferation of β cells and increased apoptosis in these fetuses of LP mothers. Islets from 21.5-day-old fetuses of LP mothers have been shown to have a reduced secre-

tory response to both leucine and arginine in vitro (Dahri *et al.* 1991). Defects in glucose-stimulated insulin secretion have also been noted in adult LP offspring when an additional dietary insult is introduced postnatally (Hughes and Wilson 1997). This creates an imbalance between the fetal and adult environments. These data support the thrifty phenotype hypothesis, which suggests that conflict between the fetal and postnatal environment leads to type 2 diabetes and the metabolic syndrome (Barker and Hales 1992). Fetal origins of adult disease are summarised in Fig. 17.1.

Studies have shown that taurine supplementation may be one possible intervention strategy. Taurine is a sulphur-containing amino acid found in almost all mammalian tissues. It is known to have an anti-diabetic action, potentiating the secretion of insulin and its hypoglycaemic effect (Tokunaga *et al.* 1983). Supplementing the diets of pregnant dams on a low-protein diet with taurine prevents the abnormal development of the fetal endocrine pancreas usually seen in LP fetuses (Cherif *et al.* 1998, Boujendar *et al.* 2002; see also Chapter 16). Further studies on taurine, for example on the time-windows for intervention, and identification of other possible supplements, may help in developing future prevention programmes for IUGR individuals.

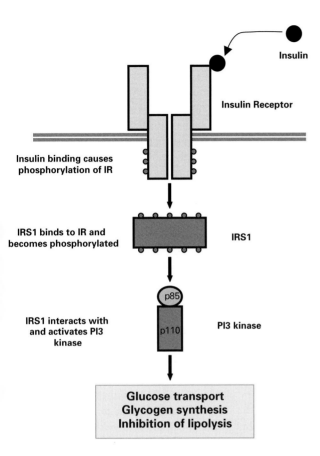

Insulin

Insulin Receptor

Insulin binding causes phosphorylation of IR

IRS1 binds to IR and becomes phosphorylated

IRS1

IRS1 interacts with and activates PI3 kinase

PI3 kinase

**Glucose transport
Glycogen synthesis
Inhibition of lipolysis**

Figure 17.2 Schematic diagram of PI3 kinase activation by insulin via the insulin receptor.

The long-term effects of maternal protein restriction on insulin-sensitive tissues (such as the liver, muscle and fat) have also been studied. In the livers of LP offspring hepatic lobule volume is twice that of controls, indicating that maternal-low-protein livers have half the normal number of lobules (Burns *et al.* 1997). Ex-vivo liver perfusions performed on 3-month-old male LP offspring have shown that they are relatively resistant to the ability of glucagon to stimulate hepatic glucose output compared to controls (Ozanne *et al.* 1996a). The observed glucagon resistance is associated with a reduction in glucagon receptor expression (Ozanne *et al.* 1996a). These ex-vivo studies also showed that livers of LP offspring have an unexpected response to

insulin, with insulin initially stimulating hepatic glucose output (Ozanne *et al.* 1996a). Similar responses have been reported in human subjects with type 2 diabetes (Frank *et al.* 1995).

Skeletal muscle of young adult LP offspring is more sensitive to insulin in terms of its ability to stimulate glucose uptake (Ozanne *et al.* 1996b). This increased sensitivity is associated with an increased expression of the insulin receptor, and may in part contribute to their better glucose tolerance compared to controls at this age.

Potential markers of growth restriction have been identified during detailed analysis of adipocytes (Ozanne *et al.* 1997). Elevated levels of basal and insulin-stimulated glucose uptake, and also increased expression of the insulin receptor, have been seen in isolated adipocytes of young adult LP offspring (Ozanne *et al.* 1997). The insulin receptor (IR) is well studied and the mechanism by which it mediates the action of insulin is well characterised (Virkamäki *et al.* 1999). Insulin binds to the IR, causing autophosphorylation of tyrosine residues. This phosphorylation causes subsequent phosphorylation of a number of IR substrates including IRS1. These phosphorylated IRS proteins then bind to downstream signalling elements which become active. One of these enzymes is phosphoinositide 3 kinase (PI3 kinase), which is known to be necessary for the action of insulin, both to stimulate glucose uptake and to inhibit lypolysis (Shepherd *et al.* 1998). The activation of PI3 kinase via the IR is summarised in Fig. 17.2. Elevated and basal IRS1 associated PI3 kinase activity has been seen in isolated adipocytes of young LP offspring. But despite having elevated levels of PI3 kinase, these adipocytes are resistant to the antilipolytic action of insulin (Ozanne *et al.* 1999). A suggested mechanistic basis for this has been proposed by investigating the structure of PI3 kinase. PI3 kinase is a heterodimeric enzyme which consists of a regulatory subunit (p85) and a catalytic subunit (p110) (Shepherd *et al.* 1998). In adipocytes, there are two isoforms of the p110 catalytic subunit (p110α and p110β). Early protein restriction leads to a dramatic reduction in expression of p110β, while p110α;

expression remains unchanged (Ozanne *et al.* 1997). Although little is known about the functional differences between these p110 isoforms, the existence of differentially regulated isoforms with different signalling roles would allow the cell to adjust its metabolic status in response to its environment. The relative expression levels of these isoforms may provide important information on the success of the fetus on achieving its growth potential. Limited data are available on the expression of these isoforms but some recent studies have indicated that expression and kinetic differences in both the p85 and p110 isoforms of PI3 kinase may contribute to the unique roles of these isoforms in cells (Meier *et al.* 2004). Obtaining this information is difficult, as studies both in LP offspring (Ozanne *et al.* 1999) and in humans with metabolic syndrome (Arner 1995) have suggested that resistance to the lipolytic action of insulin is depot-specific, with intra-abdominal fat being resistant and subcutaneous fat (the most available depot for biopsy) remaining relatively insulin-sensitive.

Maternal iron restriction

Iron deficiency is a common nutritional problem in humans and is especially prevalent in pregnant women. Initial studies have shown that when pregnant rats are fed an iron-deficient diet this leads to anaemia and growth restriction in the fetus (Shepard *et al.* 1980). Subsequent work has indicated that offspring of iron-deficient dams have decreased iron concentrations in the brain and also show behavioural differences compared to controls (Felt and Lozoff 1996). It has also been shown that 3-month-old offspring of iron-restricted dams have elevated blood pressures when compared to controls (Lewis *et al.* 2001). These animals were found to have decreased serum triacylglycerol and improved glucose tolerance, and they were growth-restricted at birth and remained smaller to 3 months of age (Lewis *et al.* 2001). Elevated blood pressures have been reported in offspring of iron-restricted dams at 40 days of age (Crowe *et al.* 1995), and

at 16 months of age these offspring show elevated systolic blood pressures and decreased triacylglycerol levels when compared to controls (Lewis *et al.* 2002). Heart weights of the offspring of anaemic dams have been shown to be increased in early postnatal life (day 20) (Crowe *et al.* 1995) and also in late adult life (Lewis *et al.* 2002). Maternal iron undernutrition in the rat therefore leads to long-term detrimental effects on the offspring such as raised systolic blood pressure and lower triacylglycerol levels. Ovine studies have also shown cardiac hypertrophy and decreased serum triacylglycerol levels in iron-restricted fetuses (Martin *et al.* 1998), suggesting that these changes may be initiated in utero. The mechanisms involved in the cardiac hypertrophy and elevation of blood pressure are unknown.

Glucocorticoid exposure

Maternal stress has long been known to induce IUGR. This stress response is thought to be partly mediated by glucocorticoids. Glucocorticoid overexposure during gestation is known to lead to a reduction in birthweight. There is therefore a growing interest in the roles of glucocorticoids in IUGR and the subsequent development of type 2 diabetes and the metabolic syndrome. Glucocorticoid treatment during pregnancy in both humans and animals is known to cause a reduction in birthweight of offspring (Reinisch *et al.* 1978). Rat offspring exposed to excess prenatal glucocorticoids undergo a catch-up growth postnatally such that their body weights are normalised by weaning (21 days of age). This rapid catch-up growth is similar to that seen in the LP model (discussed earlier) and has been shown to have adverse effects on health. In fact, the phenotypic outcome is very similar to that of the LP-model animals. Fetal glucocorticoid overexposure in rats has been shown to be associated with raised blood glucose levels (Lindsay *et al.* 1996) and elevated blood pressure (Benediktsson *et al.* 1993), both of which have been reported in the LP-model rats. This has led to the suggestion that fetal glucocorticoid overexposure may be a common mechanism linking maternal environment factors with fetal growth and programming. Treatment of pregnant rats with dexamethazone (a synthetic glucocorticoid) or carbenoxolone (an inhibitor of the placental enzyme that metabolises corticosterone to the inert 11-dehydrocorticosterone) results in a decreased body weight and also an increased blood pressure and blood glucose in adult offspring (Benediksson *et al.* 1993). Dietary protein restriction during pregnancy has been shown to reduce 11β-hydroxysteroid dehydrogenase type 2 (11β-HSD2) activity in rats, and this has also been reported to be decreased in babies with low birthweight (Stewart *et al.* 1995). 11β-HSD2 converts physiological glucocorticoids to inactive 11-keto products, forming a placental barrier which minimises fetal exposure to glucocorticoids. This low placental 11β-HSD2 activity and subsequent exposure of fetuses to high levels of glucocorticoids from maternal origin could lead to disturbances of the uterine development (Lesage *et al.* 2001).

Uterine artery ligation

A large number of cases of IUGR in humans, particularly in the Western world, are thought to be due to uteroplacental insufficiency which causes a reduction in the placental transport of nutrients to the fetus. Rat models of IUGR have therefore been developed by carrying out uterine artery ligation during late gestation (Wigglesworth 1974). Blood flow to the fetus is not ablated, but is reduced to a degree similar to that observed in human pregnancies complicated by uteroplacental insufficiency (Simmons *et al.* 2001). Growth-retarded fetuses of these animals have decreased levels of glucose, insulin, IGF1, amino acids and oxygen (Ogata *et al.* 1986, Unterman *et al.* 1990), which is very similar to the metabolic profile seen in IUGR human fetuses (Simmons *et al.* 2001). At 2 weeks of age growth-retarded offspring have a reduced nephron number, which is associated with impaired renal function despite an apparent large compensatory hypertro-

phy of nephrons in these animals (Marlet-Benichou *et al.* 1994). Changes in mitochondrial gene expression and function have also been reported in skeletal muscle from fetuses of 21-day-old offspring of dams with ligated uterine arteries. mRNA levels of the mitochondrial proteins NADH-ubiquinone-oxidoreductase subunit 4L, subunit C of the F_1F_0 ATP synthase and adenine nucleotide translocator 1 were all reduced in the fetus and at 21 days of age postnatally when compared to controls (Lane *et al.* 1998). These reductions were also associated with a reduced skeletal muscle mitochondrial $NAD^+/NADH$ ratio, indicative of an alteration in mitochondrial function (Lane *et al.* 1998). Bilateral uterine artery ligation at 19 days of gestation has also been shown to induce insulin resistance early in life, and these offspring develop diabetes by 6 months of age.

Glycogen content and insulin-stimulated glucose uptake were significantly decreased in muscle from IUGR rats (Selak *et al.* 2003). Muscle mitochondria from IUGR rats showed defects leading to a chronic reduction in the supply of ATP available for oxidative phosphorylation. Impaired ATP synthesis in muscle comprises GLUT4 recruitment, glucose transport and glycogen synthesis, which contribute to insulin resistance and hyperglycaemia of type 2 diabetes. mRNA expression levels of developmental transcription factors such as PDX1 are also reduced in the fetus and continue to decline progressively with age in the offspring (Stoffers *et al.* 2003). PDX1 is a homeobox transcription factor that is critical for early endocrine and exocrine development of the pancreas. GLP1 and Ex4 (a long-acting GLP1 analogue) have both been shown to improve glucose tolerance, increase islet size and stimulate PDX1 protein expression in the pancreas. Treating growth-retarded offspring with Ex4 in the early postnatal period completely prevents the development of diabetes in the uterine-artery-ligation rodent model (Stoffers *et al.* 2003). Other studies using a unilateral uterine-artery-ligation model to induce IUGR found no association between the low birthweight and elevated adult blood pressure (Jansson and Lambert 1999). This is in contrast with other growth-restriction models such as those caused by maternal calorie restriction, maternal LP, maternal iron restriction and maternal dexamethazone treatment, suggesting that intrauterine growth restriction per se is not sufficient to cause elevated blood pressure in adulthood. Further investigation into the exact timing of the insult or the composition of the adult diet may aid our understanding of this relationship. There is also evidence of gender differences in this uterine-artery-ligation model. In female rats, IUGR caused by unilateral uterine artery ligation is associated with impaired regulation of insulin secretion by glucose. Female offspring show increased fasting blood glucose levels but fasting insulin levels are unaltered, suggesting a degree of insulin resistance (Jansson and Lambert 1999). In males, there are similar fasting blood glucose and fasting insulin levels when compared to controls (Jansson and Lambert 1999).

High-fat feeding

High proportions of fat in the diet are contributing to the current epidemic of obesity and type 2 diabetes. A number of studies have investigated the effects of a high-fat diet during pregnancy and during adulthood in rats. Fetuses of dams fed a diet high in saturated fat during pregnancy have been shown to be insulin-resistant (Guo and Jen 1995). Young adult offspring of dams fed a diet rich in corn oil during pregnancy exhibit abnormal cholesterol metabolism (Brown *et al.* 1990) and offspring of dams fed a diet rich in coconut oil (predominantly saturated fats) during pregnancy have been shown to be hypertensive (Langley-Evans 1996). Vascular dysfunction, plasma lipid abnormalities (Koukkou *et al.* 1998) and also irregularities in the fatty acid composition of the liver (Ghebremeskel *et al.* 1999) have been seen in young adult offspring. Abnormal vascular function, plasma lipid disturbances and altered vascular fatty acid content have also been reported in female offspring of 20% saturated-fat-fed pregnant dams (Ghosh *et al.* 2001). If the high-fat diet is fed to normal adult rats for four weeks, increases in body weight and fat-pad weight are seen; increased

food intake and fasting plasma insulin levels are also observed when compared to controls (Koshinaka *et al.* 2004). High-fat feeding has also been used to induce gestational diabetes mellitus (GDM). Rats fed a high-fat diet four weeks prior to and during pregnancy show signs of glucose intolerance (Holemans *et al.* 2004). These dams also show increased fat mass and plasma leptin concentrations. Insulin resistance was also seen in high-fat-fed non-pregnant rats, and this was aggravated by pregnancy (Holemans *et al.* 2004).

Other insults

Cytokine exposure in utero has been shown to have long-term effects on insulin sensitivity (Dahlgren *et al.* 2001). Interleukin 6 administration at days 8, 10 and 12 of gestation caused an increase in body weight at 3 weeks of age even though there was no difference seen in the growth of the fetuses. Increased body fat was seen at 10 weeks of age, and this was associated with whole-body insulin resistance in males but not in females (Dahlgren *et al.* 2001).

Maternal endotoxemia has also been shown to have similar effects to increased cytokine exposure in utero. Administration of lipopolysaccharide at days 8, 10 and 12 of gestation to pregnant rat dams has no effect on fetal growth (Nilsson *et al.* 2001). However these offspring underwent greater postnatal growth such that male rats were significantly heavier than controls at 4 weeks of age. Male rats also showed whole-body insulin resistance at 12 weeks of age when compared to controls. In contrast, females showed no weight gain or insulin resistance compared to controls (Nilsson *et al.* 2001).

Sheep models

The majority of models used for studying insulin resistance and type 2 diabetes in relation to fetal growth restriction have been in rodents. Rats are known to be particularly nutritionally sensitive to either global or specific undernutrition or high-dose glucocorticoid exposure during pregnancy, due to their being a litter-bearing species. Sheep have a similar rate of pre- and postnatal growth to the human and usually produce one or two offspring. So an increasing amount of research is being carried out focusing on larger mammals such as the sheep. Both the effects of maternal protein restriction (Nishina *et al.* 2003) and global food restriction (Heasman *et al.* 1999, Hawkins *et al.* 2000, Vonnahme *et al.* 2003, Gopalakrishnan *et al.* 2004) have been used to investigate the effects of IUGR in sheep. Studies have been carried out with mild (85% normal maternal global food intake) (Hawkins *et al.* 2000) and also with more severe reductions in maternal food intake (50% of normal intake) (Heasman *et al.* 1999, Vonnahme *et al.* 2003, Gopalakrishnan *et al.* 2004). Mild maternal food restriction leads to a lower fetal blood pressure without any changes in the growth of the fetus (Hawkins *et al.* 2000, Edwards and McMillen 2002). More severe maternal food restriction has been associated with a reduction in placental weight during mid term but an increase in the weight of the placenta towards the end of gestation (Heasman *et al.* 1999). There was no effect seen on the weight of the fetus, although some differences in body dimensions have been reported (Heasman *et al.* 1999). Placental weights are unchanged if maternal nutrient restriction occurs in the first 40 days or the last 50 days of gestation, but if the maternal diet is restricted for periods of variable length between 30 and 107 days of gestation the placental weight is altered (reviewed by Heasman *et al.* 1999). Both increases and decreases in placental weight have been seen in these studies, which may be due to differences in maternal weight, body condition and breed (Heasman *et al.* 1999). Increases in fetal liver and the heart ventricle weights have also been reported in fetuses of ewes fed a 50% protein diet (Vonnahme *et al.* 2003). These compensations may be beneficial to the fetus during early nutrient restriction but may prove to be detrimental later in gestation as well as in postnatal life (Vonnahme *et al.* 2003). The long-term effects of global food restriction during pregnancy on the offspring have been investigated (Gopalakrishnan *et al.* 2004). At 3 years of age offspring of food-restricted ewes

have higher blood pressure before feeding (but not after) than controls. Undernutrition in humans and rodents has been shown to reduce 11β-HSD2 (discussed earlier), leading to overexposure of the fetus to maternal glucocorticoids (Stewart *et al.* 1995). It is possible that 11β-HSD2 levels are altered in the ovine placenta by maternal protein restriction (Nishina *et al.* 2003). Glucocorticoids have also been implicated in the programming of cardiovascular function in sheep (Dodic *et al.* 1998). One more recent study compared offspring of globally and protein-restricted mothers. Fetal and placental weights in both groups were unchanged compared to controls. But protein restriction did produce blunting of endothelial relaxation in systemic arteries from the mid-gestation fetus (Nishina *et al.* 2003).

Future prospects

There is a great need for continued investment and research into animal models that study the biological and molecular processes which link insults during pregnancy to subsequent disease in later life. Further investigation of the effects of nutrition and other insults (such as maternal stress and infection) during pregnancy, and pinpointing the critical time-windows for these insults, will be essential. Human studies can then be maximised and treatments/interventions identified. Human studies have used birthweight and ponderal index to indicate if growth restriction has occurred. Both measurements are only a very crude indicator of whether IUGR has taken place, and indeed it is becoming clear that insults during fetal life can have long-term consequences which are independent of birthweight. More reliable indications are required to identify susceptible individuals and the time frame in which this occurs. A further assessment of what potential there is for childhood nutrition and growth to exacerbate or ameliorate the long-term effects of fetal growth restriction is also necessary. When the molecular mechanisms underlying the fetal origins of adult disease are understood, rational intervention strategies will become a realistic possibility.

REFERENCES

Arner, P. (1995). Differences in lypolysis between human subcutaneous and omental adipose tissue. *Ann. Med.*, **27**, 435–8.

Barker, D. J. P. and Hales, C. N. (1992). Type 2 (non-insulin-dependent) diabetes mellitus: the thrifty phenotype hypothesis. *Diabetologia*, **35**, 595–601.

Benediktsson, R., Lindsay, R. S., Noble, J., Sekl, J. R. and Edwards, C. R. W. (1993). Glucocorticoid exposure *in utero*: a new model for adult hypertension. *Lancet*, **341**, 339–41.

Boujendar, S., Reusens, B., Merezak, S. *et al.* (2002). Taurine supplementation to a low protein diet during fetal and early postnatal life restores a normal proliferation and apoptosis of rat pancreatic islets. *Diabetologia*, **45**, 856–66.

Brown, S. A., Rogers, L. K., Dunn, J. K., Gotto, A. M. and Patsch, W. (1990). Development of cholesterol homeostatic memory in the rat is influenced by maternal diets. *Metabolism*, **39**, 468–73.

Burns, S. P., Desai, M., Cohen, R. D. *et al.* (1997). Gluconeogenesis, glucose handling, and structural changes in livers of the adult offspring of rats partially deprived of protein during pregnancy and lactation. *J. Clin. Invest.*, **100**, 1768–74.

Cherif, H., Reusens, B., Ahn, M. T., Hoet, J. J. and Remacle, C. (1998). Effects of taurine on the insulin secretion of rat fetal islets from dams fed a low-protein diet. *J. Endocrinol.*, **159**, 341–8.

Cherif, H., Reusens, B., Dahri, S. and Remacle, C. (2001). A protein-restricted diet during pregnancy alters in vitro insulin secretion from islets of fetal Wistar rats. *J. Nutr.*, **131**, 1555–9.

Crowe, C., Dandekar, P., Fox, M., Dhingra, K., Bennet, L. and Hanson, M. A. (1995). The effects of anaemia on heart, placenta and body weight, blood pressure in fetal and neonatal rats. *J. Physiol.*, **488**, 515–19.

Dahlgren, J., Nilsson, C., Jennische, E. *et al.* (2001). Prenatal cytokine exposure results in obesity and gender-specific programming. *Am. J. Physiol. Endocrinol. Metab.*, **281**, E326–34.

Dahri, S., Snoeck, A., Reusens, B., Remacle, C. and Hoet, J. J. (1991). Islet function in offspring of mothers on low-protein diet during gestation. *Diabetes*, **40**, 115–20.

Desai, M., Crowther, N. J., Lucas, A. and Hales, C. N. (1996). Organ-selective growth in the offspring of protein restricted mothers. *Br. J. Nutr.*, **76**, 591–603.

Dodic, M., May, C. N., Wintour, E. M. and Coghlan, J. P. (1998). An early prenatal exposure to excess glucocorticoid leads to hypertensive offspring in sheep. *Clin. Sci. (Lond.)*, **94**, 149–55.

Edwards, L. J. and McMillen, I. C. (2002). Vascular endothelial dysfunction. *Prog. Cardiovasc. Dis.*, **39**, 325–42.

Eriksson, J. G., Forsen, T., Tuomilehto, J., Osmond, C. and Barker, D. J. P. (2000). Fetal and childhood growth and hypertension in adult life. *Hypertension*, **36**, 790–4.

Felt, B. T. and Lozoff, B. (1996). Brain iron and behavior of rats are not normalized by treatment of iron deficiency anemia during early development. *J. Nutr.*, **126**, 693–701.

Frank, J. W., Saslow, S. B., Camilleri, M., Thomforde, G. M., Dinneen, S. and Rizza, R. A. (1995). Mechanism of accelerated gastric emptying of liquids and hyperglycaemia in patients with type 2 diabetes mellitus. *Gastroenterology*, **109**, 755–65.

Garofano, A., Czernichow, P. and Bréant, B. (1997). In utero undernutrition impairs rat β-cell development. *Diabetologia*, **40**, 1231–4.

(1999). Effect of ageing on beta-cell mass and function in rats malnourished during the perinatal period. *Diabetologia*, **42**, 711–18.

Ghebremeskel, K., Bitsanis, D., Koukkou, E., Lowy, C., Poston, L. and Crawford, M. A. (1999). Saturated fat maternal diet in the pregnant rat reduces docosahexaenoic acid in liver lipids of neonate and suckling pups. *Br. J. Nutr.*, **81**, 395–404.

Ghosh, P., Bitsanis, D., Ghebremeskel, K., Crawford, M. A. and Poston, L. (2001). Abnormal aortic fatty acid composition and small artery function in offspring of rats fed a high fat diet in pregnancy. *J. Physiol.*, **533**, 815–22.

Godfrey, K., Robinson, S., Barker, D. J. P., Osmond, C. and Cox, V. (1996). Maternal nutrition in early and late pregnancy in relation to placental and fetal growth. *BMJ*, **312**, 410–14.

Gopalakrishnan, G. S., Gardner, D. S., Rhind, S. M. *et al.* (2004). Programming of adult cardiovascular function after early maternal undernutrition in sheep. *Am. J. Physiol. Regul. Integr. Comp. Physiol.*, **287**, R12–20.

Guo, F. and Jen, K. C. L. (1995). High fat feeding during pregnancy and lactation affects offspring metabolism in rats. *Physiol. Behav.*, **57**, 681–6.

Hales, C. N. and Ozanne, S. E. (2004). Catch-up growth and obesity in male mice. *Nature*, **247**, 411–12.

Hales, C. N., Desai, M., Ozanne, S. E. and Crowther, N. J. (1996). Fishing in the stream of diabetes: from measuring insulin to the control of fetal organogenesis. *Biochem. Soc. Trans.*, **24**, 341–50.

Hawkins, P., Steyn, C., Ozaki, T., Saito, T., Noakes, D. E. and Hanson, M. A. (2000). Effect of maternal undernutrition in early gestation on ovine fetal blood pressure and cardiovascular reflexes. *Am. J. Physiol. Regul. Integr. Comp. Physiol.*, **279**, R340–8.

Heasman, L., Clarke, L., Stephenson, T. J. and Symonds, M. E. (1999). The influence of maternal nutrient restriction in early to mid-pregnancy on placental and fetal development in sheep. *Proc. Nutr. Soc.*, **58**, 283–8.

Holemans, K., Verhaeghe, J., Dequeker, J., Van Assche, F. A. (1996). Insulin sensitivity in adult female offspring of rats subjected to malnutrition during the perinatal period. *J. Soc. Gynecol. Investig.*, **3**, 71–7.

Holemans, K., Caluwarts, S., Poston, L. and Van Assche, F. A. (2004). Diet-induced obesity in the rat: a model for gestational diabetes mellitus. *Am. J. Obs. Gynecol.*, **190**, 858–65.

Holness, M. J. and Sugden, M. C. (1999). Antecedent protein restriction exacerbates development of impaired insulin action after high-fat feeding. *Am. J. Physiol.*, **276**, E85–93.

Hughes, S. J. and Wilson, M. R. (1997). The effect of maternal protein deficiency during pregnancy and lactation on glucose tolerance and pancreatic islet function in adult rat offspring. *J. Endocrinol.*, **27**, 177–85.

Jansson, T. and Lambert, G. W. (1999). Effect of intrauterine growth restriction on blood pressure, glucose tolerance and sympathetic nervous system activity in the rat at 3–4 months of age. *J. Hypotens.*, **17**, 1239–48.

Jennings, B. J., Ozanne, S. E., Dorling, M. W. and Hales, C. N. (1999). Early growth restriction determines longevity in male rats and may be related to telomere shortening in the kidney. *FEBS Lett.*, **448**, 4–9.

Koshinaka, K., Oshida, Y., Han, Y. Q. *et al.* (2004). Insulin-specific reduction in skeletal muscle glucose transport in high-fat-fed rats. *Metabolism*, **53**, 912–17.

Koukkou, E., Ghosh, P., Lowy, C. and Poston, L. (1998). Offspring of normal and diabetic rats fed saturated fat in pregnancy demonstrate vascular dysfunction. *Circulation*, **86**, 217–22.

Lane, R. H., Chandorkar, A. K., Flozak, A. S. and Simmons, R. A. (1998). Intrauterine growth retardation alters mitochondrial gene expression and function in fetal and juvenile rat skeletal muscle. *Pediatr. Res.*, **43**, 563–70.

Langley-Evans, S. C. (1996). Intrauterine programming of hypertension in the rat: nutrient interactions. *Comp. Biochem. Physiol.*, **114**, 327–33.

Langley-Evans, S. C., Sherman, R. C., Welham, S. J., Nwagwu, M. O., Gardner, D. S. and Jackson, A. A. (1999). Intrauterine programming of hypertension: the role of the rennin–angiotensin system. *Biochem. Soc. Trans.*, **27**, 88–93.

Law, C. M., Barker, D. J. P., Osmond, C., Fall, C. H. and Simmonds, S. J. (1992). Early growth and abdominal fatness in adult life. *J. Epidemiol. Community Health*, **46**, 184–6.

Leon, D., Koupilova, I., Lithell, H. O. *et al.* (1996). Failure to realize growth potential *in utero* and adult obesity in relation to blood pressure in 50 year old Swedish men. *BMJ*, **312**, 401–6.

Lesage, J., Blondeau, B., Grino, M., Bréant, B. and Dupouy, J. P. (2001). Maternal undernutrition during late gestation induces fetal overexposure to glucocorticoids and intrauterine growth retardation, and disturbs the hypothalamo-pituitary adrenal axis in the newborn rat. *Endocrinology*, **142**, 1692–702.

Lewis, R. M., Petry, C. J., Ozanne, S. E. and Hales, C. N. (2001). Effects of maternal iron restriction in the rat on blood pressure, glucose tolerance, and serum lipids in the 3-month-old offspring. *Metabolism*, **50**, 562–7.

Lewis, R. M., Forhead, A. J., Petry, C. J., Ozanne, S. E. and Hales, C. N. (2002). Long-term programming of blood pressure by maternal dietary iron restriction in the rat. *Brit. J. Nutr.*, **88**, 283–90.

Lindsay, R. S., Lindsay, R. M., Wadell, B. J. and Sekl, J. R. (1996). Prenatal glucocorticoid exposure leads to offspring hyperglycaemia in the rat; studies with the 11β-hydroxysteroid dehydrogenase inhibitor carbenoxenolone. *Diabetologia*, **39**, 1299–305.

Marlet-Benichou, C., Gilbert, T., Muffat-Joly, M., Lelievre-Pegorier, M. and Leroy, B. (1994). Intrauterine growth retardation leads to a permanent nephron deficit in the rat. *Pediatr. Nephrol.*, **8**, 175–80.

Martin, C. M., Yu, A. Y., Jiang, B. H. *et al.* (1998). Cardiac hypertrophy in chronically anemic fetal sheep: increased vascularization is associated with increased myocardial expression of vascular endothelial growth factor and hypoxia-inducible factor 1. *Am. J. Obstet. Gynecol.*, **178**, 527–34.

Meier, T. I., Cook, J. A., Thomas, J. E. *et al.* (2004). Cloning, expression, purification, and characterization of the human class 1a phosphoinositide 3-kinase isoforms. *Protein Expr. Purif.*, **35**, 218–24.

Nilsson, C., Larsson, B. M., Jennische, E. *et al.* (2001). Maternal endotoxemia results in obesity and insulin resistance in adult male offspring. *Endocrinology*, **142**, 2622–30.

Nishina, H., Green, L. R., McGarrigle, H. H. G., Noakes, D. E., Poston, L. and Hanson, M. A. (2003). Effect of nutritional restriction in early pregnancy on isolated femoral artery function in mid-gestation fetal sheep. *J. Physiol.*, **553**, 637–47.

Ogata, E. S., Bussey, M. and Finley, S. (1986). Altered gas exchange, limited glucose, branched chain amino acids, and hypoinsulinism retard fetal growth in the rat. *Metabolism*, **35**, 950–77.

Ozanne, S. E., Smith, G. D., Tikererpae, J. and Hales, C. N. (1996a). Altered regulation of hepatic glucose output in the male offspring of protein malnourished rat dams. *Am. J. Physiol.*, **270**, E55–64.

Ozanne, S. E., Wang, C. L., Coleman, N. and Smith, G. D. (1996b). Altered muscle insulin sensitivity in the male offspring of protein malnourished rats. *Am. J. Physiol.*, **271**, E1128–34.

Ozanne, S. E., Nave, B. T., Wang, C. L., Shepherd, P. R., Prins, J. and Smith, G. D. (1997). Poor fetal nutrition causes long-term changes in expression of insulin signaling components in adipocytes. *Am. J. Physiol.*, **273**, E46–51.

Ozanne, S. E., Wang, C. L., Dorling, M. W. and Petry, C. J. (1999). Dissection of the metabolic actions of insulin in adipocytes from early growth retarded male rats. *J. Endocrinol.*, **162**, 313–19.

Petrik, J., Reusens, B., Arany, C. *et al.* (1999). A low protein diet alters the balance of islet cell replication and apoptosis in the fetal and neonatal rat and is associated with a reduced pancreatic expression of insulin-like growth factor II. *Endocrinology*, **140**, 4861–73.

Petry, C. J., Ozanne, S. E., Wang, C. L. and Hales, C. N. (1997). Early protein restriction and obesity independently induce hypertension in 1-year-old rats. *Clin. Sci. (Lond.)*, **93**, 147–52.

Petry, C. J., Dorling, M. W., Pawlak, D. B., Ozanne, S. E. and Hales, C. N. (2001). Diabetes in old rat dams fed a reduced protein diet. *Int. J. Diabetes Res.*, **2**, 139–43.

Reinisch, J. M., Simon, N. G., Karwo, W. G. and Gandelman, R. (1978). Prenatal exposure to prednisone in humans and animals retards intrauterine growth, *Science*, **202**, 436–8.

Rosso, P. and Kava, R. (1980). Effects of food restriction on cardiac output and blood flow to the uterus and placenta in the pregnant rat. *J. Nutr.*, **110**, 2350–4.

Selak, M. A., Storey, B. T., Peterside, I. and Simmons, R. A. (2003). Impaired oxidative phosphorylation in skeletal muscle of intrauterine growth-retarded rats. *Am. J. Physiol. Endocrinol. Metab.*, **285**, E130–7.

Shepard, T. H., Mackler, B. and Finch, C. A. (1980). Reproductive studies in the iron-deficient rat. *Teratology*, **22**, 329–34.

Shepherd, P. R., Crowther, N. J., Desai, M., Hales, C. N. and Ozanne, S. E. (1997). Altered adipocyte proteins in the offspring of protein malnourished rats. *Br. J. Nutr.*, **78**, 121–9.

Shepherd, P. R., Withers, D. J. and Siddle, K. (1998). Phospho-inositide 3-kinase: the key switch mechanism in insulin signalling. *Biochem. J.*, **333**, 471–90.

Simmons, R. A., Templeton, L. J. and Gertz, S. J. (2001). Intrauterine growth retardation leads to the development of type 2 diabetes in the rat. *Diabetes*, **50**, 2279–86.

Snoeck, A., Remacle, C., Reusens, B. and Hoet, J. J. (1990). Effect of a low protein diet during pregnancy on the fetal rat endocrine pancreas. *Biol. Neonate*, **57**, 107–18.

Stewart, P. M., Rogerson, F. M. and Mason, J. I. (1995). Type 2 11β-hydroxysteroid dehydrogenase messenger RNA and activity in human placenta and fetal membranes: its relationship to birth weight and putative role in fetal steroidogenesis. *J. Clin. Endcrinol. Metab.*, **80**, 885–90.

Stoffers, D. A., Desai, B. M., DeLeon, D. D. and Simmons, R. A. (2003). Neonatal exendin-4 prevents the development of diabetes in the intrauterine growth retarded rat. *Diabetes*, **52**, 734–40.

Tokunaga, H., Yoneda, Y. and Kuriyama, K. (1983). Streptozotocin-induced elevation of pancreatic tau-rine content and suppressive effect of taurine on insulin secretion. *Eur. J. Pharmacol.*, **87**, 237–43.

Unterman, T., Lascon, R., Gotway, M. *et al.* (1990). Circulating levels of insulin-like growth factor binding protein-1 (IGFBP-1) and hepatic mRNA are increased in the small for gestational age fetal rat. *Endocrinology*, **127**, 2035–7.

Vickers, M. H., Breier, B. H., Cutfield, W. S., Hofman, P. L. and Gluckman, P. D. (2000). Fetal origins of hyperphagia, obesity, and hypertension and its postnatal amplification by hypercaloric nutrition. *Am. J. Physiol. Endocrinol. Metab.*, **279**, E83–7.

Vickers, M. H., Breier, B. H., McCarthy, D. and Gluckman, P. D. (2003). Sedentary behavior during postnatal life is determined by the prenatal environment and exacerbated by postnatal hypercaloric nutrition. *Am. J. Physiol. Regul. Integr. Comp. Physiol.*, **285**, R271–3.

Virkamäki, A., Ueki, K. and Kahn, C. R. (1999). Protein–protein interaction in insulin signalling and the molecular mech-anisms of insulin resistance. *J. Clin. Invest.*, **103**, 931–43.

Vonnahme, K. A., Hess, B. W., Hansen, T. R. *et al.* (2003). Maternal undernutrition from early- to mid-gestation leads to growth retardation, cardiac ventricular hypertrophy, and increased liver weight in the fetal sheep. *Biol. Reprod.*, **69**, 133–40.

Wigglesworth, J. S. (1974). Fetal growth retardation. Animal model: uterine vessel ligation in the pregnant rat. *Am. J. Pathol.*, **77**, 347–50.

18

The developmental environment and the development of obesity

Michael E. Symonds and David S. Gardner

University of Nottingham

The pandemic of obesity: what are its origins?

The incidence of childhood and adult obesity continues to increase annually worldwide within both developed and developing countries, despite substantial international research into the potential mechanisms that may underlie this pandemic. Indeed worldwide there are now as many individuals who are overnourished as are undernourished. The speed with which obesity, has risen, particularly in countries such as India and China as they adopt Western diets and lifestyles, strongly suggests that genetic factors are not the explanation. Currently nearly all research and intervention strategies are targeted towards adult obesity, which could explain the failure to reduce its incidence. Given the growing body of epidemiological and experimental evidence demonstrating that obesity is programmed in utero, this anomaly should be addressed. The potential significance of fetal programming to later health is emphasised by the fact that obesity alone is not only a major health risk itself, but is also an adverse factor contributing towards hypertension (Hall 2003) and cancer (Bray 2002).

Epidemiological evidence for fetal programming of obesity

Taken together, the overall consensus from epidemiological studies is that being either small or large at birth predicts later obesity (Law *et al.* 1992, Sorensen *et al.* 1997). Whether this is the result of changes within the adipocyte itself, or in appetite control, or a combination of both, remains an area of intense debate within the field of obesity research. With respect to the influence of fetal programming on later fat mass, the magnitude of response can be further determined by the ethnic, and thus genetic, background of an individual. For example, small thin Indian babies have poor muscle and visceral mass but higher adiposity for a given weight compared to white Caucasian infants (Yajnik 2004). Heavier mothers also have larger babies which go on to have a high body mass index in adult life (Parsons *et al.* 2001).

However, as will be emphasised later, animal studies demonstrate that fetal fat development can be significantly reprogrammed by manipulating maternal and therefore fetal nutrition. Importantly these effects occur in the absence of any effect on birthweight (Bispham *et al.*, 2003a). It should be noted that infants born small, or large, only represent the extremes of 'normality'. In these subgroups their increased or decreased size could therefore be the result of a propensity for genetic or pathological influences such as maternal diabetes (Buchanan and Kjos 1999) or pre-eclampsia (Broughton Pipkin and Roberts 2000). Under these adverse environmental conditions maternal and/or fetal nutritional constraints may not be the main determinants of size at birth. For example, pre-eclampsia, which results in a

Developmental Origins of Health and Disease, ed. Peter Gluckman and Mark Hanson. Published by Cambridge University Press.

range of maternal complications plus compromised placental function that culminates in intrauterine growth retardation (IUGR) (Broughton Pipkin and Roberts 2000), has not been shown to predispose to later obesity. Moreover, when interpreting the results from twin studies (a natural form of IUGR), which appear to indicate that size at birth does not have an influence on later obesity (Rogers 2003), it must be remembered that twins are exposed to very different metabolic and endocrine environments compared to singletons (Gardner et al. 2004a). Hormonal sensitivity of twins to nutritional challenges (Edwards and McMillen 2002) is therefore very different and it is not surprising that fat development is very different during both fetal and early life (Budge et al. 2003, Gardner et al. 2004b).

Overall, and not surprisingly, the plethora of publications from largely retrospective epidemiological studies do not provide a clear consensus as to whether obesity can be determined in utero. Animal studies provide a much better insight into the potential significance of fetal programming on later disease and will be the focus of the present chapter. We will therefore review current experimental evidence on fetal and adult fat development, and the extent to which this process may be nutritionally regulated with respect to differences between current animal models, as well as other major factors that could potentially contribute to excess fat deposition after birth.

Fetal adipose tissue function

In the fetus of the majority of species studied to date adipose tissue comprises brown and white adipocytes which have a common mesenchymal stem cell precursor lineage. The energetic requirement for lipid synthesis (39 MJ kg^{-1}) is much greater than for carbohydrate or protein (15–25 MJ kg^{-1}). Thus in an environment in which oxygen and the majority of metabolic substrates are limited, growth of fat in the fetus is usually restricted. However, despite the small amount of fat present in most species at birth, its abundance and endocrine sen-

sitivity are highly sensitive to the maternal and fetal nutritional regime throughout gestation (Bispham et al. 2003a).

The primary role of fat in the newborn relates to thermoregulation. This function is achieved either as a result of the production of very large amounts of heat following rapid activation of the brown adipocyte-specific uncoupling protein 1 (UCP1) (Clarke et al. 1997b), or by providing insulation (Symonds et al. 2001). It is also the main source of a rapidly mobilised energy-rich substrate in the form of lipid from which non-esterified fatty acids (NEFAs) are released (Alexander and Williams 1968). At birth NEFAs have several roles, including:

(1) activation of UCP1
(2) provision of a metabolic substrate for UCP1 and related mitochondrial proteins
(3) an energy source for skeletal muscle during shivering thermogenesis

The relative contribution of fat to heat production and insulation varies greatly between species, but the main function of fetal fat is to enable the newborn to meet the tremendous thermal challenge at birth. This occurs over a short time period in which the newborn has to rapidly adapt to the substantial decrease in ambient temperature whilst being surrounded by rapidly cooling intrauterine fluids (Symonds et al. 1995). The instantaneous activation of thermogenesis at birth, coincident with a near maximal metabolic rate that is seldom matched throughout the rest of the lifecycle, is an important example of the very different function of fat in fetal compared with adult life. The dramatic change in the role of fat, from one primarily concerned with heat production (and insulation, depending on the species) to a site of energy storage linked to appetite regulation, may have critical implications for the propensity, or otherwise, towards excess fat deposition in later life.

With respect to which animal model is adopted for studies on fetal programming, their predisposition to obesity under 'normal conditions' should be taken into account. In wild rodents and most domestic species, obesity is not a health problem but it can be induced by specific genetic and/or dietary manipulations. For humans and pigs that adopt a sedentary lifestyle in conjunction with consumption of excess calories and/or an unbalanced diet then obesity develops. The current scientific challenge is therefore to integrate relevant information from the diverse range of experimental models adopted in order to define the fetal mechanisms by which excess fat growth can be programmed. In this regard it is necessary to take into account differences in both pre- and postnatal fat location and development among the different animal models.

Nutritional regulation of fetal fat growth

The primary metabolic precursor for lipid synthesis is glucose (Vernon *et al.* 1981), so it is not unexpected that an increase in fetal plasma glucose as a result of either changes in maternal food intake (Symonds *et al.* 2004) or direct infusion into the fetus are accompanied by parallel effects on fetal fat mass (Stevens *et al.* 1990). Because of the critical importance of glucose with respect to the regulation of fetal fat growth, nutritional manipulations that alter glucose status of both the mother and fetus similarly influence fetal adiposity (Symonds *et al.* 2004). This close relationship appears to be limited to late gestation, when about 90% of fetal fat is deposited; but this is not accompanied by any significant change in total fetal body weight. Furthermore, the magnitude by which fetal fat mass is enhanced appears to be strongly influenced by previous exposure to nutrient restriction. Adiposity is therefore greater in term fetuses whose mothers were nutrient-restricted between early and mid gestation (Bispham *et al.* 2003a). This adaptation is accompanied by an increased abundance of mRNA for IGF1 and IGF2 receptors (Bispham *et al.* 2003a), which is predicted to enhance adipose-tissue sensitivity to anabolic effects of IGFs (Teruel *et al.* 1996). Fat deposition will then be promoted in previously nutrient-restricted fetuses (Stevens *et al.* 1990) if glucose supply to the fetus is subsequently raised (Dandrea *et al.* 2001). In contrast to the effects of caloric restriction of the mother, protein depletion (Ozanne *et al.* 1997) or supplemen-

tation (Davies *et al.* 2003) has minimal effects on fat mass in either the fetus or the resulting offspring.

Although fetal glucose supply is a main determinant of fetal adiposity in late gestation there are certain nutritional conditions under which fat mass can be enhanced in the absence of any increase in fetal plasma glucose. For example, prolonged maternal nutrient restriction extending through gestation and commencing around the time of conception results in growth-restricted fetuses with more fat (Budge *et al.* 2004). This effect is apparent in twins but not singletons and could be the result of a differential resetting in the development of the fetal hypothalamic–pituitary–adrenal (HPA) axis (Edwards and McMillen 2002). Late-gestation twin fetuses have lower plasma cortisol compared to age-matched singletons and show a delayed increase in both cortisol and ACTH with gestational age, despite no difference in length of gestation (Edwards and McMillen 2002, Gardner *et al.* 2004a). Further evidence of delayed HPA maturation in twins is the finding that the increments in fetal plasma concentration of cortisol in response both to acute hypoxaemia and to exogenous ACTH are blunted relative to singletons (Gardner *et al.* 2004a). Endocrine sensitivity of fat from twins is also up-regulated at birth, when the abundance of the class 1 cytokine receptor for the pituitary hormone prolactin is much greater than in singletons (Budge *et al.* 2003). Prolactin acting through its receptor is known to be important in promoting UCP1 abundance in the newborn (Budge *et al.* 2002) and can influence longer-term fat mass (Freemark *et al.* 2001). The composition of fat from twins is also altered in that the plasma membrane content is reduced whereas total UCP1 abundance is increased (Budge *et al.* 2003). A smaller plasma membrane in conjunction with greater receptor abundance would increase tissue sensitivity, thus resulting in more UCP1 even in the absence of any change in circulating hormone abundance. The long-term consequences are that although twins have less fat at birth than singletons they subsequently deposit appreciably more fat up to one year of age despite the same amount of food consumption (Gardner *et al.* 2004b).

It is likely that in species that have a mature HPA at birth and show precocial postnatal adaptation to birth, an increase in central endocrine responsiveness may also contribute to excess fat deposition at birth, particularly if this is accompanied by a resetting of the HPA as a result of previous nutritional manipulation. The exact nature of this interaction remains to be clarified, but it is intriguing to note that ablation of the fetal hypothalamus greatly promotes fetal adiposity (Stevens and Alexander 1986), although the extent to which this is a direct effect or related to alterations in fetal glucose homeostasis has never been determined.

Fetal programming of fat development and leptin sensitivity

A range of hormones are secreted by adipose tissue, including leptin, resistin and adiponectin, that are all strongly implicated in obesity (Steppan *et al*. 2001, Wolf 2003). These have recently been shown to be down-regulated in subcutaneous fat sampled from mice fetuses of dams that were nutrient-restricted from 10.5 to 18.5 days gestation (Itoh *et al*. 2004). Adaptations within the adipocyte may be predictive of later obesity as a consequence either of impaired metabolism and/or of dysregulation of appetite control. The role of these hormones alters dramatically following birth since leptin, for example, promotes the appearance of UCP1 before term (Yuen *et al*. 2003) but accelerates its disappearance soon after birth (Mostyn *et al*. 2002). Another key factor implicated in abnormal fat growth is the peroxisome proliferator-activated receptor γ2(PPARγ2), which promotes fat cell differentiation and hypertrophy in diabetes as well as being linked to birthweight (Eriksson *et al*. 2002). Of these, the most widely studied to date with respect to its role in fetal programming of obesity is leptin.

In the term fetus of both humans and sheep there is a good correlation between fat mass and plasma leptin despite the very different total amounts of fat between these species. This indicates that although leptin can be secreted by the placenta (Reitman

et al. 2001) this source contributes little to the plasma concentration in the fetus (Bispham *et al*. 2003a). Both leptin-synthetic capacity of fetal fat and its plasma concentration are nutritionally regulated, largely by the prevailing plasma glucose concentration (Mühlhäusler *et al*. 2003, Symonds *et al*. 2004). This is also highly dependent on the maternal nutritional environment through gestation, which may have lifelong consequences. Leptin mRNA abundance is thus enhanced near term in previously nutrient-restricted fetuses (Bispham *et al*. 2003a), which in conjunction with greater sympathetic innervation may explain a greater leptin-synthetic capacity in response to stress in later life (Gopalakrishnan *et al*. 2004). Increased sensitivity to stress could be important, as glucocorticoid receptor mRNA abundance is also enhanced in adipose tissue of nutrient-restricted offspring, in conjunction with increased mRNA for 11β-hydroxysteroid dehydrogenase (11β-HSD1) (Whorwood *et al*. 2001), an adaptation that is found in both males and females. The enzyme 11β-HSD1 acts predominantly as an 11-oxoreductase, catalysing the conversion of cortisone to bioactive cortisol (Bamberger *et al*. 1996, Stewart and Krozowski 1999). Transgenic mice, in which 11β-HSD1 is overexpressed, show substantially increased visceral adipose tissue deposition at 18 weeks of age (Masuzaki *et al*. 2001). Nutrient-restricted offspring have more fat from birth (Bispham *et al*. 2003a), a trend that is maintained as young adults (Fig. 18.1), but as discussed below it may be that it is only when they are provided with excess calories that substantial extra fat deposition occurs.

Postnatal fat growth

In humans and sheep, which are both born with a mature HPA, a marked change in fat composition occurs soon after birth (Clarke *et al*. 1997a). This follows the gradual decline in plasma concentrations of endocrine stimulatory factors including thyroid hormones, catecholamines (Symonds *et al*. 2000), prolactin (Budge *et al*. 2002), cortisol (Mostyn *et al*. 2003) and leptin (Yuen *et al*. 2003), which are all necessary for maximising the rapid appearance of UCP1. Coincident with this adaptation and the establishment of lactation, when the nutritional constraints of fetal life are no longer in place, fat becomes the most rapidly growing organ.

Not surprisingly, in those offspring in which fat mass is increased at birth this adaptation persists into later life (Symonds *et al.* 1992) (Figure 18.1). This process can be accelerated by hypothyroidism (Symonds *et al.* 1996) and is also strongly influenced by maternal fatness, age and parity (Symonds *et al.* 2004). Offspring of juvenile or thin mothers are thus similarly thin, at least as juveniles and young adults. In contrast, offspring of adult primiparous mothers that have the same amount of fat as multiparous mothers at birth subsequently lay down more fat postnatally. This adaptation occurs in conjunction with leptin resistance and increased IGF sensitivity (Bispham *et al.* 2003b, 2004). These distinct adaptations in fat growth are not accompanied by any apparent differences in appetite and are very likely to reflect changes in fetal fat development.

It is interesting to note the rapidity with which fat mass can be increased, at least in the short term, for sheep (but not, as discussed below, in rodents). This may be due in part to the rapid change in regional fat distribution over the first few weeks of postnatal life. Over this period omental fat, which is barely detectable in the fetus, grows rapidly until it constitutes 50% of total fat mass, and maintains this abundance until at least early adulthood. Given that it is excess central fat that constitutes the main health risk in obese humans, this emphasises the potential importance of the sheep as a model for future studies of fetal programming. It could well be that, as in human populations, the effects of previous nutrient restriction may be amplified after birth when nutrient availability is no longer limiting and appreciable amounts of adipose tissue are deposited (Clarke *et al.* 1997a). For example, low-birthweight sheep have a higher relative fat mass at a body weight of 20 kg when fed to appetite compared with higher-birthweight offspring (Greenwood *et al.* 1998).

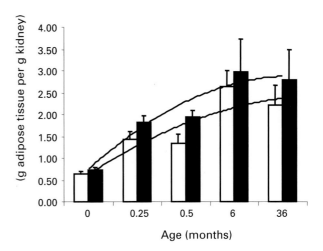

Figure 18.1 Summary of developmental persistence of increased adiposity in the perirenal abdominal region of sheep born to mothers that were either nutrient-restricted between early and mid gestation and then fed adequately (closed bars) or fed adequately throughout gestation (open bars). For full details of diet see Bispham *et al.* (2003a).

Intrauterine growth retardation and later obesity

Studies using small animals indicate that obesity can be programmed in the absence of any reported effects on fetal or postnatal fat development and may therefore reflect changes in appetite regulation. Offspring of pregnant rats that were nutrient-restricted to such an extent as to cause consistent IUGR have shown marked obesity, but only after puberty. In this model, the resulting offspring exhibit a range of adult complications including sedentary behaviour (Vickers *et al.* 2003), hyperinsulinaemia and hyperleptinaemia (Vickers *et al.* 2000, 2001). Obesity is associated with hyperphagia but is observed both on a standard and on a hypercaloric diet (Vickers *et al.* 2000). These offspring also show reduced body temperature, which may be indicative of reduced thermogenic function within brown adipose tissue. The extent to which such adaptations may be applicable to species in which brown fat is absent in later life, and which show very different regional fat distribution, remains to be clarified. It must also be noted

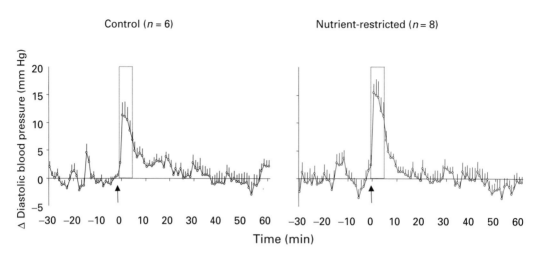

Figure 18.2 Comparison of the effect of feeding on the rise in diastolic blood pressure between 1-year-old sheep born to mothers that were either nutrient-restricted between early and mid gestation or control-fed throughout. Arrow indicates time of feeding.

that the rat appears to be particularly vulnerable to any nutritional imbalance during gestation because of its exceptional rate of protein accretion during prenatal development (estimated at 23 times that of the sheep and human fetus; McCance and Widdowson 1974) and the far larger total weight of the products of conception relative to maternal weight (25–35% vs. 7–10% in the sheep and 3–5% in humans).

Potential mechanism by which obesity contributes to impaired kidney function and hypertension

Predisposition to both obesity and hypertension can be amplified by the postnatal environment (Eriksson *et al.* 2000). For example, both a low birthweight and its associated catch-up growth after birth independently add to the risk of adult cardiovascular disease (Forsén *et al.* 1997, Cianfarani *et al.* 1999, Eriksson *et al.* 1999, Ong *et al.* 2000). The later consequences, particularly the increased risk of cardiovascular disease, are likely to be mediated through altered body composition, as catch-up growth predicts increased subcutaneous and visceral obesity in later life (Rogers 2003). This is important, as

it emphasises observations in both animals and humans which indicate that excess weight gain is associated with greater sympathetic activity, particularly in the kidney (Hall 2003). The primary mechanism by which this adaptation is mediated is through activity of the renal sympathetic nerves, which are similarly increased in obese humans (Landsberg and Krieger, 1989, Esler 2000, Hall *et al.* 2001). We therefore predict that increased fat mass and concomitant rise in plasma leptin, and thus sympathetic activity to the kidney, would have the potential to contribute directly to raised blood pressure. Critically, this adaptation would be greatest in individuals that were subjected to different feeding patterns in utero (i.e. switching from nutrient restriction to adequate nutrition) and then allowed to consume a high-calorie diet at frequent intervals in juvenile or later life. One putative hypothalamic target site is the melanocortin type 4 receptor (MC4R), as intracerebroventricular administration of leptin has been shown to activate the melanocortin system, resulting in increased renal sympathetic nerve activity (Haynes *et al.* 1999). We have further shown that, as in humans, the act of feeding in sheep is a major stimulus to raise blood pressure (Fig. 18.2), an adaptation that is enhanced in offspring of

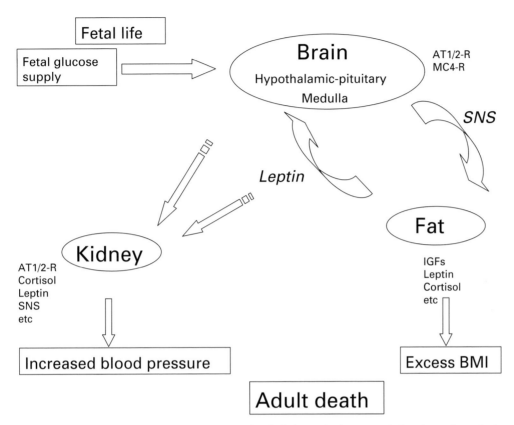

Figure 18.3 Summary of the developmental mechanisms by which changes in glucose supply from the mother to the fetus, mediated by switching from a nutrient-restricted to a normal diet, can act to adversely programme central control of blood pressure, fat and kidney development. SNS, sympathetic nervous system; AT, angiotensinogen; MC4, melanocortin type 4; R, receptor.

nutrient-restricted mothers. It could therefore be that interactions between the central regulation of blood pressure, food intake, fat mass and kidney function provide a unifying mechanism by which later cardiovascular disease is reprogrammed (Fig. 18.3).

Future perspectives

Early pregnancy and the postnatal period appear both to be critical times where the level of nutrition can have substantial consequences for long-term health. In humans it is actually the norm for maternal food intake to decrease in early pregnancy,

and this may be an important adaptive response to protect the fetus from exposure to potentially harmful compounds. This is accompanied by maternal feelings of nausea and loss of appetite that are unique to humans, although in sheep there does appear to be a substantial change in energy requirements in early pregnancy such that they are also in negative energy balance. Given the marked sensitivity of early fetal fat development to nutrient restriction, these adaptations may be geared to promoting fetal fat growth, thus ensuring sufficient reserves at birth. The potential long-term consequences are of minor importance as long as the newborn survives. It is then under conditions in which the infant, juvenile or adult is exposed to excess nutrition in conjunction with the adoption of a sedentary lifestyle that obesity-related disorders become a health problem. The challenge is therefore to identify which nutrients are critical with regard to stage of fat development. Then, in those individuals that become obese, careful consideration must be given to establishing what are the best interventions to permanently reduce and restore body weight. Given the failure of many dieting regimes, and the high costs of drug or surgical treatment of obesity, a sustainable lifelong approach to this problem has major advantages. Indeed dietary and lifestyle intervention in childhood only improves atherogenic profiles and insulin resistance if the body mass index standard deviation score is decreased by at least 0.5 over a one-year period (Reinehr and Andler 2004). In a recent study this was achieved only in 28% of subjects.

REFERENCES

Alexander, G. and Williams, D. (1968). Shivering and non-shivering thermogenesis during summit metabolism in young lambs. *J. Physiol.*, **198**, 251–76.

Bamberger, C. M., Schulte, H. M. and Chrousos, G. P. (1996). Molecular determinants of glucocorticoid receptor function and tissue sensitivity to glucocorticoids. *Endocr. Rev.*, **17**, 245–61.

Bispham, J., Gopalakrishnan, G. S., Dandrea, J. *et al.* (2003a). Maternal endocrine adaptation throughout pregnancy to nutritional manipulation: consequences for maternal plasma leptin and cortisol and the programming of fetal adipose tissue development. *Endocrinology*, **144**, 3575–85.

Bispham, J., Pearce, S., Dandrea, J., Symonds, M. E. and Stephenson, T. (2003b). The effect of maternal parity on leptin mRNA expression and perirenal adipose tissue deposition over the first month of postnatal life in sheep. *J. Physiol. Proc. Physiol. Soc.*, **555P**, C98.

Bispham, J., Pearce, S., Dandrea, J., Stephenson, T. and Symonds, M. E. (2004). The effect of maternal parity on insulin-like growth factor-I and -II receptor expression and perirenal adipose tissue deposition over the first month of postnatal life in sheep. *J. Soc. Gynecol. Investig.*, **11** (Suppl.), 254A.

Bray, G. A. (2002). The underlying basis for obesity: relationship to cancer. *J. Nur.*, **132**, 3451–5S.

Broughton Pipkin, F. and Roberts, J. M. (2000). Hypertension in pregnancy. *J. Hum. Hypertens.*, **14**, 705–24.

Buchanan, T. A. and Kjos, S. L. (1999). Gestational diabetes: risk or myth? *J. Clin. Endocrinol. Metab.*, **84**, 1854–7.

Budge, H., Mostyn, A., Wilson, V. *et al.* (2002). The effect of maternal prolactin infusion during pregnancy on fetal adipose tissue development. *J. Endocrinol.*, **147**, 427–33.

Budge, H., Dandrea, J., Mostyn, A. *et al.* (2003). Differential effects of fetal number and maternal nutrition in late gestation on prolactin receptor abundance and adipose tissue development in the neonatal lamb. *Pediatr. Res.*, **53**, 302–8.

Budge, H., Edwards, L. J., McMillen, I. C. *et al.* (2004). Nutritional manipulation of fetal adipose tissue deposition and uncoupling protein 1 abundance in the fetal sheep: differential effects of timing and duration. *Biol. Reprod.*, **71**, 359–65.

Cianfarani, S., Germani, D. and Branca, F. (1999). Low birth-weight and adult insulin resistance: the 'catch-up growth' hypothesis. *Arch. Dis. Child.*, **81**, F71–3.

Clarke, L., Buss, D. S., Juniper, D. S., Lomax, M. A. and Symonds, M. E. (1997a). Adipose tissue development during early postnatal life in ewe-reared lambs. *Exp. Physiol.*, **82**, 1015–27.

Clarke, L., Heasman, L., Firth, K. and Symonds, M. E. (1997b). Influence of route of delivery and ambient temperature on thermoregulation in newborn lambs. *Am. J. Physiol.*, **272**, R1931–9.

Dandrea, J., Wilson, V., Gopalakrishnan, G. *et al.* (2001). Maternal nutritional manipulation of placental growth and glucose transporter-1 abundance in sheep. *Reproduction*, **122**, 793–800.

Davies, D., Mostyn, A., Gardner, D. S. *et al.* (2003). Effect of protein supplementation to mother at specific stages of gestation on fetal adipose tissue. *Endocr. Abstr.*, **6**, P45.

Edwards, L. J. and McMillen, I. C. (2002). Impact of maternal undernutrition during the periconceptional period, fetal number, and fetal sex on the development of the hypothalamo-pituitary adrenal axis in sheep during late gestation. *Biol. Reprod.*, **66**, 1562–9.

Eriksson, J., Forsén, T., Tuomilehto, J., Osmond, C. and Barker, D. (2000). Fetal and childhood growth and hypertension in adult life. *Hypertension*, **36**, 790–4.

Eriksson, J. G., Forsén, T., Tuomilehto, J., Winter, P. D., Osmond, C. and Barker, D. J. P. (1999). Catch-up growth in childhood and death from coronary heart disease: longitudinal study. *BMJ*, **318**, 427–31.

Eriksson, J. G., Lindi, V., Uusitupa, M. *et al.* (2002). The effects of the Pro12Ala polymorphism of the peroxisome proliferator-activated receptor-γ2 gene on insulin sensitivity and insulin metabolism interact with size at birth. *Diabetes*, **51**, 2321–4.

Esler, M. (2000). The sympathetic nervous system and hypertension. *Am. J. Hypertens.*, **13**, 99–105S.

Forsén, T., Eriksson, J. G., Tuomilehto, J., Teramo, K., Osmond, C. and Barker, D. J. P. (1997). Mother's weight in pregnancy and coronary heart disease in a cohort of Finnish men: follow up study. *BMJ*, **315**, 837–40.

Freemark, M., Fleenor, D., Driscoll, P., Binart, N. and Kelly, P. A. (2001). Body weight and fat deposition in prolactin receptor-deficient mice. *Endocrinology*, **142**, 532–7.

Gardner, D. S., Jamall, E., Fletcher, A. J. W., Fowden, A. L. and Giussani, D. A. (2004a). Adrenocortical responsiveness is blunted in twin relative to singleton ovine fetuses. *J. Physiol.*, **557**, 1021–32.

Gardner, D. S., Pearce, S., Dandrea, J. *et al.* (2004b). The effect of feeding on leptin concentration and regional adipose tissue deposition in singleton and twin sheep at one year of age. *J. Physiol. Proc. Physiol. Soc.*, **555P**, C97.

Gopalakrishnan, G., Gardner, D. S., Rhind, S. M. *et al.* (2004). Programming of adult cardiovascular function after early maternal undernutrition in sheep. *Am. J. Physiol. Regul. Integr. Comp. Physiol.*, **287**, R12–20.

Greenwood, P. L., Hunt, A. S., Hermanson, J. W. and Bell, A. W. (1998). Effects of birth weight and postnatal nutrition on neonatal sheep. I. Body growth and composition, and some aspects of energetic efficiency. *J. Anim. Sci.*, **76**, 2354–67.

Hall, J. E. (2003). The kidney, hypertension, and obesity. *Hypertension*, **41**, 625–33.

Hall, J. E., Hilderbrandt, D. A. and Kuo, J. (2001). Obesity hypertension: role of leptin and sympathetic nervous system. *Am. J. Hypertens.*, **14**, 103–15S.

Haynes, W. G., Morgan, D. A., Djalali, A., Sivitz, W. I. and Mark, A. L. (1999). Interactions between the melanocortin system and leptin in control of sympathetic nerve traffic. *Hypertension*, **33**, 542–7.

Itoh, H., Sagawa, N., Yura, S. *et al.* (2004). Adipocytokine mRNA expression in the skin was decreased in growth restricted mice fetuses. *J. Soc. Gynecol. Investig.*, **11** (Suppl), 245A.

Landsberg, L. and Krieger, D. R. (1989). Obesity, metabolism and the sympathetic nervous system. *Am. J. Hypertens.*, **2**, 125–32S.

Law, C. M., Barker, D. J. P., Osmond, C., Fall, C. H. and Simmonds, S. J. (1992). Early growth and abdominal fatness in adult life. *J. Epidemiol. Community Health*, **46**, 184–6.

Masuzaki, H., Paterson, J., Shinyama, H. *et al.* (2001). A transgenic model of visceral obesity and the metabolic syndrome. *Science*, **294**, 2166–70.

McCance, R. A. and Widdowson, E. M. (1974). The determinants of growth and form. *Proc. R. Soc. Lond. B Biol. Sci.*, **185**, 1–17.

Mostyn, A., Bispham, J., Pearce, S. *et al.* (2002). Differential effects of leptin on thermoregulation and uncoupling protein abundance in the neonatal lamb. *FASEB J.*, **16**, 1438–40.

Mostyn, A., Pearce, S., Budge, H. *et al.* (2003). Influence of cortisol on adipose tissue development in the fetal sheep during late gestation. *J. Endocrinol.*, **176**, 23–30.

Mühlhäusler, B. S., Roberts, C. T., Yuen, B. S. J. *et al.* (2003). Determinants of fetal leptin synthesis, fat mass and circulating leptin concentrations in well nourished ewes in late pregnancy *Endocrinology*, **144**, 4947–54.

Ong, K. K., Ahmed, M. L., Emmett, P. M., Preece, M. A. and Dunger, D. B. (2000). Association between postnatal catch-up growth and obesity in childhood: prospective cohort study. *BMJ*, **320**, 967–71.

Ozanne, S. E., Nave, B. T., Wang, C. L., Shepherd, P. R., Prins, J. and Smith, G. D. (1997). Poor fetal growth causes long-term changes in expression of insulin signaling components in adipocytes. *Am. J. Physiol.*, **273**, E46–51.

Parsons, T. J., Power, C. and Manor, O. (2001). Fetal and early life growth and body mass index from birth to early adulthood in 1958 British cohort: longitudinal study. *BMJ*, **323**, 1331–5.

Reinehr, T. and Andler, W. (2004). Changes in the atherogenic risk factor profile according to degree of wieght loss. *Arch. Dis. Child.*, **89**, 419–22.

Reitman, M. L., Bi, S., Marcus-Samuels, B. and Gavrilova, O. (2001). Leptin and its role in pregnancy and fetal development: an overview. *Biochem. Soc. Trans.*, **29**, 68–72.

Rogers, I. (2003). The influence of birthweight and intrauterine environment on adiposity and fat distribution in later life. *Int. J. Obes. Relat. Metab. Disord.*, **27**, 755–77.

Sorensen, H. T., Sabroe, S., Rothman, K. J., Gillman, M., Fischer, P. and Sorensen, T. I. (1997). Relation between weight and length at birth and body mass index in young adulthood: cohort study. *BMJ*, **315**, 1137–9.

Steppan, C. M., Brown, E. J., Wright, C. M. *et al.* (2001). A family of tissue-specific resistin-like molecules. *Proc. Nat. Acad. Sci. USA*, **98**, 502–6.

Stevens, D. and Alexander, G. (1986). Lipid deposition after hypophysectomy and growth hormone treatment in the sheep fetus. *J. Dev. Physiol.*, **8**, 139–45.

Stevens, D., Alexander, G. and Bell, A. W. (1990). Effects of prolonged glucose infusion into fetal sheep on body growth, fat deposition and gestation length. *J. Dev. Physiol.*, **13**, 277–81.

Stewart, P. M. and Krozowski, Z. S. (1999). 11β-hydroxysteroid dehydrogenase. *Vitam. Horm.*, **57**, 249–324.

Symonds, M. E., Bryant, M. J., Clarke, L., Darby, C. J. and Lomax, M. A. (1992). Effect of maternal cold exposure on brown adipose tissue and thermogenesis in the neonatal lamb. *J. Physiol.*, **455**, 487–502.

Symonds, M. E., Bird, J. A., Clarke, L., Gate, J. J. and Lomax, M. A. (1995). Nutrition, temperature and homeostasis during perinatal development. *Exp. Physiol.*, **80**, 907–40.

Symonds, M. E., Andrews, D. C., Buss, D. S., Clarke, L., Darby, C. J. and Lomax, M. A. (1996). Effect of rearing temperature on perirenal adipose tissue development and thermoregulation following methimazole treatment of postnatal lambs. *Exp. Physiol.*, **81**, 995–1006.

Symonds, M. E., Bird, J. A., Sullivan, C., Wilson, V., Clarke, L. and Stephenson, T. (2000). Effect of delivery temperature on endocrine stimulation of thermoregulation in lambs born by cesarean section. *J. Appl. Physiol.*, **88**, 47–53.

Symonds, M. E., Mostyn, A. and Stephenson, T. (2001). Cytokines and cytokine-receptors in fetal growth and development. *Biochem. Soc. Trans.*, **29**, 33–7.

Symonds, M. E., Pearce, S., Bispham, J., Gardner, D. S. and Stephenson, T. (2004). Timing of nutrient restriction and programming of fetal adipose tissue development. *Proc. Nutr. Soc.*, **63**, 397–403.

Teruel, T., Valverde, A. M., Benito, M. and Lorenzo, M. (1996). Insulin-like growth factor and insulin induce adipogenic-related gene expression in fetal brown adipocyte primary cultures. *Biochem. J.*, **319**, 627–32.

Vernon, R. G., Clegg, R. A. and Flint, D. J. (1981). Aspects of adipose tissue metabolism in foetal lambs. *Biochem. J.*, **196**, 819–24.

Vickers, M. H., Breier, B. H., Cutfield, W. S., Hofman, P. L. and Gluckman, P. D. (2000). Fetal origins of hyperphagia, obesity, and hypertension and postnatal amplification by hypercaloric nutrition. *Am. J. Physiol. Endocrinol. Metab.*, **279**, E83–7.

Vickers, M. H., Reddy, S., Ikenasio, B. A. and Breier, B. H. (2001). Dysregulation of the adipoinsular axis: a mechanism for the pathogenesis of hyperleptinemia and adipogenic diabetes induced by fetal programming. *J. Endocrinol.*, **170**, 323–32.

Vickers, M. H., Breier, B. H., McCarthy, D. and Gluckman, P. D. (2003). Sedentary behavior during postnatal life is determined by the prenatal environment and exacerbated by postnatal hypercaloric nutrition *Am. J. Physiol., Regul. Integr. Comp. Physiol.*, **285**, R271–3.

Whorwood, C. B., Firth, K. M., Budge, H. and Symonds, M. E. (2001). Maternal undernutrition during early to mid-gestation programmes tissue-specific alterations in the expression of the glucocorticoid receptor, 11β-hydroxysteroid dehydrogenase isoforms and type 1 angiotensin II receptor in neonatal sheep. *Endocrinology*, **142**, 2854–64.

Wolf, G. (2003). Adiponectin: a regulator of energy homeostasis. *Nutr. Rev.*, **61**, 290–2.

Yajnik, C. S. (2004). Obesity epidemic in India: intrauterine origins? *Proc. Nutr. Soc.*, **63**, 387–96.

Yuen, B. S., Owens, P. C., Muhlhausler, B. S. *et al.* (2003). Leptin alters the structural and functional characteristics of adipose tissue before birth. *FASEB J.*, **17**, 1102–4.

19

The developmental environment and its role in the metabolic syndrome

Christopher D. Byrne and David I. W. Phillips

University of Southampton

Introduction

It has long been known that certain cardiovascular risk factors tend to cluster together in the same patients. The clustering of insulin resistance, glucose intolerance, dyslipidaemia and hypertension was originally described by Reaven (1988) and it has become evident in recent years that this clustering, now known as the metabolic syndrome, is among the most important causes of atherosclerotic vascular disease. Because of the increasing prevalence of obesity, which contributes strongly to this syndrome, the metabolic syndrome is likely to contribute markedly to the global burden of disease both in the developed and increasingly in the developing world. Despite its public-health importance, the aetiology is still poorly understood. In addition to obesity, a variety of other factors, both genetic and non-genetic, are involved, but at present these have remained poorly characterised. The demonstration over the past decade that several components of the metabolic syndrome have developmental origins offers new insights into understanding this important and common condition and may offer pointers to its prevention.

Developmental origins of the metabolic syndrome

Evidence that the metabolic syndrome might have a developmental origin came originally from a series of studies which show that several of the components of the syndrome are associated with small size at birth. In a study of 370 men born in Hertfordshire, UK, the prevalence of type 2 diabetes or glucose intolerance fell from 40% among men who weighed 5.5 lb (2.5 kg) or less at birth to 14% in those who weighed 9.5 lb (4.3 kg) or more (Hales et al. 1991). The relationship between birth size and glucose tolerance has been observed in a variety of populations, in both Europe and North America, while over 32 studies from around the world have demonstrated the association between low birthweight and raised blood pressure (Law and Shiell 1996, Newsome et al. 2003). Using a definition of the metabolic syndrome based on the occurrence of glucose intolerance, hypertension and hypertriglyceridaemia, the prevalence of the syndrome in Hertfordshire was six times higher in men aged 65 who weighed 5.5 lb (2.5 kg) or less at birth than in those who weighed 9.5 lb (4.3 kg) or more, a finding which has also been confirmed in the United States (Valdez et al. 1994) and in Sweden (Byberg et al. 2000). The metabolic syndrome is strongly associated with impaired insulin action or insulin resistance. An important finding is that low birthweight is associated with insulin resistance (Phillips et al. 1994), an observation which has been replicated in several different populations using a variety of techniques, including the hyperinsulinaemia euglycaemic clamp and the intravenous glucose tolerance test with minimal model analysis (Clausen

Developmental Origins of Health and Disease, ed. Peter Gluckman and Mark Hanson. Published by Cambridge University Press.
© P. D. Gluckman and M. A. Hanson 2006.

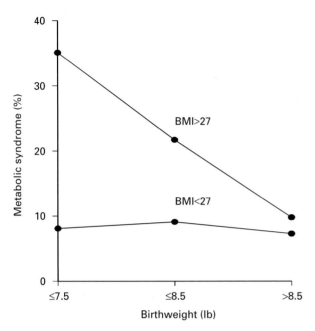

Figure 19.1 Metabolic syndrome (%) in 408 men born in Hertfordshire according to birthweight and whether the current BMI was above or below the median (27 kg m^{-2}).

syndrome. Increasing evidence suggests that early development, both intrauterine and postnatal, influences adult body composition (for review see Wild and Byrne 2004), and adult obesity adds to altered fetal growth in determining the prevalence of the metabolic syndrome (Valdez *et al.* 1994, Byberg *et al.* 2000). More recent data suggest the presence of an interaction between reduced fetal growth and adult obesity. The adverse effect of obesity is most marked in people who were of low birthweight (Lithell *et al.* 1996). This is illustrated by data from the Hertfordshire study (Fig. 19.1) showing that the effects of low birthweight on the metabolic syndrome are evident only in people who become overweight or obese in later life. Recent studies now demonstrate how the effects of prenatal growth and development combine with obesity during childhood to determine the pattern of disease in adult life. These studies show that rapid postnatal growth is linked with an increased risk of obesity, impaired glucose tolerance and diabetes in later life.

In particular, the timing of adiposity rebound appears to be an important predictor of the subsequent prevalence of obesity and diabetes. In a French study (Rolland-Cachera *et al.* 1984) individual adiposity curves assessed by BMI were drawn for 151 children from the age of 1 month to 16 years. These data showed that adiposity increases during the first year of life and thereafter decreases in childhood. A renewed rise (the adiposity rebound) occurs at about 6 years of age. This study showed a relationship between the age at adiposity rebound and final adiposity. An early rebound (before 5.5 years of age) was followed by a significantly higher degree of adiposity than a later rebound (after 7 years of age). A study from Finland suggests that the age of adiposity rebound is a key determinant of the risk of diabetes in adult life (Eriksson *et al.* 2003). The study examined records of 8760 men and women who were born at Helsinki University Central Hospital during 1934 and 1944, who attended child welfare clinics in the city of Helsinki, and who were still resident in Finland in 1971. On average each person had 18 measurements of

et al. 1996, McKeigue *et al.* 1998, Flanagan *et al.* 2000). These epidemiological studies show that the association between birthweight and the metabolic syndrome or insulin resistance seems to be independent of duration of gestation, and of possible confounding variables including cigarette smoking, alcohol consumption and social class currently or at birth. Interestingly, in addition to low birthweight, subjects with metabolic syndrome had smaller head circumference and lower ponderal index at birth, and lower weight and below-average dental eruption at 1 year of age compared with subjects who did not have metabolic syndrome. The findings from these studies suggest that the metabolic syndrome is associated with a generalised alteration in early development.

It has long been known that obesity and in particular central obesity is normally strongly associated with insulin resistance and the metabolic height and weight between birth and 12 years of age. A total of 290 individuals developed type 2 diabetes in adult life from the initial cohort of people who had birth and child welfare records. The cumulative incidence of type 2 diabetes decreased progressively from 8.6% in persons whose adiposity rebound occurred before the age of 5 years to 1.8% in those in whom it occurred after 7 years ($p < 0.001$). Interestingly, early adiposity rebound was preceded by low weight gain between birth and 1 year (Eriksson *et al.* 2003).

Given that it is now well established that South Asians are at increased risk of developing type 2 diabetes and coronary heart disease (CHD) compared with Europeans, it is significant that the effects of prenatal, infant and childhood growth are particularly evident in this racial group. In a study of nearly 1500 men and women aged 26–32, subjects with impaired glucose tolerance or diabetes typically had a low body mass index (BMI) up to the age of 2 years, followed by an early adiposity rebound and an accelerated increase in body mass index until adulthood (Bhargava *et al.* 2004). Data from Pune in India suggest that early fat deposition is greater in South Asian offspring. Small Indian newborn babies preserve subcutaneous fat (measured as skinfold thickness) much more than white European babies (Yajnik *et al.* 2003). Subscapular adiposity was better preserved than the triceps adipose tissue. These data suggest a tendency in Indian babies to truncal fat deposition during intrauterine development. Leptin levels, a marker of total body fat content, were similar in Indian and European babies. By contrast, Indian babies were small in abdominal circumference (suggesting smaller viscera) and small in mid-upper-arm circumference (suggesting smaller skeletal muscle mass). These findings suggest that Indian babies develop increased visceral adipose tissue and a reduced muscle mass compared with European offspring. Development of a reduced muscle mass may have little consequence in the presence of limited adult calorie intake and high levels of physical activity. However, persistence of this South Asian body habitus into childhood and early adulthood may have more sinister consequences for risk of CHD and type 2 diabetes, particularly if individuals consume an energy-dense Western diet and are physically inactive.

The different relationships between early development and adult obesity between ethnic groups are also illustrated by data from 267 singleton births from four Ladino Guatemalan villages. These studies show that the relationships between early growth and adult fatness are complex (Li *et al.* 2003). Although these authors showed that both prenatal and postnatal growth retardation during the first two years of life were associated with shortness and less fat-free mass in adulthood when the subjects were between 21 and 27 years, the results did not show that retardation in length during early childhood increased fatness in later life. In contrast, the findings suggested that subjects, particularly women, who were growth-retarded during early childhood were thinner as adults. Thus more data from different ethnic groups are needed to elucidate the precise relationship between early development and future levels of adiposity and lean mass in adulthood.

Mechanisms by which early development influences the prevalence of the metabolic syndrome

Because the nutrients and oxygen that a fetus receives are major determinants of its growth rate, the epidemiological observations linking growth retardation with the metabolic syndrome led to the hypothesis that the syndrome may result from fetal undernutrition. It was suggested that an imbalance between supply and demand of nutrients results in physiological adaptations which benefit the fetus in the short term but which in the longer term are maladaptive. More recent research suggests that it is these adaptations that are the key determinants of the long-term effects on the offspring, rather than low birthweight per se. Indeed, increasing evidence suggests that alterations in human physiology can occur as a result of maternal factors

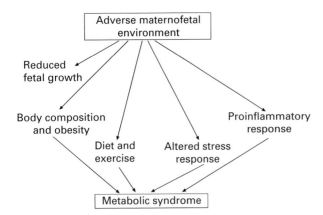

Figure 19.2 Processes by which restricted fetal growth may lead to the metabolic syndrome in adult life.

that do not alter fetal growth or result in alterations too subtle to measure with conventional techniques. For example, in the wartime famine in Holland, birth size was only slightly reduced, but there were long-term alterations in the glucose tolerance of men and women who were in utero at the time (Ravelli *et al.* 1998).

The undernutrition hypothesis is supported by a large body of data from animal experiments showing that exposure to low-protein diets during pregnancy results in high blood pressure in the offspring. In rats, maternal protein restriction using diets of low protein density (6, 9 or 12% protein compared with 18% protein control diets) reduces body weight at birth in proportion to the reduction of protein intake (Langley and Jackson 1994). Between 9 and 21 weeks of age, blood pressure is higher in the offspring exposed to low-protein diets in utero. Similar effects of moderate maternal food restriction occur in many other species, including the guinea pig and the sheep. In these species, maternal undernutrition is associated with raised blood pressure and related abnormalities including glucose intolerance (Robinson *et al.* 2001). More severe undernutrition during gestation has also been shown capable of producing features of the metabolic syndrome in the adult offspring. Using a model of severe maternal undernutrition throughout pregnancy, Vickers and colleagues (2003) investigated whether prenatal influences caused alterations in postnatal locomotor behaviour, independent of postnatal nutrition. Virgin Wistar rats were time-mated and randomly assigned to receive food either *ad libitum* (*ad libitum* group) or at 30% of *ad libitum* intake (undernourished group). The modifying influence of a hypercaloric intervention was also examined using this model. At weaning, offspring were assigned to one of two diets (a control or a hypercaloric (30% fat) diet). At ages of 35 days, 145 days and 420 days, the offspring were assessed. At all ages studied, offspring from the undernourished mothers were significantly less active than offspring of mothers on the control diet for all parameters measured, independent of postnatal nutrition. Sedentary behaviour in programmed offspring was exacerbated by the postnatal hypercaloric nutrition. Importantly, this study is the first to show that a lifestyle choice (i.e. physical inactivity, which has a powerful effect in adult humans to modify the metabolic syndrome phenotype) may have a prenatal origin. In support of the modifying effect of maternal nutrition to programme features of the adult metabolic syndrome phenotype, we have recently shown that a maternal diet enriched with unsaturated fat, and low in carbohydrate, favourably modifies hepatic lipid metabolism in the developed adult offspring (Zhang *et al.* 2005).

Clinical studies in humans, as well as animal experiments, now suggest that a number of key adaptations and physiological processes link the early environment with the metabolic syndrome, and these are summarised in Fig. 19.2. These adaptations include changes in the set-points of key endocrine axes, changes in body composition, behavioural changes and alterations in proinflammatory responses.

Endocrine programming: alterations in the behavioural response to stress

It is becoming increasingly clear that an important way in which the early environment can have long-term effects is by resetting a diverse range of hormonal systems that control growth and development, which in turn influence the predisposition to adult metabolic and cardiovascular disease (for review see Byrne and Phillips 2000, Holt and Byrne 2002). It is suggested that the evolutionary 'purpose' of these mechanisms is to adapt the organism to its environment over a much shorter timescale than is possible with genetic changes. If a pregnant animal is exposed to an unfavourable environment, such as undernutrition, it is logical that the development of the offspring should be adapted for that environment. If, however, these offspring become relatively overnourished, the prenatal alterations may be inappropriate and lead to disease.

There is increasing evidence from animal studies that the major mediating hormones of the stress response (including the adrenocortical and sympathoadrenal response) are highly susceptible to modification during development. Recent evidence from human studies suggest that alterations of these systems are found in association with low birthweight. Low-birthweight babies have raised cortisol concentrations in umbilical cord blood and raised urinary cortisol excretion in childhood (Economides *et al.* 1988, Clark *et al.* 1996). They also have increased heart rate and reduced heart-rate variability when compared with controls during sleep. A number of studies suggest that birthweight is related to increased resting pulse rate (Phillips and Barker 1997, Longo-Mbenza *et al.* 1999) and fasting adult cortisol concentrations. Fasting plasma cortisol concentrations in Hertfordshire men fell from 408 nmol^{-1} in those who weighed 5.5 lb (2.5 kg) or less to 309 nmol^{-1} among those who weighed 9.5 lb (4.3 kg) or more at birth (Phillips *et al.* 1998). A study of a subset of 205 men showed that those with lower birthweight had enhanced responses of plasma cortisol to ACTH$_{1-24}$. The secretion of cortisol in the unstressed state is not associated with birthweight, and other studies using Corticotrophin-releasing hormone (CRH) tests suggest that central regulation of the HPA axis is not disturbed in people who were small at birth, and is not comparable to the findings observed, for example, in depression. Consequently, it is likely that the previously observed relationship between birthweight and morning cortisol concentrations represents a stress response. This suggestion is supported by studies of Swedish army recruits of low birthweight, who had increased stress susceptibility at a psychological assessment, and recent evidence from a small-scale study which has suggested that low birthweight is associated with increased responses to a standard psychological stressor in young adults (Nilsson *et al.* 2001, Ward *et al.* 2004).

Relatively little is known about the relationship between infant growth and the development of the stress response. However, work in two groups of Jamaican children since infancy showed that, in comparison with controls, the growth-restricted children had higher heart rates, raised salivary cortisol concentrations and increased urinary catecholamine secretion following a psychological stressor (Fernald and Grantham-McGregor 1998, 2002). These findings did not seem to be explained by indices of social status, and the analysis suggested that the differences between groups were directly linked to growth retardation, which is strongly supported by experimental work in rats showing that undernourished pups that were rehabilitated had increased stress responses (Smart *et al.* 1975).

Alterations in body composition

Several studies have suggested that people who were light at birth have a low BMI in adult life. More detailed studies of body composition, however, suggest that birthweight correlates more strongly with measures of height, weight and non-fat mass, including muscle mass, than with measures of adiposity, suggesting that low birthweight is associated with decreased lean mass but no change in fat mass in adult life. However, an increasing body of data suggests that low birthweight is associated with truncal fat deposition. Young adult Mexicans and non-Hispanic Americans of low birthweight were found to have greater fat deposits on the trunk, as indicated by higher subscapular-to-triceps skinfold ratios (Valdez *et al.* 1994). Similarly, 7- to 12-year-old American children who were born small tended to have higher subscapular-to-triceps skinfold ratios (Malina *et al.*

1996). In both these groups, these effects were seen across the normal range of birthweight. Being fatter adds to the effect of birthweight on body fat distribution. In 14- to 16-year-old English girls, those who were smallest at birth but fattest as teenagers had the highest ratios of subscapular-to-triceps skinfolds (Barker *et al.* 1997). It has been suggested that at younger ages these measures of truncal obesity may be a better indicator of regional fat distribution than waist-to-hip ratio. In addition, data from a number of studies of cardiovascular risk suggest that the subscapular-to-triceps skinfold thickness ratio has an effect that is independent of, and additive to, abdominal adiposity.

The role of behavioural programming

Studies of wild populations of birds and experimental studies of mammals suggest that the early environment can result in lifelong adaptive behavioural changes. For example, guinea pigs exposed to exogenous steroids in utero show marked behavioural changes when exposed to standard behavioural tests such as the open field and water maize tests (Matthews 2002). As described earlier, changes in appetite and locomotor behaviour have been reported following maternal undernutrition (Vickers *et al.* 2003). This area remains relatively underexplored in terms of human health. However, behaviours such as patterns of physical activity and dietary preference, important factors in the aetiology of the metabolic syndrome, are known to be relatively stable throughout the life course and are therefore likely to be initiated in early life. Some lines of evidence now suggest that the early environment may be one of the cues leading to these behavioural changes which could impact on patterns of physical activity and dietary choices.

Inflammation and early development

There is increasing evidence to suggest that chronic subclinical inflammation is associated with insulin resistance and the metabolic syndrome (Hanley *et al.* 2004). The majority of the components of the metabolic syndrome are positively associated with inflammatory parameters, and this relationship appears to be independent of age, sex, physical activity, smoking and body mass index (Temelkova-Kurktschiev *et al.* 2002). Increased C-reactive protein (CRP) concentrations in the range traditionally accepted as 'normal', i.e. < 6 mg L^{-1}, have emerged as an independent risk factor for CHD and type 2 diabetes (Pradhan *et al.* 2001, Freeman *et al.* 2002, Pearson *et al.* 2003). Men and women with CRP concentrations in the top tertiles of the population have on average a two fold risk of myocardial infarction or type 2 diabetes compared with those in the bottom tertile after adjustment (Freeman *et al.* 2002, Pearson *et al.* 2003). Treatments known to reduce vascular and metabolic risk, such as statins, ACE inhibitors or the thiazolidenediones, possess anti-inflammatory properties. Others (Jiang *et al.* 1998, Gullestad, 1999, Palinski, 2001) suggest that the pathogenesis of vascular events and type 2 diabetes may be mediated at least in part by inflammatory processes.

It is therefore of great interest that evidence is beginning to suggest that there is a relationship between measures of inflammation in adulthood and early development. In a study of 1633 subjects participating in the MIDSPAN Family Study who had birthweight data, Sattar *et al.* (2004) measured CRP in the adults whose ages were between 30 and 59 years. After adjustment for factors known to influence CRP concentrations, including age, body mass index, smoking, socioeconomic deprivation, and hormone use in women, there was a negative association between birthweight and CRP. A 1-kg increase in birthweight was associated with a 10.7% decrease in CRP (95% CI 3.0–17.8% decrease). Thus these authors suggest that low birthweight contributes to elevated CRP concentration in adulthood. However, in contrast to the above findings, two other studies in children (Cook *et al.* 2000, Gillum 2003) failed to find a significant association between CRP and birthweight; but both studies were smaller in size. It is possible that, because CRP levels increase with age, there may have been a better chance of showing an association of CRP with birthweight caused by magnified differences over time. If the relationship between CRP and birthweight is confirmed, then potential mechanisms underlying programming of inflammatory pathways in utero need to be examined further, not least because increased concentrations of other markers of a low-grade inflammatory response such as the cytokines IL6 and TNFα have been shown to be predictive of CHD and type 2 diabetes in adulthood (Pearson et al. 2003).

It may also be relevant that pregnancy is associated with an increase in circulating cytokine and CRP concentrations (Ramsay et al. 2002), and that the increase in TNFα appears to correlate strongly with the decrease in insulin sensitivity in pregnancy (Kirwan et al. 2002). In addition, a recent study in rats demonstrates that prenatal exposure to cytokines (IL6 and TNFα) leads to a marked increase in adipose tissue mass in both male and female offspring (Dahlgren et al. 2001). The metabolic consequences of increased visceral fat mass were reduced insulin sensitivity in male offspring and hyperandrogenism in female offspring. Consequently, pregnancy-induced elevations in cytokines may be relevant to the fetal programming of the metabolic syndrome mediated by changes in visceral fat mass and insulin sensitivity.

Obesity is a major factor affecting inflammatory response in healthy individuals. Adipocytes produce inflammatory cytokines, including IL6, TNFα and other related proteins such as adiponectin and leptin. Not only does increased physical activity modulate levels of obesity, but also physical activity affects the inflammatory response. CRP concentrations are reduced with both intense and even modest levels of physical activity (Wannamethee et al. 2002, Tomaszewski et al. 2003), and it has been established that increased CRP levels are independently linked to endothelial dysfunction, dyslipidaemia, insulin resistance and increased blood pressure (Pearson et al. 2003), and to the metabolic syndrome and predict development of diabetes (Sattar et al. 2003, Ridker et al. 2003). Animal studies also provide support for the notion that altered early development is able to modify inflammatory markers later in adult life. For example, modifying the maternal diet during

gestation has been shown to influence gene expression for a key inflammatory marker, fibrinogen, in the developed adult offspring (Zhang et al. 1997, Zhang and Byrne 2000). In summary, an increasing body of evidence is now suggesting that a proinflammatory response, induced by altered early development, may increase the risk of development of the metabolic syndrome, type 2 diabetes and accelerated atherosclerosis.

Conclusion

Many Western countries are now facing an epidemic of obesity and the metabolic syndrome. The data presented in this chapter suggest that the fetal or early infant environment is an important period during the lifecycle, capable of influencing the metabolic syndrome phenotype in adulthood. We suggest this period should therefore be a priority area for research, given the worldwide epidemic of metabolic syndrome that is now developing. Although work carried out in animal models and humans over the past decade has begun to point towards the mechanisms by which the early environment can influence adult disease risk, it is hoped that these studies will define testable interventions which have the potential to improve human health.

REFERENCES

Barker, M., Robinson, S., Osmond, C. and Barker, D. J. P. (1997). Birth weight and body fat distribution in adolescent girls. *Arch. Dis. Child.*, **77**, 381–3.

Bhargava, S. K., Sachdev, H. S., Fall, C. H. *et al.* (2004). Relation of serial changes in childhood body-mass index to impaired glucose tolerance in young adulthood. *N. Engl. J. Med.*, **350**, 865–75.

Byberg, L., McKeigue, P. M., Zethelius, B. and Lithell, H. O. (2000). Birthweight and the insulin resistance syndrome: association of low birthweight with truncal obesity and raised plasminogen activator inhibitor-1 but not with abdominal obesity or plasma lipid disturbances. *Diabetologia*, **43**, 54–60.

Byrne, C. D. and Phillips, D. I. (2000). Fetal origins of adult disease: epidemiology and mechanisms. *J. Clin. Path.*, **53**, 822–8.

Clark, P. M., Hindmarsh, P. C., Shiell, A. W., Law, C. M., Honour, J. W. and Barker, D. J. P. (1996). Size at birth and adrenocortical function in childhood. *Clin. Endocrinol.*, **45**, 721–6.

Clausen, J. O., Borch-Johnsen, K. and Pedersen, O. (1996). Relation between birthweight and the insulin sensitivity index in a populaton sample of 331 young healthy caucasians. *Am. J. Epidemiol.*, **146**, 23–31.

Cook, D. G., Mendall, M. A., Whincup, P. H. *et al.* (2000). C-reactive protein concentration in children: relationship to adiposity and other cardiovascular risk factors. *Atherosclerosis*, **149**, 139–50.

Dahlgren, J., Nilsson, C., Jennische, E. *et al.* (2001). Prenatal cytokine exposure results in obesity and gender-specific programming. *Am. J. Physiol. Endocrinol. Metab.*, **281**, E326–34.

Economides, D. L., Nicholaides, K. H., Linton, E. A., Perry, L. A. and Chard, T. (1988). Plasma cortisol and adrenocorticotrophin in appropriate and small for gestational age fetuses. *Fetal Ther.*, **3**, 158–64.

Eriksson, J. G., Forsén, T., Tuomilehto, J., Osmond, C. and Barker, D. J. P. (2003). Early adiposity rebound in childhood and risk of type 2 diabetes in adult life. *Diabetologia*, **46**, 190–4.

Fernald, L. C. and Grantham-McGregor, S. M. (1998). Stress response in school-age children who have been growth retarded since early childhood. *Am. J. Clin. Nutr.*, **68**, 691–8.

(2002). Growth retardatation is associated with changes in the stress response system and behavior in school-aged Jamaican children. *J. Nutr.*, **132**, 3674–9.

Flanagan, D. E. H., Moore, V. M., Godsland, I. F., Cockington, R. A., Robinson, J. S. and Phillips, D. I. W. (2000). Fetal growth and the physiological control of glucose tolerance in adults: a minimal model analysis. *Am. J. Physiol. Endocrinol. Metab.*, **278**, E700–6.

Freeman, D. J., Norrie, J., Caslake, M. *et al.* (2002). C-reactive protein is an independent predictor of risk for the development of diabetes mellitus in the West of Scotland Coronary Prevention Study. *Diabetes*, **51**, 1596–1600.

Gillum, R. F. (2003). Association of serum C-reactive protein and indices of body fat distribution and overweight in Mexican American children. *J. Natl. Med. Assoc.*, **95**, 545–52.

Gullestad, L., Aukrust, P., Ueland, T. *et al.* (1999). Effect of high- versus low-dose angiotensin converting enzyme inhibition on cytokine levels in chronic heart failure. *J. Am. Coll. Cardiol.*, **34**, 2061–7.

Hales, C. N., Barker, D. J. P., Clark, P. M. S. *et al.* (1991). Fetal and infant growth and impaired glucose tolerance at age 64. *BMJ*, **303**, 1019–22.

Hanley, A. J., Festa, A., D'Agostino, R. B. *et al.* (2004). Metabolic and inflammation variable clusters and prediction of type 2 diabetes: factor analysis using directly measured insulin sensitivity. *Diabetes*, **53**, 1773–81.

Holt, R. I. G. and Byrne, C. D. (2002). Intrauterine growth, the vascular system and the metabolic syndrome. *Semin. Vasc. Med.*, **2**, 33–44.

Jiang, C., Ting, A. T. and Seed, B. (1998). PPAR-gamma agonists inhibit production of monocyte inflammatory cytokines. *Nature*, **391**, 82–6.

Kirwan, J. P., Hauguel-De Mouzon, S., Lepercq, J. *et al.* (2002). TNF-alpha is a predictor of insulin resistance in human pregnancy. *Diabetes*, **51**, 2207–13.

Langley, S. C. and Jackson, A. A. (1994). Increased systolic blood pressure in adult rats induced by fetal exposure to maternal low protein diets. *Clin. Sci.*, **86**, 217–22.

Law, C. M., Shiell and A. W. (1996). Is blood pressure inversely related to birthweight? The strength of evidence from a systematic review of the literature. *J. Hypertens.*, **14**, 935–41.

Li, H., Stein, A. D., Barnhart, H. X., Ramakrishnan, U. and Martorell, R. (2003). Associations between prenatal and postnatal growth and adult body size and composition. *Am. J. Clin. Nutr.*, **77**, 1498–505.

Lithell, H. O., McKeigue, P. M., Berglund, L., Mohsen, R., Lithell, U. B. and Leon, D. A. (1996). Relationship of birthweight and ponderal index to non-insulin-dependent diabetes and insulin response to glucose challenge in men aged 50–60 years. *BMJ*, **312**, 406–10.

Longo-Mbenza, B., Ngiyulu, R., Bayekula, M. *et al.* (1999). Low birthweight and risk of hypertension in African school children. *J. Cardiovasc. Risk*, **6**, 311–14.

Malina, R. M., Katzmarzyk, P. T. and Beunen, G. (1996). Birth weight and its relationship to size attained and relative fat distribution at 7 to 12 years of age. *Obes. Res.*, **4**, 385–90.

Matthews, S. G. (2002). Early programming of the hypothalamic–pituitary–adrenal axis. *Trends Endocrinol. Metab.*, **13**, 363–408.

McKeigue, P. M., Lithell, H. and Leon, D. A. (1998). Glucose tolerance and resistance to insulin-stimulated glucose uptake in men aged 70 years in relation to size at birth. *Diabetologia*, **41**, 1133–8.

Newsome, C. A., Shiell, A., Fall, C. H. D., Phillips, D. I. W., Shier, R. and Law, C. M. (2003). Is birthweight related to glucose and insulin metabolism? A systematic review. *Diabet. Med.*, **20**, 339–48.

Nilsson, P., Nyberg, P. and Ostergren, P. O. (2001). Increased susceptibility to stress at a psychological assessment of stress tolerance is associated with impaired fetal growth. *Int. J. Epidemiol.*, **30**, 75–80.

Palinski, W. (2001). New evidence for beneficial effects of statins unrelated to lipid lowering. *Arterioscler. Thromb. Vasc. Biol.*, **21**, 3–5.

Pearson, T. A., Mensah, G. A., Alexander, R. W. *et al.* (2003). Markers of inflammation and cardiovascular disease: application to clinical and public health practice. A statement for healthcare professionals from the Centers for Disease Control and Prevention and the American Heart Association. *Circulation*, **107**, 499–511.

Phillips, D. I. W. and Barker, D. J. P. (1997). Association between low birthweight and high resting pulse in adult life: is the sympathetic nervous system involved in programming the insulin resistance syndrome? *Diabet. Med.*, **14**, 673–7.

Phillips, D. I. W., Barker, D. J. P., Hales, C. N., Hirst, S. and Osmond, C. (1994). Thinness at birth and insulin resistance in adult life. *Diabetologia*, **37**, 150–4.

Phillips, D. I. W., Barker, D. J. P., Fall, C. H. D. *et al.* (1998). Elevated plasma cortisol concentrations: a link between low birth weight and the insulin resistance syndrome? *J. Clin. Endocrinol. Metab.*, **83**, 757–60.

Pradhan, A. D., Manson, J. E., Rifai, N., Buring, J. E. and Ridker, P. M. (2001). C-reactive protein, interleukin 6, and risk of developing diabetes mellitus. *JAMA*, **286**, 327–34.

Ramsay, J. E., Ferrell, W. R., Crawford, L., Wallace, A. M., Greer, I. A. and Sattar, N. (2002). Maternal obesity is associated with dysregulation of metabolic, vascular and inflammatory pathways. *J. Clin. Endocrinol. Metab.*, **87**, 4231–7.

Ravelli, A. C., van der Meulen, J. H., Michels, R. P. *et al.* (1998). Glucose tolerance in adults after prenatal exposure to famine. *Lancet*, **351**, 173–7.

Reaven, G. M. (1988). Role of insulin resistance in human disease. *Diabetes*, **37**, 1595–607.

Ridker, P. M., Buring, J. E., Cook, N. R. and Rifai, N. (2003). C-reactive protein, the metabolic syndrome, and risk of incident cardiovascular events: an 8-year follow-up of 14 719 initially healthy American women. *Circulation*, **107**, 391–7.

Robinson, J. S., McMillen, I. C., Edwards, L. J., Kind, K., Gatford, K. L. and Owens, J. (2001). Maternal and placental influences that program the fetus: experimental findings. In *Fetal Origins of Cardiovascular Disease and Lung Disease* (ed. D. J. P. Barker). New York, NY: Marcel Dekker, pp. 273–95.

Rolland-Cachera, M. F., Deheeger, M., Bellisle, F., Guilloud-Bataille, M. and Patois, E. (1984). Adiposity rebound in children: a simple indicator for predicting obesity. *Am. J. Clin. Nutr.*, **39**, 129–35.

Sattar, N., Gaw, A., Scherbakova, O. *et al.* (2003). Metabolic syndrome with and without C-reactive protein as a predictor of CHD and diabetes in the West of Scotland Coronary Prevention Study. *Circulation*, **108**, 414–19.

Sattar, N., McConnachie, A., O'Reilly, D. *et al.* (2004). Inverse association between birth weight and C-reactive protein concentrations in the MIDSPAN Family Study. *Arterioscler. Thromb. Vasc. Biol.*, **24**, 583–7.

Smart, J. L., Whatson, T. S. and Dobbing, J. (1975). Thresholds of response to electric shock in previously undernourished rats. *Br. J. Nutr.*, **34**, 511–16.

Temelkova-Kurktschiev, T., Siegert, G., Bergmann, S. *et al.* (2002). Subclinical inflammation is strongly related to insulin resistance but not to impaired insulin secretion in a high risk population for diabetes. *Metabolism*, **51**, 743–9.

Tomaszewski, M., Charchar, F. J., Przybycin, M. *et al.* (2003). Strikingly low circulating CRP concentrations in ultra-marathon runners independent of markers of adiposity: how low can you go? *Arterioscler. Thromb. Vasc. Biol.*, **23**, 1640–4.

Valdez, R., Athens, M. A., Thompson, G. H., Bradshaw, B. S. and Stern, M. P. (1994). Birthweight and adult health outcomes in a biethnic population in the USA. *Diabetologia*, **37**, 624–31.

Vickers, M. H., Breier, B. H., McCarthy, D. and Gluckman, P. D. (2003). Sedentary behavior during postnatal life is determined by the prenatal environment and exacerbated by postnatal hypercaloric nutrition. *Am. J. Physiol. Regul. Integr. Comp. Physiol.*, **285**, R271–3.

Wannamethee, S. G., Lowe, G. D., Whincup, P. H., Rumley, A., Walker, M. and Lennon, L. (2002). Physical activity and hemostatic and inflammatory variables in elderly men. *Circulation*, **105**, 1785–90.

Ward, A. M., Moore, V., Steptoe, A., Cockington, R., Robinson, J. S. and Phillips, D. I. W. (2004). Size at birth and cardiovascular responses to psychological stressors: evidence for parental programming in women. *J. Hypertens*, **22**, 2295–301.

Wild, S. H. and Byrne, C. D. (2004). Evidence for foetal programming of obesity with a focus on putative mechanisms. *Nutr. Res. Rev.*, **17**, 153–62.

Yajnik, C. S., Fall, C. H., Coyaji, K. J. *et al.* (2003). Neonatal anthropometry: the thin-fat Indian baby. The Pune Maternal Nutrition Study. *Int. J. Obes. Relat. Metab. Disord.*, **27**, 173–80.

Zhang, J. and Byrne, C. D. (2000). Differential hepatic lobar gene expression in offspring exposed to altered maternal dietary protein intake. *Am. J. Physiol. Gastrointest. Liver Physiol.*, **278**, G128–36.

Zhang, J., Desai, M., Ozanne, S. E., Doherty, C. and Hales, C. N. and Byrne C. D. (1997). Two variants of quantitative reverse transcriptase pcr used to show differential expression of fibrinogen genes in rat liver lobes. *Biochem. J.*, **321**, 769–75.

Zhang, J., Wang, C., Terroni, P. L., Cagampang, F. R., Hanson, M. and Byrne, C. D. (2005). A high unsaturated fat, high protein and low carbohydrate diet during pregnancy and lactation modulates hepatic lipid metabolism in female adult offspring. *Am. J. Physiol. Regul. Integr. Comp. Physiol.*, **288**, R112–18.

20

Programming the cardiovascular system

Kent L. Thornburg

Oregon Health and Science University

Introduction

David Barker and colleagues first trained the spotlight on the idea that the prenatal environment shapes the lifelong health of the heart. They reported that the standardised mortality for ischaemic heart disease within a large population of English men and women was much higher in babies born at the 5-pound (2.3 kg) end of the birthweight scale compared to babies at the 9-pound (4.0 kg) end (Barker *et al.*, 1989). Birthweight affected the death rate in men and women similarly across the weight range, with a significant sudden upturn in the heaviest babies studied. The latter group of heavier newborn babies may have included babies that were macrosomic and born to diabetic mothers. In a separate study, Rich-Edwards and coworkers (1997) found a similar relationship among >100 000 participants in the American Nurses study. In that study, the numbers of individuals who had symptoms for coronary disease and stroke increased with decreasing recalled birthweight.

The implications of the epidemiological findings of Barker's group are enormous. Cardiovascular disease is the most devastating disease on earth and, as a category, kills more men and women than any other disease. In the USA alone, the costs to society for cardiovascular disease currently exceed $350 billion annually. Furthermore, the rates of death due to cardiovascular events around the world are on the increase (American Heart Association 2004, World Health Organization, 2003, 2004a). Over half of all cardiovascular deaths worldwide are of women (World Health Organization 2004b, 2004c). While the death rate from ischaemic heart disease has been decreasing in Western countries for over 30 years, the number of hospitalisations due to end-stage heart failure is on the rise and increasing numbers of people are living with severe lifestyle limitations due to failing heart muscle. In developing countries, coronary disease is on the rise and is predicted to overtake infectious diseases as the primary cause of death within a decade (WHO websites).

The well-known risk factors for coronary disease are derived from statistical associations between these factors and disease prevalence. Factors that impart disease risk for coronary artery disease and that are thought to be related to personal behaviour include cigarette smoking, sedentary lifestyle, hypertension, and abnormal lipid profile. The heart associations and foundations of Western countries have been largely responsible for educating the public regarding the risk factors for heart disease and stroke as they are presently understood. There is evidence that the decrease in incidence of coronary artery disease over the past few decades has been related to changes in behaviour – like decreases in cigarette smoking, hypertension control and control of dyslipidaemias. However, the currently accepted risk factors do not explain differences in vulnerability

Developmental Origins of Health and Disease, ed. Peter Gluckman and Mark Hanson. Published by Cambridge University Press.

for adverse cardiovascular events. For example, they do not explain the apparently healthy 80-year-old man who has smoked tobacco for decades, is hypertensive and has high serum cholesterol levels but without signs of heart disease. In contrast, cardiologists regularly see the more worrisome side of the equation – the highly vulnerable 40-year-old man or woman with virtually no known risk factors who suffers coronary artery disease. At present, there is no explanation for these extremes of vulnerability within the population. The scientific community has generally relegated these cases to the 'genetic' category. Indeed, a host of specific gene defects are now known to lead to specific types of cardiac disease (Arnett *et al.* 2004) and others will, undoubtedly, be discovered. However, the role of underlying genetic diversity in affecting heart health within the human populations has not yet been determined. Furthermore, epidemiological data suggest that an adverse prenatal environment imparts a powerful influence on the cardiovascular system and leads to vulnerability for cardiovascular disease in a significant portion of the adult population. The process by which the early-life environment imparts such vulnerability for disease in later life is widely known as 'programming.'

Current dogma regarding the origins of coronary artery disease states that oxidised low-density lipoproteins are the primary source of injury to the coronary endothelium in the adult (Stocker and Keaney 2004). The evidence for this is very strong. However, there are many other factors thought to contribute to coronary vessel injury, either directly or indirectly; these include infectious agents (Kol and Santini 2004), angiotensins (Zhou *et al.* 2004), reactive oxygen species (Chen and Mehta 2004), inflammatory factors (Abrams 2003), and nitric oxide deficiency (Cooke and Oka 2001). Other factors, like high-density lipoproteins, may be protective to the endothelium (Shaul and Mineo 2004). Thus, the aetiology of coronary artery disease is highly complex and there is currently no biological explanation for how these complexities are related to the well-recognised relationship between early prenatal growth and cardiac disease.

Table 20.1 Prenatal factors associated with vulnerability to heart disease in later life.

Primary fetal stressors
Nutritional imbalances
Glucocorticoid excess
Hypoxia
Specific cardiovascular stressors
Fetal hypertension
Coronary shear stress
Low liver blood flow
Programming outcomes
Endothelial dysfunction
Myocardial dysfunction
Metabolic dysfunction
Hypothalamic–Pituitary–adrenal axis alteration

Several animal models demonstrate that specific changes in the fetal environment lead to altered physiology in offspring. For the sake of presentation, the prenatal factors associated with late-life vulnerability for heart disease will be arbitrarily divided into three categories (Table 20.1): (1) primary stressors that lead to programming of multiple organ systems in the fetus, (2) specific stressors that affect specific cardiac developmental patterns, and (3) pathologies that represent common pathways to heart disease risk in adulthood. The first primary stressor to be discussed is fetal nutrition.

Fetal nutrition

It is becoming increasingly clear that the nutritional status of the mother during the periconceptional period and throughout pregnancy can affect the growth and development of the offspring. The undernutrition models in sheep, rat and guinea pig have provided strong evidence for the programming concept in mammals (Davis and Hohimer 1991, Langley-Evans *et al.* 1996, Lingas and Matthews 2001). While the concept that the fetus gets its nutrients from maternal blood is simple enough, in fact, there can be many ways in which the nutrition supply line between the mother and fetus can be compromised. The inadequate consumption of macronutrients appears to have a gestation-specific effect. Reduction in either maternal or fetal placental blood flow can impair transplacental nutrient exchange (Godfrey 2002). Finally, the placenta itself can have transport defects along with abnormalities in endocrine function, metabolism or vascular structure and thus prevent optimal nutrient exchange. Langley-Evans and coworkers first showed that protein reduction in a maternal rat diet leads to offspring hypertension, an important risk factor for coronary artery disease. It is now clear that protein restriction during periods of nephrogenesis in the rat leads to fewer nephrons (Langley-Evans *et al.* 1996, Woods *et al.* 2004) and abnormalities in the renin-angiotensin system (Bagby *et al.* 2002, McMullen *et al.* 2004, Woods and Weeks 2004). Most nutrient-restriction animal models show adult hypertension in offspring as well as glucose regulation abnormalities (Lingas and Matthews 2001, Armitage *et al.* 2004, Taylor *et al.* 2005). Recent clinical data (Shiell *et al.* 2001) suggest that high levels of protein intake may also lead to fetal undergrowth and late-life heart disease. Thus, it is perhaps a protein–carbohydrate intake imbalance that modifies fetal development.

Glucocorticoid

Excess glucocorticoid is also an important factor in programming the cardiorenal systems. The high degree of interest in the role of exogenous glucocorticoid is obviously related to its efficacy in stimulating the maturation of the lung surfactant system in the fetal lung (Jobe 2001). This treatment has saved the lives of countless babies destined to deliver prematurely. While the long-term effects of treatment have been studied little in humans, it is known that exogenous maternal steroid use leads to growth restriction in animal models as well as delayed myelination of the central nervous system and alterations of the HPA axis (Newnham *et al.* 1999, Huang *et al.* 2001, Bloomfield *et al.* 2004). Perhaps the most profound change from exogenous steroid

administration comes from the work of Dodic and Wintour and others (Wintour *et al.* 2003), who have shown that administration of dexamethasone during early pregnancy in sheep (about day 27–29 of a 145-day gestation) leads to adult hypertension some five years later, reduced nephron number and changes in the brain renin–angiotensin system. The degree to which these experiments relate to human disease has yet to be determined. However, there is evidence that increased levels of endogenous cortisol may have untoward effects in the fetus and may lead to long-term cardiac consequences (Watterberg 2004).

Fetal hypoxia

Hypoxia is another stressor that affects the fetal cardiovascular system. Zhang and his colleagues (Li *et al.* 2003) exposed pregnant rats to a low-oxygen environment (10.5% oxygen) for six days near term (15–21 d) and studied the offspring as adults. The adult offspring appeared to be perfectly healthy. However, when the isolated hearts from these animals were studied, they had increased sensitivity to ischaemia–reperfusion injury (Fig. 20.1). An experimental ischaemic stress caused a significantly larger infarct area and severely depressed function in hearts that were exposed to hypoxia before birth in comparison to control hearts. These investigators also showed that the cardiomyocytes in the hearts that were hypoxic in utero were greatly enlarged compared to control cardiomyocytes and were also significantly reduced in number. Perhaps the most important point of this study was the silent vulnerability of the myocardium, which would have gone unnoticed without an episode of ischaemia during adult life. Thus, the experimental hearts that were hypoxic before birth were much more vulnerable to hypoxic stress damage than were normal hearts, even though they behaved in a normal fashion until stressed.

Nutrient-rich blood returning to the fetus from the placenta joins the fetal circulation in the liver, where streams divide into the inferior vena cava via the ductus venosus and also supply the left and right lobes

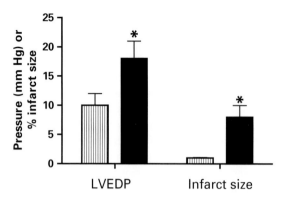

Figure 20.1 Changes in adult rat hearts as a result of ischaemia–reperfusion injury following a previous exposure to maternal hypoxia (10.5% O_2) during the last six days of gestation in utero. Note that ischaemic reperfusion injury caused exaggerated diastolic dysfunction in the previously hypoxic hearts (higher left-ventricular end diastolic pressure, LVEDP) and increased the amount of tissue that suffered infarction by some eight times over the control level.
Grey bars = control, black bars = hypoxic hearts. Mean ± SE, $p. < 0.05$. Data from Li et al. (2003).

of the liver. There is growing evidence that the distribution of umbilical venous flow through the ductus venosus is 'regulated' by dilation of the ductus venosus under hypoxaemic conditions (Kiserud et al. 2000). Thus, one can hypothesise that an enduring hypoxia may predispose a fetus to lifelong cardiac disease risk in two ways: (1) liver undergrowth and compromised hepatic function for life, which may explain abnormal lipid profiles in some adults; (2) a large ductal flow may also affect the loading conditions of the heart. Since inferior vena caval flow is directed across the foramen ovale within the heart, the left atrial inflow pattern may affect the loading conditions of the left ventricle in the form of increased kinetic energy (Anderson et al. 1985).

There is little controversy around the view that abnormal nutrient supply, excess glucocorticoid and suboptimal oxygen levels each impart a high risk for cardiovascular disease in later life. For these factors, the epidemiological findings and animal experimental data fit well. However, there may be other factors that complicate the road to programming in the cardiovascular system. Some of these

specific cardiovascular stressors will be discussed below.

Fetal anaemia

One model that has clearly shown enormous plasticity of the coronary tree is the fetal sheep anaemia model developed by Davis and colleagues (Davis and Hohimer 1991, Davis et al. 2003). The loss of fetal red blood cells lowers the viscosity of the blood and reduces its oxygen content. Thus, the model is characterised by a combination of hypoxia and increased coronary arterial shear stress. Fetal anaemia occurs rarely in humans from fetal haemorrhage but more often in the donor fetus of a twin–twin transfusion pair. In the experiments by Davis and colleagues, the fetal haematocrit of the near-term fetal sheep was reduced by ~50% over a 4–6 day period by removing red blood cells and returning plasma.

These experiments have shown that the fetal cardiovascular response to anaemia is profound. The heart of the anaemic fetus becomes larger and cardiac output and coronary blood flow increase dramatically. The slope of the flow pressure relationship under conditions of *maximal* coronary dilation with adenosine is called the conductance curve. Once the slope of a conductance curve is known, one can determine the maximal flow through the coronary tree for any given driving pressure (fetal arterial pressure – mean right atrial pressure). Normally, the driving pressure for the coronary arteries is ~40 mm Hg and coronary flow is about 300 ml min^{-1} per 100 g tissue. Davis et al. (2003), found that as haematocrit was decreased to ~28 per cent in a single fetus over a few days' time, the maximal flow at 40 mm Hg more than doubled to ~650 ml min^{-1} per 100 g. By the time the haematocrit had decreased by half to 16 per cent, blood flow had tripled to 900 ml min^{-1} per 100 g. This enormous flow was greater than the maximal flow at any pressure before the haematocrit had changed. The most likely explanation of these data is that the capacity of the coronary tree had grown enormously over a few days. Thus, these experiments showed the plasticity of the coronary tree during this critical period of coronary development.

The question remains, will a temporary decrease in the haematocrit of the fetus permanently alter the coronary tree over the life of the offspring? To answer this question, fetuses that had been anaemic, before birth were reinfused with their own red blood cells so that their haematocrit would return to normal. They were allowed to deliver along with their twin siblings that had never been anaemic, and were returned to pasture. At 6 months of age (sexual maturity), experiments were performed on the experimental animals and their control twins. The finding was surprising. Coronary arterial driving pressure in these adults was about 100 mm Hg and in a normal adult had a flow of about 300 ml min^{-1} per 100 g. However, it can be seen from Fig. 20.2 that in once-anaemic experimental adult animals the maximal coronary conductance was about twice that of the control twin; this was true in all animal pairs in the study. Thus, it is clear that anaemia is a powerful stimulant of coronary tree remodelling and that this remodelling persists into adulthood if it occurs within the critical window of coronary artery development.

When hearts from once-anaemic adult animals were studied under hypoxaemic conditions, contractile function was better maintained compared to controls (Broberg *et al.* 2003). This might suggest that building a large coronary tree before birth is beneficial. However, the jury is still out on the issue of lifelong benefit. Two factors should be considered. First, the resting blood flow of the once-anaemic adult sheep is the same as in the control animals. Since the true flow capacity of the coronary tree of the experimental animals is two times normal, one must conclude that the regulatory bed is in a constant state of relative vasoconstriction compared to control hearts. Such a constriction might affect chronic shear stress in coronary resistance vessels and therefore long-term endothelial function. Second, there is little known about the architectural changes in the coronary tree. If, for example, the vascularity of the microcirculation is altered in some way, the myocardium might be at an increased risk for ischaemia or infarction with coronary artery occlusion. This prospect is presently being tested.

Shear forces may be more important in early life than previously appreciated. Elegant experiments by

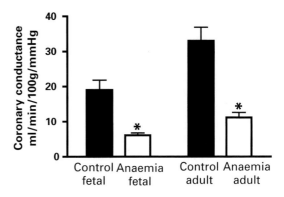

Figure 20.2 Decreased conductance of the circumflex coronary bed (slope of the maximal flow-driving pressure curve) in anaemic fetuses compared to non-anaemic fetuses (left bars), and in adults that were anaemic as fetuses compared to non-anaemic adult twins (right bars). Black bars = control, white bars = experimental. Mean ± SD. *, $p < 0.05$. Data from Davis *et al.* (2003).

Poelmann and colleagues suggest that altered shear forces in the early embryonic heart alter growth patterns and shape of the ventricles (Groenendijk *et al.* 2004). By changing inflow patterns of the venous streams through the heart, they were able to demonstrate changes in flow profiles through the heart chambers that led to apparent changes in energy transfer to the wall of the developing heart. They, and others, have shown that changes in flow pattern through the embryonic heart, can result in cardiac defects. It is likely that shear and wall deformation forces are extremely important in guiding the formation of the embryonic heart, as is well appreciated in altering vascular form and function. Thus it appears that both hypoxia and shear forces serve as programming agents for the cardiovascular system.

Cardiac anatomy: fetus versus adult

Many anatomical features of the fetal heart differ from their adult heart counterparts. In the adult heart, the left ventricular, wall is much thicker that the right ventricular wall; in contrast, the thicknesses of the two chamber free walls are similar in the fetus. However, the equatorial radius of curvature for the right ventricle, is larger than for the left ventricle even though it was long considered to be about equal (Dawes 1968). In fact, the right chamber itself is larger, which explains the larger stroke volume for the right ventricle than for the left ventricle during fetal life (Thornburg and Morton 1986). The larger right ventricular radius is important because for any given transmural pressure the wall stress is larger for the right ventricle than for the left. Wall stress can be estimated by the Laplace relationship which states that the free wall stress is the product of half the transmural pressure times the radius-to-wall-thickness ratio. In equation form:

$$S_w = (P_t/2) \times (r/h)$$

where S_w is wall stress force/area, P_t is transmural hydrostatic pressure, r is radius of curvature, h is wall thickness. The normal average ratio of radius to wall thickness for the right ventricle is ~4.6, and 2.6 for the left ventricle. This anatomic relationship means that the higher wall stress in the right ventricular wall makes the right ventricle less able to contract against increases in arterial pressure. Thus, it is the right ventricle that is most affected by increases in arterial pressure during fetal life. For example, if the fetus becomes hypoxaemic, the resultant increase in arterial pressure will depress right-ventricular stroke volume much more that left-ventricular stroke volume (Reller *et al.* 1989). Similarly, a chronic increase in arterial pressure, as would occur with high placental vascular resistance, loads the right ventricle more than the left.

Cardiac loading conditions

During fetal life, the ventricles are sensitive to changes in loading conditions – preload and afterload. **Preload** is defined by the wall stress in the ventricular wall at end – diastole (just before contraction begins) and is the result of end-diastolic transmural pressure. Preload is usually approximated in the fetus as the mean atrial pressure (either atrium, since they have similar pressures). The wall stress during ejection is known as **afterload**. It is the result

of transmural pressure generated during contraction and is determined by the pulsatile 'resistance' or input impedance of the vascular tree. Preload and afterload appear to be sensed differently by the working myocardium. Chronic changes in afterload have been studied in fetal animal models and will be discussed below. However, chronic preload changes are more difficult to characterise because few prenatal animal models have been developed. It appears that increased preload under conditions of volume overload lead to significant changes in myocardial growth through changes in cardiomyocyte maturation and proliferation (T. Karamlou *et al.*, unpublished).

Afterload

The effects of increased afterload depend upon the point in development when the load is applied. In sheep, ventricular myocytes are mononucleate and able to proliferate until about gestational day 100 (150 days is term), at which time the population gradually becomes binucleate (Burrell *et al.* 2003). Binucleate cells are able to enlarge under the influence of the α- adrenergic agonist, phenylephrine. However, they are not able to divide. Thus, as the population of binucleate cells decreases, the generative capacity of the myocardium decreases.

When right-ventricular afterload is increased in near-term fetal sheep through chronic constriction of the pulmonary artery, several changes are found. The free wall thickens and the mechanical advantage of the ventricle improves, as predicted by Laplace (Pinson *et al.* 1991, Barbera *et al.* 2000). The average cell size increases (Fig. 20.3). Perhaps the most interesting finding is that the portion of the cardiomyocyte population that is binucleated increases dramatically even in the presence of increased proliferation of mononucleate cells (Fig. 20.3). This response may occur through intracellular mechanical sensors or via specific growth factors that are known to signal within the immature myocardium (Sundgren *et al.* 2003a, 2003b). The increased loss of generative capacity suggests that loading conditions stimulate cell maturation at ages

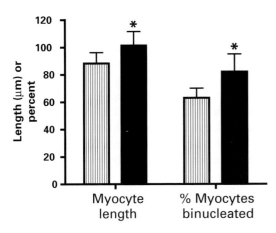

Figure 20.3 Increased length of right-ventricular myocytes following 10-day right-ventricular pressure load (101 mm Hg peak systolic pressure) in the sheep fetus. Right-hand bars show increased percentage of pressure-loaded cardiomyocytes that contain two nuclei and are thus unable to proliferate. Grey bars = control, black bars = loaded myocytes. Mean ± SD. *, $p. < 0.05$. Data from Barbera *et al.* (2000).

that precede normal maturation. The meaning of this outcome is not clear but it suggests a decreased generative capacity of the myocardium to regulate cell numbers, which would lead to lower cell numbers during adult life. This effect was clearly seen in the maternal-hypoxia experiments performed on rats in the Zhang laboratory (Li *et al.* 2003), as discussed above.

There are instances where the loading conditions of the human heart may alter the normal maturation of the fetal myocardium. This can be detected by the relationship between diastolic and systolic flow velocities in the umbilical artery (Surat and Adamson 1996). Among the population of human fetuses that are defined as undergrown, there are individuals whose diastolic flow in the umbilical artery does not increase with gestation. Ordinarily, placental vascular resistance decreases with increasing gestational age and diastolic flow increases with age. However, in some undergrown fetuses, the overall resistance to blood flow within the placental vascular bed is increased with age. In severe cases, placental vascular resistance may be depressed to levels where umbilical arterial diastolic flow is reversed. Under

such loading conditions, sheep experiments predict that the heart will remodel through premature myocardial maturation and altered coronary architecture (Pinson *et al.* 1991, Thornburg and Reller 1999, Barbera *et al.* 2000). These adaptations to systolic load will lead to vulnerability for disease in later life.

Endothelial dysfunction

The primary programming stressors may lead to vulnerability for coronary artery disease through a few common pathways. One such pathway is reduced cardiomyocyte number within the myocardium. Another likely pathway is depressed endothelial function. Endothelial function includes the ability of flow-regulating coronary arterioles to dilate under the stimulation of endothelial-cell-derived vasoactive mechanisms. These include, among other mechanisms, the release of nitric oxide and vasodilatory prostaglandins, as well as functional hyperpolarising factor. There is growing evidence that depressed endothelial function as shown by experimental test or by erectile dysfunction is a predisposing condition for human coronary artery disease (Vogel and Corretti 1998, Andersson and Stief 2000, Schachinger *et al.* 2000). Bugiardini *et al.* (2004) showed that women who had vasocontriction rather than dilation of the left coronary bed under the stimulus of acetylcholine went on to get coronary disease (Fig. 20.4). Thus, loss of endothelial function appears to be a powerful predictor of coronary disease in some populations. Endothelial dysfunction appears to be a mechanism common to animal models of programming as well. Adult rats and sheep that were exposed to protein deprivation as fetuses become hypertensive as adults. Isolated mesenteric arteries from these animals show relaxation defects compared to controls (Ozaki *et al.* 2001, Brawley *et al.* 2003, Nishina *et al.* 2003). Similar results have been found for cerebral arteries in rat (Lamireau *et al.* 2002). Fetal growth restriction in rats under the influence of reduced uterine arterial flow also leads to endothelial dysfunction.

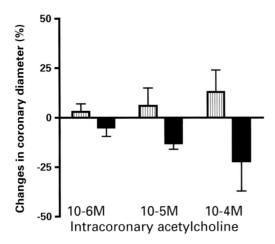

Figure 20.4 Normal coronary artery function (dilation, up bars) or cornary artery endothelial dysfunction (constriction, down bars) with intracoronary infusion of various doses of acetylcholine in 42 women with *de novo* angina (mean age 56.6 ± 8.8 years). Women who lacked the normal vasodilator response developed coronary artery disease in a 10-year follow-up. Those with a normal dilatory response showed resolution of angina and no signs of coronary disease. Grey bars = vasodilators, black bars = vasoconstrictors. Data from Bugiardini *et al.* (2004).

A number of human studies have made the connection between endothelial dysfunction and low birthweight in humans. Leeson *et al.* (1997) showed that 9–11-year-old children had impaired flow-mediated dilation in the forearm if they were born at the low end of the term birthweight spectrum. Martin and coworkers found impaired endothelial response in newborns that were born underweight (Martin *et al.* 2000a), and impaired endothelial function and increased carotid arterial stiffness in 9-year-old children who were born small (Martin *et al.* 2000b).

Postnatal pathways to cardiac disease

Very little is known regarding the growth pathways that may be unique to those who will acquire cardiovascular disease, but there are several reports from a Finnish cohort that cast light on this subject.

Eriksson and colleagues have reported on the childhood growth trajectories for both men (Forsen *et al.* 2004a) and women (Forsen *et al.* 2004b). It is clear from these studies that the men and women with disease followed a growth pattern over the course of infancy and childhood that was distinct from the non-affected population. There are several very interesting features common to those who went on to develop coronary heart disease: (1) both men and women had lower weights at birth than average; (2) boys who were thin at birth were at highest risk; (3) girls who were short at birth had highest risk; and (4) placenta – fetal weight ratios were significant factors in determining disease risk. However, the placental-ratio effect was complicated as its importance depended on the decade of birth.

The association of childhood and adult hypertension with fetal undergrowth is well known. However, the role of hypertension as a precursor to endothelial dysfunction in the coronary bed has not been studied. The fact that there are many gaps in our knowledge makes it clear that the primary biological underpinnings of programmed cardiovascular disease are not yet known. It is hard to imagine any aspect of modern medical research that would bring greater yield to human health than understanding the stressors of early life – nutrition, maternal stress and hypoxia – as they continue to impart vulnerability for cardiovascular disease to millions of people worldwide.

Summary

Based upon present evidence, it appears that there are three primary stressors that lead to growth adaptations during prenatal life: malnourishment, glucocorticoid excess and hypoxia. These stressors affect a number of organ systems depending upon their level of maturity. In addition to these, there are other intrauterine events that specifically affect the developing cardiovascular system. These include fetal hypertension, redistribution of placental blood flow through the ductus venosus and abnormal endothelial shear stress in the embryo heart and fetal coronary arteries. Fetal hypertension can arise from a decreased placental vascular resistance that may characterise a portion of the population of human fetuses that show growth restriction. Taken together, these factors lead to at least two types of vulnerability for the offspring over their lifetime: (1) endothelial dysfunction and (2) fewer and perhaps abnormal cardiomyocytes. There may, of course, be a host of other adaptations that add to the vulnerability of the heart in adult life. These might include an altered extracellular matrix, altered conduction system function and biochemical changes within the cardiomyocyte. For a characterisation of these adaptations, we must wait with anticipation for new discoveries.

REFERENCES

Abrams, J. (2003). C-reactive protein, inflammation, and coronary risk: an update. *Cardiol. Clin.*, **21**, 327–31.

American Heart Association (2004). *International Cardiovascular Disease Statistics*. www.americanheart.org/ downloadable/heart/1077185395308FS06INT4(ebook).pdf Accessed 24 November 2004.

Anderson, D. F., Faber, J. J., Morton, M. J., Parks, C. M., Pinson, C. W. and Thornburg, K. L. (1985). Flow through the foramen ovale of the fetal and new-born lamb. *J. Physiol.*, **365**, 29–40.

Andersson, K. and Stief, C. (2000). Penile erection and cardiac risk: pathophysiologic and pharmacologic mechanisms. *Am. J. Cardiol.*, **86**, 23–6F.

Armitage, J. A., Khan, I. Y., Taylor, P. D., Nathanielsz, P. W., and Poston, L. (2004). Developmental programming of metabolic syndrome by maternal nutritional imbalance: how strong is the evidence from experimental models in mammals? *J. Physiol.*, **561**, 355–77.

Arnett, D. K., de las Fuentes, L., Broeckel, U. (2004). Genes for left ventricular hypertrophy. *Curr. Hypertens. Rep.*, **6**, 36–41.

Bagby, S. P., LeBard, L. S., Luo, Z. *et al.* (2002). ANG II, AT(1) and AT(2) receptors in developing kidney of normal microswine. *Am. J. Physiol. Renal. Physiol.*, **283**, F755–64.

Barbera, A., Giraud, G. D., Reller, M. D., Maylie, J., Morton, M. J. and Thornburg, K. L. (2000). Right ventricular systolic pressure load alters myocyte maturation in fetal sheep. *Am. J. Physiol. Regul. Integr. Comp. Physiol.*, **279**, R1157–64.

Barker, D. J. P., Osmond, C., Golding, J., Kuh, D., Wadsworth, M. E. (1989). Growth in utero, blood pressure in childhood and adult life, and mortality from cardiovascular disease. *BMJ*, **298**, 564–7.

Bloomfield, F. H., Oliver, M. H., Hawkins, P. *et al.* (2004). Periconceptional undernutrition in sheep accelerates maturation of the fetal hypothalamic-pituitary-adrenal axis in late gestation. *Endocrinology*, **145**, 4278–85.

Brawley, L., Itoh, S., Torrens, C. *et al.* (2003). Dietary protein restriction in pregnancy induces hypertension and vascular defects in rat male offspring. *Pediatr. Res.*, **54**, 83–90.

Broberg, C. S., Giraud, G. D., Schultz, J. M., Thornburg, K. L., Hohimer, A. R. and Davis, L. E. (2003). Fetal anemia leads to augmented contractile response to hypoxic stress in adulthood. *Am. J. Physiol. Regul. Integr. Comp. Physiol.*, **285**, R649–55.

Bugiardini, R., Manfrini, O., Pizzi, C., Fontana, F. and Morgagni, G. (2004). Endothelial function predicts future development of coronary artery disease: a study of women with chest pain and normal coronary angiograms. *Circulation*, **109**, 2518–23.

Burrell, J. H., Boyn, A. M., Kumarasamy, V., Hsieh, A., Head, S. I. and Lumbers, E. R. (2003). Growth and maturation of cardiac myocytes in fetal sheep in the second half of gestation. *Anat. Rec.*, **274A**, 952–61.

Chen, J. and Mehta, J. L. (2004). Role of oxidative stress in coronary heart disease. *Indian Heart J.*, **56**, 163–73.

Cooke, J. P. and Oka, R. K. (2001). Atherogenesis and the arginine hypothesis. *Curr. Atheroscler. Rep.*, **3**, 252–9.

Davis, L., Roullet, J. B., Thornburg, K. L., Shokry, M., Hohimer, A. R. and Giraud, G. D. (2003). Augmentation of coronary conductance in adult sheep made anaemic during fetal life. *J. Physiol.*, **547**, 53–9.

Davis, L. E. and Hohimer, A. R. (1991). Hemodynamics and organ blood flow in fetal sheep subjected to chronic anemia. *Am. J. Physiol.*, **261**, R1542–8.

Dawes, G. S. (1968). *Foetal and Neonatal Physiology: a Comparative Study of the Changes at Birth*. Chicago, IL: Year Book Medical Publishers.

Forsen, T. J., Eriksson, J. G., Osmond, C. and Barker, D. J. P. (2004a). The infant growth of boys who later develop coronary heart disease. *Ann. Med.*, **36**, 389–92.

Forsen, T. J., Osmond, C., Eriksson, J. G. and Barker, D. J. P. (2004b). Growth of girls who later develop coronary heart disease. *Heart*, **90**, 20–4.

Godfrey, K. M. (2002). The role of the placenta in fetal programming: a review. *Placenta*, **23** (Suppl. A) S20–7.

Groenendijk, B. C., Hierck, B. P., Gittenberger-de Groot, A. C. and Poelmann, R. E. (2004). Development-related changes in the expression of shear stress responsive genes KLF-2,

ET-1, and NOS-3 in the developing cardiovascular system of chicken embryos. *Dev. Dyn.*, **230**, 57–68.

Huang, W. L., Harper, C. G., Evans, S. F., Newnham, J. P. and Dunlop, S. A. (2001). Repeated prenatal corticosteroid administration delays myelination of the corpus callosum in fetal sheep. *Int. J. Dev. Neurosci.*, **19**, 415–25.

Jobe, A. H. (2001). Glucocorticoids, inflammation and the perinatal lung. *Semin. Neonatol.*, **6**, 331–42.

Kiserud, T., Ozaki, T., Nishina, H., Rodeck, C. and Hanson, M. A. (2000). Effect of NO, phenylephrine, and hypoxaemia on ductus venosus diameter in fetal sheep. *Am. J. Physiol. Heart Circ. Physiol.*, **279**, H1166–71.

Kol, A. and Santini, M. (2004). Infectious agents and atherosclerosis: current perspectives and unsolved issues. *Ital. Heart J.*, **5**, 350–7.

Lamireau, D., Nuyt, A. M., Hou, X. *et al.* (2002). Altered vascular function in fetal programming of hypertension. *Stroke*, **33**, 2992–8.

Langley-Evans, S. C., Phillips, G. J., Benediktsson, R. *et al.* (1996). Protein intake in pregnancy, placental glucocorticoid metabolism and the programming of hypertension in the rat. *Placenta*, **17**, 169–72.

Leeson, C. P., Whincup, P. H., Cook, D. G. *et al.* (1997). Flow-mediated dilation in 9- to 11-year-old children: the influence of intrauterine and childhood factors. *Circulation*, **96**, 2233–8.

Li, G., Xiao, Y., Estrella, J. L., Ducsay, C. A., Gilbert, R. D. and Zhang, L. (2003). Effect of fetal hypoxia on heart susceptibility to ischaemia and reperfusion injury in the adult rat. *J. Soc. Gynecol. Investig.*, **10**, 265–74.

Lingas, R. I. and Matthews, S. G. (2001). A short period of maternal nutrient restriction in late gestation modifies pituitary – adrenal function in adult guinea pig offspring. *Neuroendocrinology*, **73**, 302–11.

Martin, H., Gazelius, B. and Norman, M. (2000a). Impaired acetylcholine-induced vascular relaxation in low birthweight infants: implications for adult hypertension? *Pediatr. Res.*, **47**, 457–62.

Martin, H., Hu, J., Gennser G. and Norman, M. (2000b). Impaired endothelial function and increased carotid stiffness in 9-year-old children with low birthweight. *Circulation*, **102**, 2739–44.

McMullen, S., Gardner, D. S. and Langley-Evans, S. C. (2004). Prenatal programming of angiotensin II type 2 receptor expression in the rat. *Br. J. Nutr.*, **91**, 133–40.

Newnham, J. P., Evans, S. F., Godfrey, M., Huang, W., Ikegami, M. and Jobe, A. (1999). Maternal, but not fetal, administration of corticosteroids restricts fetal growth. *J. Matern. Fetal. Med.*, **8**, 81–7.

Nishina, H., Green, L. R., McGarrigle, H. H., Noakes, D. E., Poston, L. and Hanson, M. A. (2003). Effect of nutritional restriction in early pregnancy on isolated femoral artery function in mid-gestation fetal sheep. *J. Physiol.*, **553**, 637–47.

Ozaki, T., Nishina, H., Hawkins, P., Crowe, C., Poston, L. and Hanson, M. A. (2001). Isolated systemic resistance vessel function in hypertensive male rat offspring of mildly nutritionally restricted dams. *J. Physiol.*, **513**, 118p.

Pinson, C. W., Morton, M. J. and Thornburg, K. L. (1991). Mild pressure loading alters right ventricular function in fetal sheep. *Circ. Res.*, **68**, 947–57.

Reller, M. D., Morton, M. J., Giraud, G. D., Reid, D. L. and Thornburg, K. L. (1989). The effect of acute hypoxaemia on ventricular function during beta-adrenergic and cholinergic blockade in the fetal sheep. *J. Dev. Physiol.*, **11**, 263–9.

Rich-Edwards, J. W., Stampfer, M. J., Manson, J. E. *et al.* (1997). Birthweight and risk of cardiovascular disease in a cohort of women followed up since 1976. *BMJ*, **315**, 396–400.

Schachinger, V., Britten, M. B. and Zeiher, A. M. (2000). Prognostic impact of coronary vasodilator dysfunction on adverse long-term outcome of coronary heart disease. *Circulation*, **101**, 1899–906.

Shaul, P. W. and Mineo, C. (2004). HDL action on the vascular wall: is the answer NO? *J. Clin. Invest.*, **113**, 509–13.

Shiell, A. W., Campbell-Brown, M., Haselden, S., Robinson, S., Godfrey, K. M. and Barker, D. J. P. (2001). High-meat, low-carbohydrate diet in pregnancy: relation to adult blood pressure in the offspring. *Hypertension*, **38**, 1282–8.

Stocker, R. and Keaney, J. F., Jr. (2004). Role of oxidative modifications in atherosclerosis. *Physiol. Rev.*, **84**, 1381–478.

Sundgren, N. C., Giraud, G. D., Stork, P. J., Maylie, J. G. and Thornburg, K. L. (2003a). Angiotensin II stimulates hyperplasia but not hypertrophy in immature ovine cardiomyocytes. *J. Physiol.*, **548**, 881–91.

Sundgren, N. C., Giraud, G. D., Schultz, J. M., Lasarev, M. R., Stork, P. J. and Thornburg, K. L. (2003b). Extracellular signal-regulated kinase and phosphoinositol-3 kinase mediate IGF-1 induced proliferation of fetal sheep cardiomyocytes. *Am. J. Physiol. Regul. Integr. Comp. Physiol.*, **285**, R1481–9.

Surat, D. R. and Adamson, S. L. (1996). Downstream determinants of pulsatility of the mean velocity waveform in the umbilical artery as predicted by a computer model. *Ultrasound Med. Biol.*, **22**, 707–17.

Taylor, P. D., McConnell, J., Khan, I. Y. *et al.* (2005). Impaired glucose homeostasis and mitochondrial abnormalities in offspring of rats fed a fat-rich diet in pregnancy. *Am. J. Physiol. Regul. Integr. Comp. Physiol.*, **288**, R134–9.

Thornburg, K. L. and Morton, M. J. (1986). Filling and arterial pressures as determinants of left ventricular stroke volume in fetal lambs. *Am. J. Physiol.*, **251**, H961–8.

Thornburg, K. L. and Reller, M. D. (1999). Coronary flow regulation in the fetal sheep. *Am. J. Physiol.*, **277**, R1249–60.

Vogel, R. A. and Corretti, M. C. (1998). Estrogens, progestins, and heart disease: can endothelial function divine the benefit? *Circulation*, **97**, 1223–6.

Watterberg, K. L. (2004). Adrenocortical function and dysfunction in the fetus and neonate. *Semin. Neonatol.*, **9**, 13–21.

Wintour, E. M., Moritz, K. M., Johnson, K., Ricardo, S., Samuel, C. S. and Dodic, M. (2003). Reduced nephron number in adult sheep, hypertensive as a result of prenatal glucocorticoid treatment. *J. Physiol.*, **549**, 929–35.

Woods, L. L. and Weeks, D. A. (2004). Naturally occurring intrauterine growth retardation and adult blood pressure in rats. *Pediatr. Res.*, **56**, 763–7.

Woods, L. L., Weeks, D. A. and Rasch, R. (2004). Programming of adult blood pressure by maternal protein restriction: role of nephrogenesis. *Kidney Int.*, **65**, 1339–48.

World Health Organization (2003). *World Health Report, 2003.* www.who.int/whr/2003/en. Accessed 24 November 2004.

(2004a). *Cardiovascular Diseases.* www.who.int/cardiovasculardiseases/en. Accessed 24 November 2004.

(2004b). WHO publishes definitive atlas on global heart disease and stroke epidemic. WHO Media Centre. www.who.int/mediacentre/releases/2004/pr68/en. Accessed 24 November 2004.

(2004c). Global cardiovascular infobase. WHO Collaborating Centre on Surveillance of Cardiovascular Diseases. www.cvdinfobase.ca. Accessed 24 November 2004.

Zhou, M. S., Schulman, I. H. and Raij, L. (2004). Nitric oxide, angiotensin II, and hypertension. *Semin. Nephrol.*, 24, 366–78.

21

The role of vascular dysfunction in developmental origins of health and disease: evidence from human and animal studies

Lucilla Poston,[1] Christopher Torrens,[2] James A. Armitage[1] and Mark A. Hanson[2]

[1]King's College London
[2]University of Southampton

Introduction

Early studies in population cohorts proposed that perturbation of the environment in utero and in early life gives rise to marked and permanent alteration in offspring cardiovascular homeostasis, leading to increased risk of cardiovascular and metabolic disease in later life (reviewed in this volume). Clinical outcomes focused on the incidence of heart disease and hypertension in relation to birthweight, with little detailed investigation of other parameters of cardiovascular risk or outcome. More recent studies have given insight into underlying aetiological pathways, and the development of the different animal models of developmental plasticity has provided an opportunity to assess parameters of cardiovascular function at a depth which is not feasible, or indeed practicable, in humans.

The mechanisms contributing to cardiovascular homeostasis are complex and interwoven; they range from central control of the heart rate and vascular tone to paracrine, autocrine and genomic influences on the vascular smooth muscle and function of the endothelium. Fluid and volume homeostatic pathways, as well as the intricacy of haemostatic control, also contribute to the status quo. The complexity is such that common disorders such as essential hypertension remain poorly understood despite decades of research. The scientist wishing to inves-

tigate developmental programming of, for example, metabolic syndrome faces a bewildering choice of avenues to explore. Without a firm understanding of the early aetiology of hypertension or of insulin resistance, he or she has little choice but to follow the well-trodden paths which characterise research into these disorders in humans. At this relatively early stage of investigation in this rapidly expanding field, it is inevitable that there remain many missing pieces in the largely descriptive jigsaw which forms a picture of the developmentally programmed phenotype. The novelty of research into DOHaD must lie in our understanding of how it is that relatively modest disturbance of the early environment can permanently alter the developing cardiovascular system of the embryo, fetus or neonate to have such a major impact in later life. Importantly, emerging research into the permanent alteration of gene expression and tissue composition in early development now provides an entirely novel approach to the aetiology of cardiovascular disease.

Other chapters in this book focus on the elevation of blood pressure in many of the models, and have highlighted the potential role of the renin–angiotensin system and the HPA axis. In this review we discuss how early-life environmental disturbances, particularly those relating to maternal nutrition, may give rise to permanent and sometimes deleterious influences on offspring vascular

Developmental Origins of Health and Disease, ed. Peter Gluckman and Mark Hanson. Published by Cambridge University Press.

function. Relevant studies in humans will be discussed and a description provided of the vascular phenotypes induced in the different animal models.

Parameters of vascular function which may be influenced by the environment during development

Disorders of vascular function which contribute to cardiovascular disease occur predominantly in the arteries. Developmentally programmed alteration in constrictor function of the small resistance arteries in the peripheral circulation, for example, could lead to increased peripheral resistance and thereby elevate arterial blood pressure. This could arise simply from permanent alteration in smooth muscle cell size or density or from alterations in receptor density or function, ion channel expression and activity or altered sympathetic innervation. The possibility that the distribution of vascular smooth muscle phenotypic clones is influenced by the developmental environment is being investigated (Owens *et al.* 2004), and others have proposed a developmental influence on sympathetic activity. As individuals age, cardiovascular risk increases. This in part is related to increased stiffness, or reduced compliance, of the large arteries, which leads to a rise in systolic blood pressure (Wadsworth 1990). Isolated systolic hypertension is a cardiovascular risk factor (Black 2004), as is reduced vascular compliance (Kingwell and Gatzka 2002). It has been proposed that impaired growth in early development may be linked to prematurely reduced compliance in adulthood through early and permanent alteration in structure of the aorta and other large conduit arteries. The secretion of elastin by the vascular smooth muscle occurs during development, and thus early environmental influences can induce effects on vascular compliance (Martyn and Greenwald 1997). However, the major focus of research in developmental programming has related to the function of the vascular endothelium.

The vascular endothelium

This all-important organ, which forms an unbroken layer throughout the entire vascular system, was once considered to be a passive barrier which served to limit transport of water and molecules to the extravascular compartment. The endothelium is now recognised to play a central role in cardiovascular homeostasis (Hunt and Jurd 2002). The endothelial cell expresses a range of factors which influence the tone of the underlying vascular smooth muscle, control platelet and leucocyte adhesion, and directly influence thrombogenesis and inflammatory responses. Activation of the endothelium and resultant leucocyte recruitment leads to inception of the relentless progression towards atherosclerotic plaque formation (Landmesser *et al.* 2004). Failure of endothelium-dependent dilatation may also contribute to hypertension (Panza *et al.* 1993), but is not a predominant cause. The endothelium has also been implicated in insulin resistance and type 2 diabetes (McVeigh *et al.* 1992, Yu *et al.* 2001, Hsueh *et al.* 2004).

The endothelium synthesises and releases many vasoactive agents. The most notable is nitric oxide (NO), which reduces vascular smooth muscle calcium, and thus tone, by elevation of cyclic GMP (Chan and Vallance 2002). Others include prostacyclin, evoking vasodilatation through elevation of cyclic AMP, and endothelial-derived hyperpolarising factors (EDHFs), which cause vasodilatation through hyperpolarisation of the vascular smooth muscle membrane and reduced calcium entry through voltage-gated calcium channels (Busse *et al.* 2002). The endothelium also synthesises vasoconstrictor factors including endothelin and thromboxane A_2. Synthesis is under control of local humoral and mechanical influences. The importance of normal function of the endothelium is highlighted by the observation that reduction of endothelium-dependent dilatation in coronary arteries in humans is an indicator for later development of cardiovascular disease, particularly atherosclerosis (Halcox *et al.* 2002). Endothelial cell activation, resulting in poor synthesis of NO and increased expression of cell-adhesion molecules (e.g. VCAM1) is considered to provide a proatherogenic stimulus. It is proposed that subsequent leucocyte adhesion and monocyte migration into the intima leads to a local inflammatory response and ultimately to generation of an atherosclerotic plaque (Libby 2002).

Poor endothelial function has also been implicated in insulin resistance because impairment of endothelium-dependent dilatation is a frequent accompaniment to insulin resistance and type 2 diabetes (Hsueh *et al.* 2004). Reduced endothelium-dependent dilatation, it is suggested, would reduce blood flow to skeletal muscle and lead to reduced glucose uptake. Since NO also modulates both growth and metabolism, its release upstream may have additional effects to regulate the balance of supply and demand in developing tissues and organs.

The different studies which have proposed developmental programming of vascular function are summarised in the following sections, describing separately the investigations in humans and animals.

Studies of vascular function in developmental programming in humans

Endothelial function

The in-vitro methods frequently used in the study of isolated artery function in animals are largely inappropriate for evaluation of vascular function in humans. Small arteries can be obtained by biopsy of subcutaneous fat or muscle and investigated in vitro in organ baths, as in many investigations of isolated artery function in essential hypertension (Intengan *et al.* 1999), but to our knowledge there has not been any similar investigation into the origins of vascular disorders arising from developmental processes. Investigations in humans must necessarily use less invasive measures. One of the most physiologically relevant stimuli resulting in endothelium-dependent dilatation relies on the flow of blood through the vasculature, and this can be assessed using ultrasound technology. As blood flows through an artery it leads to a tangential force on the endothelial cell, known as shear stress. This gives rise to a sequence of events which alters the synthesis

of vasoactive molecules through well-characterised mechanisms. In relation to NO, an increase in shear-stress can lead to altered phosphorylation of the NOS gene, promoting immediate NO synthesis, or in the longer term to increased NOS expression through generation of transcription factors which bind to a shear-stress response element on the promoter region of the NOS gene (Boo and Jo 2003). Endothelial dilator function may be evaluated non-invasively in humans by estimation of flow-mediated dilatation in the brachial artery. A rapid increment in flow is achieved by application of a cuff on the lower arm. Inflation and subsequent deflation of the cuff leads to a hyperaemic response and increased flow in the brachial artery. The resultant dilator response is assessed by measurement of the diameter of the artery by high-resolution ultrasound. Impairment of endothelial function in the brachial artery correlates with that in the carotid artery, a vessel more prone to development of atherosclerotic plaques (Anderson *et al.* 1995).

Using this approach, Leeson *et al.* (1997) reported that low birthweight was linked to development of a defect in endothelial-dependent dilatation. These authors found a positive association of flow-mediated dilatation with birthweight in 9- to 11-year-old children which remained after adjustment for potential confounding variables. An inverse relationship with blood HDL cholesterol concentrations was also found, and might implicate a role for the lipid environment in the origin of the defect. Low-birthweight adults have also been shown to demonstrate reduced flow-mediated dilatation (Leeson *et al.* 2001a). However, this association did not stand after correction for other risk factors. Another group showed reduced endothelium-dependent dilatation in younger subjects (fit 19- to 20-year-olds) of low birthweight (Goodfellow *et al.* 1998).

Endothelial function can also be assessed by local application of dilator stimuli. Responses to cutaneous application of the endothelium-dependent dilator acetylcholine (ACh) and to local heating have been studied in 9-year-olds; the dilator response to ACh as assessed by laser Doppler flowmetry in low-birthweight children was only 40% of that in normal-birthweight children (Martin *et al.* 2000). The same group later undertook a similar study in which they compared children born at term to those born prematurely, and found the relationship previously described was absent in the premature group (Norman and Martin 2003). A subsequent study in 3-month-old infants, by a different group but using the same methodological approach, showed the maximal hyperaemic response (which is partially endothelium-dependent) was reduced in low-birthweight children, whereas the ACh response was unaffected (Goh *et al.* 2001). A further investigation of prepubertal children, in which capillary recruitment to heating or ACh was assessed by videomicrosopy, also showed defects in responses to both stimuli in those children of low birthweight, but this was not related to any defect in insulin sensitivity (Ijzerman *et al.* 2002). Exaggerated catch-up growth has also been linked to poor endothelial function. Premature infants who showed rapid catch-up in the first two weeks of life demonstrate reduced brachial artery endothelium-dependent dilatation at age 13–16 years. Interestingly, these children were also insulin-resistant, suggesting that early endothelial dysfunction could play a role in the evolution of this condition (Singhal and Lucas 2004, Singhal *et al.* 2004a). Alteration in capillary density (capillary rarefaction) is unlikely to provide an explanation for these observations, or indeed for an elevation of blood pressure, as a recent study has shown no association between birthweight and capillary density as assessed by video capillaroscopy in dorsal index-finger skin of two cohorts: healthy 6- to 16-year-olds and healthy 24-year-olds (Irving *et al.* 2004).

Taken together, these observations make it clear that endothelial function can be altered by aspects of early development. In adults endothelial dysfunction relates to increased risk of cardiovascular and metabolic diseases. Whether the dysfunction is a cause or an effect of disease, or both, is unknown. Nor it is known whether the perturbations of the early environment affect endothelial cell phenotype directly, or via some other intervening mechanism. Despite this uncertainty, measures of endothelial cell function have an important role in diagnosis and human research.

Markers of endothelial cell activation and the inflammatory response

Few investigators of developmental programming in humans have attempted to measure endothelial or inflammatory markers, although increased expression of cell-adhesion molecules and pro-thrombotic factors are intimately linked to cardiovascular disease. Proposed stimuli include oxidised lipids, cytokines and C-reactive protein (CRP), a significant cardiovascular risk factor (Szmitko *et al.* 2003a, 2003b). Goodfellow *et al.* (1998) found no evidence of a correlation between birthweight and serum concentrations of von Willebrand factor, a marker of endothelial cell activation in fit young adults, whereas a smaller study found higher concentrations in low-birthweight subjects (McAllister *et al.* 1999). Adolescents born prematurely and fed formula feed in neonatal life have higher concentrations of CRP than those fed bank breast milk (Singhal *et al.* 2004b), indicating that fat-rich formula feed in early life may contribute to cardiovascular risk. A negative association between birthweight and adulthood CRP has also recently been reported in a large cohort of adults; the effect remained after adjustment for potential confounders, although it was relatively small as a large (1 kg) increase in birthweight was associated with only a small (10.7%) decrease in CRP (Sattar *et al.* 2004). An inverse association between low birthweight and plasma concentrations of fibrinogen (Martyn *et al.* 1995a) has also been observed, although a recent study comparing monozygotic and dizygotic twins has suggested that this relationship may depend entirely on genetic influences (Ijzerman *et al.* 2003). Others have reported an association between low birthweight and the endothelial maker plasminogen activator inhibitor 1 (PAI1) in middle-aged men (Byberg *et al.* 2000). Considerably more research is needed on the role of inflammatory processes in the changes in endothelial function associated with disease.

Vascular compliance

Studies of compliance in humans are confounded by the fact that hypertension can lead to a secondary alteration in artery stiffness (remodelling). Therefore investigations aiming to assess whether compliance can be independently influenced during development are best undertaken in young individuals before the development of hypertension, and there is some evidence of an association from such studies. One study in 9-year-old low-birthweight children has reported increased carotid artery stiffness compared with normal-birthweight controls (Martin *et al.* 2000), and another in children (mean age 8 years) has found that, amongst those born preterm, only the children that were growth-restricted for gestational age at delivery demonstrated reduced compliance (and also raised blood pressure) (Norman and Martin 2003). An investigation of 20–28-year-olds has suggested that extended breast-feeding (and therefore prolonged exposure to a fat-rich diet) is also linked to reduced arterial distensibility (Leeson *et al.* 2001b). In adult populations, an inverse association between birth size and pulse-wave velocity (PWV) of the femoral and radial arteries (an estimate of compliance) was reported in middle-aged men and women (Martyn *et al.* 1995b), but others have found no relationship (Kumeran *et al.* 2000, Montgomery *et al.* 2000). A recent study, also using PWV analysis, has investigated 281 subjects (16 women) at a mean age of 36 years. The authors reported that lower birthweight was related to reduced carotid, femoral and brachial artery compliance, but that this could only partially explain the association between low birthweight and the elevated blood pressure also found, i.e. birthweight was independently linked to both variables (Te Velde *et al.* 2004).

Studies of vascular function in developmental programming in animals

Animal models

Several animal models of developmental programming have now been employed, using a wide range of dietary manipulations of the mother. These models can vary greatly in both the severity and the duration of the insult, as well as the gestational window to which they are targeted. However, despite the existence of such a broad range of models, they are on the whole associated with cardiovascular dysfunction in adult offspring. These will now briefly be summarised.

Maternal protein restriction

The protein-restriction model during pregnancy was developed in the early 1980s and has been utilised as a model of intrauterine growth restriction (IUGR) in the rat (Resnick and Morgane 1983). Whilst protein availability is not necessarily low in the Western diet, the importance of dietary protein has been demonstrated by close regulation of its intake in both rats and humans (Simpson *et al.* 2003), and the model may mimic conditions similar to those of the developing world.

The restriction of dietary protein during pregnancy alters the maternal cardiovascular adaptations which characterise normal rat pregnancy, impairing both the rise in plasma volume and the increase in cardiac output (Rosso and Streeter 1979). Despite these maternal effects, and employment of protein deprivation in the rat dam as a model of IUGR, the restriction of dietary protein during pregnancy does not uniformly lead to reductions in birthweight (Resnick and Morgane 1983, Langley and Jackson 1994, Brawley *et al.* 2003). However, despite the inconsistent reports on birthweight, systolic blood pressure as assessed by tail cuff measurement has been seen to be consistently elevated in this model (Langley and Jackson 1994, Tonkiss *et al.* 1998, Kwong *et al.* 2000, Woods *et al.* 2001, Brawley *et al.* 2003). However, a report by Tonkiss *et al.* (1998) showed normal blood pressure by remote recording in conscious animals using radiotelemetry, and reported that the blood pressure was raised only when the animals were stressed, which may be indicative of developmental programming of an abnormal stressor response.

The renin–angiotensin system has been implicitly linked to the raised blood pressure in the protein-restriction model, with raised plasma angiotensin converting enzyme (ACE) levels noted (Langley and Jackson 1994), a more pronounced pressor response to angiotensin II (Ang II) and prevention of hypertension by pre-treatment with captopril or the AT1 receptor antagonist losartan (Langley-Evans and Jackson 1995, Sherman and Langley-Evans 2000). Furthermore, renal abnormalities, such as decreased kidney size and glomerular and nephron number, are also present (Langley-Evans et al. 1999, Woods et al. 2001, McMullen et al. 2004).

Maternal global dietary restriction

Many investigators have determined the effects of reducing the maternal dietary intake on offspring vascular function. Dietary deprivation has been used as a model for IUGR and also has relevance to the diet of developing countries.

In the late-gestation fetal sheep, HPA responses are decreased following an early-gestation dietary restriction (Hawkins et al. 1999). Fetal mean arterial blood pressure is decreased in restricted fetuses, with a lower operation point for the baroreflex (Hawkins et al. 2000a). In contrast, increased blood pressure and plasma ACTH have been reported following a later dietary challenge (Edwards and McMillen 2001, Edwards et al. 2002). Moderate restriction of maternal nutrients during gestation does not affect the birthweight of lambs (Hanson et al. 1999), although blood pressure is raised both in young lambs (Hawkins et al. 2000b) and in 3-year-old sheep, before feeding (Gopalakrishnan et al. 2004).

As is the case for protein restriction, global nutrient restriction in rats leads to an attenuation of maternal cardiovascular adaptations to pregnancy (Rosso and Kava 1980, Ahokas et al. 1984, Dandrea et al. 2002). Unlike the sheep, maternal nutrient restriction in the rat repeatedly produces IUGR and raised systolic blood pressure (Woodall et al. 1996, Vickers et al. 2000, Ozaki et al. 2001 Franco et al. 2002, 2004). How-

ever, some studies have reported no change in blood pressure in the offspring (Holemans et al. 1999). Associated with the raised blood pressure in the offspring of nutrient-restricted dams is an increased heart rate (Woodall et al. 1996, Ozaki et al. 2001) and altered HPA function (Lesage et al. 2001). Similarly in the guinea pig, undernutrition during pregnancy leads to reduced birthweight, raised blood pressure and altered glucose handling in the offspring (Kind et al. 2002, 2003).

Maternal fat feeding

Restriction protocols may mimic the challenge faced in developing nations, or that faced by the fetus in situations of maternal dieting, pre-eclampsia or placental disease, but they do not mimic dietary intakes of modern Western society, where fat accounts for approximately 40% of energy intake. Several groups have therefore investigated the effects of a diet high in fat, or a diet which invokes maternal hypercholesterolaemia, both of which may give insight into potential mechanisms for the aetiology of cardiovascular disease in Western societies (Napoli et al. 2000, Ghosh et al. 2001, Palinski et al. 2001, Khan et al. 2003, 2004). Thus diets rich in animal lard (Khan et al. 2003), saturated fat (Siemelink et al. 2002) or cholesterol (Palinski et al 2001) have been fed to rodents and the offspring cardiovascular phenotype characterised.

Birthweight in animals from fat-fed dams is not consistent; animals exposed to high saturated fat during gestation and suckling may be smaller (Langley-Evans 1996) or of the same (Siemelink et al. 2002) birthweight compared with controls. Maternal high-fat or cholesterol over-feeding protocols in rodents result in an offspring phenotype that closely resembles the human metabolic syndrome (Armitage et al. 2004a). Abnormal glucose homeostasis (Guo and Jen 1995, Taylor et al. 2004a), increased blood pressure (Langley-Evans 1996, Khan et al. 2003), abnormal serum lipid profiles (Karnik et al. 1989, Guo and Jen 1995, Khan et al. 2003), increased adiposity (Guo and Jen 1995, Khan et al. 2005), proatherogenic and atherosclerosis-like lesions (Palinski *et al.* 2001), and reduced acetylcholine-induced vasodilatation (Khan *et al.* 2003, 2004, 2005) have all been reported.

Evidence for vascular endothelial dysfunction

Protein restriction during development leads to endothelial dysfunction in adult rat offspring, as determined by endothelium-dependent vasodilator function in a Mulvany–Halpern myograph (Brawley *et al.* 2003, Torrens *et al.* 2003). Data from the low-protein feeding protocol indicate that small resistance arteries (approximately 250 µm luminal diameter) of the adult offspring are prone to endothelial dysfunction, and show blunted vasodilatation in response to ACh, but that conduit arteries such as the aorta are not affected (Torrens *et al.* 2003). Lamireau and colleagues (2002) have also shown reduced endothelium-dependent vasodilatation of cerebral microvessels (50 µm) in offspring of low-protein-fed dams. Interestingly, these reports highlight increases in smooth muscle sensitivity to NO (a key factor in endothelium-dependent vasodilatation), suggestive of compensatory mechanisms, at least in terms of vasodilatation.

Intriguing as it is, the current data do not give insight into any possible adaptive advantage served by reducing endothelium-dependent dilatation in response to protein restriction, although the endothelium is indirectly involved in the processes regulating blood flow, nutrient delivery, growth and metabolism during development (Gluckman and Hanson in press). In addition to the effects noted in adult rats, in the mid-gestation fetal sheep, femoral endothelium-dependent vasodilatation is also impaired, suggesting reduced NO bioavailability (Nishina *et al.* 2003). Impaired femoral dilatation has also been reported in the late-gestation embryonic chick in response to hypoxia (Ruijtenbeek *et al.* 2003). It could be hypothesised therefore that reduced femoral dilatation in the developing fetus is an important adaptation during conditions of nutrient stress, reducing blood flow to peripheral tissues with high metabolic activity (Giussani *et al.* 1993).

Torrens *et al.* (2002) have recently shown transgenerational transmission of risk factors for cardiovascular and metabolic disease to F_2 offspring from both male and female F_1 parentage. Poor maternal adaptation to pregnancy provides one possible explanation for these effects observed in the F_2 offspring. Raised maternal blood pressure in women is associated with reduced birthweight and higher blood pressure in the offspring (Walker *et al.* 1998). Hypertension during pregnancy alters fetal growth and development and could contribute to the influence of the female on the F_2 phenotype. Putative effects of maternal diet on oocyte development would only be relevant to transmission through the female lineage, as in males spermatogenesis is continuous throughout life (Goyal *et al.* 2003).

As fetal nutritional imbalance is unlikely to have consequences on male gametogenesis or the in-utero environment, transmission down the paternal lineage could be epigenetic and may, according to current hypothesis, reflect changes in DNA methylation status (Rees *et al.* 2000, Lillycrop *et al.* 2005). Alterations in DNA methylation are heritable, avoiding demethylation during gametogenesis as has been demonstrated in the mouse at both the *Agouti* and *Axin^{Fu}* alleles (Morgan *et al.* 1999, Rakyan *et al.* 2003). Folate can provide methyl groups for DNA methylation, and maternal dietary folate supplementation has been shown to prevent obesity, insulin resistance and cancer in the offspring of the Agouti mouse (Waterland and Jirtle 2004). Importantly, Dance *et al.* (2003) have shown that maternal folate supplementation prevents the raised blood pressure and endothelial dysfunction in the adult rat offspring of protein-restricted dams. Furthermore, there is evidence of environmental interactions in the paternal transmission of risk factors to the F_2 offspring, hinting at epigenetic inheritance (Kaati *et al.* 2002). Similar claims have been made for the transgenerational effects of glucocorticoid administration on metabolic homeostasis (Drake *et al.* 2005).

Adult offspring of maternal Wistar rats which were semi-starved (fed 50% of control diet) from mid to late gestation (when fetal growth is maximal) and through lactation demonstrated significantly reduced constrictor responses, reduced endothelium-dependent relaxation and enhanced sensitivity to the endothelium-independent dilator sodium nitroprusside (Holemans *et al.* 1999). The difference in maximal contraction reflects smaller vascular smooth-muscle mass in growth-retarded offspring, and reduced dilator responses may be indicative of reduced synthesis of NO. In a similar study (Wistar rats fed 50% of normal intake during pregnancy), increased blood pressure and decreased endothelial-derived relaxation in aortic rings were noted. Furthermore, mRNA expression of endothelial nitric oxide synthase (eNOS) was lower in restricted males compared with control males at 14 weeks (Franco *et al.* 2002), and oxidative stress (increased superoxide synthesis by NADPH oxidase activity) was increased due to activation of the angiotensin II type 1 receptor (Franco *et al.* 2003). An increase in superoxide generation, which to our knowledge has not been investigated in any other model, could contribute to reduced endothelium-dependent dilatation through reduction of bioavailable NO or tissue oxidative damage. Ozaki *et al.* (2001) found that male offspring of globally restricted dams (30% reduction) had modest vascular abnormalities (increased maximal thromboxane-mimetic-induced contraction and enhanced sensitivity to potassium) at 200 days but no alteration to endothelium-dependent vasodilatation. Taken together, these studies may suggest that the severity of maternal caloric restriction is linked to the offspring endothelial phenotype.

Maternal diets rich in animal fat also produce endothelial dysfunction in offspring, evidenced by reduced endothelium-dependent dilatation in small mesenteric resistance vessels (Ghosh *et al.* 2001, Khan *et al.* 2003), and also in aorta (Armitage *et al.* 2004b). Smooth-muscle sensitivity to nitric oxide was not altered in these studies but a primary defect in eNOS was also indicated by preliminary evidence from Affymetrix gene array analysis showing lower eNOS expression in aortas of 1-year-old offspring from lard-exposed dams compared with controls (Armitage *et al.* 2004b). The mechanism underlying endothelial dysfunction in the offspring fed the normal diet has been further characterised by our group. The blunted endothelial-dependent vasodilatation observed in small mesenteric arteries from offspring of lard-fed dams appears to be underpinned by a reduction in EDHF rather than an NO or prostacyclin deficit (Taylor *et al.* 2004b). Reduced arachidonic acid concentration in aorta (Ghosh *et al.* 2001) may underlie the EDHF defect, as arachidonic acid is a precursor of a putative EDHF.

Khan and colleagues (2004) have recently found evidence for 'predictive adaptive responses' in this model. Adult rats maintained on the same fat-rich diet that they were exposed to in utero (continued fat-feeding) demonstrated improved endothelium-dependent vasodilatation compared with animals adapted to a control diet in utero and subsequently exposed to a fat-rich diet in adulthood. A similar observation has been made in piglets. Sows were fed either a control or a pro-atherogenic diet during pregnancy and suckling, then piglets fed either the same diet as their mother or crossed to the opposite diet. Pigs exposed to the atherogenic diet in utero appeared to be protected from the development of aortic fatty streaks when fed an atherogenic diet in adulthood, compared with those that were exposed to the control diet in utero and the atherogenic diet in adulthood (Norman and LeVeen 2001).

We have also examined whether maternal fat-rich diets induce transgenerational deficits. In contrast to that observed in the low-protein model, the aortic endothelial dysfunction present in the F_1 offspring of lard-fed dams did not persist to the F_2 generation (Armitage *et al.* 2004c).

Endothelial cell activation

Endothelial cell activation has not often been studied in offspring from models of maternal nutritional intervention. This may partly reflect the relative resistance of rat endothelium to activation stimuli but requires further study given the obvious parallel between human and animal studies in relation to endothelium-dependent dilator function. One group has described increased NADPH oxidase activity (Franco *et al.* 2003) and decreased antioxidant defence (decreased superoxide dismutase activity) (Franco *et al.* 2002) in offspring of nutritionally restricted animals; these are likely accompaniments to endothelial cell activation. There is limited evidence in adult offspring of protein-malnourished dams for increased sensitivity to inflammatory stimuli; Merezak demonstrated enhanced islet cell susceptibility to a combination of the cytokines IL1B, TNFα and IFNγ in offspring of protein-malnourished (8% protein) rats (Merezak *et al.* 2004). Should this also occur at the level of the endothelium cell, endothelial cell activation might also occur. However, a recent study has assessed acute inflammatory responses to a pleurisy-inducing agent (carrageenan) in offspring of protein-restricted rat dams and these animals mounted a *reduced* inflammatory response (Barja-Fidalgo *et al.* 2003).

Without doubt endothelium-dependent relaxation is an accompaniment of most of the developmental programming models in rodents. Given the pivotal role proposed for reduced endothelium-dependent dilatation in insulin resistance and type 2 diabetes (Meigs *et al.* 2004) these observations, coupled with the evidence for insulin resistance, provide a compelling parallel to human metabolic syndrome.

Vascular compliance

Evidence for alteration in vascular compliance is limited in animal models of developmental programming. Berry and Looker (1973) demonstrated that intrauterine growth restriction (induced by maternal methotrexate administration on day 15 of pregnancy followed by folinic acid administration as a specific methotrexate antagonist 16 hours later) resulted in offspring of low birthweight without catch-up growth. Collagen and elastin content were reduced in offspring of methotrexate-treated animals at 26 weeks of age, and it was hypothesised that failure to synthesise adequate amounts of elastin during a critical period cannot be rectified later in life. Altered smooth-muscle structure, particularly in myosin heavy chain (SM_2) content may also lead to

altered compliance, but this has not been investigated. The measurement of vascular distensibility can readily be undertaken in isolated arteries, and assessment of compliance and collagen, elastin and smooth-muscle content in young and adult offspring would be worthwhile in the different animal models.

We have reported reduced passive elasticity in the aortas of offspring of lard-fed dams at 6 months of age. Aortas were mounted on an organ bath containing calcium-free physiological salt solution and subjected to cumulative stretches to assess the force generated by stretch. Offspring of the fat-fed dams demonstrated an increase in force across the incremental stretches, indicative of altered matrix or smooth-muscle elasticity (Armitage *et al.* 2004b). As there were no apparent changes to smooth-muscle morphology in these vessels (unpublished observation), and we have reported altered collagen mRNA expression in these vessels by Affymetrix microarray (Armitage *et al.* 2004b), we may hypothesise that remodelling of the extracellular matrix is responsible for the observed changes.

Other parameters of cardiovascular dysfunction

Endothelial dysfunction may play a role in elevation of the blood pressure and insulin resistance in developmental programming. However, blood pressure could also rise through enhanced constrictor responses in the vasculature, thereby increasing peripheral resistance, or from elevation of the cardiac output. Several groups have assessed constrictor function of isolated arteries, and other than one report of enhanced endothelin constrictor responses in fetal sheep exposed to glucocorticoids (Molnar *et al.* 2003) there is little evidence for a fundamental defect in constrictor function amongst the different animal models. Emerging evidence has implicated altered sympathetic activity, which has been associated with essential hypertension in humans, and which may contribute to raised blood pressure in some models. The adult offspring of nutritionally deprived sheep show altered baroreceptor responses (Gardner *et al.* 2004) and there is evidence in low-birthweight humans of altered sympathetic outflow

(Phillips and Barker 1997). Chronically hypoxic chick embryos also develop altered sympathetic function (Ruijtenbeek *et al.* 2000), and adrenergic responses are altered in the vasculature of rats subjected to antenatal stress (Young *et al.* 1985). In normotensive male offspring of rat dams fed a fat-rich diet we have also observed a reduction of basal heart rate, which may be indicative of an altered baroreceptor response (Khan *et al.* 2003).

Conclusion

Alterations in the development and function of the peripheral vasculature, induced by the quality of the early environment, are fundamental to DOHaD. It is now clear that these vascular phenotypes respond very differently to a range of stimuli in later life. Intriguingly, a common feature of the animal models used is perturbed vascular function, especially endothelial dysfunction. It appears that the endothelium is particularly sensitive to such challenges. Endothelial dysfunction is an early marker of human disease but is probably part of a vicious circle of cause and effect. Despite the gaps in our knowledge of underlying mechanisms, DOHaD research on the peripheral vasculature is now suggesting productive areas for early diagnosis and intervention.

ACKNOWLEDGMENTS

The authors are grateful to the British Heart Foundation for support.

REFERENCES

Ahokas, R. A., Reynolds, S. L., Anderson, G. D. and Lipshitz, J. (1984). Maternal organ distribution of cardiac output in the diet-restricted pregnant rat. *J. Nutr.*, **114**, 2262–8.

Anderson, T. J., Uehata, A., Gerhard, M. D. *et al.* (1995). Close relation of endothelial function in the human coronary and peripheral circulations. *J. Am. Coll. Cardiol.*, **26**, 1235–41.

Armitage, J. A., Khan, I. Y., Taylor, P. D., Nathanielsz, P. W. and Poston, L. (2004a). Developmental programming of metabolic syndrome by maternal nutritional imbalance: how strong is the evidence from experimental models in animals? *J. Physiol.*, **561**, 355–77.

Armitage, J. A., Jensen, R., Taylor, P. D. and Poston, L. (2004b). Exposure to a high fat diet during gestation and weaning results in reduced elasticity and endothelial function as well as altered gene expression and fatty acid content of rat aorta. *J. Soc. Gynecol. Investig.*, **11**, 183A.

Armitage, J. A., Ishibashi, A., Taylor, P. D. and Poston, L. (2004c). Developmental programming of aortic dysfunction by maternal fat-feeding does not persist to the second generation. *J. Physiol.*, **565P**, C165.

Barja-Fidalgo, C., Souza, E. P., Silva, S. V. *et al.* (2003). Impairment of inflammatory response in adult rats submitted to maternal undernutrition during early lactation: role of insulin and glucocorticoid. *Inflamm. Res.*, **52**, 470–6.

Berry, C. L. and Looker, T. (1973). An alteration in the chemical structure of the aortic wall induced by a finite period of growth inhibition. *J. Anat.*, **114**, 83–94.

Black, H. R. (2004). The paradigm has shifted to systolic blood pressure. *J. Hum. Hypertens.*, **18**, S3–7.

Boo, Y. C. and Jo, H. (2003). Flow-dependent regulation of endothelial nitric oxide synthase: role of protein kinases. *Am. J. Physiol. Cell. Physiol.*, **285**, C499–508.

Brawley, L., Itoh, S., Torrens, C., Barker, A., Bertram, C., Poston, L. and Hanson, M. (2003). Dietary protein restriction in pregnancy induces hypertension and vascular defects in rat male offspring. *Pediatr. Res.*, **54**, 83–90.

Busse, R., Edwards, G., Feletou, M., Fleming, I., Vanhoutte, P. M. and Weston, A. H. (2002). EDHF: bringing the concepts together. *Trends Pharmacol. Sci.*, **23**, 374–80.

Byberg, L., McKeigue, P. M., Zethelius, B. and Lithell, H. O. (2000). Birth weight and the insulin resistance syndrome: association of low birth weight with truncal obesity and raised plasminogen activator inhibitor-1 but not with abdominal obesity or plasma lipid disturbances. *Diabetologia*, **43**, 54–60.

Chan, N. and Vallance, P. (2002). Nitric oxide. In *An Introduction to Vascular Biology* (ed. B. Hunt, L. Poston, M. Schachter and A. Halliday). Cambridge: Cambridge University Press, pp. 216–58.

Dance, C. S., Brawley, L., Dunn, R. L., Poston, L., Jackson, A. A. and Hanson, M. A. (2003). Folate supplementation of a protein restricted diet during pregnancy: restoration of vascular dysfunction in small mesenteric arteries of female adult rat offspring. *Pediatr. Res.*, **53**, 19A.

Dandrea, J., Cooper, S., Ramsay, M. M. *et al.* (2002). The effects of pregnancy and maternal nutrition on the maternal renin–angiotensin system in sheep. *Exp. Physiol.*, **87**, 353–9.

Drake, A. J., Walker, B. R. and Seckl, J. R. (2005). Intergenerational consequences of fetal programming by in utero exposure to glucocorticoids in rats. *Am. J. Physiol. Regul. Integr. Comp. Physiol.*, **288**, R34–8.

Edwards, L. J. and McMillen, I. C. (2001). Maternal undernutrition increases arterial blood pressure in the sheep fetus during late gestation. *J. Physiol.*, **533**, 561–70.

Edwards, L. J., Bryce, A. E., Coulter, C. L. and McMillen, I. C. (2002). Maternal undernutrition throughout pregnancy increases adrenocorticotrophin receptor and steroidogenic acute regulatory protein gene expression in the adrenal gland of twin fetal sheep during late gestation. *Mol. Cell. Endocrinol.*, **196**, 1–10.

Franco, M. C., Arruda, R. M., Dantas, A. P. *et al.* (2002). Intrauterine undernutrition: expression and activity of the endothelial nitric oxide synthase in male and female adult offspring. *Cardiovasc. Res.*, **56**, 145–53.

Franco, M. C., Akamine, E. H., Di Marco, G. S. *et al.* (2003). NADPH oxidase and enhanced superoxide generation in intrauterine undernourished rats: involvement of the renin–angiotensin system. *Cardiovasc. Res.*, **59**, 767–75.

Franco, M. C., Akamine, E. H., Fortes, Z. B. *et al.* (2004). Tetrahydrobiopterin improves endothelial dysfunction and vascular oxidative stress in microvessels of intrauterine undernourished rats. *J. Physiol.*, **558**, 239–48.

Gardner, D. S., Pearce, S., Dandrea, J. *et al.* (2004). Periimplantation undernutrition programs blunted angiotensin II evoked baroreflex responses in young adult sheep. *Hypertension*, **43**, 1290–6.

Ghosh, P., Bitsanis, D., Ghebremeskel, K., Crawford, M. A. and Poston, L. (2001). Abnormal fatty acid composition and small artery function in offspring of rats fed a high fat diet in pregnancy. *J. Physiol.*, **533**, 815–22.

Giussani, D. A., Spencer, J. A., Moore, P. J., Bennet, L. and Hanson, M. A. (1993). Afferent and efferent components of the cardiovascular reflex responses to acute hypoxia in term fetal sheep. *J. Physiol.*, **461**, 431–49.

Gluckman, P. D. and Hanson, M. A. (in press). Endothelial dysfunction and cardiovascular disease: the role of PARs. *Heart*.

Goh, K. L., Shore, A. C., Quinn, M. and Tooke, J. E. (2001). Impaired microvascular vasodilatory function in 3-month-old infants of low birth weight. *Diabetes Care*, **24**, 1102–7.

Goodfellow, J., Bellamy, N. F., Gorman, S. T. *et al.* (1998). Endothelial function is impaired in fit young adults of low birthweight. *Cardiovasc. Res.*, **40**, 600–6.

Gopalakrishnan, G. S., Gardner, D. S., Rhind, S. M. *et al.* (2004). Programming of adult cardiovascular function after early maternal undernutrition in sheep. *Am. J. Physiol. Regul. Integr. Comp. Physiol.*, **287**, R12–20.

Goyal, H. O., Robateau, A., Braden, T. D., Williams, C. S., Srivastava, K. K. and Ali, K. (2003). Neonatal estrogen exposure of male rats alters reproductive functions at adulthood. *Biol. Reprod.*, **68**, 2081–91.

Guo, F. and Jen, K. L. (1995). High-fat feeding during pregnancy and lactation affects offspring metabolism in rats. *Physiol. Behav.*, **57**, 681–6.

Halcox, J. P. J., Schenke, W. H., Zalos, G. *et al.* (2002). Prognostic value of coronary vascular endothelial dysfunction. *Circulation*, **106**, 653–8.

Hanson, M. A., Hawkins, P., Ozaki, T. *et al.* (1999). Effects of experimental dietary manipulation during early pregnancy on the cardiovascular and endocrine function in fetal sheep and young lambs. In *Fetal Programming: Consequences for Health in Later Life* (ed. D. J. P. Barker and T. Wheeler). London: RCOG Press, pp. 365–73.

Hawkins, P., Steyn, C., McGarrigle, H. H. *et al.* (1999). Effect of maternal nutrient restriction in early gestation on development of the hypothalamic–pituitary–adrenal axis in fetal sheep at 0.8–0.9 of gestation. *J. Endocrinol.*, **163**, 553–61.

Hawkins, P., Steyn, C., Ozaki, T., Saito, T., Noakes, D. E. and Hanson, M. A. (2000a). Effect of maternal undernutrition in early gestation on ovine fetal blood pressure and cardiovascular reflexes. *Am. J. Physiol. Regul. Integr. Comp. Physiol.*, **279**, R340–8.

Hawkins, P., Steyn, C., McGarrigle, H. H. *et al.* (2000b). Cardiovascular and hypothalamic–pituitary–adrenal axis development in late gestation fetal sheep and young lambs following modest maternal nutrient restriction in early gestation. *Reprod. Fertil. Dev.*, **12**, 443–56.

Holemans, K., Gerber, R., Meurrens, K., De, Clerck, F., Poston, L. and Van Assche, F. A. (1999). Maternal food restriction in the second half of pregnancy affects vascular function but not blood pressure of rat female offspring. *Br. J. Nutr.*, **81**, 73–9.

Hsueh, W. A., Lyon, C. J. and Quinones, M. J. (2004). Insulin resistance and endothelium. *Am. J. Med.*, **117**, 109–17.

Hunt, B. J. and Jurd, K. M. (2002). The endothelium in health and disease. In *An Introduction to Vascular Biology* (ed. B. Hunt, L. Poston, M. Schachter and A. Halliday). Cambridge: Cambridge University Press , pp. 186–215.

Ijzerman, R. G., van Weissenbruch, M. M., Voordouw, J. J. *et al.* (2002). The association between birth weight and capillary recruitment is independent of blood pressure and insulin sensitivity: a study in prepubertal children. *J. Hypertens.*, **20**, 1957–63.

Ijzerman, R. G., Stehouwer, C. D., de Geus, E. J., Kluft, C. and Boomsma, D. I. (2003). The association between birth weight and plasma fibrinogen is abolished after the elimination of genetic influences *J. Thromb. Haemost.*, **1**, 239–42.

Intengan, H. D., Thibault, G., Li, J. S. and Schiffrin, E. L. (1999). Resistance artery mechanics, structure, and extracellular components in spontaneously hypertensive rats: effects of angiotensin receptor antagonism and converting enzyme inhibition. *Circulation*, **100**, 2267–75.

Irving, R. J., Shore, A. C., Belton, N. R., Elton, R. A., Webb, D. J. and Walker, B. R. (2004). Low birth weight predicts higher blood pressure but not dermal capillary density in two populations. *Hypertension*, **43**, 610–13.

Kaati, G., Bygren, L. O. and Edvinsson, S. (2002). Cardiovascular and diabetes mortality determined by nutrition during parents' and grandparents' slow growth period. *Eur. J. Hum. Genet.*, **10**, 682–8.

Karnik, H. B., Sonawane, B. R., Adkins, J. S. and Mohla, S. (1989). High dietary fat feeding during perinatal development of rats alters hepatic drug metabolism of progeny. *Dev. Pharmacol. Ther.*, **14**, 135–40.

Khan, I. Y., Taylor, P. D., Dekou, V. *et al.* (2003). Gender-linked hypertension in offspring of lard-fed pregnant rats. *Hypertension*, **41**, 168–75.

Khan, I. Y., Dekou, V., Hanson, M., Poston, L. and Taylor, P. (2004). Predictive adaptive responses to maternal high fat diet prevent endothelial dysfunction but not hypertension in adult rat offspring. *Circulation*, **110**, 1097–102.

Khan, I. Y., Dekou, V., Douglas, G. *et al.* (2005). A high-fat diet during rat pregnancy or suckling induces cardiovascular dysfunction in adult offspring. *Am. J. Physiol. Regul. Integr. Comp. Physiol.*, **288**, R127–33.

Kind, K. L., Simonetta, G., Clifton, P. M., Robinson, J. S. and Owens, J. A. (2002). Effect of maternal feed restriction on blood pressure in the adult guinea pig. *Exp. Physiol.*, **87**, 469–77.

Kind, K. L., Clifton, P. M., Grant, P. A. *et al.* (2003). Effect of maternal feed restriction during pregnancy on glucose tolerance in the adult guinea pig. *Am. J. Physiol. Regul. Integr. Comp. Physiol.*, **284**, R140–52.

Kingwell, B. A. and Gatzka, C. D. (2002). Aterial stiffness and prediction of cardiovascular risk. *J. Hypertens.*, **20**, 2337–40.

Kumeran, K., Fall, C., Martyn, C. N., Vijayakumar, M., Stein, C. and Shier, R. (2000). Blood pressure, arterial compliance and left ventricular mass: no relation to small size at birth in south Indian adults. *Heart*, **83**, 272–7.

Kwong, W. Y., Wild, A. E., Roberts, P., Willis, A. C. and Fleming, T. P. (2000). Maternal undernutrition during the preimplanta-tion period of rat development causes blastocyst abnormal-ities and programming of postnatal hypertension. *Development*, **127**, 4195–202.

Lamireau, D., Nuyt, A. M., Hou, X. *et al.* (2002). Altered vascular function in fetal programming of hypertension. *Stroke*, **33**, 2992–8.

Landmesser, U., Hornig, B. and Drexler, H. (2004). Endothelial function: a critical determinant in atherosclerosis? *Circulation*, **109**, 27–33.

Langley, S. C. and Jackson, A. A. (1994). Increased systolic blood pressure in adult rats induced by fetal exposure to maternal low protein diets. *Clin. Sci.*, **86**, 217–22.

Langley-Evans, S. C. (1996). Intrauterine programming of hyper-tension in the rat: nutrient interactions. *Comp. Biochem. Physiol. A Physiol.*, **114**, 327–33.

Langley-Evans, S. C. and Jackson, A. A. (1995). Captopril nor-malises systolic blood pressure in rats with hypertension induced by fetal exposure to maternal low protein diets. *Comp. Biochem. Physiol. A. Physiol.*, **110**, 223–8.

Langley-Evans, S. C., Welham, S. J. and Jackson, A. A. (1999). Fetal exposure to a maternal low protein diet impairs nephroge-nesis and promotes hypertension in the rat. *Life Sci.*, **64**, 965–74.

Leeson, C. P., Whincupp, P. H., Cook, D. G. *et al.* (1997). Flow-mediated dilatation in 9–11 year old children: the influ-ence of intrauterine and childhood factors. *Circulation*, **96**, 2233–8.

Leeson, C. P., Katternhorm, M., Morley, R., Lucas, A. and Dean-field, J. E. (2001a). Impact of low birthweight and cardiovas-cular risk factors on endothelial function in early adult life. *Circulation*, **103**, 1264–8.

Leeson, C. P., Katternhorm, M., Deanfield, J. E. and Lucas, A. (2001b). Duration of breast feeding and arterial distensibil-ity in early life: population based study. *BMJ*, **332**, 643–7.

Lesage, J., Blondeau, B., Grino, M., Breant, B. and Dupouy, J. P. (2001). Maternal undernutrition during late gestation induces fetal overexposure to glucocorticoids and intrauter-ine growth retardation, and disturbs the hypothalamo-pituitary adrenal axis in the newborn rat. *Endocrinology*, **142**, 1692–702.

Libby, P. (2002). Inflammation and atherosclerosis. *Nature*, **420**, 868–74.

Lillycrop, K. A., Phillips, G. S., Jackson, A. A., Hanson, M. A. and Burdge, G. C. (2005). Dietary protein restriction of preg-nant rats induces and folic acid supplementation prevents epigenetic modification of hepatic gene expression in the offspring. *J. Nutr.*, **135**, 1382–6.

Martin, H., Hu, J., Gennser, G. and Norman, M. (2000). Impaired endothelial function and increased carotid stiffness in

9-year old children with low birthweight. *Circulation*, **102**, 2739–44.

Martyn, C. N. and Greenwald, S. E. (1997). Impaired synthesis of elastin in walls of aorta and large conduit arteries during early development as an initiating event in pathogenesis of systemic hypertension. *Lancet*, **350**, 953–5.

Martyn, C. N., Meade, T. W., Stirling, Y. and Barker, D. J. P. (1995a). Plasma concentrations of fibrinogen and factor VII in adult life and their relation to intra-uterine growth. *Br. J. Haematol.*, **89**, 142–6.

Martyn, C. N., Barker, D. J. P., Jespersen, S., Greenwald, S., Osmond, C. and Berry, C. (1995b). Growth in utero, adult blood pressure, and arterial compliance. *Br. Heart J.*, **73**, 116–21.

McAllister, A. S., Atkinson, A. B., Johnston, G. D. and McCance, D. R. (1999). Relationship of endothelial function to birth weight in humans. *Diabetes Care*, **22**, 2061–6.

McMullen, S., Gardner, D. S. and Langley-Evans, S. C. (2004). Prenatal programming of angiotensin II type 2 receptor expression in the rat. *Br. J. Nutr.*, **91**, 133–40.

McVeigh, G. E., Brennan, G. M., Johnston, G. D. *et al.* (1992). Impaired endothelium-dependent and independent vasodilation in patients with type 2 (non-insulin-dependent) diabetes mellitus. *Diabetologia*, **35**, 771–6.

Meigs, J. B., Hu, F. B., Rifai, N. and Manson, J. E. (2004). Biomarkers of endothelial dysfunction and risk of type 2 diabetes mellitus. *JAMA*, **291**, 1978–86.

Merezak, S., Reusens, B., Renard, A. *et al.* (2004). Effect of maternal low-protein diet and taurine on the vulnerability of adult Wistar rat islets to cytokines. *Diabetologia*, **47**, 669–75.

Molnar, J., Howe, D. C., Nijland, M. J. and Nathanielsz, P. W. (2003). Prenatal dexamethasone leads to both endothelial dysfunction and vasodilatory compensation in sheep. *J. Physiol.*, **547**, 61–6.

Montgomery, A. A., Ben-Sholmo, Y., McCarthy, A., Davies, D., Elwood, P. and Smith, G. D. (2000). Birth size and arterial compliance in young adults. *Lancet*, **355**, 2136–7.

Morgan, H. D., Sutherland, H. G., Martin, D. I. and Whitelaw, E. (1999). Epigenetic inheritance at the agouti locus in the mouse. *Nat. Genet.*, **23**, 314–18.

Napoli, C., Witztum, J. L., Calara, F., de Nigris, F. and Palinski, W. (2000). Maternal hypercholesterolemia enhances atherogenesis in normocholesterolemic rabbits, which is inhibited by antioxidant or lipid-lowering intervention during pregnancy: an experimental model of atherogenic mechanisms in human fetuses. *Circ. Res.*, **87**, 946–52.

Nishina, H., Green, L. R., McGarrigle, H. H., Noakes, D. E., Poston, L. and Hanson, M. A. (2003). Effect of nutritional restriction in early pregnancy on isolated femoral artery function in mid-gestation fetal sheep. *J. Physiol.*, **553**, 637–47.

Norman, J. F., and LeVeen, R. F. (2001). Maternal atherogenic diet in swine is protective against early atherosclerosis development in offspring consuming an atherogenic diet postnatally. *Atherosclerosis*, **157**, 41–7.

Norman, M. and Martin, H. (2003). Preterm birth attenuates association between low birthweight and endothelial dysfunction. *Circulation*, **108**, 996–1001.

Owens, G. K., Kumar, M. S. and Wamhoff, B. R. (2004). Molecular regulation of vascular smooth muscle cell differentiation in development and disease. *Physiol. Rev.*, **84**, 767–801.

Ozaki, T., Nishina, H., Hanson, M. A. and Poston, L. (2001). Dietary restriction in pregnant rats causes gender-related hypertension and vascular dysfunction in offspring. *J. Physiol.*, **530**, 141–52.

Palinski, W., D'Armiento, F. P., Witztum, J. L. *et al.* (2001). Maternal hypercholesterolemia and treatment during pregnancy influence the long-term progression of atherosclerosis in offspring of rabbits. *Circ. Res.*, **89**, 991–6.

Panza, J. A., Casino, P. R., Kilcoyne, C. M. and Quyyumi, A. A. (1993). Role of endothelium-derived nitric oxide in the abnormal endothelium-dependent vascular relaxation of patients with essential hypertension. *Circulation*, **87**, 1468–74.

Phillips, D. I. and Barker, D. J. P. (1997). Association between low birthweight and high resting pulse in adult life: is the sympathetic nervous system involved in programming the insulin resistance syndrome. *Diabet. Med.*, **14**, 673–7.

Rakyan, V. K., Chong, S., Champ, M. E. *et al.* (2003). Transgenerational inheritance of epigenetic states at the murine *Axin^{Fu}* allele occurs after maternal and paternal transmission. *Proc. Nat. Acad. Sci. USA*, **100**, 2538–43.

Rees, W. D., Hay, S. M., Brown, D. S., Antipatis, C. and Palmer, R. M. (2000). Maternal protein deficiency causes hypermethylation of DNA in the livers of rat fetuses. *J. Nutr.*, **130**, 1821–6.

Resnick, O. and Morgane, P. J. (1983). Animal models for small-for-gestational-age (SGA) neonates and infants-at-risk (IAR). *Brain Res.*, **312**, 221–5.

Rosso, P. and Kava, R. (1980). Effects of food restriction on cardiac ouput and blood flow to the uterus and placenta in the pregnant rat. *J. Nutr.*, **110**, 2350–4.

Rosso, P. and Streeter, M. R. (1979). Effects of food or protein restriction on plasma volume expansion in pregnant rats. *J. Nutr.*, **109**, 1887–92.

Ruijtenbeek, K., le Noble, F. A., Janssen, G. M. *et al.* (2000). Chronic hypoxia stimulates periarterial sympathetic nerve development in chicken embryo. *Circulation*, **102**, 2892–7.

Ruijtenbeek, K., Kessels, L. C., De, Mey, J. G. and Blanco, C. E. (2003). Chronic moderate hypoxia and protein malnutrition both induce growth retardation, but have distinct effects on arterial endothelium-dependent reactivity in the chicken embryo. *Pediatr. Res.*, **53**, 573–9.

Sattar, N., McConnachie, A., O'Reilly, D. *et al.* (2004). Inverse association between birth weight and C-reactive protein concentrations in the MIDSPAN Family Study. *Arterioscler. Thromb. Vasc. Biol.*, **24**, 583–7.

Sherman, R. C. and Langley-Evans, S. C. (2000). Antihypertensive treatment in early postnatal life modulates prenatal dietary influences upon blood pressure in the rat. *Clin. Sci.*, **98**, 269–75.

Siemelink, M., Verhoef, A., Dormans, J. A., Span, P. N. and Piersma, A. H. (2002). Dietary fatty acid composition during pregnancy and lactation in the rat programs growth and glucose metabolism in the offspring. *Diabetologia*, **45**, 1397–403.

Simpson, S. J., Batley, R. and Raubenheimer, D. (2003). Geometric analysis of macronutrient intake in humans: the power of protein? *Appetite* **41**, 123–40.

Singhal, A. and Lucas, A. (2004). Early origins of cardiovascular disease: is there a unifying hypothesis? *Lancet*, **363**, 1642–5.

Singhal, A., Cole, T. J., Fewtrell, M. and Lucas, A. (2004a). Breast-milk feeding and lipoprotein profile in adolescents born preterm: follow-up of a prospective randomised study. *Lancet*, **15**, 1571–8.

Singhal, A., Cole, T. J. and Fewtrell, M., Deanfield, J. and Lucas, A. (2004b). Is slower early growth beneficial for long term cardiovascular health? *Circulation*, **109**, 1108–13.

Szmitko, P. E., Wang, C. H., Weisel, R. D. *et al.* (2003a). New markers of inflammation and endothelial cell activation. *Circulation*, **108**, 1917–23.

Szmitko, P. E., Wang, C. H., Weisel, R. D., Jeffries, G. A., Anderson, T. J. and Verma, S. (2003b). Biomarkers of vascular disease linking inflammation to endothelial activation. *Circulation*, **108**, 2041–48.

Taylor, P. D., McConnell, J., Khan, I. Y. *et al.* (2004a). Impaired glucose homeostasis and mitochondrial abnormalities in offspring of rats fed a fat-rich diet in pregnancy. *Am. J. Physiol. Regul. Integr. Comp. Physiol.*, **288**, R134–9.

Taylor, P. D., Khan, I. Y., Hanson, M. A. and Poston, L. (2004b). Impaired EDHF-mediated vasodilatation in adult offspring of rats exposed to a fat-rich diet in pregnancy. *J. Physiol.*, **558**, 943–51.

Te Velde, S. J., Ferreira, I., Twisk, J. W., Stehouwer, C. D., van Mechelen, W. and Kemper, H. C. (2004). Birthweight and arterial stiffness and blood pressure in adulthood: results from the Amsterdam Growth and Health Longitudinal Study. *Int. J. Epidemiol.*, **33**, 154–61.

Tonkiss, J., Trzcinska, M., Galler, J. R., Ruiz-Opazo, N. and Herrera, V. L. (1998). Prenatal malnutrition-induced changes in blood pressure: dissociation of stress and non-stress responses using radiotelemetry. *Hypertension*, **32**, 108–14.

Torrens, C., Brawley, L., Dance, C. S, Itoh, S., Poston, L. and Hanson, M. A. (2002). First evidence for transgenerational vascular programming in the rat protein restriction model. *J. Physiol.*, **543P**, 41P.

Torrens, C., Brawley, L., Barker, A. C., Itoh, S., Poston, L. and Hanson, M. A. (2003). Maternal protein restriction in the rat impairs resistance artery but not conduit artery function in pregnant offspring. *J. Physiol.*, **547**, 77–84.

Vickers, M. H., Breier, B. H., Cutfield, W. S., Hofman, P. L. and Gluckman, P. D. (2000). Fetal origins of hyperphagia, obesity, and hypertension and postnatal amplification by hypercaloric nutrition. *Am. J. Physiol. Endocrinol. Metab.*, **279**, E83–7.

Wadsworth, R. M. (1990). Calcium and vascular reactivity in aging and hypertension. *J. Hypertens.*, **8**, 975–83.

Walker, B. R., McConnachie, A., Noon, J. P., Webb, D. J. and Watt, G. C. (1998). Contribution of parental blood pressures to association between low birth weight and adult high blood pressure: cross sectional study. *BMJ*, **316**, 834–7.

Waterland, R. A. and Jirtle, R. L. (2004). Early nutrition, epigenetic changes at transposons and imprinted genes, and enhanced susceptibility to adult chronic diseases. *Nutrition*, **20**, 63–8.

Woodall, S. M., Johnston, B. M., Breier, B. H. and Gluckman, P. D. (1996). Chronic maternal undernutrition in the rat leads to delayed postnatal growth and elevated blood pressure of offspring. *Pediatr. Res.*, **40**, 438–43.

Woods, L. L., Ingelfinger, J. R., Nyengaard, J. R. and Rasch, R. (2001). Maternal protein restriction suppresses the newborn renin–angiotensin system and programs adult hypertension in rats. *Pediatr. Res.*, **49**, 460–7.

Young, J. B., Kaufman, L. N., Saville, M. E. and Landsberg, L. (1985). Increased sympathetic nervous system activity in rats fed a low-protein diet. *Am. J. Physiol.*, **248**, R627–37.

Yu, H. I., Sheu, W. H., Lai, C. J., Lee, W. J. and Chen, Y. T. (2001). Endothelial dysfunction in type 2 diabetes mellitus subjects with peripheral artery disease. *Int. J. Cardiol.*, **78**, 19–25.

22

The developmental environment and atherogenesis

C. Napoli, O. Pignalosa, L. Rossi, C. Botti, C. Guarino, V. Sica and F. de Nigris

University of Naples

Introduction

Crucial advances in our understanding of athero-genesis have been achieved during the past two decades. The historical hypothesis of pathogene-sis ('lipid accumulation') has evolved to integrate several pathogenic mechanisms contributing to the initiation and evolution of atherogenesis. Vascular inflammation and apoptosis may play pivotal roles in its progression and onset. Endothelial dysfunc-tion is considered to be one of the earliest events in atherogenesis. This chapter will discuss emerg-ing concepts in the pathogenesis of, and therapeu-tic approaches to, atherosclerosis. Some novel risk factors, including impaired fasting glucose, triglyc-erides and triglyceride-rich lipoprotein remnants, lipoprotein (a), homocysteine, and high-sensitivity C-reactive protein, might contribute to an increased risk of atherosclerosis (Fruchart et al. 2004). More-over, hypercholesterolaemia and hypertension have synergistic deleterious effects on coronary endothe-lial function (Rodriguez-Porcel et al. 2003). The pathogenesis of atherosclerosis has been related also to infiltration of immune cells, which are involved in systemic and local, innate as well as adaptive, immune responses (Zhou and Hansson 2004). As some inflammatory and autoimmune diseases could be treated by immunologically based therapy, it is of particular interest to consider whether such prin-ciples could also be applied to prevent or treat atherosclerosis.

Atherosclerosis is ultimately responsible for myo-cardial infarction, peripheral arterial disease and ischaemic stroke, and is characterised by a long lag-time between onset and clinical manifestation. The prodromal stages of human atherosclerotic lesions are already formed during fetal development (Napoli et al. 1997a, 1999a, Palinski and Napoli 2002a). Intimal thickening is also observed in fetal coronary arteries (Ikari et al. 1999). In children and young adults, fatty streaks become increasingly prevalent and some of them progress to advanced stages of atherosclerotic lesions (Stary 1989, Berenson et al. 1992, PDAY Research Group 1993, Berenson et al. 1998, Napoli et al. 1999b). Once initiated, the pro-gression of the atherogenesis is influenced by classi-cal risk factors that promote vascular inflammation and plaque rupture (Ross 1999, Napoli and Ignarro 2001, de Nigris et al. 2003a).

The pre-eminent role of hypercholesterolaemia has been suggested by the marked reduction of atherosclerosis-related clinical events by cholesterol-lowering interventions (Napoli and Sica 2004). The observation that maternal hyper-cholesterolaemia is associated with greatly enhanced fatty streak formation in human fetal arteries (Napoli et al. 1997a, 1999b, Palinski and Napoli 2002a) suggested that hypercholestero-laemia may also play a pathogenic role in fetal lesion formation. Fetal lesions occur at the same sites as more advanced lesions in adolescents and adults. However, the size of fetal lesions is minute

Developmental Origins of Health and Disease, ed. Peter Gluckman and Mark Hanson. Published by Cambridge University Press.
© P. D. Gluckman and M. A. Hanson 2006.

and there is evidence that they may partially regress during the final stages of gestation or early infancy, when cholesterol levels were low in the FELIC study (Napoli *et al.* 1999b). This post-mortem study of 156 normocholesterolaemic children showed that the progression of atherosclerosis was markedly faster in offspring of hypercholesterolaemic mothers than in those of normocholesterolaemic mothers. Establishing such pathogenic links is important, not only because it would add to our understanding of the pathogenesis of the disease, but also for clinical considerations.

Maternal hypercholesterolaemia may enhance fetal lesion formation

Direct evidence for the causal role of maternal hypercholesterolaemia and the involvement of oxidative stress has been obtained in a rabbit model (Napoli *et al.* 2000a). In this study, groups of originally normocholesterolaemic female rabbits were fed a control chow or one of two hypercholesterolaemic diets yielding average plasma cholesterol levels of about 153 or 360 mg dL^{-1} during pregnancy. Additional groups received the same two hypercholesterolaemic diets supplemented with 1–3% cholestyramine, 100 IU vitamin E, or both. Cholesterol levels significantly increased in mothers fed the hypercholesterolaemic diets. Cholestyramine reduced maternal cholesterol, whereas vitamin E had no effect. Plasma concentrations of oxidised fatty acids and other measures of lipid peroxidation, such as malondialdehyde, differed significantly between groups. Lipid peroxidation end products increased roughly in proportion to the maternal cholesterol level in offspring of hypercholesterolaemic and cholestyramine-treated mothers, and were markedly reduced in offspring of vitamin-E-treated mothers. Hypercholesterolaemia is known to be accompanied by increased lipid peroxidation both in plasma and in tissues (Napoli *et al.* 1997b, Reilly *et al.* 1998). Because plasma cholesterol levels were similar and very low in all groups of offspring, these differences are likely to reflect placental transfer of oxidised fatty acids from the mother to the fetal circulation (Hendrickse *et al.* 1985).

Lesions doubled in offspring from hypercholesterolaemic mothers. Maternal cholestyramine treatment significantly reduced fetal lesions, roughly in proportion to the reduction of maternal cholesterol levels. A regression analysis of individual animals in all groups (except those receiving vitamin E) confirmed the linear correlation between maternal cholesterol and lesions at birth ($r = 0.78$, $p < 0.0001$) (Napoli *et al.* 2000a). Vitamin-E treatment of mothers did not affect maternal hypercholesterolaemia, but reduced atherosclerosis at birth by about 40%, clearly implicating lipid oxidation or increased intracellular oxidative stress in fetal lesion formation.

Interference with oxidation-sensitive cytoplasmic and/or nuclear signalling pathways that regulate arterial gene expression or transcription constitutes an important mechanism through which oxidation may promote lesion formation (Finkel 1998, Napoli *et al.* 2001, de Nigris *et al.* 2002) (Fig. 22.1). A multitude of mechanisms involving oxidative end products, including oxidatively modified proteins and other peroxidative compounds, can affect the basic machinery of the cell. For example, oxidised low-density lipoprotein (OxLDL) modulates the expression of genes involved in cell differentiation and proliferation regulated by the nuclear factor kappa B (NFκB) (Finkel 1998, Napoli *et al.* 2001, de Nigris *et al.* 2002, Rodriguez-Porcel *et al.* 2002). An increasing body of evidence from both animal models and human specimens suggests that apoptosis (programmed cell death) is a major event in the pathophysiology of atherosclerosis (Napoli 2003). It has been proposed that apoptotic cell death contributes to plaque instability, rupture and thrombus formation. Both mildly and extensively oxidised LDL also influences the expression of apoptotic factors activated through Fas and TNF receptors (Napoli *et al.* 2000b, Napoli 2003) and c-Myc-dependent transcription factors (de Nigris *et al.* 2000, 2001), as well as genes regulated by the peroxisome proliferator activated receptor gamma (PPARγ), e.g. genes promoting inflammation or reverse cholesterol transport

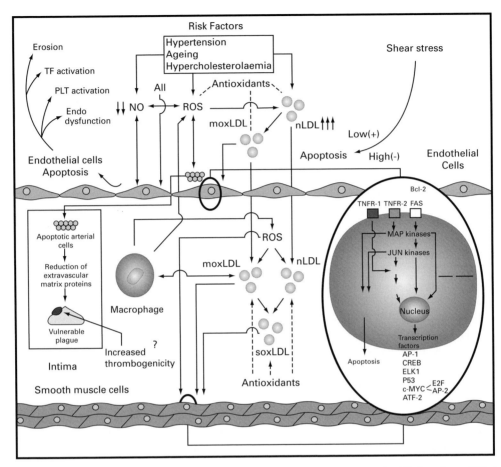

Figure 22.1 Oxidation-sensitive mechanisms in the arterial wall. ROS, reactive oxygen species; TF, tissue factor; PLT, platelets; AII, angiotensin II; TNFR, tumor necrosis factor. Adapted from de Nigris *et al.* (2003a).

(Li *et al.* 2000). Smooth-muscle cells and macrophages in atherosclerotic plaques express a different panel of apoptosis-related genes in response to proapoptotic stimuli (Napoli 2003). Although this may seem a promising starting point for the development of antiatherogenic drugs, it remains to be determined whether modulation of apoptosis can become a clinically important approach to influence plaque progression. OxLDL also triggers extensive immune responses (Wick *et al.* 2004). More recently, we have shown that glycoxidation of LDL downregulates endothelial nitric oxide synthase in cells from human coronary vessels (Napoli *et al.* 2002a).

Evidence that maternal hypercholesterolaemia or the ensuing pathogenic events in the fetus increase the susceptibility to atherosclerosis later in life was provided in the same rabbit model (Palinski *et al.* 2001). These results demonstrate that maternal hypercholesterolaemia accelerates the atherogenic response to postnatal exposure to hypercholesterolaemia and indicate that in-utero programming influences the susceptibility to atherosclerosis later in life. Great caution should be applied in extrapolating this assumption to humans. Cholesterol levels in chow-fed NZW rabbits are very low (50 mg dL^{-1}) and may actually result in lesion regression, whereas lesion sizes clearly increase with increasing age in children, even those with 'normal' cholesterol levels and lacking other classical risk factors of atherosclerosis (Napoli *et al.* 1997b).

As discussed above, numerous signalling pathways are affected by increased oxidation of LDL or intracellular formation of reactive oxygen species (Finkel 1998, Li *et al.* 2000, de Nigris *et al.* 2000, 2001, Napoli *et al.* 2000b, 2001, Rodriguez-Porcel *et al.* 2002). The first evidence for persistent differences in arterial gene expression was obtained in LDL-receptor-deficient (LDLR$^{-/-}$) mice (Napoli *et al.* 2002a). A murine model was selected for the fetal studies because the murine genome is far better characterised than that of the rabbit, and because microarrays encompassing a large segment of the murine genome are commercially available. Groups of female mice were fed regular chow or high-fat diets supplemented with 0.075% or 1.25% cholesterol, starting three weeks prior to pregnancy. Offspring were fed regular chow until the age of 3 months and had nearly identical cholesterol levels of about 260 mg dL^{-1}. At the age of 3 months, lesions at the root of the aorta were indeed markedly greater in male offspring of both hypercholesterolaemic groups than in the control group. Confirmation of an atherogenic effect of maternal hypercholesterolaemia in a second animal model lends weight to the concept that it also contributes to enhanced lesion formation in humans. Aortic RNA was extracted from individual or pooled aortic segments or entire aortas and subjected to analysis by Affymetrix gene chips (Napoli *et al.* 2002b, 2003a).

Microarrays have been extensively used for studies of cultured cells, but their application to cardiovascular tissues is only just beginning (Napoli *et al.* 2003a). Microarray analysis of the expression of 11 000 murine genes and ESTs in the non-atherosclerotic aortic media and intima (Napoli *et al.* 2002b) indicated that 135 genes/ESTs were significantly up or down-regulated in offspring of hypercholesterolaemic mothers. Four of these genes were found to be up-regulated more than 1.7-fold (fibroblast growth factor binding protein (*FGFbp*), flavin containing monooxidase 3 (*FCMo3*), NPAS2 (*MOP4*),

and the potassium channel (*MERG1*)). Comparison of the expression of one of these genes, *FCMo3*, in individual mice by quantitative PCR yielded qualitatively similar differences (Napoli *et al.* 2002c). Immunocytochemistry of lesion-free segments of the aortic origin of the same mice also indicated consistently more MERG, FGFbp and NPAS2 protein in the offspring of hypercholesterolaemic mothers than in controls (Napoli *et al.* 2002c). Future studies investigating the expression of genes affected by fetal programming in animals exposed to hypercholesterolaemic diets after birth, in which atherosclerotic lesions are present, will have to rely on laser dissection microscopy to isolate intimal tissues or specific cell types (Bonner *et al.* 1997). This is increasingly attractive, due to the smaller amounts of RNA required for the microarrays and technical advances in laser capture microscopes.

Intervention experiments in experimental models may also answer the question whether in-utero programming affects genes promoting or inhibiting lipid peroxidation in the arterial wall. A first indication that differences in the vascular activity of antioxidant enzymes (Mn-superoxide dismutase, catalase or glutathione peroxidase) may influence lesion formation was provided in human fetuses (Napoli *et al.* 1999b). In this study, intracranial arteries showed greater antioxidant activity and a much smaller atherogenic response to (maternal) hypercholesterolaemia than extracranial arteries. Another study also supports this, by showing that when the antioxidant activity in intracranial arteries declines to that of comparable-sized extracranial arteries in adult and elderly subjects, their atherogenesis accelerates (D'Armiento *et al.* 2001).

A multitude of drugs affecting nitric oxide (NO) bioactivity are now available which not only have direct beneficial effects on endothelial function, but may also contribute to reduced formation of reactive oxygen species (ROS) and asymmetric dimethyl-methylarginine (ADMA) (Ignarro *et al.* 1999, Napoli and Ignarro 2003, Ignarro and Napoli 2004) (Fig. 22.2). Indeed, NO released by nitroaspirin may decrease experimental atherosclerosis (Napoli *et al.* 2002c).

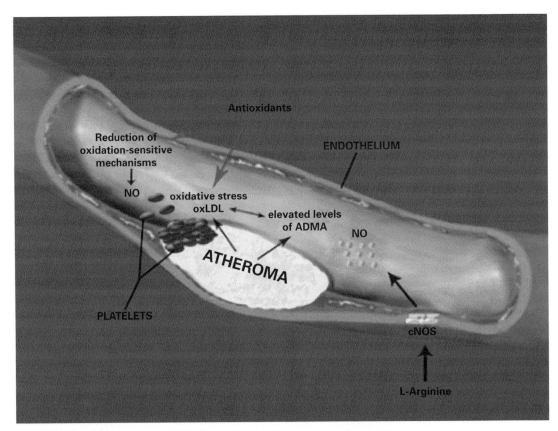

Figure 22.2 Nitric-oxide-related mechanisms in the pathogenesis of vascular damage. ADMA, asymmetric dimethyl-methylarginine; NO, nitric oxide; eNOS, endothelial nitric oxide synthase; oxLDL, oxidised low-density lipoprotein.

Based on extensive in-vitro evidence, it is presumed that accumulation of OxLDL in fatty streaks and enhanced oxidative stress in plasma affect multiple oxidation-sensitive signalling pathways in the arterial wall of the fetus. These in turn modulate expression of many genes that affect endothelial function and promote lesion formation.

Maternal cholesterol levels increase during the third trimester, even in 'normal' mothers (Martin *et al.* 1999), and preliminary data indicate that this increase may be much greater in hypercholesterolaemic mothers. Placental functions and permeability can also be assumed to change over time, if only as a result of rapid growth. During adolescence and in adulthood, atherogenesis is clearly driven by

conventional risk factors and becomes an extraordinarily complex process (Ross 1999, Napoli and Ignarro 2001, de Nigris *et al.* 2003a). To date, accelerated progression of atherosclerosis in human offspring of hypercholesterolaemic mothers has only been established for children and adolescents (Napoli *et al.* 1999b).

Novel diagnostic and therapeutic implications

If it can be established that fetal pathogenic events linked to maternal hypercholesterolaemia contribute significantly to atherosclerosis-related

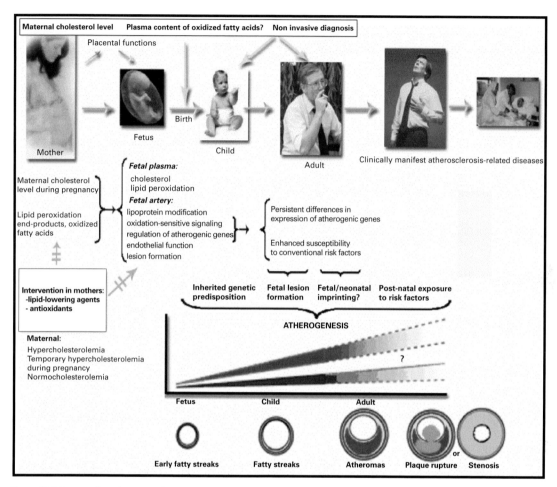

Figure 22.3 Proposed mechanisms of the natural history of atherosclerosis-related diseases. Modified from Palinski and Napoli (2002a).

morbidity and mortality, an early recognition of the risk would be desirable. Maternal hypercholesterol-aemia should therefore be added to the list of risk factors justifying such steps (National Cholesterol Education Program 1992, Spinler *et al.* 2001, Smith *et al.* 2001) (Fig. 22.3). The diagnostic approaches to estimate lesion progression in children and young adults have been the subject of an earlier review (Napoli and Palinski 2001) and will not be discussed here. There has been great interest in the possibility of identifying plaques that might be the site of future acute coronary events. These plaques are termed vulnerable and the majority are lipid-rich with an abundance of inflammatory cells and a thin fibrous cap. Several techniques developed to identify these plaques are in various stages of development (including ultrasound, magnetic resonance imaging, electron beam CT and both novel nuclear medicine and molecular imaging approaches) and in the near future one might employ a strategy to potentially identify and therapeutically modify such lesions. Although this approach of identifying the vulnerable plaque seems promising, there are significant potential limitations. The natural history of a vulnerable plaque is unknown, and clinical trials utilising this strategy of identification and therapeutic intervention are lacking. Moreover, in any given patient, multiple vulnerable plaques are likely to be present.

Of even greater importance are the therapeutic implications of the hypothesis. Cholesterol lowering in hypercholesterolaemic mothers is indicated, and dietary means (McMurry *et al.* 1982), cholestyramine or other hypocholesterolaemic drugs that are safe during pregnancy are obvious candidates. Cholesterol lowering also reduces oxidative stress (Martinet *et al.* 2001, Palinski and Napoli 2002b, Bonetti *et al.* 2003). More important, experimental studies show that the deletion of *p66shc* gene increases the resistance to oxidative stress and vascular damage (Napoli *et al.* 2003b). Another protective approach would be the association of L-arginine with antioxidants (de Nigris *et al.* 2003b) or graduated physical exercise and antioxidants/L-arginine (Napoli *et al.* 2004). Overwhelming evidence indicates that structurally unrelated antioxidants inhibit conventional atherosclerosis in animal models, but human trials have yielded conflicting results (Stephens *et al.* 1996, HOPE Study Investigators 1996, Gruppo Italiano per lo Studio della Sopravvivenza nell'Infarto Miocardico 1999, Boaz *et al.* 2000, Pryor 2000). The majority of these trials measured clinical outcomes in adult subjects with pre-existing and often advanced lesions, in whom multiple risk factors were present and who were treated for a limited time period and often with relatively low doses of antioxidants. Moreover, the time of follow-up (one to four years) was probably too short to assess the clinical outcome of a chronic disease. It is therefore doubtful that they provide useful indications on the efficacy of high doses of vitamin E in human fetuses, where the prevention of pathogenic effects on oxidation-sensitive regulatory pathways may be more important than the reduction of other atherogenic or thrombogenic effects of OxLDL. Novel molecular therapeutic approaches against atherosclerosis may include gene therapy (George *et al.* 2003).

Barker postulated a correlation between reduced birthweight and hypertension and atherosclerosis-related diseases later in life (Barker *et al.* 1989, Martyn *et al.* 1998). This challenges the view that predisposition to atherosclerosis is an exclusive consequence of inherited genetic traits, and has therefore been the subject of acerbic controversy (Susser and Levin, 1999) which even very large epidemiological studies have not been able to resolve (Smith *et al.* 2001). The most convincing evidence, supported by a recent report (Adair *et al.* 2001), points to a long-term effect of maternal diet on blood pressure, but the large number of genes, postnatal risk factors (some of which are influenced by inherited genes) and age-dependent factors make it extraordinarily complicated to disentangle genetic from environmental influences on atherosclerosis. Another major obstacle has been that many pathogenically distinct factors can lead to a reduced birthweight. Therefore, experimental verification of the Barker hypothesis is only in its infancy (Radunovic *et al.* 2000). The maternofetal cholesterol hypothesis differs from the Barker hypothesis in that there is little evidence for a significant role of reduced birthweight. The FELIC study noted an inverse correlation between birthweight and atherosclerosis in children, but only in offspring of normocholesterolaemic mothers (Napoli *et al.* 1999b).

ACKNOWLEDGMENTS

We would like to dedicate this chapter to the memory of Dr Russel Ross, a pioneer in the study of atherosclerosis, who died in March 1999. We thank our colleagues Drs Louis J. Ignarro (UCLA, USA), Joseph Loscalzo (Boston University, USA), Wulf Palinski (UCSD, USA), Lilach and Amir Lerman (Mayo Clinic at Rochester, USA) and Francesco P. D'Armiento (Naples, Italy), for fruitful discussions in the field and collaboration during the last 10 years. Studies quoted in this work were funded by National Institutes of Health (NIH), Mayo Clinic Foundation, Whitaker Cardiovascular Institute, Regione Campania, and National Funds from the Italian Ministry of University (MIUR).

REFERENCES

Adair, L. S., Kuzawa, C. W. and Borja, J. (2001). Maternal energy stores and diet composition during pregnancy program adolescent blood pressure. *Circulation*, **104**, 1034–9.

Barker, D. J. P., Winter, P. D., Osmond, C., Margetts, B. and Simmonds, S. J. (1989). Weight in infancy and death from ischaemic heart disease. *Lancet*, **2**, 577–80.

Berenson, G. S., Wattigney, W. A., Tracy, R. E. *et al.* (1992). Atherosclerosis of the aorta and coronary arteries and cardiovascular risk factors in persons aged 6 to 30 years and studied at necropsy (the Bogalusa Heart Study). *Am. J. Cardiol.*, **70**, 851–8.

Berenson, G. S., Srinivasan, S. R., Bao, W., Newman, W. P., Tracy, R. E. and Wattigney, W. A. (1998). Association between multiple cardiovascular risk factors and atherosclerosis in children and young adults: the Bogalusa Heart Study. *N. Engl. J. Med.* **338**, 1650–6.

Boaz, M., Smetana, S., Weinstein, T. *et al.* (2000). Secondary prevention with antioxidants of cardiovascular disease in endstage renal disease (SPACE): randomised placebo-controlled trial. *Lancet*, **356**, 1213–18.

Bonetti, P. O., Lerman, L. O., Napoli, C. and Lerman, A. (2003). Statin effects beyond lipid lowering. *Eur. Heart J.*, **24**, 225–48.

Bonner, R. F., Emmert-Buck, M., Cole, K. *et al.* (1997). Laser capture microdissection: molecular analysis of tissue. *Science*, **278**, 1481–3.

D'Armiento, F. P., Bianchi, A., de Nigris, F. *et al.* (2001). Age-related effects on atherogenesis and scavenger enzymes of intracranial and extracranial arteries in men without classic risk factors for atherosclerosis. *Stroke*, **32**, 2472–80.

de Nigris, F., Youssef, T., Ciafré, S. A. *et al.* (2000). Evidence for oxidative activation of c-Myc-dependent nuclear signaling pathways in cultured human coronary SMC and in early atherosclerotic lesions of WHHL rabbits: protective effects of vitamin E. *Circulation*, **102**, 2111–17.

de Nigris, F., Lerman, L. O., Rodriguez-Porcel, M., De Montis, M. P., Lerman, A. and Napoli, C. (2001). c-myc activation in early coronary lesions in experimental hypercholesterolemia. *Biochem. Biophys. Res. Commun.* **281**, 945–50.

de Nigris, F., Lerman, L. O. and Napoli, C. (2002). New insights in the transcriptional activity and coregulator molecules in the arterial wall. *Int. J. Cardiol.*, **86**, 153–68.

de Nigris, F., Lerman, A., Ignarro, L. J. *et al.* (2003a). Oxidation-sensitive mechanisms, vascular apoptosis, and atherosclerosis. *Trends Mol. Med.*, **9**, 351–9.

de Nigris, F., Lerman, L. O., Williams-Ignarro, S. *et al.* (2003b). Beneficial effects of antioxidants and L-arginine on oxidation-sensitive gene expression and endothelial nitric oxide synthase activity at the sites of disturbed shear stress. *Proc. Natl. Acad. Sci. USA*, **100**, 1420–5.

Finkel, T. (1998). Oxygen radicals and signaling. *Curr. Opin. Cell Biol.* **10**, 248–53.

Fruchart, J. C., Nierman, M. C., Stroes, E. S., Kastelein, J. J. and Duriez, P. (2004). New risk factors for atherosclerosis and patient risk assessment. *Circulation*, **109** (Suppl. III), 15–19.

George, S. J., de Nigris, F., Baker A. H. and Napoli, C. (2003). Gene therapy for vascular diseases. *Gene Ther. Mol. Biol.*, **7**, 135–51.

Gruppo Italiano per lo Studio della Sopravvivenza nell'Infarto Miocardico (1999). Dietary supplementation with n-3 polyunsaturated fatty acids and vitamin E after myocardial infarction: results of the GISSI-Prevenzione trial. *Lancet.* **354**, 447–55.

Hendrickse, W., Stammers, J. P. and Hull, D. (1985). The transfer of free fatty acids across the human placenta. *Br. J. Obstet. Gynaecol.* **92**, 945–52.

HOPE Study Investigators (1996). The HOPE (Heart Outcomes Prevention Evaluation) Study: the design of a large, simple randomized trial of an angiotensin-converting enzyme inhibitor (ramipril) and vitamin E in patients at high risk of cardiovascular events. *Can. J. Cardiol.* **12**, 127–37.

Ignarro, L. J. and Napoli, C. (2004). Novel features of nitric oxide, endothelial nitric oxide synthase and atherosclerosis. *Curr. Atheroscler. Rep.*, **6**, 281–7.

Ignarro, L. J., Cirino, G. and Napoli, C. (1999). Nitric oxide as a signaling molecule in the vascular system: an overview. *J. Cardiovasc. Pharmacol.*, **34**, 879–86.

Ikari, Y., McManus, B. M., Kenyon, J. and Schwartz, S. M. (1999). Neonatal intima formation in the human coronary artery. *Arterioscler. Thromb. Vasc. Biol.*, **19**, 2036–40.

Li, A. C., Brown, K. K., Silvestre, M. J., Willson, T. M., Palinski, W. and Glass, C. K. (2000). Peroxysome proliferator-activated receptor γ ligands inhibit development of atherosclerosis in LDL receptor-deficient mice. *J. Clin. Invest.* **106**, 523–31.

Martin, U., Davies, C., Hayavi, S., Hartland, A. and Dunne, F. (1999). Is normal pregnancy atherogenic? *Clin. Sci.* **96**, 421–5.

Martinet, W., Knaapen, M. W., De Meyer, G. R., Herman, A. G. and Kockx, M. M. (2001). Oxidative DNA damage and repair in experimental atherosclerosis are reversed by dietary lipid lowering. *Circ. Res.* **88**, 733–9.

Martyn, C. N., Gale, C. R., Jespersen, S. and Sherriff, S. B. (1998). Impaired fetal growth and atherosclerosis of carotid and peripheral arteries. *Lancet*, **352**, 173–8.

McMurry, M. P., Connor, W. E. and Goperud, C. P. (1982). The effects of dietary cholesterol upon the hypercholesterolemia of pregnancy. *Metabolism*, **30**, 869–79.

Napoli, C. (2003). Oxidation of LDL, atherogenesis and apoptosis. *Ann. NY. Acad. Sci.*, **1010**, 698–709.

Napoli, C. and Ignarro, L. J. (2001). Nitric oxide and atherosclerosis. *Nitric Oxide* **5**, 88–97.

(2003). Nitric oxide-releasing drugs. *Ann. Rev. Pharmacol. Toxicol.*, **47**, 97–123.

Napoli, C. and Palinski, W. (2001). Maternal hypercholesterolemia during pregnancy influences the later development of atherosclerosis: clinical and pathogenic implications. *Eur. Heart J.* **22**, 4–9.

Napoli, C. and Sica, V. (2004). Statin treatment and the natural history of atherosclerotic-related diseases: pathogenic mechanisms and the risk–benefit profile. *Curr. Pharm. Design*, **10**, 425–32.

Napoli, C., D'Armiento, F. P., Mancini, F. P., Witztum, JL., Palumbo, G. and Palinski W. (1997a). Fatty streak formation occurs in human fetal aortas and is greatly enhanced by maternal hypercholesterolemia: intimal accumulation of LDL and its oxidation precede monocyte recruitment into early atherosclerotic lesions. *J. Clin. Invest.* **100**, 2680–90.

Napoli, C., Ambrosio, G., Scarpato, N. *et al.* (1997b). Decreased low-density lipoprotein oxidation after repeated selective apheresis in homozygous familial hypercholesterolemia. *Am. Heart J.* **133**, 585–95.

Napoli, C., Witztum, J. L., de Nigris, F., Palumbo, G., D'Armiento, F. P. and Palinski, W. (1999a). Intracranial arteries of human fetuses are more resistant to hypercholesterolemia-induced fatty streak formation than extracranial arteries. *Circulation*, **99**, 2003–10.

Napoli, C., Glass C. K., Witztum J. L., Deutsch R., D'Armiento F. P. and Palinski, W. (1999b). Influence of maternal hypercholesterolaemia during pregnancy on progression of early atherosclerotic lesions in childhood: Fate of Early Lesions in Children (FELIC) study. *Lancet*, **354**, 1234–41.

Napoli, C., Witztum, J. L., Calara, F., de Nigris, F. and Palinski, W. (2000a). Maternal hypercholesterolemia enhances atherogenesis in normocholesterolemic rabbits, which is inhibited by antioxidant or lipid-lowering intervention during pregnancy: an experimental model of atherogenic mechanisms in human fetuses. *Circ. Res.*, **87**, 946–52.

Napoli, C., Quehenberger, O., de Nigris, F., Abete, P., Glass, C. K. and Palinski, W. (2000b). Apoptosis induced by mildly oxidized LDL involves multiple apoptotic signaling pathways in human coronary cells. *FASEB J.*, **14**, 1996–2007.

Napoli, C., de Nigris, F. and Palinski, W. (2001). Multiple role of reactive oxygen species in the arterial wall. *J. Cell. Biochem.* **82**, 674–82.

Napoli, C., Lerman, L. O., de Nigris, F., Loscalzo, J. and Ignarro, L. J. (2002a). Glycoxidized low-density lipoprotein downregulates endothelial nitric oxide synthase in human coronary cells. *J. Am. Coll. Cardiol.*, **40**, 1515–22.

Napoli, C., de Nigris, F., Welch, J. *et al.* (2002b). Maternal hypercholesterolemia during pregnancy promotes early atherogenesis in LDL receptor-deficient mice and alters aortic gene expression determined by microarray. *Circulation*, **105**, 1360–7.

Napoli, C., Ackah, E., de Nigris, F. *et al.* (2002c). Chronic treatment with nitric oxide-releasing aspirin inhibits plasma LDL oxidation and oxidative stress, oxidation-specific epitopes in the arterial wall, and atherogenesis in hypercholesterolemic mice. *Proc. Natl. Acad. Sci. USA*, **99**, 12467–70.

Napoli, C., Lerman, L. O., Sica, V., Lerman, A., Tajana, G. and de Nigris, F. (2003a). Microarray analysis: a novel reasearch tool for cardiovascular scientists and physicians. *Heart*, **89**, 597–604.

Napoli, C., Martin-Padura, I., de Nigris, F. *et al.* (2003b). Deletion of the p66Shc longevity gene reduces systemic and tissue oxidative stress, vascular cell apoptosis, and early atherogenesis in mice fed high-fat diet. *Proc. Natl. Acad. Sci. USA*, **100**, 2112–16.

Napoli, C., Williams-Ignarro, S., de Nigris, F. *et al.* (2004). Long-term combined beneficial effects of physical training and metabolic treatment on atherosclerosis in hypercholesterolemic mice. *Proc. Natl. Acad. Sci. USA*, **101**, 8797–802.

National Cholesterol Education Program. (1992). Report of the Expert Panel on Blood Cholesterol Levels in Children and Adolescents. *Pediatrics*, **89**, 525–84.

Palinski, W. and Napoli, C. (2002a). The fetal origins of atherosclerosis: maternal hypercholesterolemia and cholesterol-lowering or antioxidant treatment during pregnancy influence in utero programming and post-natal susceptibility to the disease. *FASEB J.*, **16**, 1348–60.

(2002b). Unraveling pleiotropic effects of statins on plaque rupture. *Arterioscler. Thromb. Vasc. Biol.*, **22**, 1745–50.

Palinski, W., D'Armiento, F. P., Witztum, J. L., de Nigris, F., Casanada, F. and Napoli, C. (2001). Maternal hypercholesterolemia and treatment during pregnancy influence the long term progression of atherosclerosis in offspring of rabbits. *Circ. Res.*, **89**, 991–6.

Pathobiological Determinants of Atherosclerosis in Youths (PDAY) Research Group (1993). Natural history of aortic and coronary atherosclerotic lesions in youth: findings from the PDAY study. *Arterioscler. Thromb.*, **13**, 1291–8.

Pryor, W. A. (2000). Vitamin E and heart disease: basic science to clinical intervention trials. *Free Rad. Biol. Med.*, **28**, 141–64.

Radunovic, N., Kuczynski, E., Rosen, T., Dukanac, J., Petkovic, S. and Lockwood, C. J. (2000). Plasma apolipoprotein A-I and B concentrations in growth-retarded fetuses: a link between low birth weight and adult atherosclerosis. *J. Clin. Endocrinol. Metab.*, **85**, 85–8.

Reilly, M. P., Praticò, D., Delanty, N. *et al.* (1998). Increased formation of distinct F2 isoprostanes in hypercholesterolemia. *Circulation*, **98**, 2822–8.

Rodriguez-Porcel, M., Lerman, L. O., Holmes, D. R., Richardson, D., Napoli, C. and Lerman, A. (2002). Chronic antioxidant supplementation attenuates nuclear factor-κB activation and preserves endothelial function in hypercholesterolemic pigs. *Cardiovasc. Res.*, **53**, 1010–18.

Rodriguez-Porcel, M., Lerman, L. O., Herrmann, J., Sawamura, T., Napoli, C. and Lerman, A. (2003). Hypercholesterolemia and hypertension have synergistic deleterious effects on coronary endothelial function. *Arterioscler. Thromb. Vasc. Biol.*, **23**, 885–91.

Ross, R. (1999). Atherosclerosis: an inflammatory disease. *N. Engl. J. Med.*, **340**, 115–26.

Smith, G. C., Pell, J. P. and Walsh, D. (2001). Pregnancy complications and maternal risk of ischaemic heart disease: a retrospective cohort study of 129,290 births. *Lancet*, **357**, 2002–6.

Smith, S. C. Jr., Blair, S. N., Bonow, R. O. *et al.* (2001). AHA/ACC guidelines for preventing heart attack and death in patients with atherosclerotic cardiovascular disease: 2001 update. A statement for healthcare professionals from the American Heart Association and the American College of Cardiology. *Circulation*, **104**, 1577–9.

Spinler, S. A., Hilleman, D. E., Cheng, J. W. *et al.* (2001). New recommendations from the 1999 American College of Cardiology/American Heart Association acute myocardial infarction guidelines. *Ann. Pharmacother.*, **35**, 589–617.

Stary, H. C. (1989). Evolution and progression of atherosclerotic lesions in coronary arteries of children and young adults. *Arteriosclerosis*, **9** (Suppl. 1), 19–32.

Stephens, N. G., Parsons, A., Schofield, P. M., Kelly, F., Cheeseman, K. and Mitchinson, M. J. (1996). Randomised controlled trial of vitamin E in patients with coronary disease: Cambridge Heart Antioxidant Study (CHAOS). *Lancet*, **347**, 781–6.

Susser, M. and Levin, B. (1999). Ordeals for the fetal programming hypothesis: the hypothesis largely survives one ordeal but not another. *BMJ*, **318**, 885–6.

Wick, G., Knoflach, M. and Xu, Q. (2004). Autoimmune and inflammatory mechanisms in atherosclerosis. *Annu. Rev. Immunol.*, **22**, 361–403.

Zhou, X. and Hansson, G. K. (2004). Immunomodulation and vaccination for atherosclerosis. *Expert Opin. Biol. Ther.*, **4**, 599–612.

23

The developmental environment, renal function and disease

Karen M. Moritz, E. Marelyn Wintour and Miodrag Dodic

Monash University

Introduction

Chronic renal disease is a major health problem in many societies. In some populations, including the Australian Aborigine, the Pima Indians of the USA, and certain populations of African-Americans, diseased kidneys due to chronic hypertension progress into end-stage renal disease, with a particularly high incidence (Hoy *et al.* 1999, Kett and Bertram 2004). The American Kidney Foundation estimates that as many as 20 million Americans, or approximately 10% of adults in the population, have some form of renal disease. Not only is it the ninth leading cause of death in Americans, but treatment for patients with chronic renal failure is amongst the most expensive for any chronic disease. The causes of kidney disease are numerous, including inherited and congenital renal defects, but by far the greatest risk factors are diabetes and hypertension. Similar to other adult-onset diseases, such as hypertension and diabetes mellitus, lifestyle factors such as a high-fat/high-salt diet, smoking and lack of exercise can contribute significantly to the development of renal disease. Epidemiological and experimental evidence is accumulating to suggest that, as with hypertension and diabetes, the susceptibility of an individual to develop renal disease may be increased if that person has been exposed to a poor or suboptimal intrauterine environment. If a substantive link can be proven between abnormal kidney development and the later development of hypertension and renal disease, then measures can be recommended which could decrease significantly the incidence of adult hypertension.

Kidney development

During development in utero two sets of temporary kidneys are present for a period during early gestation. A very primitive organ, the pronephros, is the first 'kidney' that is present in the human embryo. This is thought to be a non-functional organ in the mammal and is soon replaced by the mesonephros. The permanent kidney, the metanephros, begins to develop whilst the mesonephros is still present. Of particular importance in terms of fetal programming, the period of nephrogenesis is completed before birth in the human and sheep but continues postnatally in rodent species (Moritz and Wintour 1999). Correct formation of the pronephros and mesonephros is absolutely essential for the normal growth and development of the permanent metanephric kidney.

The mesonephros

By day 24–26 post conception in the human, the primitive mesonephric tubules begin to form on the lateral and ventral sides of the nephrogenic ridges and develop into a longitudinal duct. This

Developmental Origins of Health and Disease, ed. Peter Gluckman and Mark Hanson. Published by Cambridge University Press.
© P. D. Gluckman and M. A. Hanson 2006.

mesonephric or Wolffian duct extends the length of the nephrogenic ridge and opens into the cloaca by day 28 of gestation (de Martino and Zamboni 1966). By the eighth week the mesonephros is fully developed and consists of glomeruli and tubules (Moritz and Wintour 1999). In comparison to the permanent metanephros, the glomeruli are relatively large and the tubules lack a loop of Henle, macula densa and juxtaglomerular apparatus (de Martino and Zamboni 1966). There are considerably fewer glomeruli in the mesonephros compared to the metanephros (<100 compared to >500 000). The glomeruli receive their blood supply from branches of the dorsal aorta. The tubules open into the mesonephric duct that in turn connects to the urogenital sinus that has been formed by division of the cloaca into two compartments. Development of the tubules progresses from the cranial to the caudal end such that degeneration of tubules at the cranial end is occurring simultaneously with formation of tubules at the caudal end. In the human, the mesonephros has completely regressed by week 16 of gestation (Moritz and Wintour 1999). The mesonephros is an excretory organ is some species (sheep and pig) but also may be a site of haemopoiesis, and may contribute to the development of the adrenal and gonad as well as function as an endocrine gland (Moritz and Wintour 1999).

The metanephros

The metanephros begins as an outgrowth from the lower end of the mesonephric duct. This growth, termed the ureteric bud, is essential for metanephric kidney formation. The process of nephrogensis is one of reciprocal induction between two distinct tissues: the ureteric bud and the renal (or metanephric) mesenchyme. The ureteric bud causes the metanephric mesenchyme to differentiate and form nephrons whilst the mesenchyme causes the ureteric bud to bifurcate and go on to form the collecting ducts (for review see Bard 2002). The ureteric bud dilates at its growing tip to form an ampulla and becomes surrounded by a mass of cells of the nephrogenic ridge which form the nephrogenic cap

or blastema. Induction signals from the ureteric bud cause the metanephric mesenchyme to condense and form a closed tube of epithelial cells called the nephrogenic vesicle. The tip of the ureteric bud then continues to divide dichotomously, with one arm of each division inducing the condensation of mesenchyme and initiating the formation of a nephrogenic vesicle, whilst the other arm continues to divide. At the periphery, the branching of the ureteric bud continues rapidly. However, the first two to three branches start to dilate and go on to form the pelvis of the kidney and the major calices. At this stage, urine can be secreted. The next few generations of branches will form the minor calices and the main collecting ducts, whilst the cells forming the nephrogenic caps become the nephrons. Meanwhile, the nephrogenic vesicle, which is a hollow tube of epithelial cells, forms firstly a comma, then an S-shaped tubule which goes on to form the glomerulus and the proximal and distal tubules. The sequential branching eventually leads to the formation of hundreds of thousands of nephrons. The expression of many growth factors, receptors and peptides has been demonstrated to regulate branching morphogenesis as well as controlling development and differentiation of the metanephric mesechyme (Bard 2002). Thus, final nephron number is dependent on factors regulating both ureteric bud growth and nephrogenesis, and any factor altering expression of these factors will ultimately affect nephron endowment. When assessing nephron endowment, appropriate and high-quality methodology is critical in the assessment of glomerular number. Unbiased stereology remains the 'gold standard' for determining nephron number but has only been used in a limited number of studies (Kett and Bertram 2004).

Functional development of the fetal kidney

The metanephric kidney can produce urine from soon after it can first be identified, although accurate estimations of volume are not possible early in gestation. The fetus, in contrast to the adult, produces a large volume of dilute urine and only

Table 23.1 Comparison of adult and fetal renal function.

	Adult kidney (60 kg adult)	Fetal kidney (2 kg fetus)
Blood flow	20% cardiac output	3% cardiac output
Glomerular filtration rate	180 L day^{-1}	3.5 L day^{-1}
Urine volume	1 L day^{-1}	0.5 L day^{-1}
Urine osmolality, normal	~800 mOsm kg^{-1} water	60–100 mOsm kg^{-1} water
Urine osmolality, maximal	1200 mOsm kg^{-1} water	400 mOsm kg^{-1} water
Fractional sodium reabsorption	99.9% filtered load	95% filtered load

reabsorbs approximately 95% of the filtered sodium. A comparison between the renal function in the adult and fetus is shown in Table 23.1. The major function of fetal urine production is to provide a constant source of hypotonic fluid inflow to the fluid compartments surrounding the fetus (amniotic in the human; amniotic and allantoic in sheep, cow etc.). Thus a relatively large proportion of filtrate is excreted: 14% versus ~0.5% in the adult (Table 23.1). Factors known to alter fetal renal function include natriuretic peptides, adrenal steroids and arginine vasopressin (Wintour *et al.* 1999). The renin–angiotensin system (RAS) is critical for the normal morphological and functional development of the kidney. As described below, the sodium transporters and water channels responsible for controlling fluid homeostasis are expressed at different levels in the fetus and adult.

Sodium transporters

Sodium transporters and water channels in the developing kidney

Although many systems can influence blood pressure in the short term, long-term blood pressure control ultimately depends on renal sodium handling (Hall 2003). High dietary sodium (salt) intake can increase plasma volume, due to expansion of total extracellular fluid volume. It has been speculated

that failure to suppress intrarenal Ang II activity during chronic salt loading may lead to salt-sensitive hypertension, resulting primarily from salt and water retention. The bulk of the reabsorption of sodium is carried out in the proximal tubule of the nephron, and the fine control of sodium reabsorption is carried out in the distal nephron and collecting duct, suggesting that the epithelial sodium channel (ENaC) plays a key role in controlling sodium balance and blood pressure. In Table 23.2 are listed the major sodium transporters of the adult kidney, and the major regulation; the ontogeny of each form, in so far as it is known, is also indicated (Burrow *et al.* 1999, Knepper *et al.* 2003, Beutler *et al.* 2003, Holtback and Aperia 2003, Baum and Quigley 2004, Matsubara 2004). The newborn kidney has both an inability to excrete a sodium load, and an inability to conserve sodium maximally. It is worth noting that while there are several isoforms of Na, K-ATPase β, the dominant forms show changed expression after birth. In general the total level of expression is lower in the fetus than in the adult, and this accounts for the higher percentage of sodium excreted in fetal urine (5% vs. 1%) even though fetal urine is normally hypotonic in the unstressed mammalian fetus (Wintour *et al.* 1999).

Water channels

The major water channels in the adult kidney are aquaporin 1 (AQP1) in the proximal tubules and descending limb of the loop of Henle, and in the descending vasa recta; aquaporin 2 in the cytoplasm and apical membrane of the principal cells of the collecting duct; aquaporins 3, 4 in the basolateral membranes of the principal cells of the collecting duct; aquaporin 6 in intracellular membranes of the intercalating cells of the collecting duct (Verkman 2002). AQP1 is present before birth in species in which nephrogenesis is complete before birth (human, sheep), and at term values are approximately half those in the adult (Wintour *et al.* 1998, 1999), AQP2, which is essential for the action of vasopressin to concentrate urine, is present at very low levels (~4% of adult) at mid gestation in sheep, and

Table 23.2 Expression and regulation of the major sodium channels in the kidney.

Segment	Sodium transporter	Regulation
Basolateral		
All	Sodium–potassium ATPase (Na, K-ATPase α_1) rate-limiting increased 5–10-fold postnatally; ↑80% at birth in sheep; effect of glucocorticoid	↑ by sodium deficiency, aldosterone, angiotensin II, noradrenaline (α receptor) ↓ by dopamine (D_1) atrial natriuretic factor
	Na, K-ATPase $\beta_{1(2\ before\ birth)}$	↓ by aldosterone, angiotensin II, sodium deficiency
	Na, K-ATPase γ Regulatory on activity	MW of protein form changed by sodium deficiency (85 KD to 70 KD)
Apical		
Proximal convoluted tubule (PCT); proximal straight tubule (PST)	Sodium hydrogen exchanger (NHE $_{3\ (1,2,4\ before\ birth)}$) Major Na transporter	↑ by noradrenaline (α) angiotensin II ↓ by dopamine, parathyroid hormone (PTH)
Thick ascending limb of loop of Henle (TAL); macula densa (MD)	Na, K-2Cl cotransporter (NKCC2) present in fetal life (? active)	Inhibited by furosemide, bumetanide
Distal tubule (DT)	Na/Cl cotransporter	Inhibited by thiazide
	NCC	Protein but not mRNA ↑ by aldosterone, sodium deficiency
Cortical connecting tubule (CNT); collecting duct-cortical (CCD); outer medullary (OMCD)	ENaC α Lower levels in fetus vs. adult	Inhibited by amiloride mRNA and protein ↑ by aldosterone, sodium deficiency, angiotensin II ↑ relocation to membrane
	ENaC β Higher levels in fetus vs. adult	Protein but not mRNA ↓ by sodium deficiency, aldosterone, angiotensin II
	ENaC γ Higher levels in fetus	As for ENaC β

at ~40% at term (Butkus *et al.* 1999). The same is true for the human fetus (Devuyst *et al.* 1996). The newborn kidney thus has limited sodium transporters to create a hypertonic medullary gradient, and a limited ability to save water in the collecting duct, so a limited capacity to concentrate urine maximally.

How can kidney development be altered?

Normal renal development can be impaired by a wide variety of causes, both genetic and environmental (Vanderheyden *et al.* 2003). A list of some factors known to impair mammalian nephrogenesis is given in Table 23.3. The kidney has been implicated in the programming of adult disease predominantly through studies in which a low or reduced nephron number resulting from maternal intervention is associated with elevated blood pressure in the adult offspring. Much interest has focused on the so-called 'Brenner hypothesis', which states that a reduction in nephron endowment at birth contributes to the development of hypertension (Brenner and Mackenzie 1997). There are many fetal exposures that have been shown in the human and experimental models to cause an alteration in glomerular (and thus nephron) number, although

Table 23.3 Factors known to affect renal development in humans and experimental models.

Treatment	Reference	Type/experiment
Undernutrition	do Carmo Pinho Franco *et al.* 2003	Global
	Langley-Evans *et al.* 2003a	Protein
	Burrow 2000	Vitamin A deficiency
	Yang *et al.* 2003	Iron-deficiency anaemia
	Pham *et al.* 2003	Uterine artery ligation
	Godfrey 2002	Placental malfunction
	Silver 2003	?? Aetiology
Maternal drug intake	Tabacova *et al.* 2003	Inhibitors of renin–angiotensin system
	Chan 2004	
	Sawdy *et al.* 2003	Inhibitors of cyclo-oxygenases
	Mitra *et al.* 2000	Cocaine
Twin–twin transfusion syndrome	Mahieu-Caputo *et al.* 2001	
Genetic	Glassberg 2002	GDNF heterozygote mice
	Cullen-McEwen *et al.* 2003	
Urinary tract obstruction	Chevalier 2004	
Maternal disease	Nelson 2003	Diabetes
Maternal stress	Moritz *et al.* 2003	Endogenous glucocorticoids
	Dodic *et al.* 2002b	Exogenous glucocorticoids

one of the difficulties in comparing the effects of various models/studies on glomerular number is that not all studies have used appropriate methodology. It is of interest that uninephrectomy during nephrogenesis results in altered development of the remaining kidney and hypertension in the adult (Woods 1999, Woods *et al.* 2001b, Douglas-Denton *et al.* 2002, Moritz *et al.* 2002b). Other studies have shown that there may be permanent changes in expression in some genes, particularly those involved in sodium transport and fluid homeostasis. Thus, the simple hypothesis of Brenner has been modified to the following. Any factor which results in decreased nephron endowment **during nephrogenesis**, and causes compensatory changes in the remaining kidney(s), will result in hypertension in the adult.

Is low birthweight a risk for kidney disease? Effects of undernutrition in the human fetus

Moderately low birthweight (<2.5 kg, taken as an index of compromised intrauterine environment),

has been shown to contribute to early-onset end-stage renal disease (ESRD) in children from the southern USA (Lackland *et al.* 2000) as well as in the Australian Aboriginal population (Hoy *et al.* 1999). Growth-restricted fetuses have been shown to have smaller kidneys (Silver *et al.* 2003), indicating a role of altered renal development. Much of the evidence for programming of adult disease comes from human epidemiological studies and animal models where the offspring is of low birthweight due to maternal undernutrition or placental insufficiency. Low birthweight has been cited as a 'progression promoter' for renal disease (Alebiosu 2003). Other studies have found no association between low birthweight and renal parameters. One study demonstrated that males of low birthweight did not have impaired renal function despite having elevated blood pressure and elevated natriuresis (Vasarhelyi *et al.* 2000), and in females born at term but small for gestational age, neither blood pressure nor renal function were altered (Kistner *et al.* 2000). Low birthweight was not found to be a risk factor in the progression of diabetic nephropathy in type 1 diabetic patients (Jacobsen *et al.* 2003).

Table 23.4 Effects of maternal undernutrition/low protein on nephron number. Result = % of nephrons compared to control group. M = male, F = female, NC = no change.

Authors	Species	Time in pregnancy	Diet	Technique and age	Result
Merlet-Benichou et al. 1994	Rat (Sprague–Dawley)	8–21	5% protein	Maceration, 2 weeks	68% nephrons (?M/F)
Langley-Evans et al. 1999	Rat (Wistar)	All preg 0–7 8–14 15–22	9% protein	Biased stereology, 4 weeks	88% NC 88% 88% (?M/F)
Paixao et al. 2001	Rat (Wistar)	All preg Preg + lact	Multidef- 9% protein	Maceration, adult	69% (M) 67% (M)
Vehaskari et al. 2001	Rat (Sprague–Dawley)	12–term	6% protein	Maceration, 8 weeks	72% (M) 71% (F)
Welham et al. 2002	Rat(Wistar)	All preg	6% protein 9% protein	Maceration, 2 weeks	60% 70%
do Carmo Pinho Franco et al. 2003	Rat (SHR)	All preg	50% ad lib	Biased stereology, 14 weeks	89% (M) 86% (F)
Woods et al. 2001a	Rat (Sprague–Dawley)	All preg	8.5% protein	Unbiased stereology, adult	74% (M)
Woods et al. 2004	Rat (Sprague–Dawley)	All preg 1–11 11–term	5% protein	Unbiased stereology, adult	55% (M/F) NC 70% (M)

Undernutrition: results from animal studies

Maternal undernutrition/protein restriction has been the most commonly used experimental protocol to initiate programming effects. Table 23.4 shows the studies that demonstrate alterations in nephron number. It is of importance to note that not all treatments that cause a decrease in nephron number result in offspring with hypertension (Zimanyi et al. 2004), although blood pressure measurements made using tail-cuff methods may not reflect true basal blood pressure. Rats exposed to low-protein diets but supplemented with additional nitrogen sources had a normal nephron number but still developed hypertension. Only the addition of glycine could reverse the hypertensive effects of the low-protein diet (Langley-Evans et al. 2003b). These data suggest other compensatory mechanisms play an important role. As discussed later, one of these appears to be the renin–angiotensin system.

Maternal diabetes

The level of diabetes, worldwide, was 2.8% in 2000, and is projected to rise to 4.4% by 2030 (Wild et al. 2004). Of the 171 million people with diabetes in 2000, the majority had type 2, and a substantial number (30 million) were in the reproductive age group of 22–44 years. There is substantial evidence that the embryo which develops in an environment of maternal hyperglycaemia, particularly during the third to seventh week, has a two- to four-fold incidence of malformations, including those of the genitourinary tract (Chugh et al. 2003). The risk of stillbirth is increased in prediabetic and diabetic pregnancies (Wood et al. 2003, Carrapato and Marcelino 2001, Di Cianni et al. 2003). Diabetic nephropathy is a serious complication associated with greatly increased risk of cardiovascular disease (Parving et al. 2004). Not all type 2 diabetes is genetic; there is evidence that the intrauterine environment can play a role (Sobngwi *et al.* 2003). It has been shown, in rats, that a mild increase in maternal blood glucose levels, to ~10 mmol L^{-1}, from day 12 to day 16 of development, is sufficient to cause a significant decrease in nephron number in the offspring (Amri *et al.* 1999, 2001, Duong Van Huyen *et al.* 2003). This is associated with an increase in the quantity and duration of expression of the IGF2/mannose-6-phosphate receptor. IGF2 is a major growth factor for the developing kidney, and this receptor is thought to function as a 'clearance' receptor, so one might expect the net effect of exposure to maternal hyperglycaemia to be a decrease in the effectiveness of IGF2. It is of interest that the period in which the treatment is effective corresponds to the time when the ureteric bud is first branching and the first glomeruli are starting to form (Bertram *et al.* 2000). Diabetic Pima Indians who were exposed to a diabetic intrauterine environment are at increased risk of albuminuria compared to diabetic Pima Indians exposed to a normal intrauterine environment (Nelson *et al.* 1998). This just reaffirms the notion that individuals born to diabetic mothers can potentially suffer long-term renal consequences.

Anaemia and vitamin A deficiency

Whilst some drop in haemoglobin (Hb) concentration occurs normally in pregnancy (to ~105g L^{-1}), due to a greater expansion of plasma volume than red cell mass, half the pregnant women of the world are estimated to suffer some degree of true anaemia, with haemoglobin levels of 80–100g L^{-1} (van den Broek 2003). Estimations of mild vitamin A deficiency (<0.7 mmol L^{-1} = <20 microgram L^{-1} serum retinol), assessed by the incidence of night blindness, is thought to affect 250 million people, of whom approximately 20 million are pregnant women (Christian 2003). There is some evidence from animal experiments that iron deficiency impairs mobilisation of liver retinol (the vitamin A precursor), exacerbating the problems (Strube *et al.* 2002). In fact, in developing countries, micronutrient deficiencies are probably the major problem in undernutrition during pregnancy, contributing

to the increased mortality and morbidity seen in mother and baby (Fall *et al.* 2003). The offspring of iron-deficient pregnant rats are known to be hypertensive (Crowe *et al.* 1995, Lisle *et al.* 2003). There was also the suggestion that nephron number was decreased in female offspring, though the method used to count nephrons was not ideal (Lisle *et al.* 2003). Retinol (vitamin A) is converted to retinoic acid and acts via binding to dimers of retinoic acid receptors (RARs) and retinoid X receptors (RXRs) to influence many developmental processes (Wei 2004). Mild vitamin A deficiency is associated with decreased nephron number (Lelievre-Pegorier *et al.* 1998, Burrow 2000). The effects of vitamin A deficiency could be exerted at numerous levels, including placental function, but two important genes, expressed in the developing kidney are definitely affected. Glial-derived neurotrophic factor, GDNF, is a critical molecule in branching nephrogenesis, and acts in part by binding to a receptor, c-ret, in the tips of the ureteric buds. This c-ret receptor is down-regulated in vitamin-A-deficient animals (Batourina *et al.* 2001). Another gene, midkine, encoding a heparin-binding growth/differentiation factor, involved in mesenchyme/epithelium transformation, is also down-regulated in vitamin A deficiency (Vilar *et al.* 2002). The action of vitamin A deficiency on midkine is independent of the effects via c-ret.

Elevated maternal steroids

A summary of animal studies in which maternal glucocorticoids have been shown to affect nephron number is shown in Table 23.5. In sheep exposed to elevated levels of glucocorticoids for 48 hours very early in pregnancy (26–28 days out of a 150 day pregnancy) a reduction in nephron number of ~30% is found in the adult (Wintour *et al.* 2003). Offspring of both sexes develop high blood pressure from 4 months of age (Dodic *et al.* 2002a). This hypertension worsens with age and animals develop left ventricular hypertrophy by 7 years of age (Dodic *et al.* 2001). This is particularly interesting as at the time of the treatment the branching of the ureteric bud

Table 23.5 Effects of maternal steroid administration on nephron number. Dex = dexamethasone. Result = % of nephrons compared to control group, NC = no change.

Reference	Species	Time of treatment	Steroid (dose)	Technique and age	Result
Celsi *et al.* 1998	Rat	All pregnancy	Dex (100 mg kg^{-1})	Maceration	60%
			Cortisol		NC
Ortiz *et al.* 2001	Rat	11,12	Dex (0.2 mg kg^{-1})	Maceration,	NC
		13,14		2 months	NC
		15,16			70%
		17,18			80%
		19,20			NC
		20,21			NC
Ortiz *et al.* 2003	Rat	11,12	Dex (0.2 mg kg^{-1})	Maceration,	NC
		13,14		6–9 months	NC
		15,16			80%
		17,18			83%
		19,20			NC
Wintour *et al.* 2003	Sheep	26–28 d	Dex (0.48 mg h^{-1})	Unbiased stereology, adult (7 years)	60%
Moritz, Wintour and	Sheep	26–28 d	Dex (0.48 mg h^{-1})	Unbiased Stereology, fetus (140 days)	75%
Dodic (unpublished)			Cortisol (5 mg h^{-1})		65%

(which will develop into the permanent metanephric kidney) has just occurred. In the rat, maternal glucocorticoid treatment also affects final nephron number and may cause hypertension when the insult is early in the development of the kidney, around E15–E18 (Ortiz *et al.* 2001, 2003, Langley-Evans *et al.* 2003a). It is also of great significance that undernutrition/protein restriction may in fact cause programming effects through elevation of glucocorticoids (Dodic *et al.* 2002c).

The exposure of the fetus to maternal glucocorticoids is largely dependent upon placental transfer. The placenta is the interface between the mother and fetus, and many factors shown to alter fetal development may do so via altering placental transport of nutrients/hormones or placental hormone production itself (Godfrey 2002). For example, if the maternal renin–angiotensin system is up-regulated, say by vitamin D deficiency, the fetal exposure to maternal steroids may be increased because elevated angiotensin II concentrations can decrease the expression of the placental 11β-hydroxysteroid dehydrogenase 2 gene (11β-HSD2), which normally inactivates maternal glucocorticoid hormone (Lanz *et al.* 2003). As the placenta is partly of fetal origin,

the level of placental hormone production can vary with the gender of the fetus (Chellakooty *et al.* 2002). In the human placenta the level of expression of both the 11β-HSD2 gene and the glucocorticoid receptor (GR) are higher, at term, if the fetus is female (Clifton and Murphy 2004). Alcohol ingestion during pregnancy in rats causes left ventricular hypertrophy in adult female offspring only, and this is dependent on there being an intact maternal adrenal gland; placental 11β-HSD2 mRNA is decreased by alcohol exposure only when the fetus is female (Wilcoxon *et al.* 2003). These are but a few examples to show that the exposure of the female fetus to any change in maternal glucocorticoid is likely to be greater than that of the male fetus, due to gender-specific placental effects.

Compensatory changes in the kidney

As discussed above, a decrease in nephron number is hypothesised to be the major mechanism through which in-utero events programme the fetal kidney. However, the situation is likely to be more complex. A decreased nephron endowment will likely cause compensatory changes within the kidney in order to maintain normal renal function. As yet, the RAS is the most thoroughly examined system, but changes in sodium transporters have also been identified in some models.

Sodium channels

There have been two reports of 'programmed' changes in renal sodium transporters. Bertram *et al.* (2001) reported that the kidneys of 12-week-old off-spring of rats, which had been protein-deprived (9% vs. 18%) during pregnancy, had higher levels of mRNA for both α_1 and β_1 subunits of Na/K/ATPase than their controls. This may signify that the tubules were more 'adult-like' in these offspring; when kidneys are stimulated to increase sodium retention, by aldosterone or angiotensin II, they normally increase the α subunit but decrease the β subunit (Knepper *et al.* 2003, Beutler *et al.* 2003). In the second study, however, both the NKCC2 and NCC transporters were up-regulated in the 4-week-old offspring of rats treated with a lower protein intake (6%) from day 12 to parturition, without changes in NHE3, or any ENaC channels (Manning *et al.* 2002).

Renin–angiotensin system (RAS)

In numerous models of undernutrition and gluco-corticoid exposure, components of the RAS, especially the AT1 and AT2 receptors, are significantly altered. During the period of nephrogenesis, expression of these receptors is often decreased, but after completion of nephrogenesis there is a compensatory increase in receptor expression. In the sheep, early prenatal glucocorticoid exposure had not affected arterial pressure when examined at 130 days, but it had led to increased gene expression of renal angiotensin II type 1 and type 2 receptors and angiotensinogen in dexamethasone-exposed animals, as well as renal AT1 and AT2 receptors in cortisol-exposed animals (Moritz *et al.* 2002a). Recently, we have shown that expression of these receptors is decreased at mid gestation (75 days) after early prenatal glucocorticoids

(Moritz, Dodic and Wintour, unpublished). In a maternal-undernutrition model in sheep (from day 28 to day 77 of pregnancy) expression of the AT1 receptor was elevated in the fetal kidneys at birth (Whorwood *et al.* 2001). This early-gestation undernutrition has been reported, recently, to decrease nephron number (Langley-Evans *et al.* 2003b). Exposure of rats to a low-protein diet was found to have up-regulated the angiotensin II type 1A receptor in offspring at 4 weeks, although it had been lower than normal in the newborn kidney (Vehaskari *et al.* 2004). Thus the evidence strongly suggests that components of the RAS are down-regulated during nephrogenesis during maternal low protein/malnutrition/stress, but are up-regulated in compensation after nephrogenesis is complete.

Important questions and areas for future research

Research in the field is moving rapidly, with the development of new animal models to test hypotheses. In all studies it is essential that optimal methodologies are employed, especially when determining nephron number and blood pressure. Blood pressure measurement in conscious, unstressed animals using telemetry or indwelling catheters is critical to obtain 'normal' basal values. These should be carried out over at least 24 hours for optimal information to be obtained. Adequate analysis of both males and females is also necessary, as outcomes (and mechanisms) may vary between sexes. There are still many questions to be answered. In animal models where a nephron deficit has been observed, such as the rat vitamin A deficiency, what is the blood pressure of the offspring? What happens to renal function in many of these models? Is there an additive effect of high salt or lifestyle factors that contribute to adult disease? The compensatory changes made by the kidney at completion of nephrogenesis also warrant intensive investigation.

Finally, in order to develop early intervention strategies, it is necessary to be able to identify individuals born with a low nephron endowment who may be predisposed to later renal disease. In an important study, birthweight in humans was found to be significantly correlated with nephron number, with a predictive increase of 250 000 nephrons for each 1 kg increase in birthweight (Hughson *et al.* 2003). Thus, should low-birthweight individuals be considered a high risk for developing early renal failure? If so, what can be measured or examined to detect this? Guidelines developed by the National Kidney Foundation's Kidney Disease Outcomes Quality Initiative suggest that the two most critical tests are the measurement of protein-to-creatinine ratios in spot urines and estimation of glomerular filtration rate (GFR) from serum creatinine using predictive equations (Hogg *et al.* 2003). Recently, it has also been reported that a high urine output and low urine osmolality are risk factors for rapid progression of renal disease (Hebert *et al.* 2003).

REFERENCES

Alebiosu, C. O. (2003). An update on 'progression promoters' in renal diseases. *J. Natl. Med. Assoc.*, **95**, 30–42.

Amri, K., Freund, N., Vilar, J., Merlet-Benichou, C. and Lelievre-Pegorier, M. (1999). Adverse effects of hyperglycemia on kidney development in rats: in vivo and in vitro studies. *Diabetes*, **48**, 2240–5.

Amri, K., Freund, N., Van Huyen, J. P., Merlet-Benichou, C. and Lelievre-Pegorier, M. (2001). Altered nephrogenesis due to maternal diabetes is associated with increased expression of IGF-II/mannose-6-phosphate receptor in the fetal kidney. *Diabetes*, **50**, 1069–75.

Bard, J. B. (2002). Growth and death in the developing mammalian kidney: signals, receptors and conversations. *Bioessays*, **24**, 72–82.

Batourina, E., Gim, S., Bello, N. *et al.* (2001). Vitamin A controls epithelial/mesenchymal interactions through Ret expression. *Nat. Genet.*, **27**, 74–8.

Baum, M. and Quigley, R. (2004). Ontogeny of renal sodium transport. *Semin. Perinatol.*, **28**, 91–6.

Bertram, C., Trowern, A. R., Copin, N., Jackson, A. A. and Whorwood, C. B. (2001). The maternal diet during pregnancy programs altered expression of the glucocorticoid receptor and type 2 11beta-hydroxysteroid dehydrogenase: potential molecular mechanisms underlying the programming of hypertension in utero. *Endocrinology*, **142**, 2841–53.

Bertram, J. F., Young, R. J., Spencer, K. and Gordon, I. (2000). Quantitative analysis of the developing rat kidney: absolute and relative volumes and growth curves. *Anat. Rec.*, **258**, 128–35.

Beutler, K. T., Masilamani, S., Turban, S. *et al.* (2003). Long-term regulation of ENaC expression in kidney by angiotensin II. *Hypertension*, **41**, 1143–50.

Brenner, B. M. and Mackenzie, H. S. (1997). Nephron mass as a risk factor for progression of renal disease. *Kidney Int. Suppl.*, **63**, S124–7.

Burrow, C. R. (2000). Retinoids and renal development. *Exp. Nephrol.*, 8, 219–25.

Burrow, C. R., Devuyst, O., Li, X., Gatti, L. and Wilson, P. D. (1999). Expression of the beta2-subunit and apical localization of Na+−K+−ATPase in metanephric kidney. *Am. J. Physiol.*, **277**, F391–403.

Butkus, A., Earnest, L., Jeyaseelan, K. *et al.* (1999). Ovine aquaporin-2: cDNA cloning, ontogeny and control of renal gene expression. *Pediatr. Nephrol.*, **13**, 379– 90.

Carrapato, M. R. and Marcelino, F. (2001). The infant of the diabetic mother: the critical developmental windows. *Early Pregnancy*, **5**, 57–8.

Celsi, G., Kistner, A., Aizman, R. *et al.* (1998). Prenatal dexamethasone causes oligonephronia, sodium retention, and higher blood pressure in the offspring. *Pediatr. Res.*, **44**, 317–22.

Chan, V. S. (2004). A mechanistic perspective on the specificity and extent of COX-2 inhibition in pregnancy. *Drug. Saf.*, **27**, 421–6.

Chellakooty, M., Skibsted, L., Skouby, S. O. *et al.* (2002). Longitudinal study of serum placental GH in 455 normal pregnancies: correlation to gestational age, fetal gender, and weight. *J. Clin. Endocrinol. Metab.*, **87**, 2734–9.

Chevalier, R. L. (2004). Perinatal obstructive nephropathy. *Semin. Perinatol.*, **28**, 124–31.

Christian, P. (2003) Micronutrients and reproductive health issues: an international perspective. *J. Nutr.*, **133**, 1969–73S.

Chugh, S. S., Wallner, E. I. and Kanwar, Y. S. (2003). Renal development in high-glucose ambience and diabetic embryopathy. *Semin. Nephrol.*, **23**, 583–92.

Clifton, V. L. and Murphy, V. E. (2004). Maternal asthma as a model for examining fetal sex-specific effects on maternal physiology and placental mechanisms that regulate human fetal growth. *Placenta*, **25** (Suppl. A), S45–52.

Crowe, C., Dandekar, P., Fox, M., Dhingra, K., Bennet, L. and Hanson, M. A. (1995). The effects of anaemia on heart, placenta and body weight, and blood pressure in fetal and neonatal rats. *J. Physiol.*, **488**, 515–19.

Cullen-McEwen, L. A., Kett, M. M., Dowling, J., Anderson, W. P. and Bertram, J. F. (2003). Nephron number, renal function, and arterial pressure in aged GDNF heterozygous mice. *Hypertension*, **41**, 335–40.

de Martino, C. and Zamboni, L. (1966). A morphologic study of the mesonephros of the human embryo. *J. Ultrastruct. Res.*, **16**, 399–427.

Devuyst, O., Burrow, C. R., Smith, B. L., Agre, P., Knepper, M. A. and Wilson, P. D. (1996). Expression of aquaporins-1 and -2 during nephrogenesis and in autosomal dominant polycystic kidney disease. *Am. J. Physiol.*, **271**, F169–83.

Di Cianni, G., Volpe, L., Lencioni, C. *et al.* (2003). Prevalence and risk factors for gestational diabetes assessed by universal screening. *Diabetes Res. Clin. Pract.*, **62**, 131–7.

do Carmo Pinho Franco, M., Nigro, D., Fortes, Z. B. *et al.* (2003). Intrauterine undernutrition: renal and vascular origin of hypertension. *Cardiovasc. Res.*, **60**, 228–34.

Dodic, M., Samuel, C., Moritz, K. *et al.* (2001). Impaired cardiac functional reserve and left ventricular hypertrophy in adult sheep after prenatal dexamethasone exposure. *Circ. Res.*, **89**, 623–9.

Dodic, M., Abouantoun, T., O'Connor, A., Wintour, E. M. and Moritz, K. M. (2002a). Programming effects of short prenatal exposure to dexamethasone in sheep. *Hypertension*, **40**, 729–34.

Dodic, M., Hantzis, V., Duncan, J. *et al.* (2002b). Programming effects of short prenatal exposure to cortisol. *FASEB J.*, **16**, 1017–26.

Dodic, M., Moritz, K., Koukoulas, I. and Wintour, E. M. (2002c). Programmed hypertension: kidney, brain or both? *Trends Endocrinol. Metab.*, **13**, 403–8.

Douglas-Denton, R., Moritz, K. M., Bertram, J. F. and Wintour, E. M. (2002). Compensatory renal growth after unilateral nephrectomy in the ovine fetus. *J. Am. Soc. Nephrol.*, **13**, 406–10.

Duong Van Huyen, J. P., Amri, K., Belair, M. F. *et al.* (2003). Spatiotemporal distribution of insulin-like growth factor receptors during nephrogenesis in fetuses from normal and diabetic rats. *Cell Tissue Res.*, **314**, 367–79.

Fall, C. H., Yajnik, C. S., Rao, S., Davies, A. A., Brown, N. and Farrant, H. J. (2003). Micronutrients and fetal growth. *J. Nutr.*, **133**, 1747–56S.

Glassberg, K. I. (2002). Normal and abnormal development of the kidney: a clinician's interpretation of current knowledge. *J. Urol.*, **167**, 2339–51.

Godfrey, K. M. (2002). The role of the placenta in fetal programming: a review. *Placenta*, **23** (Suppl. A), S20–7.

Hall, J. E. (2003). The kidney, hypertension, and obesity. *Hypertension*, **41**, 625–33.

Hebert, L. A., Greene, T., Levey, A., Falkenhain, M. E. and Klahr, S. (2003). High urine volume and low urine osmolality are risk factors for faster progression of renal disease. *Am. J. Kidney Dis.*, **41**, 962–71.

Hogg, R. J., Furth, S., Lemley, K. V. *et al.* (2003). National Kidney Foundation's Kidney Disease Outcomes Quality Initiative clinical practice guidelines for chronic kidney disease in children and adolescents: evaluation, classification, and stratification. *Pediatrics*, **111**, 1416–21.

Holtback, U. and Aperia, A. C. (2003). Molecular determinants of sodium and water balance during early human development. *Semin. Neonatol.*, **8**, 291–9.

Hoy, W., Kelly, A., Jacups, S. *et al.* (1999). Stemming the tide: reducing cardiovascular disease and renal failure in Australian Aborigines. *Aust. NZ J. Med.*, **29**, 480–3.

Hughson, M., Farris, A. B., Douglas-Denton, R., Hoy, W. E. and Bertram, J. F. (2003). Glomerular number and size in autopsy kidneys: the relationship to birth weight. *Kidney Int.*, **63**, 2113–22.

Jacobsen, P., Rossing, P., Tarnow, L., Hovind, P. and Parving, H. H. (2003). Birth weight: a risk factor for progression in diabetic nephropathy? *J. Intern. Med.*, **253**, 343–50.

Kett, M. M. and Bertram, J. F. (2004). Nephron endowment and blood pressure: what do we really know? *Curr. Hypertens. Rep.*, **6**, 133–9.

Kistner, A., Celsi, G., Vanpee, M. and Jacobson, S. H. (2000). Increased blood pressure but normal renal function in adult women born preterm. *Pediatr. Nephrol.*, **15**, 215–20.

Knepper, M. A., Kim, G. H. and Masilamani, S. (2003). Renal tubule sodium transporter abundance profiling in rat kidney: response to aldosterone and variations in NaCl intake. *Ann. NY Acad. Sci.*, **986**, 562–9.

Lackland, D. T., Bendall, H. E., Osmond, C., Egan, B. M. and Barker, D. J. P. (2000). Low birth weights contribute to high rates of early-onset chronic renal failure in the southeastern United States. *Arch. Intern. Med.*, **160**, 1472–6.

Langley-Evans, S. C., Welham, S. J. and Jackson, A. A. (1999). Fetal exposure to a maternal low protein diet impairs nephrogenesis and promotes hypertension in the rat. *Life Sci.*, **64**, 965–74.

Langley-Evans, S. C., Langley-Evans, A. J. and Marchand, M. C. (2003a). Nutritional programming of blood pressure and renal morphology. *Arch. Physiol. Biochem.*, **111**, 8–16.

Langley-Evans, S. C., Fahey, A. and Buttery, P. J. (2003b). Early gestation is a critical period in the nutritional programming of nephron number in the sheep. *Pediatr. Res.*, **53** (Suppl.), 30A.

Lanz, B., Kadereit, B., Ernst, S. *et al.* (2003). Angiotensin II regulates 11beta-hydroxysteroid dehydrogenase type 2 via AT2 receptors. *Kidney Int.*, **64**, 970–7.

Lelievre-Pegorier, M., Vilar, J., Ferrier, M. L. *et al.* (1998). Mild vitamin A deficiency leads to inborn nephron deficit in the rat. *Kidney Int.*, **54**, 1455–62.

Lisle, S. J., Lewis, R. M., Petry, C. J., Ozanne, S. E., Hales, C. N. and Forhead, A. J. (2003). Effect of maternal iron restriction during pregnancy on renal morphology in the adult rat offspring. *Br. J. Nutr.*, **90**, 33–9.

Mahieu-Caputo, D., Muller, F., Joly, D. *et al.* (2001). Pathogenesis of twin–twin transfusion syndrome: the renin–angiotensin system hypothesis. *Fetal Diagn. Ther.*, **16**, 241–4.

Manning, J., Beutler, K., Knepper, M. A. and Vehaskari, V. M. (2002). Upregulation of renal BSC1 and TSC in prenatally programmed hypertension. *Am. J. Physiol. Renal Physiol.*, **283**, F202–6.

Matsubara, M. (2004). Renal sodium handling for body fluid maintenance and blood pressure regulation. *Yakugaku Zasshi*, **124**, 301–9.

Merlet-Benichou, C., Gilbert, T., Muffat-Joly, M., Lelievre-Pegorier, M. and Leroy, B. (1994). Intrauterine growth retardation leads to a permanent nephron deficit in the rat. *Pediatr. Nephrol.*, **8**, 175–80.

Mitra, S. C., Seshan, S. V., Salcedo, J. R. and Gil, J. (2000). Maternal cocaine abuse and fetal renal arteries: a morphometric study. *Pediatr. Nephrol.*, **14**, 315–18.

Moritz, K. M. and Wintour, E. M. (1999). Functional development of the meso- and metanephros. *Pediatr. Nephrol.*, **13**, 171–8.

Moritz, K. M., Johnson, K., Douglas-Denton, R., Wintour, E. M. and Dodic, M. (2002a). Maternal glucocorticoid treatment programs alterations in the renin–angiotensin system of the ovine fetal kidney. *Endocrinology*, **143**, 4455–63.

Moritz, K. M., Wintour, E. M. and Dodic, M. (2002b). Fetal uninephrectomy leads to postnatal hypertension and compromised renal function. *Hypertension*, **39**, 1071–6.

Moritz, K. M., Dodic, M. and Wintour, E. M. (2003). Kidney development and the fetal programming of adult disease. *Bioessays*, **25**, 212–20.

Nelson, R. G. (2003). Intrauterine determinants of diabetic kidney disease in disadvantaged populations. *Kidney Int. Suppl.*, **83**, S13–16.

Nelson, R. G., Morgenstern, H. and Bennett, P. H. (1998). Intrauterine diabetes exposure and the risk of renal disease in diabetic Pima Indians. *Diabetes*, **47**, 1489–93.

Ortiz, L. A., Quan, A., Weinberg, A. and Baum, M. (2001). Effect of prenatal dexamethasone on rat renal development. *Kidney Int.*, **59**, 1663–9.

Ortiz, L. A., Quan, A., Zarzar, F., Weinberg, A. and Baum, M. (2003). Prenatal dexamethasone programs hypertension and renal injury in the rat. *Hypertension*, **41**, 328–34.

Paixao, A. D., Maciel, C. R., Teles, M. B. and Figueiredo-Silva, J. (2001). Regional Brazilian diet-induced low birth weight is correlated with changes in renal hemodynamics and glomerular morphometry in adult age. *Biol. Neonate*, **80**, 239–46.

Parving, H. H., Andersen, S., Jacobsen, P. *et al.* (2004). Angiotensin receptor blockers in diabetic nephropathy: renal and cardiovascular end points. *Semin. Nephrol.*, **24**, 147–57.

Pham, T. D., MacLennan, N. K., Chiu, C. T., Laksana, G. S., Hsu, J. L. and Lane, R. H. (2003). Uteroplacental insufficiency increases apoptosis and alters p53 gene methylation in the full-term IUGR rat kidney. *Am. J. Physiol. Regul. Integr. Comp. Physiol.*, **285**, R962–70.

Sawdy, R. J., Lye, S., Fisk, N. M. and Bennett, P. R. (2003). A double-blind randomized study of fetal side effects during and after the short-term maternal administration of indomethacin, sulindac, and nimesulide for the treatment of preterm labor. *Am. J. Obstet. Gynecol.*, **188**, 1046–51.

Silver, L. E., Decamps, P. J., Korst, L. M., Platt, L. D. and Castro, L. C. (2003). Intrauterine growth restriction is accompanied by decreased renal volume in the human fetus. *Am. J. Obstet. Gynecol.*, **188**, 1320–5.

Sobngwi, E., Boudou, P., Mauvais-Jarvis, F. *et al.* (2003). Effect of a diabetic environment in utero on predisposition to type 2 diabetes. *Lancet*, **361**, 1861–5.

Strube, Y. N., Beard, J. L. and Ross, A. C. (2002) Iron deficiency and marginal vitamin A deficiency affect growth, hematological indices and the regulation of iron metabolism genes in rats. *J. Nutr.*, **132**, 3607–15.

Tabacova, S., Little, R., Tsong, Y., Vega, A. and Kimmel, C. A. (2003). Adverse pregnancy outcomes associated with maternal enalapril antihypertensive treatment. *Pharmacoepidemiol. Drug. Saf.*, **12**, 633–46.

van den Broek, N. (2003). Anaemia and micronutrient deficiencies. *Br. Med. Bull.*, **67**, 149–60.

Vanderheyden, T., Kumar, S. and Fisk, N. M. (2003). Fetal renal impairment. *Semin. Neonatol.*, **8**, 279–89.

Vasarhelyi, B., Dobos, M., Reusz, G. S., Szabo, A. and Tulassay, T. (2000). Normal kidney function and elevated natriuresis in young men born with low birth weight. *Pediatr. Nephrol.*, **15**, 96–100.

Vehaskari, V. M., Aviles, D. H. and Manning, J. (2001). Prenatal programming of adult hypertension in the rat. *Kidney Int.*, **59**, 238–45.

Vehaskari, V. M., Stewart, T., Lafont, D., Soyez, C., Seth, D. and Manning, J. (2004). Kidney angiotensin and angiotensin receptor expression in prenatally programmed hypertension. *Am. J. Physiol. Renal. Physiol.*, **287**, F262–7.

Verkman, A. S. (2002). Physiological importance of aquaporin water channels. *Ann. Med.*, **34**, 192–200.

Vilar, J., Lalou, C., Duong, V. H. *et al.* (2002). Midkine is involved in kidney development and in its regulation by retinoids. *J. Am. Soc. Nephrol.*, **13**, 668–76.

Wei, L. N. (2004). Retinoids and receptor interacting protein 140 (RIP140) in gene regulation. *Curr. Med. Chem.*, **11**, 1527–32.

Welham, S. J., Wade, A. and Woolf, A. S. (2002). Protein restriction in pregnancy is associated with increased apoptosis of mesenchymal cells at the start of rat metanephrogenesis. *Kidney Int.*, **61**, 1231–42.

Whorwood, C. B., Firth, K. M., Budge, H. and Symonds, M. E. (2001). Maternal undernutrition during early to midgestation programs tissue-specific alterations in the expression of the glucocorticoid receptor, 11beta-hydroxysteroid dehydrogenase isoforms, and type 1 angiotensin II receptor in neonatal sheep. *Endocrinology*, **142**, 2854–64.

Wilcoxon, J. S., Schwartz, J., Aird, F. and Redei, E. E. (2003). Sexually dimorphic effects of maternal alcohol intake and adrenalectomy on left ventricular hypertrophy in rat offspring. *Am. J. Physiol. Endocrinol. Metab.*, **285**, E31–9.

Wild, S., Roglic, G., Green, A., Sicree, R. and King, H. (2004). Global prevalence of diabetes: estimates for the year 2000 and projections for 2030. *Diabetes Care*, **27**, 1047–53.

Wintour, E. M., Earnest, L., Alcorn, D., Butkus, A., Shandley, L. and Jeyaseelan, K. (1998). Ovine AQP1: cDNA cloning, ontogeny, and control of renal gene expression. *Pediatr. Nephrol.*, **12**, 545–53.

Wintour, E. M., Dodic, M., Johnston, H., Moritz, K. and Peers, A. (1999). Kidney and urinary tract. In *Fetal Medicine: Basic Science and Clinical Practice* (ed. C. H. Rodeck and M. J. Whittle). London: Churchill Livingstone, pp. 155–71.

Wintour, E. M., Moritz, K. M., Johnson, K., Ricardo, S., Samuel, C. S. and Dodic, M. (2003). Reduced nephron number in adult sheep, hypertensive as a result of prenatal glucocorticoid treatment. *J. Physiol.*, **549**, 929–35.

Wood, S. L., Jick, H. and Sauve, R. (2003). The risk of stillbirth in pregnancies before and after the onset of diabetes. *Diabet. Med.*, **20**, 703–7.

Woods, L. L. (1999). Neonatal uninephrectomy causes hypertension in adult rats. *Am. J. Physiol.*, **276**, R974–8.

Woods, L. L., Ingelfinger, J. R., Nyengaard, J. R. and Rasch, R. (2001a). Maternal protein restriction suppresses the newborn renin–angiotensin system and programs adult hypertension in rats. *Pediatr. Res.*, **49**, 460–7.

Woods, L. L., Weeks, D. A. and Rasch, R. (2001b). Hypertension after neonatal uninephrectomy in rats precedes glomerular damage. *Hypertension*, **38**, 337–42.

(2004). Programming of adult blood pressure by maternal protein restriction: role of nephrogenesis. *Kidney Int.*, **65**, 1339–48.

Yang, J., Mori, K., Li, J. Y. and Barasch, J. (2003). Iron, lipocalin, and kidney epithelia. *Am. J. Physiol. Renal Physiol.*, **285**, F9–18.

Zimanyi, M. A., Bertram, J. F. and Black, M. J. (2004.) Does a nephron deficit in rats predispose to salt-sensitive hypertension? *Kidney Blood Press. Res.*, **27**, 239–47.

24

The developmental environment: effect on fluid and electrolyte homeostasis

Mostafa A. El-Haddad and Michael G. Ross

University of California, Los Angeles

Introduction

Body fluid and electrolytes in adults are maintained under tight control by complex central and peripheral mechanisms. A relatively minor increase in plasma osmolality, or somewhat larger decrease in plasma volume, triggers counter-regulatory mechanisms in the hypothalamus and kidneys to restore plasma osmolality and/or plasma volume to normal values. Arginine vasopressin (AVP) synthesised in the hypothalamic paraventricular nucleus (PVN) and released into systemic circulation from the posterior pituitary plays a key role in fluid and electrolyte regulation by acting upon renal water channels to conserve water. Other important hypothalamic nuclei, namely the circumventricular organs (CVOs), which are located along the anteroventral wall of the third ventricle, are responsible for regulation of body water and salt content by modulating water and salt intake. CVOs also play a critical role in cardiovascular regulation via efferent connections with brainstem centres regulating sympathetic nervous system responses. The renin–angiotensin system (RAS) is highly expressed within brain centres regulating water and electrolytes and cardiovascular homeostasis. RAS is also highly expressed in the fetal and adult kidney, contributing to normal kidney development in the former.

Programming of water and electrolyte regulatory systems is defined as a perinatal 'insult' inflicted to the fetus/neonate during critical developmental period(s) which will impact on the water and electrolyte regulatory systems in the offspring. As reviewed, there are significant data demonstrating the perinatal programming of offspring hypothalamopituitary and AVP responses, renal water regulatory mechanisms, thirst and salt appetite, and blood pressure homeostasis in numerous species.

Fluid and electrolyte changes during pregnancy

A number of critical maternal physiological pregnancy adaptations, including plasma volume (pVol) expansion, increased cardiac output, reduced systemic vascular resistance and a decrease in maternal plasma osmolality (pOsm) contribute to successful pregnancy, and ultimately impact on normal fetal development. In normal pregnancy, pVol expansion begins as early as 6 weeks' gestation (Duvekot et al. 1993) and continues to 24–34 weeks. Adequate pVol expansion is necessary for normal pregnancy outcome, as a lack or loss of adequate pVol expansion has been associated with a high risk of pre-eclampsia, intrauterine growth restriction (IUGR), premature labour and oligohydramnios (Goodlin et al. 1983). In addition to pVol expansion, early human pregnancy is notable for marked reductions in maternal pOsm (Duvekot et al. 1993) as pOsm decreases

Developmental Origins of Health and Disease, ed. Peter Gluckman and Mark Hanson. Published by Cambridge University Press.

approximately 10 mOsm kg^{-1} by 6 weeks of pregnancy (Davison *et al.* 1980). Plasma hypotonicity is maintained via central resetting of the osmotic threshold for arginine vasopressin (AVP) secretion to a lower level. Thus, hypothalamic osmoreceptors sense the relative pregnancy plasma hypotonicity as normal (Davison *et al.* 1984). As in humans, pregnant rats demonstrate a marked decrease in plasma tonicity (Atherton *et al.* 1982). In contrast, sheep demonstrate only modest reductions in pOsm during pregnancy, and the osmotic threshold for arginine vasopressin (AVP) secretion is not reset (Keller-Wood 1994). Notably, the increase in maternal pVol in sheep (10%) (Metcalfe and Parer 1966) is also less than in humans (30%).

Fetal water is ultimately derived from the maternal compartment, a result of placental water exchange. Driven by both osmotic (i.e. maternal plasma hypotonicity) and hydrostatic (maternal blood pressure) forces, maternal water crosses to the fetus. Thus, maternal hypo- and hypertonicity may alter placental water exchange. Our studies have demonstrated that maternal [desamino, D-Arg8]-AVP (dDAVP; desmopressin)-induced plasma hypotonicity facilitates the transfer of water to the fetus, and induces relative fetal plasma hypotonicity (Roberts *et al.* 1999). Conversely, exposure to maternal plasma hypertonicity, as a result of hyperemesis, exercise or dehydration, results in increased fetal pOsm, stimulation of fetal AVP secretion, and reduced amniotic fluid (AF) volume (oligohydramnios) (Ross *et al.* 1988).

Maternal plasma volume expansion and plasma hypotonicity are of great clinical significance to the developing fetus. A lack of these fluid and osmoregulatory changes may adversely impact upon short-term pregnancy outcomes. Equally important, chronic fetal hypertonicity may programme osmoregulatory and cardiovascular mechanisms in the newborn and adult offspring, as discussed below.

Development of fetal osmoregulatory and dipsogenic mechanisms

Body fluid regulation is mediated via two principal mechanisms: osmolality and intravascular volume. As noted above, small increases in extracellular fluid osmolality (~2%) stimulate AVP secretion (with resultant urinary antidiuresis) and thirst, thus returning extracellular fluid osmolality towards normal values. Although there is species variation, a dual system of central nervous system (CNS) osmoreceptors and Na$^+$ sensors mediates these responses (McKinley *et al.* 1978). Somewhat larger decreases (~10%) in circulating volume initiate AVP-mediated antidiuresis and likely angiotensin II (AngII) mediated thirst (Ross *et al.* 1986). Neuroanatomical studies in adults of several species indicate that systemic osmotic effects are mediated via sites within brain CVOs, small midline organs positioned on the anterior surface of the third cerebral ventricles. Having fenestrated capillaries, the CVOs are in a unique position in the central nervous system to function as receptor sites for central neural signals, cerebrospinal fluid (CSF) signals (Thrasher *et al.* 1980), and transduction of blood-borne signals to neural signals. CVOs are known to participate in the central control of salt and water balance, and probably regulate autonomic, endocrine and even behavioural functions of fluid homeostasis.

Although fetal pOsm is maintained parallel to maternal levels (via placental equilibration), functional osmoregulatory mechanisms develop in utero in sheep and humans. Although prior studies suggested that osmoregulatory responses develop during the newborn period in altricial species (e.g. rat) (Wirth and Epstein 1976), we have demonstrated central osmotic responsiveness in the near-term fetal rat (Xu and Ross 2000). In the more precocial sheep fetus, systemic and central osmotic–dipsogenic mechanisms are functional near term, as swallowing activity is stimulated in response to intravenous or intracarotid hypertonic saline (Ross *et al.* 1992). Similarly, intracerebroventricular (ICV) hypertonic saline and AngII in the near-term ovine fetus stimulate fetal swallowing and AVP secretion (Ross *et al.* 1994, 1995). Although fetal osmotic–dipsogenic responses are intact near term, the regulation of fetal swallowing may be fundamentally different from the adult, in part a result of the pattern of neural development. Spontaneous fetal swallowing is exaggerated, as the fetus normally swallows 5 to 10 times the volume of fluid intake of the adult, relative to body weight (Sherman *et al.* 1990). Significant differences in osmotic sensitivity also are apparent; whereas a 2–3% pOsm increase stimulates adult water intake (Davison *et al.* 1984), fetal stimulation requires a 6% increase (Xu *et al.* 2001). Behavioural studies in the adult rat have demonstrated important roles for central AngII and glutamate N-methyl-D-aspartate (NMDA) receptors, and neuronal nitric oxide synthase (nNOS) in the regulation of stimulated, though not spontaneous, adult drinking (Zhu and Herbert 1997, Blair-West *et al.* 1998, Lewis *et al.* 2001, El-Haddad *et al.* 2001a). We have recently explored the neuronal mechanisms underlying the high rate of in-utero fetal swallowing (El-Haddad *et al.* 1999, 2000, 2001a). Unlike adult rat basal drinking, we have demonstrated that central AngII (El-Haddad *et al.* 2001a), glutamate (El-Haddad *et al.* 2001b) and nNOS (El-Haddad *et al.* 1999, 2000) contribute to the high rate of basal fetal swallowing. Although speculative, chronic fetal hyperosmolality may programme abnormal levels of these and other neurotransmitters and their receptors within hypothalamic dipsogenic neurons, leading to abnormal osmoregulatory mechanisms in the offspring (discussed below).

Fetal renal development

A functioning kidney is essential for fluid regulation both during intrauterine life and post delivery. During intrauterine life, the kidney produces large volumes of dilute urine, which serves to maintain amniotic fluid volume, essential for normal fetal development. The fetus produces hypotonic urine, as fetal AVP secretion occurs at a relatively higher plasma osmolality than in the adult (Xu *et al.* 2000). Furthermore, the fetal kidney is relatively resistant to antidiuretic action of AVP due to a relative lack of water channel aquaporin 2 (AQP2)(Butkus *et al.* 1999).

Understanding of the normal pattern of fetal kidney development is important, as recent evidence has demonstrated that intrauterine insults during critical times of renal development may programme hypertension and fluid abnormalities in offspring (Langley-Evans *et al.* 1999, Dodic *et al.* 1999, Ortiz *et al.* 2001) (see also Chapter 23). In mammals, the pronephros and mesonephros appear during embryonic and early fetal life. These organs regress and the metanephros becomes the permanent adult kidney (Wintour *et al.* 1998). In rats and pigs, nephrogenesis of the permanent metanephros is not complete until eight days and three weeks after birth, respectively (Friis 1980, Moritz and Wintour 1999), while in human and sheep, nephrogenesis is complete before birth at 36 weeks and 130 days gestation, respectively (Moritz and Wintour 1999, Solhaug *et al.* 2004). Normal kidney development is greatly dependent upon the renin–angiotensin system (RAS) produced locally within the metanephros. Components of RAS are synthesised and expressed within the metanephros as early as 41 and 56 days gestation in sheep and human fetuses, respectively (Wintour *et al.* 1996, Schutz *et al.* 1996). Accordingly, both angiotensin AT1 receptor and angiotensinogen-gene knockout mice demonstrate severe kidney abnormalities (Niimura *et al.* 1995, Hilgers *et al.* 1997, Tsuchida *et al.* 1998).

Programming of fetal dipsogenic and osmoregulatory mechanisms

The in-utero environment has long been recognised as contributing to offspring behaviour, though it was not until the late 1980s that Barker *et al.* (1989) expanded the concept of in-utero programming to an association of low birthweight with risks of adult cardiovascular disease, diabetes mellitus and dyslipidaemia (Barker *et al.* 1993, Ravelli *et al.* 1998). Human adult blood pressure is elevated among growth-restricted fetuses (Leon and Koupilova 2001). Studies in rat, sheep, piglets and baboons, at varying gestational periods, degrees and types of nutrient deficiency (Holemans *et al.* 1999, Nwagwu *et al.* 2000, Sherman and Langley-Evans 2000, Calzone *et al.* 2001, Jones *et al.* 2001, Regina *et al.* 2001, Vehaskari *et al.* 2001, Woods *et al.* 2001), have confirmed a link, albeit sometimes inconsistent, between intrauterine growth restriction and adult hypertension or metabolic disease.

Although pOsm or plasma sodium has rarely been measured, there was no change in maternal plasma sodium of nutritionally deprived dams (Leizea *et al.* 1999).

Programming of osmoregulation (AVP and thirst) (Handelmann and Sayson 1984) has been demonstrated in the fetal and neonatal rat (Mouw *et al.* 1978, Galaverna *et al.* 1995). Extracellular dehydration during pregnancy increases salt appetite (Nicolaidis *et al.* 1990) and blood pressure (Arguelles *et al.* 1996) of offspring rats. Renal responsiveness to AVP also may be programmed as neonatal rat exposure to AVP results in a long-lasting decrease in renal AVP responsiveness (Handelmann *et al.* 1983) due to a reduction in AVP binding sites in the adult kidney (Handelmann and Sayson 1984). AVP administration during the first month of life increases 24-hour water intake and decreases urine osmolality in diabetes insipidus rats six weeks after cessation of treatment (Wright and Kutscher 1977). In adult rats, prolonged tonicity alterations alter hypothalamic AVP mRNA content (Robinson *et al.* 1990). More importantly, similar studies of young rats suggest a permanent programming of AVP synthesis in response to tonicity alterations (Fitzsimmons *et al.* 1994). Recent human studies also suggest the programming of neonatal osmoregulatory/salt appetite systems as a result of the maternal pregnancy osmotic environment; although hypertonic exposure occurs earlier in human pregnancy as compared to the ovine model (see below). Mothers with moderate/severe emesis during pregnancy, likely to result in maternal dehydration and plasma hypertonicity, have infants with significantly enhanced salt preference at 16 weeks of age (Crystal and Bernstein 1998, Leshem 1998).

Our laboratory has developed an ovine model of gestational hypertonicity resulting in the development of plasma hypertonicity, hypertension, and haemoconcentration in 1-month-old offspring. Furthermore, programming of AVP secretory responses is demonstrated by an elevated threshold for AVP secretion in response to plasma hypertonicity. These responses are in sharp distinction to phenotypes from those of periconceptional,

early- or late-pregnancy malnutrition, or early-pregnancy glucocorticoids. Notably, offspring of glucocorticoid-exposed fetuses have normal AVP secretory responses (Dodic *et al.* 2002a).

We initially explored the programming of AVP/osmoregulatory mechanisms, first by examining the maturation of normal fetal pituitary AVP content and hypothalamic AVP mRNA expression (Zhao *et al.* 1998). Hypothalamic AVP mRNA expression was significantly greater in ewes versus preterm (110 days) and near-term (135 days) fetuses. Pituitary AVP content was significantly greater in 110-day fetuses versus maternal ewes and 135-day fetuses, suggesting that the greater pituitary AVP content in the 110-day fetuses may suppress AVP mRNA expression. In response to subacute (four days) maternal tonicity alterations, near-term (135 days) ovine hypothalamic AVP mRNA expression and pituitary AVP content did not change (Zhao *et al.* 1998). However, AVP mRNA expression was significantly negatively correlated with pituitary AVP content ($r^2 = 0.684$; $p < 0.006$), suggesting a dynamic AVP synthesis-content feedback relationship in the near-term fetus.

To determine the potential programming effect of chronic gestational hyperosmolality on offspring AVP gene expression and pituitary content, pregnant ewes were water-restricted to maintain plasma hypertonicity (10–20 mOsm kg^{-1} above baseline level) from 119 days until normal term delivery. Newborns were provided with *ad libitum* maternal nursing. Within 24 hours after birth, study and age-matched control neonatal lambs were euthanised and the pituitary and hypothalamus removed. Total pituitary AVP content was greater (8.3 ± 2.8 µg vs. 1.6 ± 1.3 µg; $p < 0.05$) and hypothalamic AVP mRNA was lower (AVP/β-actin ratio 0.29 ± 0.01 vs. 0.68 ± 0.15; $p < 0.05$) in gestational hyperosmolality than in control newborns (Ramirez *et al.* 2002). More prolonged effects of gestational hyperosmolality were determined by following *ad libitum* nursed lambs until 28 days of age. Study lambs had higher total pituitary AVP content (6.5 ± 1.0 vs. 2.8 ± 1.2 µg; $p < 0.05$), though there was no difference in hypothalamic AVP mRNA levels between study and control lambs (Wang *et al.* 2003). Thus prolonged prenatal exposure to plasma hypertonicity may programme the fetal hypothalamic–pituitary AVP regulatory system.

In response to these studies suggesting osmoregulatory programming, we sought to explore the osmoregulatory systems of offspring of gestational-hyperosmolality ewes. Our results conclusively demonstrate the programming of newborn hypertonicity and hypertension. Prenatally dehydrated (as described above) and control singleton lambs were normally delivered and nursed by ewes provided *ad libitum* food and water after delivery. At the time of birth, prenatally dehydrated lambs weighed 18% less than controls, though the offspring demonstrated catch-up growth to equivalent weight as controls by 3 weeks of age. Furthermore, at 3 weeks of age, prenatally dehydrated lambs had significantly increased plasma osmolality, sodium and haematocrit, though normal plasma AVP levels. Moreover, the prenatally dehydrated offspring demonstrated markedly elevated systolic, diastolic and mean arterial pressures, with values 10 mm Hg above control levels (Desai *et al.* 2003). The increase in basal plasma osmolality and sodium levels suggested an altered plasma osmolality threshold for AVP secretion. Accordingly, we performed an intravenous infusion of hypertonic saline to the offspring to assess the relation between AVP and plasma osmolality. Throughout the hypertonic saline infusion, prenatally dehydrated offspring maintained persistently elevated plasma osmolality, sodium and haematocrit, as well as elevated systolic, diastolic and mean arterial pressures. The prenatally dehydrated offspring demonstrated an increased plasma osmolality threshold for AVP secretion as compared to the controls (290 vs. 280 mOsm kg^{-1}). Further evaluation of the AVP secretory responses demonstrated that the prenatally dehydrated offspring have an increased slope of the AVP vs. pOsm relationship (0.28 ± 0.07 vs. 0.13 ± 0.04; $p < 0.05$).

As noted above, gestational malnutrition may result in an increased risk of offspring hypertension. In sheep, maternal nutrient reduction (50%) from 115 days until term increased fetal blood pressure and a heightened pressor response to angiotensin II

(AngII) at 115–125 days (Edawards and McMillen 2001). In view of the association of AngII with renal development and function, we have explored the effects of nutrient restriction on offspring fluid homeostasis. In sheep, natural twin gestation was utilised as a model of nutrient restriction during pregnancy, while twin nursing by the maternal ewe was utilised to continue nutrient restriction throughout the 3 weeks of lactation. Twin lambs were 30% smaller at birth than control singletons, and demonstrated a further relative weight reduction, to 50% of singletons following twin nursing at 3 weeks of age. When studied at 3 weeks, twins demonstrated significantly increased plasma sodium (144 vs. 140 mEq L^{-1}) as compared to singletons, though similar plasma osmolality, plasma AVP levels and arterial haematocrit. At 3 weeks, twins demonstrated elevated arterial systolic, diastolic and mean arterial blood pressure, with the mean arterial pressures approximately 5 mm Hg greater than in singletons. We performed a determination of the plasma osmolality threshold for AVP secretion in twin offspring (as described above). The plasma osmolality threshold for AVP secretion was greater in twins than in singletons (285 vs. 280 mOsm kg^{-1}), though intermediate between prenatally dehydrated singletons and singleton controls.

These results suggest that both hypertonicity and perhaps nutrition reduction (i.e. dehydration anorexia) contribute to offspring programming (Desai *et al.* 2003). Notably, none of the previously described models of malnutrition or glucocorticoid-induced programming simulate our consistently observed effects of gestational hyperosmolality on offspring: the marked degree of plasma hypertonicity hypertension and increased haematocrit in offspring of gestational-hyperosmolality ewes are unique findings consistent with programmed AVP/osmoregulatory and cardiovascular alterations. We hypothesise that chronic gestational hyperosmolality alters offspring central osmoreceptors, AVP secretory and sympathetic nervous system regulatory responses, and potentially the HPA axis and RAS responses. Central or systemic hyperosmolality is well known to activate the splanchnic, adrenal and lumbar sympathetic nervous system, with resulting elevation of blood pressure (Bealer *et al.* 1996, Weiss *et al.* 1996, Doda 1997, Seki *et al.* 1997, Scrogin *et al.* 1999, McKinley *et al.* 2001, Toney *et al.* 2003). These studies suggest that activation of fetal fluid regulatory mechanisms within the gestational environment initiate events which permanently alter the offspring and perhaps mature animal. Consistent with studies in fetal and neonatal rats, programming is most likely to occur during the functional maturation of endocrine systems. Human and ovine fetal development is markedly more precocial than that of the rat, with marked development during the last third of gestation. Consequently, we hypothesise that this represents a critical period of exposure to altered tonicity.

Programming of the central renin–angiotensin system

Fluid and electrolyte homeostasis is regulated via both the kidneys and selective forebrain centres. In this section of the review we will focus mainly upon the brain RAS and its potential programming in response to prolonged fetal hyperosmolality. Components of the RAS and its receptors are highly expressed within hypothalamic and forebrain centres involved in fluid homeostasis and brainstem centres involved in cardiovascular regulation (McKinley *et al.* 1986, Allen *et al.* 1987). Central AngII may influence arterial pressure at numerous brain sites, including the anteroventral third ventricle, paraventricular nucleus (PVN), forebrain regions, nucleus tractus solitarius (NTS), area postrema, and subfornical organ (SFO), with both pressor and depressor pathways, acting via both AT1 and AT2 receptors, respectively (McKinley *et al.* 2003). In the adult and fetus, central angiotensin sites in the anteroventral third ventricle mediate dipsogenic responses and release of AVP via AT1 receptors (El-Haddad *et al.* 2003, McKinley *et al.* 2003). There is evidence for the role of brain RAS in offspring programming in the ovine fetus. Dodic *et al.* (2002b),

utilising pregnant sheep treated with IV dexamethasone at 26–28 days gestation, demonstrated up-regulation of angiotensinogen gene in the hypothalamus, and AT1 receptor in the medulla oblongata at 130 days gestation. The effects on medullary AT1 expression were still evident in female offspring at 7 years of age. These authors also noted programmed hypertension at 2 years of age in both male and female offspring. Although dexamethasone treatment in the very-early-gestation ovine fetus has been shown to up-regulate RAS factors in central dipsogenic and cardiovascular regulatory centres, and programme hypertension in the offspring, the role of the central RAS in response to gestational hyperosmolality remains unknown.

Programming of central sympathetic nervous system (SNS)

SNS activation may be critical to programmed hypertension resulting from gestational hypertonicity, in a manner similar to hypertension associated with increased sodium intake (Brooks *et al.* 2001). At rest, sympathetic nerves exhibit tonic activity which contributes to arterial blood pressure maintenance. Both hypertonicity and AngII act as sympathoexcitatory factors via osmo- or AngII AT1 receptors in the organ vasculosum lamina terminalis (OVLT) and/or SFO (McKinley *et al.* 2001). Neural pathways from the median preoptic nucleus (MnPO) and PVN, to the rostral ventrolateral medulla (rVLM) and spinal intermediolateral cell column, and finally the sympathetic preganglionic neurons (Badoer 2001, Oldfield *et al.* 2001, Toney *et al.* 2003), increase SNS activity.

Significant evidence suggests that the absolute level of sympathetic tone is altered under conditions of increased salt intake or plasma hypertonicity (Brooks *et al.* 2001). In normal individuals, increased salt intake reduces plasma AngII, though arterial blood pressure is maintained by a balance of reduced AngII-mediated and increased osmo- or sodium-receptor-mediated SNS activity. However, in salt-sensitive individuals or animals, hypertonicity-induced sympathoexcitatory actions dominate, possibly due to decreases in the levels or actions of AngII. Reduced AVP secretory responses may be expected to potentiate hypertonicity-induced pressor responses, as AVP acts as a sympatho-inhibitory stimulus. Thus, AVP V1 receptor antagonism may result in salt-dependent hypertension (Osborn 1997).

Arterial baroreceptors also may be primarily acute mediators, as baroreceptor responses rapidly adapt to sustained changes in pressure; that is, baroreceptor firing rates return rapidly (i.e. reset) towards original levels despite continued pressure changes (Brooks and Osborn 1995). Although alternative systems (e.g. renal SNS, baroreceptor responses) may respond to acute hypertonicity or salt intake to maintain normal blood pressure, these mechanisms may be primarily acute, rather than chronic modulators. Whereas acute hypertonicity induces renal sympathoinhibition and promotes sodium excretion, chronic hypertonicity may induce renal sympathoexcitation and increased pressor responses (Scrogin et al. 1999, Chen and Toney 2001).

Programming of the kidney and renal renin–angiotensin system

The kidney acts in close harmony with the brain, via neuroendocrine mechanisms, to achieve body fluid and cardiovascular homeostasis. Evidence is accumulating that intrauterine insults at critical periods of nephrogenesis cause permanent reduction of the nephron number and programme late-onset hypertension (Dodic et al. 1999, Langley-Evans et al. 1999, Ortiz et al. 2001). In rats, in which nephrogenesis is completed only after birth, protein undernutrition throughout or only in the second half of pregnancy (total gestational period ~22 days) has been shown to reduce the nephron number by ~30% and cause hypertension in adult offspring (Ortiz et al. 2001). The mechanism of protein undernutrition causing reduction of fetal nephron number is likely

due, in part, to fetal exposure to excess glucocorticoid at a critical developmental period. Undernutrition of both rats and guinea pigs increases maternal and potentially fetal glucocorticoid production (Dwyer and Stickland 1992, Lesage et al. 2001). Protein deprivation further decreases placental 11β-hydroxysteroid dehydrogenase 2 (11β-HSD2) enzyme, which protects the fetus from relatively higher levels of maternal corticosteroid, therefore allowing increased access of endogenous maternal corticosteroid to the fetus (Langley-Evans et al. 1996). Treatment of pregnant rats with dexamethasone on days 15–16 of gestation reduced nephron number, while treatment at other time periods had less dramatic or no effect on nephron number (Celsi et al. 1998, Bertram et al. 2000, Ingelfinger and Woods 2002). In pregnant sheep, in which nephrogenesis is complete before birth, dexamethasone treatment given for a brief period early in gestation (days 26–28; total gestational period ~150 days), when the permanent metanephric kidney is just starting to form, was associated with a 40% reduction of nephron number at 7 years of age and adult-onset hypertension (Wintour et al. 2003).

The RAS plays important roles in the development and function of the fetal kidney in utero (Lumbers 1995, Moritz and Wintour 1999). All components of the RAS (angiotensinogen, renin, angiotensin-converting enzyme, AT1 and AT2 receptors) are expressed from very early in gestation in the mesonephros and metanephros of human (Schutz et al. 1996), and sheep (Wintour et al. 1996) gestation. There is good evidence that either excess or deficiency of intrarenal RAS may lead to reduction of nephron number and abnormal development of the kidney, with programming of adult-onset hypertension. In rats maintained on a low-protein diet during pregnancy, AT1 receptors were overexpressed in the kidney at birth and at 16 weeks of age (Trowern et al. 2000). Blocking AT1 overactivity with losartan treatment between week 2 and 4 after birth prevented the development of hypertension (Langley-Evans 1997). Up-regulation of intrarenal RAS components occurred in fetal sheep treated with dexamethasone

(Moritz *et al.* 2002), or exposed to undernutrition (Langley-Evans 1997, Trowern *et al.* 2000), early in gestation. The resulting offspring of glucocorticoid-exposed fetuses showed reduction of nephron number at 7 years of age (Wintour *et al.* 2003). In humans, the growth-restricted fetus has smaller kidneys and higher expression of renin gene within the kidney (Kingdom *et al.* 1999), suggesting up-regulation of renal RAS. Up-regulation of renal RAS likely results in premature maturation of metanephric nephrogenesis with resulting reduction of total nephron number. In the ovine model treated with dexamethasone early in gestation, the expression of renal AT1 receptors at 130 days gestation was similar to neonatal expression at 2 days of age, indicating premature metanephros maturation (Butkus *et al.* 1997). The ovine fetal kidney with up-regulated RAS is not only structurally mature but, functionally, it reacts to AngII infusion in a way similar to neonatal kidney, namely, aldosterone secretion and water and sodium retention (Moritz *et al.* 2002). The timing of intrauterine events is critical for programming of renal RAS, as evidence suggests that the insult must occur at a very primitive stage of metanephric development for programming of adult hypertension, low nephron number and up-regulation of renal RAS (Ortiz *et al.* 2001, Wintour *et al.* 2003).

Conclusion

In summary, in-utero programming of fluid and electrolyte homeostasis may be accomplished via central and/or peripheral mechanisms. Studies of gestational hyperosmolality in the ovine model suggest an alteration of offspring AVP regulatory mechanisms, as demonstrated by an elevated plasma osmolality threshold for AVP secretion and an increased AVP secretory response (i.e. slope). We propose the following model (Fig. 24.1): maternal water restriction induces maternal plasma hypertonicity, moderately reduced nutrient intake due to dehydration-induced anorexia, and increased glucocorticoids. Chronic fetal hypertonicity programmes increased osmoreceptors and AVP secretory set-points, accounting

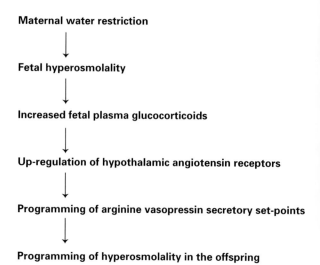

Maternal water restriction

↓

Fetal hyperosmolality

↓

Increased fetal plasma glucocorticoids

↓

Up-regulation of hypothalamic angiotensin receptors

↓

Programming of arginine vasopressin secretory set-points

↓

Programming of hyperosmolality in the offspring

Figure 24.1 Hyperosmolality model.

for the elevated pOsm threshold for AVP-secretion in offspring. Fetal glucocorticoid exposure, perhaps a result of fetal AVP-mediated ACTH stimulation (Zehnder *et al.* 1995) or secondary to elevated maternal glucocorticoids, may up-regulate central Ang AT1 receptors (Dodic *et al.* 2002c) and thus alter the offspring HPA axis. In the offspring, elevated sympathetic nervous system excitation, potentially a result of chronic hypertonicity as well as activation of central AT1 receptors, contributes to systemic hypertension (Bealer *et al.* 1996, Weiss *et al.* 1996, Doda 1997, Seki *et al.* 1997, Scrogin *et al.* 1999, Chen and Toney 2001, McKinley *et al.* 2001, Toney *et al.* 2003).

The programming of AVP–osmoregulatory effects may have developed as a result of species survival advantage. Throughout evolution and development, humans and animals have been exposed to environmental stresses, with drought and famine representing two of the most frequent conditions. Notably, drought-induced water deprivation is associated with dehydration anorexia, and thus a concomitant potential nutrient stress. It is well recognised that genetic mutations within species may provide a survival advantage, either to promote population growth under static environmental conditions or to assure survival under a long-term environmental alteration. Genetic mutations generally require pro-longed, evolutionary time periods to influence the species population. Furthermore, mutations are not likely to be reversible or rapidly adaptable to altering environmental conditions. Conversely, perinatal programming may provide a species survival benefit, facilitating varying offspring phenotypes that are adaptable to environmental condition changes which may resolve or reverse frequently. Should drought occur during the gestational period, developmental programming of specific offspring phenotypes may be of value in adapting the offspring to survival in this environment: for offspring born into an epoch of drought, an elevated slope of AVP secretion in response to dehydration may result in more efficient antidiuresis and water conservation. Further studies exploring the long-term effects of gestational hypertonicity programming and the potential for intergenerational impact are necessary to fully understand the clinical consequences of maternal fluid alterations during pregnancy.

REFERENCES

Allen, A. M., Chai, S. Y., Sexton, P. M. *et al.* (1987). Angiotensin II receptors and angiotensin converting enzyme in the medulla oblongata. *Hypertension*, **9**, III198–205.

Arguelles, J., Lopez-Sela, P., Brime, J. I., Costales, M. and Vijande, M. (1996). Changes of blood pressure responsiveness in rats exposed in utero and perinatally to a high-salt environment. *Regul. Pept.*, **66**, 113–15.

Atherton, J. C., Dark, J. M., Garland, H. O., Morgan, M. R. A., Pidgeon, J. and Soni, S. (1982). Changes in water and electrolyte balance, plasma volume and composition during pregnancy in the rat. *J. Physiol.*, **330**, 81–93.

Badoer, E. (2001). Hypothalamic paraventricular nucleus and cardiovascular regulation. *Clin. Exp. Pharmacol. Physiol.*, **28**, 95–9.

Barker, D. J. P., Osmond, C., Golding, J., Kuh, D. and Wadsworth, M. E. (1989). Growth in utero, blood pressure in childhood and adult life, and mortality from cardiovascular disease. *BMJ*, **298**, 564–7.

Barker, D. J. P., Hales, C. N., Fall, C. H., Osmond, C., Phipps, K. and Clark, P. M. (1993). Type 2 (non-insulin-dependent) diabetes mellitus, hypertension and hyperlipidaemia (syndrome X): relation to reduced fetal growth. *Diabetologia*, **36**, 62–7.

Bealer, S. L., Delle, M., Skarphedinsson, J. O., Carlsson, S. and Thoren, P. (1996). Differential responses in adrenal and renal nerves to CNS osmotic stimulation. *Brain Res. Bull.*, **39**, 205–9.

Bertram, J. F., Young, R. J., Spencer, K. and Gordon, I. (2000). Quantitative analysis of the developing rat kidney: absolute and relative volumes and growth curves. *Anat. Rec.*, **258**, 128–35.

Blair-West, J. R., Carey, K. D., Denton, D. A., Weisinger, R. S. and Shade, R. E. (1998). Evidence that brain angiotensin II is involved in both thirst and sodium appetite in baboons. *Am. J. Physiol.*, **275**, R1639–46.

Brooks, V. L. and Osborn, J. W. (1995). Hormonal–sympathetic interactions in long-term regulation of arterial pressure: an hypothesis. *Am. J. Physiol.*, **268**, R1343–58.

Brooks, V. L., Scrogin, K. E. and McKeogh, D. F. (2001). The interaction of angiotensin II and osmolality in the generation of sympathetic tone during changes in dietary salt intake: an hypothesis. *Ann. NY Acad. Sci.*, **940**, 380–94.

Butkus, A., Albiston, A., Alcorn, D. *et al.* (1997). Ontogeny of angiotensin II receptors, types 1 and 2, in ovine mesonephros and metanephros. *Kidney Int.*, **52**, 628–36.

Butkus, A., Earnest, L., Jeyaseelan, K. *et al.* (1999). Ovine aquaporin-2: cDNA cloning, ontogeny and control of renal gene expression. *Pediatr. Nephrol.*, **13**, 379–90.

Calzone, W. L., Silva, C., Keefe, D. L. and Stachenfeld, N. S. (2001). Progesterone does not alter osmotic regulation of AVP. *Am. J. Physiol. Regul. Integr. Comp. Physiol.*, **281**, R2011–20.

Celsi, G., Kistner, A., Aizman, R. *et al.* (1998). Prenatal dexamethasone causes oligonephronia, sodium retention, and higher blood pressure in the offspring. *Pediatr. Res.*, **44**, 317–22.

Chen, Q. H., Toney, G. M. (2001). AT (1)-receptor blockade in the hypothalamic PVN reduces central hyperosmolality-induced renal sympathoexcitation. *Am. J. Physiol. Regul. Integr. Comp. Physiol.*, **281**, R1844–53.

Crystal, S. R., and Bernstein, I. L. (1998). Infant salt preference and mother's morning sickness. *Appetite.*, **30**, 297–307.

Davison, J. M., Valloton, M. B., and Lindheimer, M. D. (1980). Alterations in plasma osmolality (Posm) during human pregnancy. *Clin. Res.*, **281**, 442A.

Davison, J. M., Gilmore, E. A., Durr, J., Robertson, G. L. and Lindheimer, M. D. (1984). Altered osmotic thresholds for vasopressin secretion and thirst in human pregnancy. *Am. J. Physiol.*, **246**, F105–9.

Desai, M., Guerra, C., Wang, S. and Ross, M. G. (2003). Programming of hypertonicity in neonatal lambs: resetting of the threshold for vasopressin secretion. *Endocrinology*, 144, 4332–7.

Doda, M. (1997). Role of different subtypes of adrenoceptors in pressor responses to catecholamines released from sympathetic nerve endings. *Brain Res. Bull.*, 42, 51–7.

Dodic, M., Peers, A., Coghlan, J. P. *et al.* (1999). Altered cardiovascular haemodynamics and baroreceptor–heart rate reflex in adult sheep after prenatal exposure to dexamethasone. *Clin. Sci.*, 97, 103–9.

Dodic, M., Peers, A., Moritz, K., Hantzis, V. and Wintour, E. M. (2002a). No evidence for HPA reset in adult sheep with high blood pressure due to short prenatal exposure to dexamethasone. *Am. J. Physiol. Regul. Integr. Comp. Physiol.*, 282, R343–50.

Dodic, M., Abouantoun, T., O'Connor, A., Wintour, E. M. and Moritz, K. M. (2002b). Programming effects of short prenatal exposure to dexamethasone in sheep. *Hypertension*, 40, 729–34.

Dodic, M., Hantzis, V., Duncan, J. *et al.* (2002c). Programming effects of short prenatal exposure to cortisol. *FASEB J.*, 16, 1017–26.

Duvekot, J. J., Cheriex, E. C., Pieters, F. A. A., Menheere, P. C. A. and Peeters, L. L. H. (1993). Early pregnancy changes in hemodynamics and volume homeostatis are consecutive adjustments triggered by a primary fall in systemic vascular tone. *Am. J. Obstet. Gynecol.*, 169, 1382–92.

Dwyer, C. M. and Stickland, N. C. (1992). The effects of maternal undernutrition on maternal and fetal serum insulin-like growth factors, thyroid hormones and cortisol in the guinea pig. *J. Dev. Physiol.*, 18, 303–13.

Edwards, L. J. and McMillen, I. C. (2001). Maternal undernutrition increases arterial blood pressure in the sheep fetus during late gestation. *J. Physiol.*, 533, 561–70.

El-Haddad, M. A., Chao, C. R., Ma, S. X. and Ross, M. G. (1999). Nitric oxide modulates spontaneous swallowing behavior in near-term ovine fetus. *Am. J. Physiol.*, 277, R981–6.

(2000). Nitric oxide modulates angiotensin II-induced drinking behavior in the near-term ovine fetus. *Am. J. Obstet. Gynecol.*, 182, 713–19.

El-Haddad, M. A., Chao, C. R., Sayed, A. A., El-Haddad, H. and Ross, M. G. (2001a). Effects of central angiotensin II receptor antagonism on fetal swallowing and cardiovascular activity. *Am. J. Obstet. Gynecol.*, 185, 828–33.

El-Haddad, M. A., Chao, C. and Ross, M. G. (2001b). N-methyl-d-aspartame glutamate receptors mediates spontaneous and angiotensin II-stimulated fetal swallowing. *J. Soc. Gynecol. Investig.*, 8, 62A.

El-Haddad, M. A., Ismail, Y., Guerra, C., Day, L. and Ross, M. G. (2003). Angiotensin II AT1 receptors mediate the high rate of both spontaneous and stimulated fetal swallowing activities in near term ovine fetus. *J. Soc. Gynecol. Investig.* 10, (Suppl. 2).

Fitzsimmons, M. D., Roberts, M. M. and Robinson, A. G. (1994). Control of posterior pituitary vasopressin content: implications for the regulation of the vasopressin gene. *Endocrinology*, 134, 1874–8.

Friis, C. (1980). Postnatal development of the pig kidney: ultrastucture of the glomerulus and the proximal tubule. *J. Anat.*, 130, 513–26.

Galaverna, O., Nicolaidis, S., Yao, S. Z., Sakai, R. R. and Epstein, A. N. (1995). Endocrine consequences of prenatal sodium depletion prepare rats for high need-free NaCl intake in adulthood. *Am. J. Physiol.*, 269, R578–83.

Goodlin, R. C., Dobry, C. A., Anderson, J. C., Woods, R. E. and Quaife, M. (1983). Critical signs of normal plasma volume expansion during pregnancy. *Am. J. Obstet. Gynecol.*, 145, 1001–10.

Handelmann, G. E. and Sayson, S. C. (1984). Neonatal exposure to vasopressin decreases vasopressin binding sites in the adult kidney. *Peptides*, 5, 1217–19.

Handelmann, G. E., Russell, J. T., Gainer, H., Zerbe, R. and Bayorh, M. (1983). Vasopressin administration to neonatal rats reduces antidiuretic response in adult kidneys. *Peptides*, 4, 827–32.

Hilgers, K. F., Reddi, V., Krege, J. H., Smithies, O. and Gomez, R. A. (1997). Aberrant renal vascular morphology and renin expression in mutant mice lacking angiotensin-converting enzyme. *Hypertension*, 29, 216–21.

Holemans, K., Gerber, R., Meurrens, K., De Clerck, F., Poston, L. and Van, Assche F. A. (1999). Maternal food restriction in the second half of pregnancy affects vascular function but not blood pressure of rat female offspring. *Br. J. Nutr.*, 81, 73–9.

Ingelfinger, J. R. and Woods, L. L. (2002). Perinatal programming, renal development, and adult renal function. *Am. J. Hypertens.*, 15, 46–9S.

Jones, S. E., Bilous, R. W., Flyvbjerg, A. and Marshall, S. M. (2001). Intra-uterine environment influences glomerular number and the acute renal adaptation to experimental diabetes. *Diabetologia*, 44, 721–8.

Keller-Wood, M. (1994). Vasopressin responses to hyperosmolality and hypotension during ovine pregnancy. *Am. J. Physiol.*, 266, R188–93.

Kingdom, J. C., Hayes, M., McQueen, J., Howatson, A. G. and Lindop, G. B. (1999). Intrauterine growth restriction is associated with persistent juxtamedullary expression of renin in the fetal kidney. *Kidney Int.*, **55**, 424–9.

Langley-Evans, S. C. (1997). Hypertension induced by foetal exposure to a maternal low-protein diet, in the rat, is prevented by pharmacological blockade of maternal glucocorticoid synthesis. *J. Hypertens.*, **15**, 537–44.

Langley-Evans, S. C., Phillips, G. J., Benediktsson, R. *et al.* (1996). Protein intake in pregnancy, placental glucocorticoid metabolism and the programming of hypertension in the rat. *Placenta*, **17**, 169–72.

Langley-Evans, S. C., Welham, S. J. and Jackson, A. A. (1999). Fetal exposure to a maternal low protein diet impairs nephrogenesis and promotes hypertension in the rat. *Life Sci.*, **64**, 965–74.

Leizea, J. P., Gonzalez, C. G., Garcia, F. D., Patterson, A. M. and Fernandez, S. F. (1999). The effects of food restriction on maternal endocrine adaptations in pregnant rats. *J. Endocrinol. Invest* **22**, 327–32.

Leon, D. A. and Koupilova, I. (2001). Birth weight, blood pressure, and hypertension: epidemiological studies. In *Fetal Origins of Cardiovascular and Lung Disease*. (ed. D. J. P. Barker). New York, NY: Marcel Dekker, pp. 23–48.

Lesage, J., Blondeau, B. and Grino, M., Breant, B., Dupouy, J. P. (2001). Maternal undernutrition during late gestation induces fetal overexposure to glucocorticoids and intrauterine growth retardation, and disturbs the hypothalamo-pituitary adrenal axis in the newborn rat. *Endocrinology*, **142**, 1692–702.

Leshem, M. (1998). Salt preference in adolescence is predicted by common prenatal and infantile mineralofluid loss. *Physiol. Behav.*, **63**, 699–704.

Lewis, K., Li, C., Perrin, M. H. *et al.* (2001). Identification of urocortin III, an additional member of the corticotropin-releasing factor (CRF) family with high affinity for the CRF2 receptor. *Proc. Natl. Acad. Sci. USA*, **98**, 7570–5.

Lumbers, E. R. (1995). Functions of the renin–angiotensin system during development. *Clin. Exp. Pharmacol. Physiol.*, **22**, 499–505.

McKinley, M. J., Denton, D. A. and Weisinger, R. S. (1978). Sensors for antidiuresis and thirst: osmoreceptors or CSF sodium detectors? *Brain Res.*, **141**, 89–103.

McKinley, M. J., Allen, A., Clevers, J., Denton, D. A. and Mendelsohn, F. A. (1986). Autoradiographic localization of angiotensin receptors in the sheep brain. *Brain Res.*, **375**, 373–6.

McKinley, M. J., Allen, A. M., May, C. N. *et al.* (2001). Neural pathways from the lamina terminalis influencing cardiovascular and body fluid homeostasis. *Clin. Exp. Pharmacol. Physiol.*, **28**, 990–2.

McKinley, M. J., Albiston, A. L., Allen, A. M. *et al.* (2003). The brain renin-angiotensin system: location and physiological roles. *Int. J. Biochem. Cell Biol.*, **35**, 901–18.

Metcalfe, J. and Parer, J. T. (1966). Cardiovascular changes during pregnancy in ewes. *Am. J. Physiol.*, **210**, 821–5.

Moritz, K. M. and Wintour, E. M. (1999). Functional development of the meso- and metanephros. *Pediatr. Nephrol.*, **13**, 171–8.

Moritz, K. M., Johnson, K., Douglas-Denton, R., Wintour, E. M. and Dodic, M. (2002). Maternal glucocorticoid treatment programs alterations in the renin–angiotensin system of the ovine fetal kidney. *Endocrinology.*, **143**, 4455–63.

Mouw, D. R., Vander, A. J. and Wagner, J. (1978). Effects of prenatal and early postnatal sodium deprivation on subsequent adult thirst and salt preference in rats. *Am. J. Physiol.*, **234**, F59–63.

Nicolaidis, S., Galaverna, O. and Metzler, C. H. (1990). Extracellular dehydration during pregnancy increases salt appetite of offspring. *Am. J. Physiol.*, **258**, R281–3.

Niimura, F., Labosky, P. A., Kakuchi, J. *et al.* (1995).Gene targeting in mice reveals a requirement for angiotensin in the development and maintenance of kidney morphology and growth factor regulation. *J. Clin. Invest.*, **96**, 2947–54.

Nwagwu, M. O., Cook, A. and Langley-Evans, S. C. (2000). Evidence of progressive deterioration of renal function in rats exposed to a maternal low-protein diet in utero. *Br. J. Nutr.*, **83**, 79–85.

Oldfield, B. J., Davern, P. J., Giles, M. E., Allen, A. M., Badoer, E. and McKinley, M. J. (2001). Efferent neural projections of angiotensin receptor (AT1) expressing neurones in the hypothalamic paraventricular nucleus of the rat. *J. Neuroendocrinol.*, **13**, 139–46.

Ortiz, L. A., Quan, A., Weinberg, A. and Baum, M. (2001). Effect of prenatal dexamethasone on rat renal development. *Kidney Int.*, **59**, 1663–9.

Osborn, J. W. (1997). Hormones as long-term error signals for the sympathetic nervous system: importance of a new perspective. *Clin. Exp. Pharmacol. Physiol.*, **24**, 109–15.

Ramirez, B. A., Wang, S., Kallichanda, N. and Ross, M. G. (2002). Chronic in utero plasma hyperosmolality alters hypothalamic arginine vasopressin synthesis and pituitary arginine vasopressin content in newborn lambs. *Am. J. Obstet. Gynecol.*, **187**, 191–6.

Ravelli, A. C., van der Meulen, J. H., Michels, R. P. *et al.* (1998). Glucose tolerance in adults after prenatal exposure to famine *Lancet*, **351**, 173–7.

Regina, S., Lucas, R., Miraglia, S. M., Zaladek, G. F. and Machado, C. T. (2001). Intrauterine food restriction as a determinant of nephrosclerosis. *Am. J. Kidney Dis.*, **37**, 467–76.

Roberts, T. J., Nijland, M. J. M., Curran, M. and Ross, M. G. (1999). Maternal 1-deamino-8-D-arginine-vasopressin-induced sequential decreases in plasma sodium concentration: ovine fetal renal responses. *Am. J. Obstet. Gynecol.*, **180**, 82–90.

Robinson, A. G., Roberts, M. M., Evron, W. A., Verbalis, J. G. and Sherman, T. G. (1990). Hyponatremia in rats induces downregulation of vasopressin synthesis. *J. Clin. Invest.*, **86**, 1023–9.

Ross, M. G., Ervin, M. G., Leake, R. D., Humme, J. A. and Fisher, D. A. (1986). Continuous ovine fetal hemorrhage: sensitivity of plasma and urine arginine vasopressin. *Am. J. Physiol.*, **251**, E464–9.

Ross, M. G., Sherman, D. J., Ervin, M. G., Castro, R. and Humme, J. (1988). Maternal dehydration–rehydration: fetal plasma and urinary responses. *Am. J. Physiol.*, **255**, E674–9.

Ross, M. G., Agnew, C., Fujino, Y., Ervin, M. and Day, L. (1992). Concentration thresholds for fetal swallowing and vasopressin secretion. *Am. J. Physiol.*, **262**, R1057–63.

Ross, M. G., Kullama, L. K., Ogundipe, A., Chan, K. and Ervin, M. G. (1994). Central angiotensin II stimulation of ovine fetal swallowing. *J. Appl. Physiol.*, **76**, 1340–5.

(1995). Ovine fetal swallowing response to intracerebroventricular hypertonic saline. *J. Appl. Physiol.*, **78**, 2267–71.

Schutz, S., Le, Moullec J. M., Corvol, P. and Gasc, J. M. (1996). Early expression of all the components of the renin–angiotensin system in human development. *Am. J. Pathol.*, **149**, 2067–79.

Scrogin, K. E., Grygielko, E. T. and Brooks, V. L. (1999). Osmolality: a physiological long-term regulator of lumbar sympathetic nerve activity and arterial pressure. *Am. J. Physiol.*, **276**, R1579–86.

Seki, K., Aibiki, M. and Ogura, S. (1997). 3.5% hypertonic saline produces sympathetic activation in hemorrhaged rabbits. *J. Auton. Nerv. Syst.*, **64**, 49–56.

Sherman, D. J., Ross, M. G., Day, L. and Ervin, M. G. (1990). Fetal swallowing: correlation of electromyography and esophageal fluid flow. *Am. J. Physiol.*, **258**, R1386–94.

Sherman, R. C. and Langley-Evans, S. C. (2000). Antihypertensive treatment in early postnatal life modulates prenatal dietary influences upon blood pressure in the rat. *Clin. Sci.* **98**, 269–75.

Solhaug, M. J., Bolger, P. M. and Jose, P. A. (2004). The developing kidney and environmental toxins. *Pediatrics*, **113**, 1084–91.

Thrasher, T. N., Jones, R. G., Keil, L. C., Brown, C. J. and Ramsay, D. J. (1980). Drinking and vasopressin release during ventricular infusions of hypertonic solutions. *Am. J. Physiol.*, **238**, R340–5.

Toney, G. M., Chen, Q. H., Cato, M. J. and Stocker, S. D. (2003). Central osmotic regulation of sympathetic nerve activity. *Acta Physiol. Scand.*, **177**, 43–55.

Trowern, A. R., Bertram, C. and Whorwood, C. B. (2000). The intra-uterine environment programmes hypertension. *Fetal and Neonatal Physiological Society 27th Annual Meeting*, **35**.

Tsuchida, S., Matsusaka, T., Chen, X. *et al.* (1998). Murine double nullizygotes of the angiotensin type 1A and 1B receptor genes duplicate severe abnormal phenotypes of angiotensinogen nullizygotes. *J. Clin. Invest.*, **101**, 755–60.

Vehaskari, V. M., Aviles, D. H. and Manning, J. (2001). Prenatal programming of adult hypertension in the rat. *Kidney Int.*, **59**, 238–45.

Wang, S., Chen, J., Kallichanda, N., Azim, A., Calvario, G. and Ross, M. G. (2003). Prolonged prenatal hypernatremia alters neuroendocrine and electrolyte homeostasis in neonatal sheep. *Exp. Biol. Med.*, **228**, 41–5.

Weiss, M. L., Claassen, D. E., Hirai, T. and Kenney, M. J. (1996). Nonuniform sympathetic nerve responses to intravenous hypertonic saline infusion. *J. Auton. Nerv. Syst.*, **57**, 109–15.

Wintour, E. M., Alcorn, D., Butkus, A. *et al.* (1996). Ontogeny of hormonal and excretory function of the meso- and metanephros in the ovine fetus. *Kidney Int.*, **50**, 1624–33.

Wintour, E. M., Alcorn, D. and Rockell, M. D. (1998). Development and function of the fetal kidney. In *Fetus and Neonate: Physiology and Clinical Applications* (ed. R. A. Brace, M. A. Hanson, and C. H. Rodeck). Cambridge: Cambridge University Press, pp. 3–56.

Wintour, E. M., Moritz, K. M., Johnson, K., Ricardo, S., Samuel, C. S. and Dodic, M. (2003). Reduced nephron number in adult sheep, hypertensive as a result of prenatal glucocorticoid treatment. *J. Physiol.* **549**, 929–35.

Wirth, J. B. and Epstein, A. N. (1976). Ontogeny of thirst in the infant rat. *Am. J. Physiol.*, **230**, 188–98.

Woods, L. L., Ingelfinger, J. R., Nyengaard, J. R. and Rasch, R. (2001). Maternal protein restriction suppresses the newborn renin–angiotensin system and programs adult hypertension in rats. *Pediatr. Res.*, **49**, 460–7.

Wright, W. A. and Kutscher, C. L. (1977). Vasopressin administration in the first month of life: effects on growth and water metabolism in hypothalamic diabetes insipidus rats. *Pharmacol. Biochem. Behav.*, **6**, 505–9.

Xu, Z. and Ross, M. G. (2000). Appearance of central dipsogenic mechanisms induced by dehydration in near-term rat fetus. *Brain Res. Dev. Brain Res.*, **121**, 11–18.

Xu, Z., Glenda, C., Day, L., Yao, J. and Ross, M. G. (2000). Osmotic threshold and sensitivity for vasopressin release and fos expression by hypertonic NaCl in ovine fetus. *Am. J. Physiol. Endocrinol. Metab.*, **279**, E1207–15.

Xu, Z., Nijland, M. J. and Ross, M. G. (2001). Plasma osmolality dipsogenic thresholds and c-fos expression in the near-term ovine fetus. *Pediatr. Res.*, **49**, 678–85.

Zehnder, T. J., Valego, N. K., Schwartz, J., White, A. and Rose, J. C. (1995). Regulation of bioactive and immunoreactive ACTH secretion by CRF and AVP in sheep fetuses. *Am. J. Physiol.*, **269**, E1076–82.

Zhao, X., Nijland, M. J., Ervin, M. G. and Ross, M. G. (1998). Regulation of hypothalamic arginine vasopressin messenger ribonucleic acid and pituitary arginine vasopressin content in fetal sheep: effects of acute tonicity alterations and fetal maturation. *Am. J. Obstet. Gynecol.*, **179**, 899–905.

Zhu, B. and Herbert, J. (1997). Angiotensin II interacts with nitric oxide–cyclic GMP pathway in the central control of drinking behaviour: mapping with c-fos and NADPH-diaphorase. *Neuroscience*, **79**, 543–53.

25

The developmental environment: effects on lung structure and function

Richard Harding,[1] Megan L. Cock[1] and Gert S. Maritz[2]

[1] Monash University
[2] University of the Western Cape

Introduction

Epidemiological studies have provided strong evidence that a suboptimal intrauterine environment can have long-term effects on postnatal lung function and respiratory symptoms or illness. Prenatal factors that have been causally related to long-term changes in respiratory function and health include impaired fetal nutrition and growth (Harding *et al.* 2004), maternal tobacco smoking and nicotine exposure (Joad 2004, Maritz 2004) and preterm birth (Albertine and Pysher 2004). Evidence is accruing that a number of common respiratory illnesses of childhood and adulthood may have their origins in fetal life, or that predisposing conditions may be laid down at the time (Shaheen and Barker 1994). Similarly, it is now recognised that alterations to the early postnatal environment can lead to persistent alterations in lung structure and function later in life.

Lung development and maturation are characterised by several distinct phases, namely the embryonic phase followed by the pseudoglandular, canalicular, saccular and alveolar phases. These are followed by the phase of equilibrated lung growth, the final stage of lung maturation (Kauffman *et al.* 1974). During each phase, specific structural changes occur which eventually result in a lung that can effectively fulfil its role as a gas exchanger, with an ability to resist infection and damage by inhaled toxic agents. Interference with the developmental programme of the lung during any of these phases may render the lung less effective as a gas exchanger or may render it more susceptible to disease.

Effect of undernutrition on lung development

Evidence from epidemiological, clinical and experimental studies indicates that nutritional and oxygen status during development can induce both immediate and long-term alterations in the structure and function of many organs including the lung. In particular, it has been shown that intrauterine growth restriction (IUGR) or being small for gestational age (SGA), both of which are regarded as indicators of impaired fetal nutrition and/or oxygenation, are associated with adverse outcomes, including alterations of respiratory function at all stages of postnatal life. In addition to affecting lung development, it is likely that impaired nutrition or oxygenation during development can influence the rate of pulmonary ageing. It has become apparent that the early nutritional/oxygen environment, as well as the endocrine environment, may be important for the entire life-cycle of the lung (Harding *et al.* 2004).

Fetal growth restriction (or SGA) implies that fetal weight falls below the 10th percentile for gestational age. Normally, growth has been restricted by factors

Developmental Origins of Health and Disease, ed. Peter Gluckman and Mark Hanson. Published by Cambridge University Press.

affecting the intrauterine environment or the delivery of nutrients to the fetus (Nicolaides *et al.* 1989, Resnik 2002). The underlying aetiology is varied and can include maternal, fetal or placental causes. Factors that can adversely affect the nutrient supply from the mother to the fetus and thus fetal growth include maternal undernutrition, maternal drug use (tobacco, ethanol, heroine, cocaine, corticosteroids), maternal vascular diseases (renal disease, diabetes, chronic hypertension), placental pathology and maternal hypoxia (high altitude, anaemia).

Effects of intrauterine growth restriction on postnatal lung function

A number of studies have shown that IUGR/SGA increases the risk of metabolic and respiratory complications in the early postnatal period. In both term and preterm neonates, IUGR increases the risk of respiratory insufficiency and the need for respiratory support after birth (Tyson *et al.* 1995, Minior and Divon 1998). The reasons for the impaired gas exchange in IUGR infants are unclear at present, but they could include delayed clearance of lung liquid from the airways, impaired pulmonary perfusion or pulmonary structural abnormalities; they are unlikely to involve surfactant deficiency (Gagnon *et al.* 1999). Several studies have shown that restricted nutrition during fetal life leading to low birthweight can alter lung development such that lung function is impaired from childhood (Rona *et al.* 1993, Nikolajev *et al.* 1998, 2002) through to adult life (Barker *et al.* 1991, Stein *et al.* 1997): specifically, airway and alveolar development appear to be adversely affected (Harding *et al.* 2004). There is also evidence in humans that fetal undernutrition can alter airway function at birth, and it has been suggested that alterations may be long-lasting, potentially accounting for alterations in adult lung function (Lopuhaä *et al.* 2000).

Restricted growth and nutrition after birth

Few data are available regarding the effect of *postnatal* nutrient restriction on human lung development and function. During infancy and childhood there are numerous potential causes of inadequate nutrition. Severe protein deficiency may occur in infancy and childhood in some developing countries in situations of poverty and during times of famine. Nutrition may also be impaired during disease states, such as infections, and in association with congenital anomalies such as cystic fibrosis. Altered nutrition associated with illness during early life may contribute to the later effects of these illnesses on respiratory function (Pullan and Hey 1982, Shaheen *et al.* 1998). This is supported by the finding that size at 1 year was a significant predictor of later deaths from respiratory causes (Ryan 1998). Effects of malnutrition on lung function have been documented in undernourished children. For example, in Indian children aged 6–12 years, evidence of current malnutrition and body wasting, indicated by low weight for height, was associated with lower than expected peak expiratory flow rates (Primhak and Coates 1988). More recently it was found that wasted and stunted children have lower lung volumes and reduced forced expiratory flow rates (Nair *et al.* 1999), indicating that nutrition influences aspects of lung development in children other than lung size (Ong *et al.* 1998).

A group that is particularly vulnerable to inadequate nutrition during early development is preterm infants, who represent about 7–10% of all births. Impaired nutrition can occur in these infants as a result of limited fat deposits, parenteral feeding, poor feeding ability or gut immaturity. It is considered likely that undernutrition, both before and after birth, contributes to the aetiology of neonatal chronic lung disease or bronchopulmonary dysplasia. It has therefore been suggested that preterm infants require particular nutritional management (Ong *et al.* 1998). Owing to ongoing lung development in preterm infants, undernutrition, or a lack of the necessary minerals or micronutrients, could have detrimental effects on lung antioxidant and defence mechanisms, surfactant production and alveolar formation.

In undernutrition it is likely that respiratory muscle function may also be impaired, contributing to reduced flow rates. Studies in humans and animals have shown that undernutrition can impair the function and structure of major respiratory muscles. It is considered possible that nutritional factors resulting in weight loss may contribute to respiratory illness such as chronic obstructive lung disease (Lewis and Belman 1988, Schols 2000), although it is recognised that increased energy expenditure due to airway obstruction may be involved. A study in rats showed that prolonged undernutrition leads to reduced oxidative capacity in the diaphragm, secondary to a reduced production of NADH in the Krebs cycle (Matecki *et al.* 2002). Biopsies of adult human intercostal muscle indicate that nutritional status, as well as gender, is related to altered fibre morphometry, although no relation was found between muscle structure and lung function or respiratory muscle strength (Hards *et al.* 1990).

Undernutrition may also affect other aspects of the lungs, such as defence mechanisms. In animal and human studies it was found that malnutrition causes a reduction in macrophage function, mucociliary clearance, and specific B- and T-cell responses to infection (Bellanti *et al.* 1997). Such effects may explain the elevated incidence of respiratory infections in undernourished infants and children.

Effects of impaired nutrition on the developing lung

Several studies have explored the relation between early impairment of nutrition or oxygen availability and lung development. Oxygen is an essential nutrient since it is required for the oxidation of nutrients such as glucose and fatty acids to satisfy the energy demands of the developing lung. It therefore plays an important role in the development of the lung from the embryonic stage through to the final stages, during which alveoli are formed and the lung becomes an effective gas exchanger. Throughout fetal lung development, the future airways and airspaces are not collapsed but contain a unique liquid secreted by the epithelial cells lining the future airways. This liquid plays an important role in lung development

as it maintains the fetal lungs in an expanded state, which is essential for normal lung growth and structural development (Harding and Hooper 1996). As lung liquid secretion depends on the metabolic activity of the airway epithelial cells, it is likely that this process is affected by restricted nutrient and oxygen availability. It has been shown that both acute and chronic hypoxia and hypoglycaemia, induced in fetal sheep by the restriction of placental blood flow, inhibit the secretion of lung liquid and alter its composition (Albuquerque *et al.* 1998), although they do not affect its volume within the future pulmonary airspaces (Cock *et al.* 2001a).

Fetal breathing movements (FBM) are critical for normal lung growth and structural maturation by maintaining the appropriate degree of lung expansion (Harding and Hooper 1996). In humans, IUGR is associated with a reduced incidence of FBM, which may be due to increased adenosine concentrations in the fetal brain (Koos *et al.* 2001). Thus it appears that IUGR, perhaps due to chronic hypoxaemia, hypoglycaemia and elevated adenosine levels, may have an inhibitory effect on FBM. However, an inhibition of FBM is unlikely to be a cause of impaired lung development in IUGR, as in fetal sheep with IUGR there was no alteration, relative to body weight, in fetal lung weight or lung liquid volume (Cock *et al.* 2001).

Several animal studies have shown that restriction of nutrient supply during fetal life can alter lung development. The effects vary according to the nature and gestational timing of the nutritional intervention. IUGR induced in sheep by pre-pregnancy removal of placental attachment sites has been shown to reduce (Maloney *et al.* 1982) or have no effect (Rees *et al.* 1991) on lung weights, relative to fetal body weight, in the near-term fetus. In sheep, 10 days of maternal undernutrition during late gestation reduced lung weight, although fetal body weight was unaffected (Harding and Johnston 1995). More prolonged periods of fetal undernutrition, induced by chronic placental insufficiency, restricted fetal growth, but lung growth relative to body growth was not impaired (Duncan *et al.* 2000, Cock *et al.* 2001). Similarly in the rat, four days of gestational undernutrition did not affect fetal lung weight or DNA content (Rhoades and Ryder 1981).

However, it has been shown in several species that undernutrition during development can interfere with alveolar formation. In rats, intermittent starvation during the late saccular and early alveolar phases of lung development resulted in enlarged alveoli with thicker septa and an apparent reduction in elastin deposition (Das 1984). Protein deficiency in the rat during postnatal development led to changes in lung morphometry which were mostly attributable to growth restriction and smaller lung volume, with normal lung parenchymal maturity being apparent at weaning (Kalenga *et al.* 1995). Therefore, it appears that the degree and type of nutrient restriction during development, as well as its timing, may determine the form of structural alteration in the lungs.

In sheep the effects of fetal hypoxaemia and nutritional restriction during late gestation, a time of rapid fetal growth coinciding with pulmonary saccular and alveolar formation, have been studied in the near-term fetus, 8-week-old lamb and 2-year-old sheep. In these studies, fetal growth was restricted by repeated umbilical–placental embolisation (Joyce *et al.* 2001, Maritz *et al.* 2001, 2004, Wignarajah *et al.* 2002). At eight weeks after term birth, but not in near-term fetuses, there was a reduction in the number of alveoli per respiratory unit, an increase in the mean diameter of alveoli and a thickening of the interalveolar septa and blood–air barrier in IUGR lambs (Fig. 25.1) (Maritz *et al.* 2001). The thickening of the interalveolar septa was due to increased extracellular matrix between adjacent interstitial cells in the alveolar wall (Plate 2). The reduction in alveolar number and increase in blood–air barrier thickness were still evident in 2-year-old adult IUGR sheep (Maritz *et al.* 2004); in addition, increased numbers of alveolar fenestrations were apparent (Plate 3). Thus it appears that adequate nutrition during early development is necessary for normal alveolar formation, and that the effects of impaired nutrition can persist into adulthood. Similar effects on alveolar formation have been observed in undernourished postnatal rats (Das 1984) and in guinea pigs

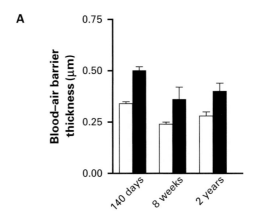

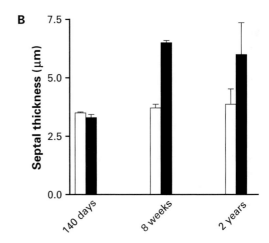

Figure 25.1 The effect of hypoxaemia and nutritional restriction during late gestation on the thicknesses of (A) the blood–air barrier and (B) the alveolar septa of the lungs of 140-day-old sheep fetuses and 8-week- and 2-year-old sheep. The blood–air barrier of the control lambs was thinner ($P>0.05$) than that of the experimental animals of all age groups. The alveolar septa of the 8-week- and 2-year-old controls were thinner than those of the experimental animals. White bars, controls; black bars, experimental animals. Data from Maritz *et al.* (2001, 2004).

following undernutrition late in gestation and during the neonatal period (Lechner 1985).

The development of airways is also affected by IUGR. In an ovine model of IUGR induced by placental restriction, tracheal wall structure was affected in the near-term fetus, such that there was less cartilage, impaired development of submucosal glands and evidence of reduced ciliation of epithelial cells (Rees *et al.* 1991). A more recent study in which IUGR was induced for 20 days during late ovine gestation also affected the structure of cartilaginous airways near to term; the walls were thinner and the submucosal glands less developed (Wignarajah *et al.* 2002). In this study, however, there was postnatal recovery of airway wall thickness by eight weeks after birth, but changes in mucus secretory structures were still evident.

In rats, early postnatal undernutrition was shown to affect bronchiolar epithelium, such that cell division was reduced, conversion of Clara cells to ciliated cells was reduced and there was a persistent abnormality of bronchiolar epithelial cells (Massaro *et al.* 1988). Such changes could underlie long-term effects of early postnatal undernutrition on lung function.

The effects of maternal smoking

In developed countries, up to one-third of women smoke while pregnant, and hence approximately one-third of infants are exposed before or after birth to components of tobacco smoke (Hofhuis *et al.* 2003). A number of studies have shown that cigarette smoking during pregnancy is associated with an increased incidence of impaired lower respiratory function in offspring (Cunningham *et al.* 1994, Pierce and Nguyen 2002, Hofhuis *et al.* 2003). Pulmonary mechanics in children whose mothers smoked during pregnancy differ from those of control children, suggesting that gestational smoking affects lung development in utero (Pierce and Nguyen 2002). Decreases in lung function due to maternal smoking are especially prevalent and long-lasting in children exposed in utero or in early childhood (Cunningham *et al.* 1994). In-utero cigarette smoke exposure could be considered as a distinct form of passive smoking in that the fetus is not directly exposed to cigarette smoke. Therefore, any effects of maternal smoking on fetal development are a result of indirect expo-

sure to components of cigarette smoke following placental transfer of these components from mother to fetus. Nicotine, which readily crosses the placenta, is likely to be the primary mediator of many of these effects of maternal smoking during pregnancy. In experimental models, maternal nicotine exposure alone elicits many of the same effects on neonates as maternal direct or side-stream tobacco smoke exposure (Pierce and Nguyen 2002).

Animal studies show that exposure to cigarette smoke during pregnancy leads to a reduction in the incidence of FBM, which is likely to result in reduced expansion and hypoplasia of the fetal lung (Harding and Hooper 1996, Harding 1997). Airway function in particular may be adversely affected. For example, infants born to mothers who smoked during pregnancy had a reduction of ~10% in expiratory flow parameters when compared to infants whose mothers did not smoke during pregnancy (Tager *et al.* 1993). Infants whose mothers smoked during pregnancy had increased airway responsiveness to inhaled histamine four weeks after delivery (Young *et al.* 1991). This observation was supported by controlled studies on pregnant guinea pigs exposed to cigarette smoke at a level equivalent to humans smoking 5–10 cigarettes per day: the offspring displayed increased airway responsiveness, a hallmark of asthma (Elliot *et al.* 2001). Epidemiological studies suggest that the increased responsiveness in smoke-exposed infants is primarily associated with in-utero cigarette smoke exposure (Hanrahan *et al.* 1992). The exact mechanism by which this occurs is not clear. However, the distances between alveolar attachment points in membranous and small cartilaginous airways are increased, resulting in smaller number of alveolar attachments to the surrounding airway adventitia (Elliot *et al.* 2001). Reduced numbers of alveolar attachments are also found in active smokers, and this reduction is associated with a reduction in lung elastic recoil (Saetta *et al.* 1985). One of the major loads that airway smooth muscle must overcome when shortening in vivo is the load imparted on the muscle by the recoil pressure of the lung parenchyma (Robinson *et al.* 1996). This elastic load on the muscle is translated to the airway wall through alveolar attachments to the airway. Therefore a reduced number of alveolar attachments to the small airways may reduce the loads opposing smooth-muscle shortening and allow increased shortening for the same stimulus (Bai *et al.* 1994). In addition to increasing airway responsiveness, in-utero tobacco exposure also decreases airway calibre, which likely decreases airflow during the first days of life in infants of smoking mothers (Fauroux 2003). Studies in developing rats have shown that the timing of exposure to tobacco smoke is key to the development of airway hyper-reactivity. When rats were exposed *both* pre- and postnatally, lungs were less compliant, and the airways were more reactive compared to controls. When rats were exposed either before *or* after birth, pulmonary function and airway reactivity were not altered. The hyper-reponsiveness persisted into adulthood (Joad 2004).

Apart from changes in the airways, studies have shown that the lung volume of fetuses of pregnant rats exposed to mainstream or environmental tobacco smoke (ETS) was reduced (Collins *et al.* 1985). The mean number of saccules was reduced, with an increase in their size, and the elastic tissue and collagen were poorly developed (Collins *et al.* 1985). Since the saccules develop into alveoli it is clear that these animals' lungs will have fewer alveoli than the lungs of the animals not exposed to cigarette smoke in utero. This would result in a reduced surface area for gas exchange during adult life.

Developmental exposure to gestational tobacco smoking is associated with accelerated maturation of the fetal lung, impairment of lung growth, and shortening of the plateau phase of FEV_1; furthermore, the age-related declines in FVC and FEV_1 were increased, indicative of premature ageing of the lung (Green and Pinkerton 2004). Prenatal smoke exposure most likely has a greater effect on lung function in childhood and long-term respiratory health than postnatal and childhood exposure. It is clear that maternal smoking during pregnancy is a major cause of impaired adult lung function and respiratory health, and hence is likely to be a major factor involved in respiratory programming in fetal life (Vidic 1991).

Effect of maternal nicotine exposure

Experimentally, nicotine has been widely used to study the impact of tobacco smoke exposure upon the developing lung. Nicotine has been implicated as the causative agent and is arguably responsible for more adverse health consequences than any other single compound in tobacco smoke (Meyer *et al.* 1971, Joad *et al.* 1999). Some studies have shown that maternal smoking results in the accumulation of nicotine (Szuts *et al.* 1978) and cotinine (Jauniaux *et al.* 1999) in fetal tissues, and an extensive epidemiological study demonstrated a positive correlation between the concentration of nicotine in maternal blood and the degree of fetal growth restriction (Bardy *et al.* 1993). It has also been shown that lung tissue of infants dying from the sudden infant death syndrome (SIDS) had higher tissue levels of nicotine compared with non-SIDS cases (McMartin *et al.* 2002).

Nicotine is typically absorbed into the body via tobacco smoke inhalation, transdermal patches, gums, nasal sprays and chewing tobacco (Luck *et al.* 1985). Although the daily intake is not different between men and women, blood nicotine concentrations may differ as men metabolise nicotine faster than women (Benowitz *et al.* 1991). Elevated levels of nicotine occur in the amniotic fluid and placental tissue of women who smoke (Van Vunakis *et al.* 1974). Nicotine crosses the placenta rapidly from mother to fetus, and considerable amounts of nicotine enter the fetal blood (Luck and Nau 1984). The levels of nicotine reach higher concentrations in the fetal circulation than in the mother's because the disappearance of nicotine from the fetal blood is slower than from the maternal circulation. Fetal skin is readily permeable to nicotine in amniotic fluid, contributing to the rapid uptake of nicotine into the fetal blood. Due to the rapid uptake of nicotine and its slower degradation in the fetal tissues it reaches high concentrations in the fetal lung (Wang *et al.* 1983). The higher concentration of nicotine together with its slower elimination from the fetal tissues could enhance the toxicity of nicotine to the fetus (Wang *et al.* 1983). After birth, elevated levels of nicotine occur in the maternal milk and nicotine is rapidly absorbed by the infant, as determined by its presence in the saliva ($166 \, ng \, ml^{-1}$) of breast-fed infants (Greenberg *et al.* 1984).

Effects of maternal nicotine exposure during gestation and lactation on lung development in the offspring

Several studies have shown that nicotine exposure during gestation interferes with the transition from the saccular to the alveolar stage of lung development, during which there is a fourfold increase in the number of interstitial fibroblasts in neonatal rat lung (Maritz 2002). Some of the effects include structural changes such as decreased elastin content in lung parenchyma (Maritz and Dolley 1996), up-regulation of collagen expression together with an increase in collagen surrounding large airways and vessels (Sekhon *et al.* 2002), decreased alveolar numbers, increased alveolar volumes (Fig. 25.2) and alveolar wall fenestrations, and a decreased surface area available for gas exchange; together, these pathologies are indicative of emphysematous changes in lung structure (Linhartova 1983, Maritz and Windvogel 2003).

The finding that fetal nicotine exposure alters alveolar development in both monkeys and rodents makes it highly likely that prenatal exposure to nicotine will affect human lung development similarly. Recent studies in the rat showed that nicotine exposure from the onset of the alveolar phase of lung development had the same effect on alveolarisation as when nicotine exposure occurred during all the phases of lung development (Maritz and Windvogel 2003). It was also shown that the lungs of the animals exposed to nicotine gradually deteriorated as the postnatal animals aged, even though they were not exposed to nicotine after weaning (Maritz and Windvogel 2003). It appears that nicotine had no effect on the control of alveolarisation, but resulted in an inability to maintain the structural and functional integrity of the lungs as the animal aged (Linhartova 1983). The increased rate at which

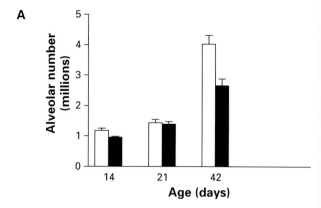

A

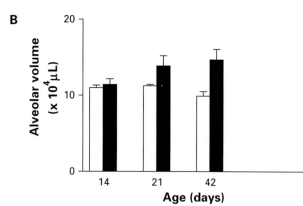

B

Figure 25.2 The effect of maternal nicotine exposure during gestation and lactation on (A) the alveolar number and (B) alveolar volumes of rat pups aged 14, 21 and 42 days. The alveolar number and volumes of the 42-day-old control rats were higher ($P < 0.001$) than those of the nicotine-exposed rats of the same age. White bars, controls; black bars, experimental animals. Adapted from Maritz and Windvogel (2003).

the lungs of the nicotine-exposed animals developed signs of pulmonary ageing (larger alveoli, more fenestrations, reduced surface available for gas exchange) indicates that nicotine interfered with the 'programming' of lung ageing. Since maternal nicotine intake had no effect on the body weight of the mother or the neonate, it is apparent that maternal nutrition and offspring nutrient supply via the placenta and milk were sufficient to sustain normal growth of the offspring (Maritz and Dolley 1996). This implies that the observed effects of maternal nicotine exposure on neonatal lung development were not due to inadequate placental supply of nutrients to the fetus, but can be attributed to direct effects of nicotine and/or products of nicotine metabolism. It is clear that nicotine exposure during gestation and the neonatal period results in gradual deterioration of the lungs with time, resembling premature ageing of the lungs. This can be attributed to an adjustment of the programming of the lung in utero, rendering the respiratory system more susceptible to disease. The use of nicotine replacement therapies by pregnant and lactating women to quit smoking may not, therefore, be advisable.

Preterm birth and lung development

Preterm birth is a major cause of low birthweight and presents an immediate physiological challenge for the neonate, as the immature lung may not be sufficiently developed to meet the infant's respiratory requirements. Even mild prematurity has been associated with adverse consequences for subsequent respiratory health, which may be due to changes in lung structure and function. A recent study of 32 healthy preterm infants, born at a mean gestational age of 29.5 weeks, showed reductions in functional residual capacity (FRC) and specific lung compliance, impaired gas mixing efficiency and higher dead space ventilation when studied at term equivalence (Hjalmarson and Sandberg 2002). This suggests that even mild preterm birth, in the absence of ventilatory support, affects alveolarisation and elastic fibre deposition (Hjalmarson and Sandberg 2002). Similarly, preterm birth has been associated with wheeze and reduced expiratory flows in 5- to 11-year-old children born at about 35 weeks of gestation (Rona et al. 1993). In more severe prematurity, respiratory insufficiency necessitating prolonged ventilatory support has been associated with respiratory diseases such as hyaline membrane disease, bronchopulmonary dysplasia (BPD) and permanent lung injury (Northway et al. 1967, Coalson 1997). Other studies have linked preterm birth with long-term

respiratory ailments such as asthma and chronic obstructive pulmonary disease (COPD) (Speer and Silverman 1998).

Prematurely born infants who develop chronic lung disease (CLD) today are those born at early gestational ages (23–26 weeks) with extremely low birthweight (<1000 gm). The radiological and pathological findings include lung hyperinflation, emphysema and interstitial densities, and the principal pathological findings at autopsy are dilated simplified distal air sacs (Hislop and Haworth 1990, Margraf et al. 1991). Prematurely born baboons and lambs that are ventilated for three weeks or more also have simplified distal air sacs (Coalson et al. 1995, Albertine et al. 1999). Simplification is related to failure of alveolar secondary septa to sprout into distal air sacs. A consequence of failed septation is a reduced surface area for gas exchange, particularly the capillary surface area (Bland et al. 2000). In 10-year-old survivors of BPD there was increased airways resistance, air trapping, blood gas abnormalities and persistent reactive airways disease (Smyth et al. 1981). Such children had increased lung volumes, airway obstruction and increased transcutaneous pCO_2 (Bader et al. 1987). These abnormalities do not seem to disappear later in life, even though symptoms were infrequently evident (Northway et al. 1990). Morphometric analysis of lungs of infants of up to 28 months of age, with persistent BPD, and who died, show a decrease in alveolar number and a decrease in the area available for gas exchange; an increase in the bronchiolar smooth muscle and glands also occurred (Margraf et al. 1991).

In recent studies using sheep it has been shown that preterm birth that did not necessitate mechanical ventilation or oxygen supplementation was associated with alterations in lung structure, some of which persisted into postnatal life (Cock et al. 2005, Sozo et al. in press). In these studies, preterm birth was induced 14 days before term (147 days), during the saccular/alveolar phase of lung development, and was considered to be mild–moderate in that sustained ventilatory support was not required. At the equivalent of full term, there was a reduction in pulmonary tropoelastin expression, and increased thicknesses of the alveolar wall, airway epithelium and blood–air barrier compared to lambs born at term (Cock *et al.* 2005). By eight weeks after preterm birth, these structural alterations had mostly resolved but the increased thickness of the airway epithelium persisted. There was also evidence that mild preterm birth results in a persistent delay in the changes in alveolar epithelial cell proportions that normally occur after birth (Sozo *et al.* in press); in particular, the proportion of type ll alveolar epithelial cells did not increase after birth as much as in controls (Flecknoe *et al.* 2003) and this was associated with an initial decrease in surfactant protein expression. However, by 8 weeks after birth, surfactant protein expression was not different to that in term controls of the same post-conceptional age (Sozo *et al.* in press).

Combination of preterm birth and IUGR

Recent evidence indicates that many preterm infants have been exposed to placental insufficiency and IUGR (Lackman *et al.* 2001, Gilbert and Danielsen 2003); hence the lungs of individuals who are born prematurely may be affected by both IUGR and preterm birth. Many of these infants may have also been affected by maternal tobacco smoking, which is a significant risk factor for both IUGR and preterm birth (Harding *et al.* 2004). In lambs, preterm birth in the presence of late-gestational placental insufficiency and IUGR resulted in a reduced diffusion capacity and thus impaired pulmonary gas exchange (Cock *et al.* 2001b). Given the effects of IUGR in lambs born at term (Maritz *et al.* 2001, Maritz *et al.* 2004), it is possible that the blood–air barriers of the lungs of the IUGR lambs born prematurely were thicker, and that the surface area for gas exchange was reduced, thereby contributing to the lower diffusion capacity than that in control lambs born at term. A common mechanism for altered lung development in both IUGR and preterm birth could be hypoxia and/or impaired nutrition, as both have been shown to have specific persistent effects on the developing lung.

The lungs may be particularly affected by the hypoxia associated with IUGR and preterm birth (and perhaps maternal smoking), as fetal hypoxaemia has been shown to reduce rates of cell division in the lung more than in other organs (Hooper *et al.* 1991), which would be expected to depress rates of cellular remodelling in the alveolar walls, for example. It is also possible that nutrient restriction in both IUGR and preterm birth affect extracellular matrix components such as elastin (Rucker and Dubick 1984), which could permanently alter alveolar properties.

Conclusions

There is now an abundance of experimental evidence showing that gestational exposure to environmental factors that restrict fetal growth and lead to a low birthweight can have long-term effects on lung development, lung function and respiratory health. Some of the major causal factors have been identified as impaired nutrient and oxygen availability, maternal tobacco smoking and preterm birth. While it is often the case that infants may have been exposed to more than one of these environmental factors, each is likely to affect the developing lung in a different manner and effects are likely to be additive. Effects will differ according to the severity of the exposure and its gestational timing. The aim of animal studies in the future should be to determine at a molecular level the mechanisms by which each of these factors adversely affects lung development, and whether such effects can be blocked or reversed. Ultimately, however, the major goal should be to avoid prenatal exposures through maternal education and by clinical monitoring and intervention, thereby ensuring that each fetus has the best possible environment in which to develop. In this way, postnatal respiratory health will be improved and the deterioration of lung function with age may be slowed.

REFERENCES

Albertine, K. H. and Pysher, T. J. (2004). Pulmonary consequences of preterm birth. In *The Lung: Development, Aging and the Environment* (ed. R. Harding, K. E. Pinkerton and C. G. Plopper). London: Academic Press, pp. 237–51.

Albertine, K. H., Jones, G. P., Starcher, B. C. *et al.* (1999). Chronic lung injury in preterm lambs: disordered respiratory tract development. *Am. J. Respir. Crit. Care Med.*, **159**, 945–58.

Albuquerque, C., Boland, R., Cock, M. L., Hooper, S. B. and Harding, R. (1998). Lung fluid composition in the chronically hypoxemic ovine fetus. *Am. J. Obstet. Gynecol.*, **178**, S37.

Bader, D., Ramos, A. D., Lew, C. D., Platzker, A. C., Stabile, M. W. and Keens, T. G. (1987). Childhood sequelae of infant lung disease: exercise and pulmonary function abnormalities after bronchopulmonary dysplasia. *J. Pediatr.*, **110**, 693–9.

Bai, A., Eidelman, D. H., Hogg, J. C. *et al.* (1994). Proposed nomenclature for quantifying subdivisions of the bronchial wall. *J. Appl. Physiol.*, **7**, 1011–14.

Bardy, A. H., Seppala, T., Lillsunde, P. *et al.* (1993). Objectively measured tobacco exposure during pregnancy: neonatal effects and relation to maternal smoking. *Br. J. Obstet. Gynaecol.*, **100**, 721–6.

Barker, D. J. P., Godfrey, K. M., Fall, C., Osmond, C., Winter, P. D. and Shaheen, S. O. (1991). Relation of birth weight and childhood respiratory infection to adult lung function and death from chronic obstructive airways disease. *BMJ*, **303**, 671–5.

Bellanti, J. A., Zeligs, B. J. and Kulszycki, L. L. (1997). Nutrition and development of pulmonary defense mechanisms. *Pediatr. Pulmonol. Suppl.*, **16**, 170–1.

Benowitz, N. L., Chan, K., Denaro, C. P. and Jacob, P., III. (1991). Stable isotope method for studying transdermal drug absorption: the nicotine patch. *Clin. Pharmacol. Ther.*, **50**, 286–93.

Bland, R. D., Albertine, K. H., Carlton, D. P. *et al.* (2000). Chronic lung injury in preterm lambs: abnormalities of the pulmonary circulation and lung fluid balance. *Pediatr. Res.*, **48**, 64–74.

Coalson, J. J. (1997). Experimental models of bronchopulmonary dysplasia. *Biol. Neonate*, **71**, 35–8.

Coalson, J. J., Winter, V. and deLemos, R. A. (1995). Decreased alveolarization in baboon survivors with bronchopulmonary dysplasia. *Am. J. Respir. Crit. Care Med.*, **152**, 640–6.

Cock, M. L., Albuquerque, C. A., Joyce, B. J., Hooper, S. B. and Harding, R. (2001a). Effects of intrauterine growth restriction on lung liquid dynamics and lung development in fetal sheep. *Am. J. Obstet. Gynecol.*, **184**, 209–16.

Cock, M. L., Camm, E. J., Louey, S., Joyce, B. J. and Harding, R. (2001b). Postnatal outcomes in term and preterm lambs following fetal growth restriction. *Clin. Exp. Pharmacol. Physiol.*, **28**, 931–7.

Cock, M. L., Hanna, M., Sozo, F. *et al.* (2005). Pulmonary function and structure following mild preterm birth in lambs. *Pediatr. Pulmonol.*, **40**, 336–48.

Collins, M. H., Moessinger, A. C., Kleinerman, J. *et al.* (1985). Fetal lung hypoplasia associated with maternal smoking: a morphometric analysis. *Pediatr. Res.*, **19**, 408–12.

Cunningham, J., Dockery, D. W. and Speizer, F. E. (1994). Maternal smoking during pregnancy as a predictor of lung function in children. *Am. J. Epidemiol.*, **139**, 1139–52.

Das, R. M. (1984). The effects of intermittent starvation on lung development in suckling rats. *Am. J. Pathol.*, **117**, 326–32.

Duncan, J. R., Cock, M. L., Harding, R. and Rees, S. M. (2000). Relation between damage to the placenta and fetal brain following late-gestational placental embolisation and fetal growth restriction in fetal sheep. *Am. J. Obstet. Gynecol.*, **183**, 1013–22.

Elliot, J., Carroll, N., Bosco, M., McCrohan, M. and Robinson, P. (2001). Increased airways responsiveness and decreased alveolar attachment points following in utero smoke exposure in the guinea pig. *Am. J. Respir. Crit. Care Med.*, **163**, 140–4.

Fauroux, B. (2003). Smoking, fetal pulmonary development and lung disease in children. *J. Gynecol. Obstet. Biol. Reprod. (Paris)*, **32**, S17–22.

Flecknoe, S. J., Wallace, M. J., Cock, M. L., Harding, R. and Hooper, S. B. (2003). Changes in alveolar epithelial cell proportions during fetal and postnatal development in sheep. *Am. J. Physiol. Lung Cell. Mol. Physiol.*, **285**, L664–70.

Gagnon, R., Langridge, J., Inchley, K., Murotsuki, J. and Possmayer, F. (1999). Changes in surfactant-associated protein mRNA profile in growth-restricted fetal sheep. *Am. J. Physiol.*, **276**, L459–65.

Gilbert, W. M. and Danielsen, B. (2003). Pregnancy outcomes associated with intrauterine growth restriction. *Am. J. Obstet. Gynecol.*, **188**, 1596–9.

Green, F. H. Y. and Pinkerton, K. E. (2004). Environmental determinants of lung ageing. In *The Lung: Development, Aging and the Environment* (ed. R. Harding, K. E. Pinkerton and C. G. Plopper). London: Academic Press, pp. 377–95.

Greenberg, R. A., Haley, N. J., Etzel, R. A. and Loda, F. A. (1984). Measuring the exposure of infants to tobacco smoke: nicotine and cotinine in urine and saliva. *N. Engl. J. Med.*, **310**, 1075–78.

Hanrahan, J. P., Tager, I. B., Segal, M. R. *et al.* (1992). The effect of maternal smoking during pregnancy on early infant lung function. *Am. Rev. Respir. Dis.*, **145**, 1129–35.

Harding, J. E. and Johnston, B. M. (1995). Nutrition and fetal growth. *Reprod. Fertil. Dev.*, **7**, 539–47.

Harding, R. (1997). Fetal pulmonary development: the role of respiratory movements. *Equine Vet. J.*, **24** (suppl.), 32–9.

Harding, R. and Hooper, S. B. (1996). Regulation of lung expansion and lung growth before birth. *J. Appl. Physiol.*, **81**, 209–24.

Harding, R., Cock, M. L. and Albuquerque, C. A. (2004). Role of nutrition in lung development before and after birth. In *The Lung: Development, Aging and the Environment* (ed. R. Harding, K. E. Pinkerton and C. Plopper). London: Academic Press, pp. 253–66.

Hards, J. M., Reid, W. D., Pardy, R. L. and Pare, P. D. (1990). Respiratory muscle fiber morphometry: correlation with pulmonary function and nutrition. *Chest*, **97**, 1037–44.

Hislop, A. A. and Haworth, S. G. (1990). Pulmonary vascular damage and the development of cor pulmonale following hyaline membrane disease. *Pediatr. Pulmonol.*, **9**, 152–61.

Hjalmarson, O. and Sandberg, K. (2002). Abnormal lung function in healthy preterm infants. *Am. J. Respir. Crit. Care Med.*, **165**, 83–7.

Hofhuis, W., de Jongste, J. C. and Merkus, P. J. (2003) Adverse health effects of prenatal and postnatal tobacco smoke exposure on children. *Arch. Dis. Child.*, **88**, 1086–90.

Hooper, S. B., Bocking, A. D., White, S., Challis, J. R. G. and Han, V. K. (1991). DNA synthesis is reduced in selected fetal tissues during prolonged hypoxemia. *Am. J. Physiol.*, **261**, R508–14.

Jauniaux, E., Gulbis, B., Acharya, G., Thiry, P. and Rodeck, C. (1999). Maternal tobacco exposure and cotinine in fetal fluids in the first half of pregnancy. *Obstet. Gynecol.*, **93**, 25–9.

Joad, J. (2004). Tobacco smoke and lung development. In *The Lung: Development, Ageing and the Environment* (ed. R. Harding, K. E. Pinkerton and C. Plopper. London: Academic Press, pp. 292–5.

Joad, J. P., Bric, J. M., Peake, J. L. and Pinkerton, K. E. (1999). Perinatal exposure to aged and diluted sidestream cigarette smoke produces airway hyperresponsiveness in older rats. *Toxicol. Appl. Pharmacol.*, **155**, 253–60.

Joyce, B. J., Louey, S., Davey, M. G., Cock, M. L., Hooper, S. B. and Harding, R. (2001). Compromised respiratory function in postnatal lambs after placental insufficiency and intrauterine growth restriction. *Pediatr. Res.*, **50**, 641–9.

Kalenga, M., Tschanz, S. A. and Burri, P. H. (1995). Protein deficiency and the growing rat lung. II. Morphometric analysis and morphology. *Pediatr. Res.*, **37**, 789–95.

Kauffman, S. L., Burri, P. H. and Weibel, E. R. (1974). The postnatal growth of the rat lung. II. Autoradiography. *Anat. Rec.*, **180**, 63–76.

Koos, B. J., Maeda, T. and Jan, C. (2001). Adenosine A(1) and A(2A) receptors modulate sleep state and breathing in fetal sheep. *J. Appl. Physiol.*, **91**, 343–50.

Lackman, F., Capewell, V., Richardson, B., daSilva, O. and Gagnon, R. (2001). The risks of spontaneous preterm delivery and perinatal mortality in relation to size at birth according to fetal versus neonatal growth standards. *Am. J. Obstet. Gynecol.*, **184**, 946–53.

Lechner, A. J. (1985). Perinatal age determines the severity of retarded lung development induced by starvation. *Am. Rev. Respir. Dis.*, **131**, 638–43.

Lewis, M. I. and Belman, M. J. (1988). Nutrition and the respiratory muscles. *Clin. Chest Med.*, **9**, 337–48.

Linhartova, A. (1983). Fenestration of the pulmonary septa as a sign of early destruction in emphysema. *Ceskoslovenska Patologie*, **19**, 211–21.

Lopuhaä, C. E., Roseboom, T. J., Osmond, C. *et al.* (2000). Atopy, lung function, and obstructive airways disease after prenatal exposure to famine. *Thorax*, **55**, 555–61.

Luck, W. and Nau, H. (1984). Exposure of the fetus, neonate, and nursed infant to nicotine and cotinine from maternal smoking. *N. Engl. J. Med.*, **311**, 672.

Luck, W., Nau, H., Hansen, R. and Steldinger, R. (1985). Extent of nicotine and cotinine transfer to the human fetus, placenta and amniotic fluid of smoking mothers. *Dev. Pharmacol. Ther.*, **8**, 384–95.

Maloney, J. E., Bowes, G., Brodecky, V., Dennett, X., Wilkinson, M. and Walker, A. (1982). Function of the future respiratory system in the growth retarded fetal sheep. *J. Dev. Physiol.*, **4**, 279–97.

Margraf, L. R., Tomasherski, J. F. Jr., Bruce, M. C. and Dahms, B. B. (1991). Morphometric analysis of the lung in bronchopulmonary dysplasia. *Am. Rev. Respir. Dis.*, **143**, 391–400.

Maritz, G. S. (2002). Maternal nicotine exposure during gestation and lactation of rats induce microscopic emphysema in the offspring. *Exp. Lung Res.*, **28**, 391–403.

　(2004). Nicotine exposure during early development: effects on the lung. In *The Lung: Development, Ageing and the Environment* (ed. R. Harding, K. E. Pinkerton and C. Plopper). London: Academic Press, pp. 301–9.

Maritz, G. S. and Dolley, L. (1996). The influence of maternal nicotine exposure on the status of the connective tissue framework of the developing rat lung. *Pathophysiology*, **3**, 212–20.

Maritz, G. S. and Windvogel, S. (2003). Chronic maternal nicotine exposure during gestation and lactation and the development of the lung parenchyma in the offspring: response to nicotine withdrawal. *Pathophysiology*, **10**, 69–75.

Maritz, G. S., Cock, M. L., Louey, S., Joyce, B. J., Albuquerque, C. A. and Harding, R. (2001). Effects of fetal growth restriction on lung development before and after birth: a morphometric analysis. *Pediatr. Pulmonol.*, **32**, 201–10.

Maritz, G. S., Cock, M. L., Louey, S., Suzuki, K. and Harding, R. (2004). Fetal growth restriction has long-term effects on postnatal lung structure in sheep. *Pediatr. Res.*, **55**, 287–95.

Massaro, G. D., McCoy, L. and Massaro, D. (1988). Postnatal undernutrition slows development of bronchiolar epithelium in rats. *Am. J. Physiol.*, **255**, R521–6.

Matecki, S., Py, G., Lambert, K. *et al.* (2002). Effect of prolonged undernutrition on rat diaphragm mitochondrial respiration. *Am. J. Respir. Cell Mol. Biol.*, **26**, 239–45.

McMartin, K. I., Platt, M. S., Hackman, R. *et al.* (2002). Lung tissue concentrations of nicotine in sudden infant death syndrome (SIDS). *J. Pediatr.*, **140**, 205–9.

Meyer, D. H., Cross, C. E., Ibrahim, A. B. and Mustafa, M. G. (1971). Nicotine effects on alveolar macrophage respiration and adenosine triphosphatase activity. *Arch. Environ. Health*, **22**, 362–5.

Minior, V. K. and Divon, M. Y. (1998). Fetal growth restriction at term: myth or reality? *Obstet. Gynecol.*, **92**, 57–60.

Nair, R. H., Kesavachandran, C. and Shashidhar, S. (1999). Spirometric impairments in undernourished children. *Indian J. Physiol. Pharmacol.*, **43**, 467–73.

Nicolaides, K. H., Economides, D. L. and Soothill, P. W. (1989). Blood gases, pH, and lactate in appropriate- and small-for-gestational-age fetuses. *Am. J. Obstet. Gynecol.*, **161**, 996–1001.

Nikolajev, K., Heinonen, K., Hakulinen, A. and Lansimies, F. (1998). Effects of intrauterine growth retardation and prematurity on spirometric flow values and lung volumes at school age in twin pairs. *Pediatr. Pulmonol.*, **25**, 367–70.

Nikolajev, K., Korppi, M., Remes, K., Lansimies, E., Jokela, V. and Heinonen, K. (2002). Determinants of bronchial responsiveness to methacholine at school age in twin pairs. *Pediatr. Pulmonol.*, **33**, 167–73.

Northway, W. H., Rosan, R. C. and Porter, D. Y. (1967). Pulmonary disease following respirator therapy of hyaline-membrane disease: bronchopulmonary dysplasia. *N. Engl. J. Med.*, **276**, 357–68.

Northway, W. H., Moss, R. B., Carlisle, K. B. *et al.* (1990). Late pulmonary sequelae of bronchopulmonary dysplasia. *N. Engl. J. Med.*, **323**, 1793–9.

Ong, T. J., Mehta, A., Ogston, S. and Mukhopadhyay, S. (1998). Prediction of lung function in the inadequately nourished. *Arch. Dis. Child.*, **79**, 18–21.

Pierce, R. A. and Nguyen, N. M. (2002). Prenatal nicotine exposure and abnormal lung function. *Am. J. Respir. Cell Mol. Biol.*, **26**, 10–13.

Primhak, R. and Coates, F. S. (1988). Malnutrition and peak expiratory flow rate. *Eur. Respir. J.*, **1**, 801–3.

Pullan, C. R. and Hey, E. N. (1982). Wheezing, asthma, and pulmonary dysfunction 10 years after infection with respiratory syncitial virus in infancy. *Br. Med. J.*, **284**, 1665–9.

Rees, S., Ng, J., Dickson, K., Nicholas, T. and Harding, R. (1991). Growth retardation and the development of the respiratory system in fetal sheep. *Early Hum. Dev.*, **26**, 13–27.

Resnik, R. (2002). High-risk pregnancy series: an expert's view. *Obstet. Gynecol.*, **99**, 490–6.

Rhoades, R. A. and Ryder, D. A. (1981). Fetal lung metabolism response to maternal fasting. *Biochim. Biophys. Acta*, **663**, 621–9.

Robinson, P. J., Hegele, R. G. and Schellenberg, R. R. (1996). Increased airway reactivity in human RSV bronchiolitis in the guinea pig is not due to increased wall thickness. *Pediatr. Pulmonol.*, **22**, 248–54.

Rona, R. J., Gulliford, M. C. and Chinn, S. (1993). Effects of prematurity and intrauterine growth on respiratory health and lung function in childhood. *BMJ*, **306**, 817–20.

Rucker, R. B. and Dubick, M. A. (1984). Elastin metabolism and chemistry: potential roles in lung development and structure. *Environ. Health Perspect.*, **55**, 179–91.

Ryan, S. (1998). Nutrition in neonatal chronic lung disease. *Eur. J. Pediatr.*, **157** (suppl. 1), S19–22.

Saetta, M., Ghezzo, H., Kim, W. D. *et al.* (1985). Loss of alveolar attachments in smokers. *Am. Rev. Resp. Dis.*, **132**, 894–900.

Schols, A. M. (2000). Nutrition in chronic obstructive pulmonary disease. *Curr. Opin. Pulmonol. Med.*, **6**, 110–15.

Sekhon, H. S., Keller, J. A., Proskocil, B. J., Martin, E. L. and Spindel, E. R. (2002). Maternal nicotine exposure upregulates collagen gene expression in fetal monkey lung: association with alpha7 nicotinic acetylcholine receptors. *Am. J. Resp. Cell. Mol. Biol.*, **26**, 31–41.

Shaheen, S. O. and Barker, D. J. P. (1994). Early lung growth and chronic airflow obstruction. *Thorax*, **49**, 533–6.

Shaheen, S. O., Sterne, J. A., Tucker, J. S. and Florey, C. D. (1998). Birth weight, childhood lower respiratory tract infection, and adult lung function. *Thorax*, **53**, 549–53.

Smyth, J. A., Tabachnik, E., Duncan, W. J., Reilly, B. J. and Levison, H. (1981). Pulmonary function and bronchial hyperreactivity in long-term survivors of bronchopulmonary dysplasia. *Pediatrics*, **68**, 336–40.

Sozo, F., Wallace, M. J., Hanna, M. R. *et al.* (in press). Alveolar epithelial cell differentiation and surfactant protein expression after mild preterm birth in sheep. *Pediatr. Res.*

Speer, C. P. and Silverman, M. (1998). Issues relating to children born prematurely. *Eur. Resp. J.*, **27**, 13–16s.

Stein, C. E., Kumaran, K., Fall, C. H., Shaheen, S. O., Osmond, C. and Barker, D. J. P. (1997). Relation of fetal growth to adult lung function in south India. *Thorax*, **52**, 895–9.

Szuts, T., Olsson, S., Lindquist, N. G., Ullberg, S., Pilotti, A. and Enzell, C. (1978). Long-term fate of [14C]nicotine in the mouse: retention in the bronchi, melanin-containing tissues and urinary bladder wall. *Toxicology*, **10**, 207–20.

Tager, I. B., Hanrahan, J. P., Tosteson, T. D. *et al.* (1993). Lung function, pre- and post-natal smoke exposure, and wheezing in the first year of life. *Am. Rev. Resp. Dis.*, **147**, 811–17.

Tyson, J. E., Kennedy, K., Broyles, S. and Rosenfeld, C. R. (1995). The small for gestational age infant: accelerated or delayed pulmonary maturation? Increased or decreased survival? *Pediatrics*, **95**, 534–8.

Van Vunakis, H., Langone, J. J. and Milunsky, A. (1974). Nicotine and cotinine in the amniotic fluid of smokers in the second trimester of pregnancy. *Am. J. Obstet. Gynecol.*, 120, 64–6.

Vidic, B. (1991). Transplacental effect of environmental pollutants on interstitial composition and diffusion capacity for exchange of gases of pulmonary parenchyma in neonatal rat. *Bull. Assoc. Anat.*, **75**, 153–5.

Wang, N.-S., Schraufnagel, D. E. and Chen, M. F. (1983). The effect of maternal oral intake of nicotine on the growth and maturation of fetal and baby mouse lungs. *Lung*, **161**, 27–38.

Wignarajah, D., Cock, M. L., Pinkerton, K. E. and Harding, R. (2002). Influence of intra-uterine growth restriction on airway development in fetal and postnatal sheep. *Pediatr. Res.*, **51**, 681–8.

Young, S., Le Souef, P. N., Geelhoed, G. C., Stick, S. M., Turner, K. J. and Landau, L. I. (1991). The influence of a family history of asthma and parental smoking on airway responsiveness in early infancy. *N. Engl. J. Med.*, **324**, 1168–73.

26

Developmental origins of asthma and related allergic disorders

J. O. Warner

University of Southampton

Introduction

Asthma is a chronic disorder affecting the conducting airways, in which genetic and environmental factors interact to produce both inflammation and structural changes in the airway wall (Tattersfield *et al.* 2002). The consequence of these pathological changes is variable airflow limitation which is manifested by recurrent cough and wheeze. Recent asthma guidelines have emphasised the importance of treating the underlying inflammatory response as well as relieving the symptoms of asthma, but beyond the use of inhaled corticosteroids (ICS) and beta-2 adrenoceptor agonists, which were introduced 30–40 years ago, there has been very little new to add to the therapeutic algorithm (British Thoracic Society 2003). While utilisation of these two pharmacotherapies is highly effective in controlling symptoms and improving quality of life, there is no evidence that these therapies either alter the natural history of the disease or ever effect a cure (Martinez 2003). With the possible exception of immunotherapy no treatment has been shown to modify the natural course of the disease and no cure has been identified (Durham *et al.* 1999).

Most asthma has its origins in early life, and the best predictors of continuation into adulthood are an early age of onset, sensitisation to house dust mites (in environments where this is the major allergen), reduced lung function, and increased bronchial

hyper-responsiveness (BHR) in early life (Sears *et al.* 2003). Even employment of ICS at a very early stage in the disease evolution does not influence outcomes (Covar *et al.* 2004). Thus it becomes imperative to understand the early-life origins of the disease in order to identify targets for prevention and early intervention.

There has been a progressively increasing prevalence of asthma and related allergic diseases such as atopic eczema and allergic rhinoconjunctivitis over the last 30–40 years. The increases have occurred far too rapidly for this to be accounted for by a genetic change in the population. It is more likely to have been due to a shift in environmental influences acting on a pre-existing genetic susceptibility (Holgate 1998). While there are two basic components which contribute to airflow limitation in asthma, namely airway inflammation and altered airway wall structure, most studies of the environmental influences on the disease have concentrated on allergic sensitisation. It has now become clear that concentrating on the cellular and mediator pathways producing an allergic inflammatory response falls short of explaining the full pathology of the disease (Holgate *et al.* 2004). Hitherto it has been assumed that allergic inflammation is the main cause of the structural changes and that one follows the other. However, genetic and environmental factors can affect the airway-wall structure independent of allergic sensitisation. Indeed increased BHR, which may well

Developmental Origins of Health and Disease, ed. Peter Gluckman and Mark Hanson. Published by Cambridge University Press.

represent changes to airway wall structure, can be detected as early as 4 weeks of age and its presence is predictive of asthma at 6 years of age independent of allergic sensitisation (Palmer *et al.* 2001). The origins of asthma will therefore be discussed both in relation to the early-life origins of allergy and its influence on airway inflammation, and in relation to the evolution of changes to airway wall structure. While there are distinct genetic and environmental influences on the two components of the disease, common pathways exist for environmental factors to affect both components simultaneously, thereby leading to the disease we know as asthma.

Epidemiology of allergy

It has long been known that allergy is one of the most important risk factors for asthma. Its presence is associated with an increased risk of developing the disease (Van Asperen and Mukhi 1994), and once the disease is manifest it predicts persistence from childhood through adolescence and into adulthood (Ross *et al.* 1995). Successive studies have demonstrated that both the prevalence and the severity of asthma has increased in many countries around the world. In the United Kingdom surveys amongst 12- to 14-year-olds have shown an increase in point prevalence from 1973 to 1988 and finally to 1996 of 4%–9%–20.9% respectively (Burr *et al.* 1989, Kaur *et al.* 1998). This increase has occurred simultaneously with increases in all other allergic diseases. Thus eczema over the same time period has increased 5%–16%–16.4%, and hay fever 9%–15%–18.2% (Austin *et al.* 1999). Similar increases have been seen in four consecutive studies conducted on children aged 9–11 years in Aberdeen, UK (Fig. 26.1) (Ninan *et al.* 2000). Diagnostic transfer does not explain this as studies had used virtually identical ascertainments at each time-point. There has also been a considerable increase in hospital admissions for childhood asthma over the last 15 years with no reduction in severity on admission, no increase in readmission ratio and no evidence of diagnostic transfer (Anderson 1989). A relatively small shift in popu-

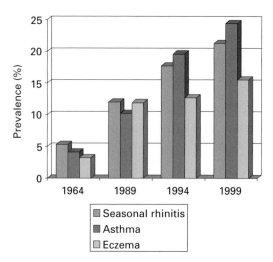

Figure 26.1 There has been a considerable increase in the prevalence rates of all allergic conditions over the last 30 years. This is shown for seasonal rhinitis, asthma and eczema between 1964 and 1999 in four successive studies conducted on Aberdeen schoolchildren aged 9–11 years. From Ninan *et al.* (2000).

lation susceptibility due to changes in the environment could account for the increased frequency of disease and particularly of severe disease. It is, however, important to note that very recent studies are suggesting that the increase in prevalence of asthma may be coming to an end (Hess and de Jongste 2004), at least in developed countries.

Many environmental factors which have been linked to the rising trends of allergic diseases have embraced the concept of an alteration in the balance of immune responses between (a) those which are associated with an allergic pattern, (b) those associated with protection against infection and (c) those which regulate all responses.

The allergic immune response

The immunological paradigm associated with allergic disease is the expression of T-lymphocyte cell-mediated immunity to common environmental allergens that is biased towards T-helper 2 (Th2) lymphocyte activity. Th2 lymphocytes release peptide regulatory factors (cytokines) which orchestrate the production of immunoglobulin E (IgE), which is the archetypal allergy-promoting antibody, and activate inflammatory cells such as eosinophils which are commonly associated with allergic inflammation. The relevant cytokines and their effects are shown in Fig. 26.2, namely interleukins (IL)4, IL5, IL9 and IL13. The counter-regulatory pathways include those generated by a normal immune response to infection orchestrated by the T-helper 1 (Th1) lymphocytes which generate the cytokines interferon gamma (IFNγ) and IL2 (Romagnani 1991). The other pathway involves a group of T-lymphocyte regulators which have an influence on both Th1 and Th2 activity by either cell–cell contact or the generation of IL10 and transforming growth factor beta (TGFβ) (Romagnani 2004) (Fig. 26.2). Based on this paradigm it becomes clear that either overexpression of Th2 activity or a failure of control by Th1 or T-regulatory function will result in a higher probability of the development of allergy and allergic inflammation.

The pattern of response of T lymphocytes is dictated by the nature of the signalling from antigen-presenting cells (APCs). APCs are affected by the nature of the antigen exposure (Rothoeft *et al.* 2003), which influences their interaction with T lymphocytes (Kruse *et al.* 2003). These cells generate IL12, 15, 18 and 23 which predominantly though not exclusively stimulate Th1 responses, while IL10 from regulatory T cells inhibits IL12 and therefore favours Th2 activity.

Genetic polymorphisms and allergy

Twin and family studies have shown that asthma is highly heritable (Duffy *et al.* 1990). A plethora of single nucleotide polymorphisms (SNPs) have been associated with allergy and are clearly associated with effects on Th2 pathways. The greatest focus has been on the cytokine gene cluster on the long arm of chromosome 5 (5q31–33) (Liu *et al.* 2003). This chromosome region contains the genes for many Th2 cytokines, IL 3, 5, 9 and 13, GM-CSF and also the gene for an endotoxin recep-

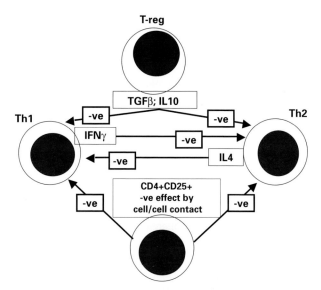

Figure 26.2 The relationship between T-helper 1, T-helper 2 and T-regulatory cells. The T-helper 1 cells generate interferon gamma which down-regulates the activity of T-helper 2 cells. Conversely IL4 from Th2 cells down-regulates Th1 activity. Regulatory T-cells either control both Th1 and Th2 activity via the generation of the cytokines transforming growth at the beta (TGFβ) or IL10. Additionally T-cell regulation can be effected by cell–cell contact with regulatory cells which express the surface markers CD4 and CD25.

tor known as CD14 (Baldini *et al.* 1999). This latter molecule will be discussed in relation to the hygiene hypothesis. However, the associations between polymorphisms in this chromosome region are much more strongly associated with allergy rather than asthma (Holloway and Holgate 2004). Other associations have been with a common subunit of the IL4 and IL13 receptor on chromosome 16p12; those for IFNγ on 12q; the major histocompatability complex molecules, tumour necrosis factor alpha and beta, on 6p21; the IgE receptor on 11q12–13; and IL18 on 11q22 (Holloway and Holgate 2004). The latter is particularly interesting because IL18 has complex interactions in initiating both Th1 and Th2 activity, dependent on the antigenic stimulus (Kruse *et al.* 2003). Thus all these polymorphisms have a credible mechanistic association with a higher probability of developing allergy and allergic inflammation.

The impact of the polymorphisms may only be apparent at critical stages during development of the immune response as their presence does not inevitably mandate the development of allergy. Relatively minor perturbations of the balance between Th1 and Th2 activity, particularly in early life, is likely to have significant effects on outcomes.

Ontogeny of immune responses in the fetus

Observations of an altered immune response at birth in children at risk of developing allergy by virtue of a family history of allergic disease, and similar alterations in the subset who go on to develop allergy and disease, highlights the contribution of fetal life (Jones *et al.* 2000). There has been a commonly held misconception that the newborn baby is immunologically naive. However, it is very clear that the capacity to mount a significant immune response is present from very early gestation. There are stem cells present in the human yolk sack at 21 days, with the first lymphocytes being seen in the thymus by the ninth week of gestation. The lymphocytes are detectable in many organs including the lungs and gut by 14 weeks, and by 16 weeks circulating B cells can be detected with surface immunoglobulin M (Hayward 1998).

The neonate is known to be able to mount an antibody response to a wide array of antigens following specific exposure of the mother during pregnancy. Fetal IgM antibody responses have been demonstrated after maternal immunisation with tetanus toxoid (Gill *et al.* 1983), and of course they are well recognised by paediatricians in association with maternal infection with rubella, toxoplasmosis, cytomegalovirus and human immunodeficiency virus early in pregnancy (Naot *et al.* 1981, Daffos *et al.* 1984, Clerici *et al.* 1993, Jones *et al.* 2002a). Studies have shown that direct immunisation of the baboon fetus with recombinant hepatitis B surface antigen can initiate a specific fetal IgG antibody response where there is no such response detected in the mother. The resulting baboon infant has an enhanced responsiveness to hepatitis B surface anti-

gen when immunised again postnatally (Watts *et al.* 1999). This indicates that the complete process of immune sensitisation must have occurred, commencing with the pickup and processing of antigen by APCs. The subsequent presentation of the antigen to T lymphocytes and thereafter stimulation of the B lymphocyte to produce specific immunoglobulin has also occurred. Thus the ability to detect antigen-specific responses at birth should not be considered unusual.

It has, therefore, been possible to demonstrate that circulating blood mononuclear cells are capable of mounting a specific proliferative response to allergens such as ovalbumin from hens' eggs and even the major allergen of house dust mite from as early as 22 weeks gestation (Jones *et al.* 1996). As the pregnancy proceeds a progressively higher percentage of fetuses mount specific responses to common environmental factors. By birth the majority, if not all, demonstrate such responses (Prescott *et al.* 1998). Furthermore, a number of studies have shown that a high proliferative response to an allergen at birth is associated with a higher probability of allergic reaction to that factor and of allergic disease later in childhood (Kondo *et al.* 1992).

The immunology of pregnancy

Normal pregnancy can only proceed if the maternal cell-mediated immune response to fetopaternal antigens is suppressed. Initial studies of murine pregnancies (Wegmann *et al.* 1993), but more recently also in humans, have shown that a range of tissues in the fetoplacental unit produce cytokines which have a profile similar to that associated with the Th2 phenotype (Tang *et al.* 1992, Warner *et al.* 1994, Piccinni *et al.* 1996, Jones *et al.* 2000). These cytokines shift the balance of the maternal immune response away from cell-mediated activity towards a less damaging humoral immune response (Raghupathy 1997). Such cytokines almost certainly also have additional properties in promoting fetal growth. Thus it has been shown that granulocyte-macrophage colony-stimulating factor (GM-CSF) has an effect on surfactant homeostasis by stimulating differentiation and proliferation of the type 2 pneumonocytes (Whitsett and Wert 1998). Based on the Th1/Th2 paradigm, it is very likely that the Th2-cytokine bias of normal pregnancy promotes a successful outcome by suppressing Th1 responses. The latter are clearly associated with pregnancy loss or intrauterine growth retardation (Raghupathy 1997, Piccinni *et al*. 1998). IL4 and the regulatory cytokine IL10 have an effect on cell maturation and therefore directly and indirectly affect lung structure and function. IL10 is worthy of specific mention because of its regulatory properties. It will diminish the production of a range of cytokines including IL12 from antigen-presenting cells which would otherwise increase IFNγ production (Fickenscher *et al*. 2002).

Decidual tissues have been shown to be a source of IL1 alpha and beta, IL6, GM-CSF, IL4, IL10 and IL13 (Jones *et al*. 1998a). IL13 immune reactivity can be detected in the placenta between 16 and 27 weeks gestation but not thereafter. From 27 weeks until 34 weeks IL13 can be found spontaneously released from fetal mononuclear cells. Thereafter it is only released on stimulation of cells (Williams *et al*. 2000). Thus there must be a very subtle regulation of production of this and other cytokines with an interaction between the mother, the placenta and fetus. These Th2 and regulatory cytokines will not only modulate the maternal immune response but will also have an impact on the fetus. It is, therefore, not surprising that there is a universally Th2-biased immune response to antigens detectable in all newborn babies. Rapid postnatal maturation of Th1 responsiveness normally counterbalances this (Prescott *et al*. 1999).

The Th2 and T-regulatory cytokines IL4, IL10, IL13 and TGFβ can be detected in amniotic fluid during the second trimester of pregnancy (Jones *et al*. 1998a). Such cytokines will be swallowed by the fetus. Indeed the protein turnover in amniotic fluid occurs at a rate of 70% each day, with much of this removal being via fetal swallowing (Gitlin *et al*. 1972). The fetus, of course, also has a highly permeable skin (Hardman *et al*. 1999) and there is some aspiration of amniotic fluid into the respiratory tract during fetal respiratory movements (Schittny *et al*. 2000). Thus factors in the amniotic fluid have the capacity to gain access to mucosal surfaces and to influence immune responses at that level.

The fetal gut has been well studied. There are many HLA-DR-positive cells comprising macrophages, B lymphocytes and dendritic cells detectable in the submucosa from as early as 11–12 weeks gestation. By 14 weeks gestation HLA-DR-positive APCs are found in lymphoid follicles of the rudimentary Peyer's patches of the fetus. Surface markers on these cells suggest that antigen presentation can occur with appropriate costimulatory signals in order to promote a sensitising immune response in T lymphocytes. Both T lymphocytes and B lymphocytes can be detected in the lymphoid follicles from 14–16 weeks gestation. They contain the relevant ligands for costimulatory signalling. Furthermore, the location of such receptors to one side of the cells, a phenomenon known as capping, suggests that communication is occurring between APCs and T cells (Jones *et al*. 2001). The mere presence of dendritic cells (the most professional of APCs) in lymphoid follicles expressing maturation markers implies that these cells have already picked up antigen and migrated to the follicles. The only likely route of exposure to antigen will have been through swallowed amniotic fluid. It has been possible to demonstrate both food and inhalant allergen in some amniotic fluids. Hen-egg ovalbumin and the major allergen of house dust mites have been detected at levels of about 10% of those levels found in the maternal circulation (Holloway *et al*. 2000). Thus all the ingredients for allergen sensitisation with a Th2 bias are present within the fetal gut. To date it has not been possible to demonstrate similar maturity of immune active cells in the fetal skin, airway or circulation. It is likely that the maturation of cells in the fetal gut is a consequence of exposure to the cytokines in the amniotic fluid.

Amniotic fluid also contains IgG and IgE antibodies of maternal origin, at levels about 10% of that found in the maternal circulation, from as early as 16 weeks gestation. IgG and IgE receptors can be detected on cells within the lamina propria of the fetal gut (Thornton *et al.* 2003). Therefore there is the potential for these immunoglobulins to facilitate the pick-up of antigen by APCs. This is a phenomenon known as antigen focusing. With IgE on relevant low- or high-affinity IgE receptors it is possible to achieve sensitisation to concentrations of allergen 100–1000 times lower than would be achieved without the immunoglobulin present (Maurer *et al.* 1995).

While the likely route of primary sensitisation to allergen in pregnancy is via the fetal gut during the second trimester, there is also exposure to allergen via the fetal circulation in the third trimester. This is predominantly as a consequence of active transport of IgG antibody across the placenta complexed with antigens and allergens. What evidence exists would suggest that the higher the IgG antibody to specific allergens the less the likelihood of subsequent sensitisation to those allergens (Casas and Björksten 2001). This indicates that the timing of exposure to allergen in pregnancy and the concentration of exposure will have subtly different influences on outcome (Jenmalm and Björksten 2000). Thus one study of birch and timothy grass pollen exposure via the pregnant mother suggested that the fetus only mounted a sensitising cellular response if the pollen season occurred during the first six months of pregnancy, with later exposure resulting in tolerance (Van Duren-Schmidt *et al.* 1997).

Environmental factors influencing antenatal immune responses

It is well known from many studies that if the mother is allergic herself the infant is far more likely to show allergy and allergic disease from an early stage in life, compared with merely inheriting allergy genes from the father, where the subsequent prevalence of disease is lower (Ruiz *et al.* 1992). This implies that maternal allergy in some way primes the fetus to be more likely to react in an allergic way. Clearly if the mother is allergic she has a higher level of IgE in her circulation. This in turn means there is more IgE in the amniotic fluid and therefore a greater probability of antigen focusing producing sensitisa-

tion to very-low-concentration allergen exposure in the second trimester of pregnancy. Furthermore, the amniotic fluid of allergic mothers has higher levels of IL10 than that of non-allergic mothers (Warner *et al.* 1997). It is interesting to speculate why such a sophisticated immune response should be in place so early in gestation. It is likely that it facilitates a fetal response to maternal helminth infection (Jones *et al.* 1998b). Certainly infants born to helminth-infected mothers have specific Th2-biased immune responses to helminth antigen and detectable IgE antibodies to those antigens at birth (Malhotra *et al.* 1997). Furthermore, although the newborn baby has an obligate exposure to its mother's parasites it is exceedingly rare for the infant to become infected by those parasites, implying a very mature immune response preventing such infection (D'Alauro *et al.* 1985). In this era of low parasite infestation it is likely that certain properties of allergens have counterparts of parasite antigens leading to stimulation of the same immune response (Stewart and Thompson 1996). These mechanisms would certainly explain the higher probability of IgE-sensitisation of the baby born to an IgE-sensitised (i.e. allergic) mother.

As suggested, the timing and concentration of allergen exposure during pregnancy could also influence outcomes. Low-dose exposure in the second trimester appears to be more likely to sensitise, while high-dose exposure has the converse effect. The latter might be explained by the generation of high levels of IgG allergen-specific antibody in the mother (Vance *et al.* 2004). One study of the children of mothers who had undergone rye-grass-allergen immunotherapy during pregnancy and consequently had high IgG antibody levels compared to children born to rye-grass-allergic mothers not receiving immunotherapy showed fewer positive skin tests to rye-grass 3–12 years later in the offspring (Glovsky *et al.* 1991). Newborn babies with high levels of IgG antibody to cats and/or pollens have been shown to have a lower probability of generating IgE antibodies to those allergens up to eight years later (Jenmalm and Björksten 2000). This might explain the recent observations that children born into families where there is a high exposure to dogs have less subsequent sensitisation to these allergens

(Gern *et al.* 2004). These observations imply that attempts to reduce allergen exposure in pregnancy might have an adverse rather than a favourable effect. Indeed two recent publications have suggested that this may be the case. While at 1 year of age house-mite avoidance has been shown to be associated with somewhat less wheezing, by 3 years of age there was increased sensitisation to house dust mite (Custovic and Simpson 2004). Most studies have failed to demonstrate any consistent effect of house-mite avoidance in preventing sensitisation or asthma, and low-level exposure to house mite has been associated with a greater risk of IgE sensitisation and asthma than higher levels (Cullinan *et al.* 2004). Studies from my own lab have suggested that there is a bell-shaped curve of risk of allergic sensitisation in relation to allergen exposure in pregnancy. Thus very low and very high-dose exposure protects, and it is in the middle range of exposures that sensitisation occurs (Vance *et al.* 2004). Any attempt to reduce exposure will shift those in the high-dose tolerance range into the sensitising range and will of course also move a number from the sensitising range into the very-low-dose no-sensitisation range. However in the majority of circumstances the overall result for a population will be of no effect on the prevalence of sensitisation and disease (Fig. 26.3).

Fetal growth and nutrition may well also have an impact on the ontogeny of immune responses. There have been some unexpected associations between large head circumference at birth and levels of total IgE at birth (Oryszczyn *et al.* 1999), in childhood (Gregory *et al.* 1999) and even in adulthood (Godfrey *et al.* 1994). More importantly, there is an association between large head circumference at birth and asthma requiring medical attention (Gregory *et al.* 1999). It has been hypothesised that large head circumference at birth is indicative of a rapid fetal growth trajectory, because of good nutrient supplies in early pregnancy. The fetus is subsequently programmed to continue on a rapid growth trajectory, but of course also retains a high nutrient demand. If this is not met in the later stages of pregnancy there is continuing head growth at the expense of relatively poor nutrition to the body, with consequent effects on immune responses (Fig. 26.4). The key ques-

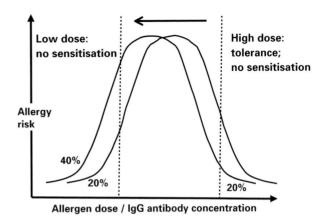

Figure 26.3 The potential effects of allergen avoidance, based on the assumption that there is a bell-shaped distribution of risk of allergy in relation to the dose of allergen exposure. The 20% of the population having either very low-dose or very high-dose exposure are not sensitised. Shifting the population by half a standard deviation results in the majority in the high-dose tolerance range moving into the lower-dose sensitisation range, with an equivalent number moving from the mid-range into the very-low-dose no-sensitisation range. The end result on the whole population is to achieve no reduction in allergy prevalence.

tion raised by these observations is whether there are any specific nutrients of importance in protecting immune responsiveness. The focus has hitherto been on antioxidants. Certainly reduced intake of fresh fruit and vegetables is associated with a higher rate of allergic sensitisation when different populations around Europe are compared (Butland *et al.* 1999). However, the prevailing view is that reduced antioxidant intake has an impact on asthma severity rather than on asthma prevalence. Low cord-blood selenium and iron have been associated with a higher subsequent risk of persistent wheeze for the former, and both wheeze and eczema for the latter nutrient (Shaheen *et al.* 2004). Trials of supplementation in pregnancy are now required.

Recent studies have focused on lipids as perhaps also being important in immune ontogeny (Peat *et al.* 2004). Indeed fatty acids have a crucial role as a source of energy, as the principal component of cell membranes, and as signalling molecules for synthesis of prostaglanadins and leukotrienes. Minor

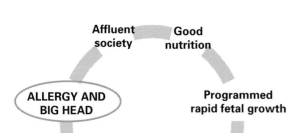

Figure 26.4 A hypothesis to explain the association between a large head circumference at birth and allergy. Affluent societies where good nutrition predominates have an impact on programming of fetal growth. Early in pregnancy, with good nutrient delivery, the fetus begins a rapid growth trajectory. This must be sustained throughout life. Nutrient need exceeds delivery in the third trimester, resulting in a brain-sparing reflex with continued growth of the brain and head but selected compromise of rapidly growing tissues, which will have a particular impact on immune responsiveness and may selectively compromise Th1 activity. This leads to the association between a big head and allergy and could explain some of the demographic trends in allergy prevalence.

variations in levels could have a profound effect on immune responses (Yaqoob 2003). Two studies are currently investigating this hypothesis (Dunstan *et al.* 2003a, Peat *et al.* 2004) and one has already demonstrated that fish oil supplementation in pregnancy does alter the neonatal immune response (Dunstan *et al.* 2003a, 2003b). To what extent this will affect subsequent allergic sensitisation and disease remains to be established. A recent very large birth cohort study has investigated the association of cord-blood red cell fatty acids and subsequent eczema and asthma. There were differences in the ratio of arachidonic to eicosapentaenoic acid in eczema and also of linoleic acid to alpha-linolenic acid in late-onset wheezing. However the associations did not remain significant when adjusting for multiple comparisons. The conclusion of the study was that it is unlikely that prenatal exposure to different ratios of n-6 : n-3 fatty-acids is an important determinant of

wheezing and atopic disease in childhood. However, further studies are clearly indicated (Newson *et al.* 2004).

One other hypothesis related to nutrition has appeared, suggesting that vitamin D supplementation increases the risk of allergic sensitisation. The geographical distribution of allergy prevalence can to a certain extent be associated with vitamin D supplementation usage during pregnancy and postnatally (Wjst 2004). Vitamin D receptors have been identified on immune active cells and there may therefore be a novel immunoregulatory function to this nutrient. Dendritic cell production of IL12 is inhibited and IL10 increased by exposure to vitamin D (Feldman *et al.* 1997). This in turn would down-regulate T-helper 1 responses and allow T-helper 2 activity to predominate, which, based on the Th1/Th2 paradigm, would be associated with greater probability of allergy and allergic disease.

Postnatal influences on allergic immune responses

Studies have shown that newborn infants have allergen-reactive T cells which are of fetal and not maternal origin (Prescott *et al.* 1998). The responses are characterised by the dominant production of Th2 rather than Th1 cytokines. Postnatally these responses are modulated, with a progressive increase in Th1 activity and associated reduction in Th2 activity. However, those infants that go on to have allergic symptoms have a very different pattern of response with an age-associated increase in Th2 activity (Prescott *et al.* 1999). Figure 26.5 shows the different outcomes arising from the interaction of postnatal allergen exposure and infection. It is also possible to detect differences in allergen-induced cytokine production at birth in infants who have subsequently developed allergic disease (Kondo *et al.* 1992). There is a generally reduced capacity in such infants to generate both IFNγ, the archetypal Th1 cytokine (Warner *et al.* 1994), and IL13, a characteristic Th2 cytokine (Williams *et al.* 2000). To what extent this represents a form of immunological immaturity or immune suppression as a consequence of

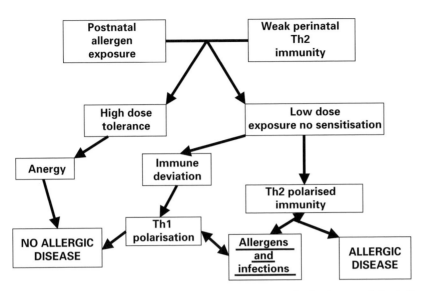

Figure 26.5 The role of postnatal allergen exposure and infection on the development of allergic disease. High-dose exposure to allergen postnatally can lead to anergy and therefore no allergic disease. Low-dose exposure can lead through a phenomenon of immune deviation to Th1 polarisation and no disease; or to a Th2 polarised response. Association of the allergen exposure with particular infections may still switch the response back to a more normal Th1 activity, whereas the absence of exposure to infection will lead on to a committed Th2 response and allergic disease.

overactive regulatory T cells remains to be established. Factors that are thought to influence the evolution of the allergic immune response postnatally include the route and dose of allergen exposure, and exposure to the adjuvantising effect of infection or particular gut flora (Holt *et al.* 2004).

Longitudinal cohort studies following atopic and non-atopic children through early childhood have demonstrated a biphasic pattern of change in IgE antibodies with significant differences in responses to dietary allergens which does not occur in response to inhalant allergens. There is an initial peak of IgE antibody production against foods in infancy followed by a decline by 1–2 years of age, but with higher peak levels in those who are allergic. There is an implication that very high levels of dietary allergen exposure will eventually stimulate so-called high-zone tolerance by mechanisms involving T-cell depletion and/or anergy. In contrast, the IgE antibody response to inhalants is much slower and takes many years to decline, with a significant percentage having a persistence of the antibody, particularly

those who manifest inhalant allergy and asthma (Holt *et al.* 1995). Clearly exposure to inhalants, predominantly in the respiratory rather than the gastointestinal tract, is at much lower concentrations and therefore is unlikely to reach the levels associated with high-zone tolerance. Again, therefore, the implication is that rather than allergen avoidance, high-dose allergen exposure as a form of immunotherapy may be more appropriate. This indeed is borne out by a few immunotherapy trials. One such study involved the administration of pollen immunotherapy to children with allergic rhinitis but not asthma. This was associated with a lower period prevalence of asthma over the three yeas of the study compared with contemporaneous controls who were not given immunotherapy (Möller *et al.* 2002). Furthermore, studies have shown that children given immunotherapy when they have a single inhalant allergy have a much lower probability of subsequently developing new inhalant allergies, again compared with untreated contemporaneous controls (Des Roches *et al.* 1997).

- Birth order
- Early day care
- Early antibiotics
- Farmers' children
- Early cat or dog ownership
- Inverse relationship with measles, tuberculin positivity etc
- Gut flora

Figure 26.6 Factors which have been suggested as explaining the so-called 'hygiene hypothesis', which states that early exposure to microbial factors is associated with a lower subsequent prevalence of allergy and allergic disease.

The hygiene hypothesis

One of the most compelling explanations for the increasing prevalence of allergic diseases in the developed world is the so-called 'hygiene hypothesis' (Fig. 26.6). Exposure to microbes might be expected to up-regulate Th1 activity, and therefore reduced exposure to microbes might be predicted to be associated with a persistence of Th2 activity and a higher probability of allergy and allergic disease (Folkerts *et al.* 2000). Many studies have shown an inverse relationship between the prevalence of certain infections and allergy (Strachan 2000). For example the infectious diseases typhoid and tuberculosis occur rarely in countries with a high prevalence of allergic disease, and it has been suggested that this explains the geographical variation in disease prevalence.

The hypothesis was first proposed in 1989 with the demonstration of an inverse relationship between birth order in families and the subsequent prevalence of allergic rhinoconjunctivitis (Strachan 1989). Whether this is an ante- or a postnatal effect could be disputed, as the sibling effect may also have an impact on cord-blood IgE levels (van Gool *et al.* 2004, Karmaus *et al.* 2001). Studies have also shown an inverse relationship between tuberculin responsiveness, previous hepatitis A or measles infection and allergy (Shaheen *et al.* 1996, Shirakawa *et al.* 1997). This is further reinforced by the observation that BCG, which will produce a positive tuberculin

test, can suppress local Th2 immune responses in a murine model (Folkerts *et al.* 2000). However BCG (Annus *et al.* 2004) has not been shown to have a significant effect on the subsequent development of allergy in Europe, although it may have an effect in developing countries (Aaby *et al.* 2000).

The hygiene hypothesis has been used to explain differences in the development of allergy and allergic disease in children born and raised on farms (Radon *et al.* 2004) or adopting an anthroposophic lifestyle (Alm *et al.* 1999). It has been suggested that the farming effect is a consequence of exposure to *Toxoplasma gondii* (Radon *et al.* 2004).

There is an inverse relationship between antibiotic usage, both during pregnancy (McKeever *et al.* 2002) and in infancy (Farooqi and Hopkin 1998), and the prevalence of allergy. Such antibiotic usage will have a potent influence on the type of organisms in the maternal gastrointestinal tract, which in turn will lead to a difference in those organisms colonising the newborn infant's gut. The composition of gastrointestinal flora has been shown to be different in allergic compared with non-allergic infants (Björksten *et al.* 1999). This has led to one study administering probiotics in a pregnancy cohort study where parents had allergy and therefore the infant was at high risk of developing allergic sensitisation and disease (Kalliomaki *et al.* 2001). In a parallel-group double-blind placebo-controlled study where the probiotic *Lactobacillus* GG was administered to the mother during pregnancy and the infant postnally there was less atopic eczema up to 2 years of age than in the group receiving placebo. Unexpectedly, however, there was no difference in the degree of allergic sensitisation between the two groups. Many more and larger studies are required to elaborate on this. It is perhaps naive to think that the administration of a single so-called probiotic organism will change outcomes. The gut flora is a complex combination of up to 200 different bacteria. The range of colonising organisms varies with age and at present it is not possible to say which are more or less important in relation to modulating immune responses (Berg 1996). Furthermore, as probiotic bacteria do not achieve long-lasting colonisation it may also be important to modulate the diet in order to achieve permanent colonisation, utilising so-called prebiotics (Gibson and Roberfroid 1995). Children brought up in families with an anthroposophic lifestyle, where there is avoidance of immunisations and indeed many medical treatments, as well as a diet consisting mainly of fermented vegetables, have a very different gut flora and a much lower prevalence of IgE-mediated allergic disease (Alm *et al.* 1999). It is, however, imperative to point out that there is no evidence that the conventional immunisation programme in any way contributes to the increasing burden of allergic disease. Indeed, in children with a high vaccine coverage there is transiently a better protection against the development of allergy in the first years of life. This is a most important public health message (Grüber *et al.* 2003).

Other proposed interventions to negate the effect of 'hygiene' have included the use of potent Th1 immune stimulators using *Mycobacterium vaccae* vaccines or bacterial CpG oligonucleotides, which have proved highly effective as Th1 selective adjuvants in experimental murine allergies (Kline *et al.* 1998). Trials with these interventions are awaited, but safety will need to be established before proceeding in humans. An additional interest in epidemiological studies has been exposure to endotoxin or lipopolysaccharide in early life and the subsequent diminished risk of IgE-mediated disease. This may be the key factor to which pregnant women and infants are exposed on farms (Oberle *et al.* 2003, Gern *et al.* 2004). It may also explain the fact the children exposed to dogs and/or cats in early infancy have less subsequent allergy. It may also explain why children with more siblings, and those who are enrolled early into day nurseries, have fewer allergies (Ball *et al.* 2000).

It is pertinent to note in relation to the 'hygiene hypothesis' that the mechanism by which microbes provide a Th1 stimulation is through pattern-recognition molecules. CD14 is one such molecule which specifically recognises lipopolysaccharide. Recent studies have identified a polymorphism in the CD14 gene manifesting as diminished levels of the soluble component of CD14 and associated increased intensity of allergy expression in American, British and Japanese but not German populations (Baldini *et al.* 1999, Gao *et al.* 1999, Sengler *et al.* 2003). CD14 is poorly expressed by fetuses and neonates but is present in a soluble form in amniotic fluid and at very high levels in human breast milk. A reduced supply of this molecule from the mother either in amniotic or breast milk is associated with a higher probability of early-onset atopic eczema (Jones *et al.* 2002b). Another pattern-recognition molecule known as toll-like receptor 4 (TLR4) is also important in binding endotoxin when complexed with CD14 to initiate a cytoplasmic signal leading to IL12 production. A study in Swedish schoolchildren has shown a polymorphism of the TLR4 gene to be associated with a fourfold higher prevalence of asthma (Bottcher *et al.* 2004). To what extent these polymorphisms can be overcome by relevant microbial exposure remains to be established. There has been a suggestion that the levels of soluble CD14 in breast milk might be correlated with levels of n-3 polyunsaturated fatty acids (Dunstan *et al.* 2004). Thus supplementation could conceivably raise levels, though this has not been shown as yet by intervention studies.

Exposure to early infection may be a two-edged sword. Some infections particularly associated with bacteria are also associated with less subsequent allergy (Williams *et al.* 2004), but it is important to note that viral respiratory tract infection may have a positive association with subsequent asthma (Resh *et al.* 2004). Whether this is a consequence of the underlying immunological aberration increasing the risk of infection, and also of allergy and asthma, remains to be established. Thus infants infected with respiratory syncitial virus (RSV) are more likely to develop bronchiolitis if they come from atopic families and are themselves atopic (Sigurs *et al.* 2000). Furthermore the immune response to RSV in those who develop bronchiolitis is Th2-biased compared with those who have an upper respiratory tract infection alone, who are more likely to generate IFNγ in response to the infection (Legg *et al.* 2003). Thus the same abnormality of immune responsiveness that leads to bronchiolitis also leads to allergy and may provide an explanation for the link between the two conditions. A severe infection-induced wheeze in infancy increases the risk of persistent asthma. It is possible that the inflammation caused by the infection adjuvantises a Th2-mediated allergic response. The more severe infection may in turn have been a consequence of an impaired maturation of Th1 responsiveness. There are, however, genetic predispositions to bronchiolitis and post-bronchiolitis wheezing independent of allergy involving the I1–8 promotor region (Goetghebuer *et al.* 2004).

Infant feeding allergy in asthma

Many studies have shown a reduced prevalence of allergy and allergic diseases with the use of human compared to cow's milk in infancy. The predominant effect has been associated with food allergy and atopic eczema in infancy rather than asthma, although the data are conflicting (Peat *et al.* 1999). There appear to be differential effects depending on whether the mother has evidence of asthma herself or not. Thus, while large birth cohorts show that breast feeding can reduce asthma rates at least in early to mid-childhood, the effect would appear to be stronger in children born into families without any first-degree relative with allergy (Kull *et al.* 2004). Indeed, if the mother herself has asthma one study showed a significantly increased risk of asthma, particularly if the child was breast-fed for more than four months compared with being breastfed for less than four months or never being breast-fed (Wright *et al.* 2001). Furthermore, in the studies of children born on farms there would appear to have been a protective effect from the administration of cow's milk to infants in reducing allergy, asthma, and rhinitis risk. However, this may have been a consequence of using unpasteurised milk with a different microbial load (Von Ehrenstein *et al.* 2000). It remains to be established whether the use of so-called hypoallergenic milk formulae will be protective in the long run. Extensively hydrolysed caseine formulae do reduce the prevalence of atopic eczema up to 1 year of age,

particularly in those who have a family history of atopic disease (von Berg *et al.* 2003).

Speed of weaning has also been considered to have an impact on outcomes. Old studies suggested that the early introduction of solids at less then 4 months of age had no effect on asthma at 4 years of age (Fergusson *et al.* 1990), but a more recent study suggested early introduction of diverse solids in preterm infants increased the risk of eczema at 1 year of age (Morgan *et al.* 2004). In contrast to this, delayed introduction of egg was associated with more eczema at 5 years of age in another study (Zutavern *et al.* 2004), and the use of full-cream milk at 2 years of age was associated with less asthma at 3 years of age (Wijga *et al.* 2003). To what extent these dietary practices were influenced by the family history of allergy or were representative of some other pattern of environmental exposures is not fully investigated. Overall, therefore, the concept of reducing allergen exposure, whether dietary or inhalant, in order to reduce allergic sensitisation and disease is fraught with problems and should probably not be attempted. There are some positive benefits to be achieved by the use of human breast milk, probably because of immune adjuvantising effects rather than anything to do with avoidance of dietary allergen. The relative benefits of human milk, however, will be appreciably affected by the health and nutrition of the mother, and particularly by her allergic status (Schoetzau *et al.* 2002).

Airway remodelling

Airway remodelling is a constellation of histopathological features characteristic of asthma, including the hypertrophy of airway smooth muscle and the deposition of collagen within the lamina propria and also below the true epithelium basement membrane in the lamina reticularis. This abnormality occurs in parallel with the characteristic eosinophilic inflammation associated with allergy (Pohunek *et al.* 2005). Hitherto it has been considered that the inflammation damages the epithelium and thereby induces a repair process which leads to remodelling.

However, remodelling can occur independently of eosinophilic inflammation and has for instance been described in élite cross-country skiers who have no allergy and primarily neutrophilic rather than eosinophilic airway inflammation (Karjalainen *et al.* 2000). It is interesting to note that many asthmatics with more severe disease both in infancy and adulthood have a predominance of neutrophils in their airways (Marguet *et al.* 1999). Neutrophils, par excellence, generate a specific matrix metalloproteinase 9 (MMP9) which disrupts the collagen matrix. This in turn will release mediators within the matrix, of which TGFβ is particularly important (Cundall *et al.* 2003). This acts as a direct trigger of fibroblast activity to lay down matrix and also to induce a fibroblast transformation to a myofibroblast, which may in turn contribute to the smooth muscle hypertrophy (Blobe *et al.* 2000). This implicates neutrophils in the pathogenesis of the remodelling process rather more than eosinophils.

Bronchial hyper-responsiveness (BHR) is the one non-invasive measure that has been associated with the pathological changes of remodelling. It is notable that the presence of increased BHR at 4 weeks of age is associated with asthma at 6 years of age independent of atopy (Palmer *et al.* 2001). From the same cohort, reduced airway function at 4 weeks was also associated with persistent wheeze at 11 years, and this was independent of both atopy and increased BHR (Turner *et al.* 2004). Furthermore, increased specific airway resistance and allergic sensitisation at 3 years of age in children who had wheezed before 3 years were independent predictors of persistent wheeze at 5 years (Lowe *et al.* 2005). One potential interpretation of these observations is that the remodelling process is present long before the onset of disease or any evidence of allergic inflammation. Indeed it is even possible that the changes had occurred antenatally. TGFβ is a key factor involved in the regulation of lung branching morphogenesis during the pseudo-glandular stage of lung development. There is a variable spatial expression of the isoforms of TGFβ during lung development. TGFβ1 colocalises to the branch clefts with collagen 1 and 3 and fibronectin. TGF2 and TGF3 are expressed in epithelial cells at the tips of the growing lung buds (Gatherer *et al.* 1990). This has led to the proposal that the asthmatic state results from a reactivation of fetal airway modelling processes to generate an inappropriate remodelling response postnatally (Davies *et al.* 2003). The other possibility is that the modelling process in utero has already been adversely affected by the intrauterine environment interacting with genetic factors, thereby setting the scene for later asthma.

Genetic polymorphisms and airway structure and function

The first candidate gene that has been associated purely with structure and function rather than allergic inflammation has been that coding for the beta-2 adrenoceptor, where polymorphisms have been associated with susceptibility to subsensitisation on continuous beta-agonist usage and a probability of BHR and increased disease severity (D'Amato *et al.* 1998). More recently a wide range of novel genes associated with airway epithelium and fibroblasts rather than with inflammatory cells have been identified. There is strong linkage between markers on the short arm of chromosome 11 (11p13) and BHR with asthma. Research has focused on two related proteins, designated ESE2 and ESE3, which are members of a transcription factor family whose basal expression is restricted to epithelial cells with a secretory capacity such as those in the airway. ESE3 is thought to be involved in epithelial cell differentiation towards a mucus-secreting phenotype. It has also been shown to be up-regulated in fibroblasts and smooth muscle when they are exposed to proinflammatory cytokines (Zamel *et al.* 1996, Silverman *et al.* 2002). In addition to the cytokine gene cluster on 5q31–34, many other genes likely to be of importance to asthma are also located in the same region, including the beta-2 adrenoceptor and corticosteroid receptor. Recently, however, a gene encoding a serine protease inhibitor, Kazal type 5 (SPINK5) has also been identified. Several mutations of this gene have been associated with a condition known as Netherton syndrome, which is characterised in part by eczema (Chavanas *et al.* 2000). SNPs in the same gene have been strongly associated with asthma and eczema (Walley *et al.* 2001). SPINK5 expression is in epithelial cells, and it has a protective function against proteases such as those produced by mast cells and those that are present in some allergen extracts such as those of house dust mite which might otherwise cause cell desquamation (Komatsu *et al.* 2002).

Another very important development has been the identification of a disintegrin and metalloproteinase 33 (ADAM33), as a major candidate gene for asthma and BHR found on chromosome 20 (20p13). The strength of associations of polymorphisms in this gene is increased when BHR is included in the definition of asthma and is weakest if the total IgE is raised or if there are specific IgE antibodies (Van Eerdewegh *et al.* 2002). Expression of the gene product is restricted to mesenchymal cells such as fibroblasts and smooth muscle, where its likely function is to influence smooth-muscle hypertrophy and airway wall remodelling, and it thereby manifests as BHR. The mouse equivalent of polymorphisms in this gene have been linked to BHR (Yoshinaka *et al.* 2002). This gene is also preferentially expressed during branching morphogenesis in mouse lung development, thereby linking concepts of airway modelling during embryonic development with the remodelling associated with asthma. Furthermore, polymorphisms of the ADAM33 gene are associated with more rapid decline in lung function in adult asthmatics (Jongepier *et al.* 2004).

One other gene selectively expressed in epithelium is mucin 8 (MUC8). This is found in similar families to those where ADAM33 was first identified. Finally a novel candidate gene linked to asthma whose product is also expressed on epithelial cells is DPP4 (CD26). It is expressed on epithelial cells where it functions as an adhesion receptor for collagen and fibronectin-associated epithelial repair. These data suggest that the range of polymorphisms may be associated with susceptibility to epithelial damage, or may be involved with repair processes and/or the processes associated with modelling of the airways in embryonic life. It is interesting to note that cells expressing ADAM33 are those whose maturation is directed by growth factors such as TGFβ. Indeed, ADAM33 is up-regulated during TGFβ-induced myofibroblast differentiation (Holloway and Holgate 2004).

Another genetic polymorphism associated with BHR in asthmatic children is in the Clara cell protein 16 (CC16) gene on 11q12–13. Polymorphisms have been associated with lower serum levels of CC16 and with asthma (Laing *et al.* 1998). The protein has sometimes been known as uteroglobulin or CC10, and it is expressed on bronchiolar epithelium. It has several immunomodulatory and antiinflammatory functions, and lower levels have been found in patients with chronic obstructive pulmonary disease.

Finally, on investigating gene–environment interactions there have been interesting associations between polymorphisms in the glutathione S-transferase M and T genes, *GSTM1* and *GSTT1*. The null genotype for these has been associated with greater reductions in lung function in asthmatic children, and supplementation of a child's diet with the antioxidants vitamin C and vitamin E may protect against an interaction between the null gene and ozone exposure (Romieu *et al.* 2004). While the null genotype may lead to reduced protection of the airway against postnatal oxidative stress, there is a suggestion that there may also be an impact on the developing lung, with an interaction between antenatal exposure to environmental tobacco smoke and wheezing in childhood (Kabesch *et al.* 2004).

Environment and airway structure

Maternal smoking severely compromises fetal health and has a clear impact on postnatal lung function. Significant differences in lung function are found in 4-week-old infants born to smoking mothers compared with non-smoking mothers (Dezateux *et al.* 1999). This in turn is associated with a significantly higher risk of wheezing illnesses in early life. It remains to be seen whether this antenatal compromise, in association with particular genetic polymorphisms, will be associated with more persistent

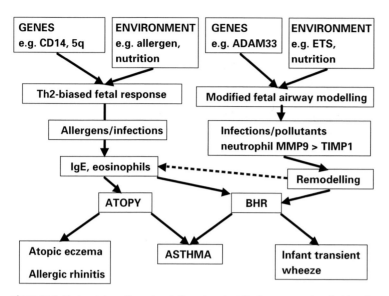

Figure 26.7 Factors interacting antenatally and postnatally that are associated with asthma, transient wheeze of infancy, or other allergic conditions.

ongoing wheezing illnesses such as asthma. Hitherto the effect of maternal smoking during pregnancy has only been associated with early rather than later wheezing, and with non-allergic rather than atopic asthma (Strachan and Cook 1998). However, maternal pregnancy smoking has been associated with modification of fetal immune responses, which might be extrapolated to an increased risk of allergy with higher cord-blood mononuclear cell release of IL13 on stimulation with allergens (Noakes *et al.* 2003). It remains to be established whether exposure to other pollutants such as ozone might also have an interactive effect, promoting susceptibility to asthma.

In a murine model, mild maternal vitamin A deficiency has been associated with reduced expression of lung surfactant and delayed maturation of lung function (Chailley-Heu *et al.* 1999). A host of other dietary factors have been associated with an increased risk either of allergy or of asthma. These include the antioxidants, selenium, vitamin E, sodium and lipids (Fogarty and Britton 2000, Devereux *et al.* 2002, Calder 2003).

There has been an interest in the association between obesity and asthma, with a number of stud-

ies reporting a strong relationship between body mass index and asthma risk in children and adults (Schachter *et al.* 2003, Tantisira *et al.* 2003). One study has shown improved asthma control following weight reduction in obese asthmatic patients (Stenius-Aarniala *et al.* 2000). However, there is also a possibility that the relationship has its origins in fetal life. A study has shown that smaller size at birth, even within the normal range of birthweight, was associated with lower lung function represented by airway calibre at 6–13 weeks of age. At all levels of birthweight, higher early weight gain was also associated with reduced lung function (Lucas *et al.* 2004). This latter phenomenon may well represent catch-up growth as a consequence of late gestational faltering of growth. Rapid postnatal weight gain following lower birthweight may well translate into later obesity and explain the relationship between obesity and asthma.

Summary

There are two components of asthma, both of which are under genetic influence (Fig. 26.7). Some genetic polymorphisms increase the risk of allergic sensitisation in association with environmental factors such as concentration of allergen exposure and variations in nutrition of the mother during pregnancy and lactation. Postnatally, further exposure to allergens in the absence of any infection polarises immune responses towards an allergic phenotype, while in the presence of infection there is a reduced risk of subsequent allergic diseases such as eczema or rhinitis. There are additional gene–environment interactions that affect the airway modelling, which in association with allergy will lead to asthma. Thus a different set of genes, in association with environmental factors such as maternal nutrition and smoking during pregnancy, modifies the fetal airway. Postnatally infections and pollutants promote an inflammatory immune response associated with the neutrophil, which induces further abnormalities in airway structure and therefore bronchial hyper-responsiveness. This, together with atopy, leads to ongoing asthma. In the absence of atopy it is associated with transient infant wheeze.

REFERENCES

Aaby, P., Shaheen, S. O., Heyes, C. B. et al. (2000). Early BCG vaccination and reduction in atopy in Guinea-Bissau. Clin. Exp. Allergy, **30**, 644–50.

Alm, J. S., Schwartz, J., Lilja, G. et al. (1999). Atopy in children of families with an anthroposophic lifestyle. Lancet, **353**, 1485–8.

Anderson, H. R. (1989). Increase in hospital admissions for childhood asthma: trends in referral, severity and re-admissions from 1970–1985 in a health region of the United Kingdom. Thorax, **44**, 614–19.

Annus, T., Mongomery, S. M., Riikjärv, M. A. and Björksten, B. (2004). Atopic disorders among Estonian school children in relation to tuberculin reactivity and the age of the BCG vaccination. Allergy, **59**, 1068–73.

Austin, J. B., Kaur, B., Anderson, R. H. et al. (1999). Hay fever, eczema and wheeze: a national UK survey (International Study of Asthma and Allergies in Childhood, ISAAC). Arch. Dis. Child., **81**, 225–30.

Baldini, M. Lohman, I. C., Halonen, M. et al. (1999). A polymorphism on the 5′-flanking region of the CD-14 gene is associated with circulating soluble CD-14 levels and with total serum immunoglobulin-E. Am. J. Respir. Cell. Mol. Biol., **20**, 976–83.

Ball, T. M., Castro-Rodriguez, J. A., Griffiths, K. A. et al. (2000). Siblings, day care and the risk of asthma and wheeze during childhood. N. Engl. J. Med., **343**, 538–43.

Berg, R. D. (1996). The indigenous gastrointestinal microflora. Trends Microbiol., **4**, 430–5.

Björksten, B., Naaber, P., Sepp, E. and Mikelsaar, M. (1999). The intestinal microflora in allergic Estonian and Swedish two-year-old children. Clin. Exp. Allergy. **29**, 342–6.

Blobe, G. C., Schiemann, W. P. and Lodish, H. F. (2000). Role of transforming growth factor beta in human disease. N. Engl. J. Med., **342**, 1350–8.

Bottcher, M F., Hmani-Aifa, M., Lindstrom, A. et al. (2004). A TLR4 polymorphism is associated with asthma and reduced lipo-poly-saccharide-induced IL20 (p70) responses in Swedish children. J. Allergy Clin. Immunol., **114**, 561–7.

British Thoracic Society. (2003). Scottish Intercollegiate Guidelines Network. British guideline on the management of asthma. Thorax, **58** (suppl.), i1–94.

Burr, M. L., Butland, B. K., King, S. and Vaughan-Williams, E. (1989). Changes in asthma prevalence: two surveys 15 years apart. Arch. Dis. Child., **64**, 1452–6.

Butland, B. K., Strachan, D. P. and Anderson, H. R. (1999). Fresh fruit intake and asthma symptoms in young British adults: confounding or effect modification by smoking. Eur. Respir. J., **13**, 744–50.

Calder, P. C. (2003). Polyunsaturated fatty acids and cytokine profiles: a clue to the changing prevalence of atopy. Clin. Exp. Allergy.,**33**, 412–15.

Casas, R. and Björksten, B. (2001). Detection of Fel d 1-immunoglobulin immune complexes of cord blood and sera from allergic and non-allergic mothers. Pediatr. Allergy Immunol., **12**, 59–64.

Chailley-Heu, B., Chelly, N., Lelievre-Pegorier, M. et al. (1999). Mild vitamin A deficiency delays fetal lung maturation in the rat. Am. J. Respir. Cell. Mol. Biol., **21**, 89–96.

Chavanas, S., Bodener, C., Rochat, A. et al. (2000). Mutations in SPINK5, encoding a serine protease inhibitor, cause Netherton syndrome. Nat. Genet., **25**, 141–2.

Clerici, M., Sison, A. V., Berzofsky, J. A. et al. (1993). Cellular immune factors associated with mother to infant transmission of HIV. AIDS, **7**, 1427–33.

Covar, R. A., Spahn, J. D., Murphy, J. R. et al. (2004). Progression of asthma measured by lung function in the childhood asthma management program. Am. J. Respir. Crit. Care Med. **170**, 234–41.

Cullinan, P., MacNeill, S. J., Harris, J. M. et al. (2004). Early allergen exposure, skin prick responses, and atopic wheeze at age 5 in English children: a cohort study. *Thorax*, **59**, 855–61

Cundall, M., Sun, Y., Miranda, C. *et al.* (2003). Neutrophil-derived matrix metallo-proteinase-9 is increased in severe asthma and poorly inhibited by glucocorticoids. *J. Allergy Clin. Immunol.*, **112**, 1064–71.

Custovic, A. and Simpson, A. (2004). Environmental allergen exposure, sensitisation and asthma: from whole populations to individuals with risk. *Thorax*, **59**, 825–7.

Daffos, F., Forestier, F., Graneot-Keros, L. *et al.* (1984). Prenatal diagnosis of congenital rubella. *Lancet*, **2**, 1–3.

D'Alauro, F., Lee, R. V., Pao-in, K. and Khairallah, M. (1985). Intestinal parasites and pregnancy. *Obstet. Gynecol.*, **66**, 639–43

D'Amato, M., Vitiani, L. R., Petrelli, G. *et al.* (1998). Association of persistent bronchial hyperresponsiveness with beta2-adrenoceptor (ADRB2) haplotypes: a population study. *Am. J. Respir. Crit. Care. Med.* **158**, 1968–73.

Davies, D. E., Wicks, J., Powell, R. M. *et al.* (2003). Airway remodeling in asthma: new insights. *J. Allergy Clin. Immunol.*, **111**, 215–25.

Des Roches, A., Paradis, L., Menardo, J. L. *et al.* (1997). Immunotherapy with a standardized *Dermatophagoides pteronyssinus* extract. VI. Specific immunotherapy prevents the onset of new sensitizations in children. *J. Allergy Clin. Immunol.* **99**, 450–3.

Devereux, G., Barker, R. N. and Seaton, A. (2002). Antenatal determinants of neonatal immune responses to allergens. *Clin. Exp. Allergy*, **32**, 43–50.

Dezateux, C., Stocks, J., Dundas, I. *et al.* (1999). Impaired airway function and wheezing in infancy: the influence of maternal smoking and a genetic pre-disposition to asthma. *Am. J. Respir. Crit. Care Med.*, **159**, 403–10.

Duffy, D. L., Martin, N. G., Battistutta, D. *et al.* (1990). Genetics of asthma and hay fever in Australian twins. *Am. Rev. Respir. Dis.*, **142**, 1351–8.

Dunstan, J. A., Mori, T. A., Barden, A. *et al.* (2003a). Maternal fish oil supplementation in pregnancy reduces interleukin-13 levels in cord blood of infants at high risk of atopy. *Clin. Exp. Allergy*, **33**, 442–8.

(2003b). Fish oil supplementation in pregnancy modifies neonatal allergen-specific immune responses and clinical outcomes in infants at high risk of atopy: a randomized, controlled trial. *J. Allergy Clin. Immunol.*, **112**, 1178–84.

Dunstan, J. A., Roper, J., Mitoulas, L. *et al.* (2004). The effect of supplementation with fish oil during pregnancy on breast milk immunoglobulin A, soluble CD14 cytokine levels and fatty acid composition. *Clin. Exp. Allergy*, **34**, 1237–42.

Durham, S. R., Walker, S. M., Varga, E. M. *et al.* (1999). Long term clinical efficacy of grass pollen immunotherapy. *N. Engl. J. Med.*, **341**, 468–75.

Farooqi, I. S. and Hopkin, J. M. (1998). Early childhood infection and atopic disorder. *Thorax*, **53**, 927–32.

Feldman, D., Glorieux, F. and Wesley Pike, J. eds. (1997). *Vitamin D*. London: Academic Press.

Fergusson, D. M., Horwood, L. J. and Shannon, F. T., (1990). Early solid feeding and recurrent childhood eczema: a 10 year longitudinal study. *Pediatrics*, **86**, 541–6.

Fickenscher, H., Hör, S., Küpers, H. *et al.* (2002). The interleukin-10 family of cytokines. *Trends Immunol.*, **23**, 89–96.

Fogarty, A. and Britton, J. (2000). The role of diet in the aetiology of asthma. *Clin. Exp. Allergy*, **30**, 615–27.

Folkerts, G., Walzl, G. and Openshaw, P. J. M., (2000). Do childhood infections 'teach' the immune system not to be allergic? *Immunol. Today*, **21**, 118–20.

Gao, P. S., Mao, X. Q., Baldini, M. *et al.* (1999). Serum in total IgE levels and CD-14 on chromosome 5q31. *Clin. Genet.*, **56**, 164–5.

Gatherer, D., Ten Dijke, P., Baird, D. T. and Akhurst, R. J. (1990). Expression of TGF-beta isoforms during the first trimester human embryogenesis. *Development*, **110**, 445–60.

Gern, J. E., Reardon, C. L., Hoffjan, S. *et al.* (2004). Effects of dog ownership and genotype on immune development and atopy in infancy. *J. Allergy Clin. Immunol.*, **113**, 307–14.

Gibson, G. R. and Roberfroid, M. B., (1995). Dietary modulation of the human colonic microbiota: introducing the concept of prebiotics. *J. Nutr.*, **125**, 1401–12.

Gill, T. J., Repetti, C. F., Metaly, L. A. *et al.* (1983). Transplacental immunisation of the human fetus to tetanus by immunisation of the mother. *J. Clin. Invest.*, **72**, 987–96.

Gitlin, D., Kumate, J., Morales, C. *et al.* (1972). The turnover of amniotic fluid protein in the human conceptus. *Am. J. Obstet. Gynecol.*, **113**, 632–45.

Glovsky, M. M., Ghekiere, L. and Rejzek, E. (1991). Effect of maternal immunotherapy on immediate skin test reactivity, specific Rye-1 IgG and IgE antibody and total IgE of the children. *Ann. Allergy*, **67**, 21–4.

Godfrey, K. M., Barker, D. J. P. and Osmond, C., (1994). Disproportionate fetal growth and raised IgE concentration in adult life. *Clin. Exp. Allergy*, **24**, 641–8.

Goetghebuer, T., Isles, K., Moore, C. *et al.* (2004). Genetic pre-disposition to wheeze following respiratory syncitial virus bronchiolitis. *Clin. Exp. Allergy*, **34**, 801–3.

Gregory, A., Doull, I., Pearce, N. *et al.* (1999). The relationship between anthropometric measurements at birth: asthma and atopy in childhood. *Clin. Exp. Allergy*, **29**, 330–3.

Grüber, C., Illi, S., Lau, S. *et al.* (2003). Transient suppression of atopy in early childhood is associated with high vaccination coverage. *Pediatrics*, **111**, 282–8.

Hardman, M. J., Moore, L., Byrne, C. and Ferguson, M. W. (1999). Barrier formation in the human fetus is patterned. *J. Invest. Dermatol.*, **113**, 1106–13.

Hayward, A. R. (1998). Ontogeny of the immune system. In *The Cambridge Encyclopedia of Growth and Development* (ed. S. J. Ulijaszek, F. E. Johnston and M. A. Preece). Cambridge: Cambridge University Press, pp. 166–9.

Hess, J. and de Jongste, J. C. (2004). Epidemiological aspects of paediatric asthma. *Clin. Exp. Allergy*, **34**, 680–5.

Holgate, S. T. (1998). Asthma and allergy: disorders of civilization? *Q. J. Med.*, **91**, 171–84.

Holgate, S.T., Puddicombe, S. M., Mullings, R. E. *et al.* (2004). New insights into asthma pathogenesis. *Allergy. Clin. Immunol. Int.*, **16**, 196–201.

Holloway, J. W. and Holgate, S. T. (2004). Genetics. (Prevention of allergy and allergic asthma, ed. S. G. O. Johansson and T. Haahtela. World Allergy Organization Project Report and Guidelines.) *Chem. Immunol. Allergy*, **84**, 1–35.

Holloway, J. A, Warner, J. O., Vance, G. H. S. *et al.* (2000). Detection of house-dust-mite allergen in amniotic fluid and umbilical-cord blood. *Lancet*, **356**, 1900–2.

Holt, P., Naspitz, C. and Warner, J. O. (2004). Early immunological influences. (Prevention of allergy and allergic asthma, ed. S. G. O. Johansson and T. Haahtela. World Allergy Organization Project Report and Guidelines.) *Chem. Immunol. Allergy*, **84**, 102–27.

Holt, P. G., O'Keeffe, P., Holt, B. J. *et al.* (1995). T-cell 'priming' against environmental allergens in human neonates: sequential deletion of food antigen specificities during infancy with concomitant expansion of responses to ubiquitous inhalant allergens. *Pediatr. Allergy Immunol.*, **6**, 85–90.

Jenmalm, M. C. and Björksten, B., (2000). Cord blood levels of immunoglobulin G subclass antibodies to food and inhalant allergens in relation to maternal atopy and the development of atopic disease during the first 8 years of life. *Clin. Exp. Allergy*, **30**, 34–40.

Jones, A. C., Miles, E A., Warner, J. O. *et al.* (1996). Fetal peripheral blood mononuclear cell proliferative responses to mytogenic and allergenic stimuli during gestation. *Pediatr. Allergy and Immunol.*, **7**, 109–16.

Jones, C. A., Kilburn, S., Warner, J. A. and Warner, J. O. (1998a). Intrauterine environment and fetal allergic sensitisation. *Clin. Exp. Allergy*, **28**, 655–9.

Jones, C. A., Warner, J. A. and Warner, J. O. (1998b). Fetal swallowing of IgE. *Lancet*, **351**, 1859.

Jones, C. A., Holloway, J. A. and Warner, J. O. (2000). Does atopic disease start in foetal life? *Allergy*, **55**, 2–10.

Jones, C. A., Vance, G. H. S., Power, L. L. *et al.* (2001). Costimulatory molecules in the developing human gastrointestinal tract: a pathway for fetal allergen priming. *J. Allergy Clin. Immunol.*, **108**, 235–41.

Jones, C. A. Holloway, J. A. and Warner, J. O. (2002a). Phenotype of fetal monocytes and B lymphocytes during the third trimester of pregnancy. *J. Reprod. Immunol.*, **56**, 45–60.

Jones, C. A., Holloway, J. A., Popplewell, E. J. *et al.* (2002b). Reduced soluble CD14 levels in amniotic fluid and breast milk are associated with subsequent development of atopy, eczema, or both. *J. Allergy Clin. Immunol.*, **109**, 858–66.

Jongepier, H., Boezen, H. M., Dijkstra, A. *et al.* (2004). Polymorphisms of the *ADAM33* gene are associated with accelerated lung function decline in asthma. *Clin. Exp. Allergy*, **34**, 757–60.

Kabesch, M., Hoefler, C., Car, D. *et al.* (2004). Glutathione-S transferase deficiency and passive smoking increase childhood asthma. *Thorax*, **59**, 569–73.

Kalliomaki, M., Salminen, S. and Arvilommi, H. (2001). Probiotics in primary prevention of atopic disease: a randomised placebo controlled trial. *Lancet*, **357**, 1076–9.

Karjalainen, E. M., Laitinen, A., Sue-Chu, M. *et al.* (2000). Evidence of airway inflammation and remodeling in ski athletes with and without bronchial hyper-responsiveness to methacholine. *Am. J. Respir. Crit. Care Med.*, **161**, 2086–91.

Karmaus, W., Arshad, H. and Mattes, J. (2001). Does the sibling effect have its origin *in utero*? Investigating birth order, cord blood immunoglobulin E concentration and allergic sensitization at age 4 years. *Am. J. Epidemiol.*, **154**, 909–15.

Kaur, B., Anderson, H. R., Austin, J. *et al.* (1998). Prevalence of asthma symptoms, diagnosis, and treatment in 12–14 year old children across Great Britain. (international study of asthma and allergies in childhood, ISAAC UK). *BMJ*, **316**, 118–24.

Kline, J. N., Waldschmidt, T. J., Businga, T. R. *et al.* (1998). Modulation of airway inflammation by CpG: oligodeoxynucleotides in a murine model of asthma. *J. Immunol.*, **160**, 2555–9.

Komatsu, N., Takata, M., Otsuki, N. *et al.* (2002). Elevated stratum corneum hydrolytic activity in Netherton syndrome suggests an inhibitory regulation of desquamation by SPINK5-derived peptides. *J. Invest. Dermatol.*, **118**, 436–43.

Kondo, N., Kobayashi, Y., Shinoda, S. *et al.* (1992). Cord blood lymphocyte responses to food antigens for the prediction of allergic disease. *Arch. Dis. Child.*, **67**, 1003–7.

Kruse, S., Kuehr, J., Moseler, M. *et al.* (2003). Polymorphisms in the IL18 gene are associated with specific sensitisation to common allergens and allergic rhinitis. *J. Allergy Clin. Immunol.* 111, 117–22.

Kull, I., Almqvist, C., Lilja, G. *et al.* (2004). Breast feeding reduces the risk of asthma during the first four years of life. *J. Allergy Clin. Immunol.*, 114, 755–60.

Laing, I. A., Goldblatt, J., Eber, E. *et al.* (1998). A polymorphism of the CC16 gene is associated with an increased risk of asthma. *J. Med. Genet.*, 35, 463–7.

Legg, J. P., Hussain, I. R., Warner, J. A. *et al.* (2003). Type 1 and type 2 cytokine imbalance in acute respiratory syncitial virus bronchioles. *Am. J. Respir. Crit. Care. Med.*, 168, 633–8.

Liu, X., Beaty, T. H., Deindl, P. *et al.* (2003). Associations between total IgE levels and six potentially functional variants within the genes IL-4, IL-13 and IL-4RA in German children: the German Multicentre Atopy Study. *J. Allergy Clin. Immunol.*, 112, 382–8.

Lowe, L. A., Simpson, A., Woodcock, A. *et al.* (2005). Wheeze phenotypes and lung function in preschool children. *Am. J. Respir. Crit. Care Med.*, 171, 231–7.

Lucas, J. S., Inskip, H. M., Godfrey, K. M. *et al.* (2004). Small size at birth and greater postnatal weight gain: relationships to diminished infant lung function. *Am. J. Respir. Crit. Care. Med.*, 170, 534–40.

Malhotra, I., Ouma, J., Wamachi, A. *et al.* (1997). In utero exposure to helminth and microbial antigens generates cytokine responses similar to that observed in adults. *J. Clin. Invest.*, 99, 1759–66.

Marguet, C., Jouen-Boedes, F., Dean, T. P. and Warner, J. O. (1999). Bronchoalveolar cell profiles in children with asthma, infantile wheeze, chronic cough or cystic fibrosis. *Am. J. Respir. Crit. Care Med.*, 159, 1533–40.

Martinez, F. D. (2003). Towards asthma prevention: does all that really matters happen before we learn to read? *N. Engl. J. Med.*, 349, 1473–5.

Maurer, D., Ebner, C., Reininger, B. *et al.* (1995). The high affinity IgE receptor (Fc epsilon R1) mediates IgE-dependent allergen presentation. *J. Immunol.*, 154, 6285–90.

McKeever, T. M., Lewis, S. A., Smith, C. and Hubbard, R. (2002). The importance of prenatal exposures and the development of allergic disease. *Am. J. Respir. Crit. Care. Med.*, 166, 827–32.

Möller, C., Dreborg, S., Ferdousi, H. A. *et al.* (2002). Pollen immunotherapy reduces the development of asthma in children with seasonal rhino-conjunctivitis (the PAT Study). *J. Allergy Clin. Immunol.*, 109, 251–6.

Morgan, J., Williams, P., Norris, F. *et al.* (2004). Eczema and early solid feeding in pre-term infants. *Arch. Dis. Child.*, 89, 309–14.

Naot, Y., Desmonts, G. and Remington, J. S. (1981). IgM enzyme linked immunosorbent assay test for the diagnosis of congenital toxoplasma infection. *J. Pediatr.*, 98, 32–6.

Newson, R. B., Shaheen, S. O., Henderson, J. *et al.* (2004). Umbilical cord and maternal blood red cell fatty acids and early childhood wheezing and eczema. *J. Allergy Clin. Immunol.*, 114, 531–7.

Ninan, T., Russell, G., Devenney, A. *et al.* (2000). Changes in the prevalence of respiratory symptoms and atopy in Aberdeen school children. *Europ. Respir. J.*, 16 (Suppl. 31), 342s.

Noakes, P. S., Holt, P. G. and Prescott, S. L. (2003). Maternal smoking in pregnancy alters neonatal cytokine responses. *Allergy*, 58, 1053–8.

Oberle, D., von Mutius, E. and von Kries, R., (2003). Childhood asthma and continuous exposure to cats since the first year of life with cats allowed in the child's bedroom. *Allergy*, 58, 1033–6.

Oryszczyn, M. P., Annesi-Maesano, I., Campagno, D. *et al.* (1999). Head circumference at birth and maternal factors related to cord blood total IgE. *Clin. Exp. Allergy*, 29, 334–41.

Palmer, L. J., Rye, P. J., Gibson, N. A. *et al.* (2001). Airway responsiveness in early infancy predicts asthma, lung function, and respiratory symptoms by school age. *Am. J. Respir. Crit. Care. Med.*, 163, 37–42.

Peat, J. K., Allen, J. and Oddy, W. (1999). Beyond breast-feeding. *J. Allergy Clin. Immunol.* 104, 526–9.

Peat, J. K., Mihrshahi, S., Kemp, A. S. *et al.* (2004). Three-year outcomes of dietary fatty-acid modification and house dust mite reduction in the childhood asthma prevention study. *J. Allergy Clin. Immunol.*, 114, 807–13.

Piccinni, M. P., Beloni, L., Giannarini L. *et al.* (1996). Abnormal production of T-helper 2 cytokines, interleukin 4 and interleukin 5 by T-cells from newborns with atopic parents. *Eur. J. Immunol.*, 26, 2293–8.

Piccinni, M. P., Beloni, L., Livi, C. *et al.* (1998). Defective production of both leukemia inhibitory factor and type 2 T-helper cytokines by decidual T-cells in unexplained recurrent abortions. *Nat. Med.*, 4, 1020–4.

Pohunek, P., Warner, J. O., Turzikova, J. Kudrmann, J. and Roche, W. R. (2005). Markers of eosinophilic inflammation and tissue re-modelling in children before clinically diagnosed bronchial asthma. *Pediatr. Allergy Immunol.*, 16, 43–51.

Prescott, S. L., Macaubas, C., Holt, B. T. *et al.* (1998). Transplacental priming of the human immune system to environmental allergens: universal skewing of initial T cell responses towards Th2 cytokine profile. *J. Immunol.*, 160, 4730–7.

Prescott, S. L., Macaubas, C., Smallacombe, T. *et al.* (1999). Development of allergen-specific T-cell memory in atopic and normal children. *Lancet*, **353**, 196–200.

Radon, K., Windsletter, D. and Eckart, J. (2004). Farming exposure in childhood, exposure to markers of infection and the development of atopy in rural subjects. *Clin. Exp. Allergy*, **34**, 1178–83.

Raghupathy, R. (1997). Th1 type immunity is incompatible with successful pregnancy. *Immunol. Today*, **18**, 478–82.

Resh, A., Schlipkotter, U., Crispin, A. *et al.* (2004). Atopic disease and its determinants: a focus on the potential role of childhood infection. *Clin. Exp. Allergy*, **34**, 1184–91.

Romagnani, S. (1991). Human Th1 and Th2 sub-sets: doubt no more. *Immunol. Today*, **12**, 256–7.

(2004). Immunologic influences on allergy and TH1/TH2 balance. *J. Allergy Clin. Immunol.*, **113**, 395–400.

Romieu, I., Sienra-Monge, J. J., Ramirez-Aguilar, M. *et al.* (2004). Genetic polymorphism of GSTM 1 and antioxidant supplementation influence lung function in relation to ozone exposure in asthmatic children in Mexico City. *Thorax*, **59**, 8–10.

Ross, S., Abdalla, M., Godden, D. J. *et al.* (1995). Outcome of wheeze in childhood: the influence of atopy. *Eur. Respir. J.*, **8**, 2081–7.

Rothoeft, T., Gronschorek, A., Bartz, H. *et al.* (2003). Antigen dose, type of antigen presenting cell and time of differentiation contribute to the T-alpha-1/T-alpha-2 polarization of naive T-cells. *Immunology*, **110**, 1–10.

Ruiz, R. G. G., Kemeny, D. M. and Price, J. F. (1992). Higher risk of infantile atopic dermatitis from maternal atopy rather than paternal atopy. *Clin. Exp. Allergy*, **22**, 762–66.

Schachter, L. M., Peat, J. K. and Salome, C. M. (2003). Asthma and atopy in overweight children. *Thorax*. **58**, 1031–5.

Schittny, J. C., Miserocchi, G. and Sparrow, M. P. (2000). Spontaneous peristaltic airway contractions propel lung liquid through the bronchial tree of intact and fetal lung explants. *Am. J. Respir. Cell. Mol. Biol.*, **23**, 11–18.

Schoetzau, A., Filipiak-Pittroff, B., Franke, K. *et al.* (2002). Effect of exclusive breast-feeding and early solid food avoidance on the incidence of atopic dermatitis in high-risk infants at 1 year of age. *Pediatr. Allergy Immunol.*, **13**, 234–42.

Sears, M. R., Greene, J. M., Willan, A. R. *et al.* (2003). Longitudinal, population based, cohort study of childhood asthma followed to adulthood. *N. Engl. J. Med.*, **349**, 1414–22.

Sengler, C., Haider, A., Sommerfield, C. *et al.* (2003). Evaluation of the CD-14 C-159 T polymorphism in the German multi-center allergy study cohort. *Clin. Exp. Allergy*, **33**, 166–9.

Shaheen, S. O., Aaby, P., Hall, A. J. *et al.* (1996). Measles and atopy in Guinea-Bissau. *Lancet*, **347**, 1792–6.

Shaheen, S. O., Newson, R. B., Henderson, A. J. *et al.* (2004). Umbilical cord trace elements and minerals and risk of early childhood wheezing and eczema. *Eur. Respir. J.*, **24**, 292–7.

Shirakawa, T., Enomoto, T., Shimazu, S. and Hopkin, J. M. (1997). Inverse association between tuberculin responses and atopic disorder. *Science*, **275**, 77–9.

Sigurs, N., Bjarnason, R., Sigurbergsson, F. and Kjellman, B. (2000). Respiratory syncytial virus bronchiolitis in infancy is an important risk factor for asthma and allergy at age 7. *Am. J. Respir. Crit. Care Med.*, **161**, 1501–7.

Silverman, E. S., Baron, R. M., Palmer, L. J. *et al.* (2002). Constitutive and cytokine-induced expression of the ETS transcription factor ESE-3 in the lung. *Am. J. Respir. Cell. Mol. Biol.*, **27**, 697–704.

Stenius-Aarniala, B., Poussa, T., Kvarnström, J. *et al.* (2000). Immediate and long term effects of weight reduction in obese people with asthma: randomised controlled study. *BMJ*, **320**, 827–32.

Stewart, G. A. and Thompson, P. J. (1996). The biochemistry of common aeroallergens. *Clin. Exp. Allergy*, **26**, 1020–44.

Strachan, D. P. (1989). Hay fever, hygiene and household size. *BMJ*, **299**, 1259–60.

(2000). Family size, infection and atopy: the first decade of the 'hygiene hypothesis'. *Thorax*, **55** (Suppl.1), S2–10.

Strachan, D. P. and Cook, D. G. (1998). Parental smoking and childhood asthma: longitudinal and case–control studies. *Thorax*, **53**, 204–12.

Tang, M. L. K., Kemp, A. S., Thorburn, J. and Hill, D. J. (1992). Reduced interferon-gamma secretion in neonates and subsequent atopy. *Lancet*, **344**, 983–5.

Tantisira, K. G., Litonjua, A. A., Weiss, S. T. *et al.* (2003). Association of body mass with pulmonary function in the Childhood Asthma Management Programme (CAMP). *Thorax*, **58**, 1036–41.

Tattersfield, A. E., Knox, A. J., Britton, J. R. *et al.* (2002). Asthma. *Lancet*, **360**, 1313–22.

Thornton, C. A., Holloway, J. A., Popplewell, E. J. *et al.* (2003). Fetal exposure to intact immunoglobulin E occurs via the gastrointestinal tract. *Clin. Exp. Allergy*, **33**, 306–11.

Turner, S. W., Palmer, L. J., Rye, P. J. *et al.* (2004). The relationship between infant airway function, childhood airway responsiveness, and asthma. *Am. J. Respir. Crit. Care Med.*, **169**, 921–7.

Van Asperen, P. P. and Mukhi, A. (1994). Role of atopy in the natural history of wheeze and bronchial hyper-responsiveness in children. *Pediatr. Allergy. Immunol.*, **5**, 178–83.

Vance, G. H. S., Grimshaw, K. E. C., Briggs, R. *et al.* (2004). Serum ovalbumin-specific immunoglobulin G responses during pregnancy reflect maternal intake of dietary egg and relate to the development of allergy in early infancy. *Clin. Exp. Allergy*, **34**, 1855–61.

Van Duren-Schmidt, K., Pichler, J., Ebner, C. *et al.* (1997). Prenatal contact with inhalant allergens. *Pediatr. Res.*, **41**, 128–31.

Van Eerdewegh, P., Little, R. D., Dupuis, J. *et al.* (2002). Association of the ADAM33 gene with asthma and bronchial hyperresponsiveness. *Nature*, **418**, 426–30.

Van Gool, C. J. A. W., Thijs, C., Dagnelie, P. C. *et al.* (2004). Determinants of neonatal IgE level: parity, maternal age, birth season and perinatal essential fatty acid status in infants of atopic mothers. *Allergy*, **59**, 961–8.

von Berg, A., Koletzko, S., Grübl, A. *et al.* (2003). The effect of hydrolyzed cow's milk formula for allergy prevention in the first year of life: the German Infant Nutritional Intervention Study, a randomized double-blind trial. *J. Allergy Clin. Immunol.*, **111**, 533–40.

Von Ehrenstein, O. S., Von Mutius, P., Illi, S. *et al.* (2000). Reduced risk of hay fever and asthma among children of farmers. *Clin. Exp. Allergy*, **30**, 187–93.

Walley, A J., Chavanas, S., Moffatt, M. F. *et al.* (2001). Gene polymorphism in netherton and common atopic disease. *Nat. Genet.*, **29**, 175–8.

Warner, J. A., Miles, E. A., Jones, A. C. *et al.* (1994). Is deficiency of interferon gamma production by allergen triggered cord blood cells predictor of atopic eczema? *Clin. Exp. Allergy*, **24**, 423–30.

Warner, J. A., Jones, C. A., Jones, A. C. *et al.* (1997) Immune responses during pregnancy and the development of allergic disease. *Pediatr. Allergy Immunol.*, **8** (Suppl. 10), 5–10.

Watts, A. M., Stanley, J. R., Shearer, M. H. *et al.* (1999). Fetal immunization of baboons induces a fetal specific antibody response. *Nat. Med.*, **5**, 427–30.

Wegmann, T. G., Lin, H., Guilbert, L. and Mosmann, T. R. (1993). Bi-directional cytokine interactions in the maternal–fetal relationship: is successful pregnancy a Th2 phenomenon. *Imunol. Today*, **14**, 353–6.

Whitsett, J. A. and Wert, S. E. (1998). Molecular determinants of lung development. In *Kendig's Disorders of the Respiratory Tract in Children*, 6th Edn. (ed. V. Chernick and T. F. Boat) Philadelphia, PA: Saunders, pp. 1–19.

Wijga, A H., Smit, H. A., Kerkhof, M. *et al.* (2003). Association of consumption of products containing milk fat with reduced asthma risk in pre-school children: the PIAMA birth cohort study. *Thorax*, **58**, 567–72.

Williams, L. K., Peterson, E. L., Ownby, D. R. and Johnson, C. C. (2004). The relationship between early fever and allergic sensitisation at 6–7 years. *J. Allergy Clin. Immunol.*, **113**, 291–6.

Williams, T. J., Jones, C. A., Miles, E. A. *et al.* (2000). Fetal and neonatal IL-13 production during pregnancy and at birth and subsequent development of atopic symptoms. *J. Allergy Clin. Immunol.*, **105**, 951–9.

Wjst, M. (2004). The triple T allergy hypothesis. *Clin. Dev. Immunol.*, **11**, 175–80.

Wright, A. L., Holberg, C. J., Taussig, L. M. and Martinez, F. D. (2001). Factors influencing the relation of infant feeding to asthma and recurrent wheeze in childhood. *Thorax* **56**, 192–7.

Yaqoob, P. (2003). Fatty acids as gatekeepers of immune cell regulation. *Trends. Immunol.*, **24**, 639–45.

Yoshinaka, T., Nishii, K., Yamada, K. *et al.* (2002). Identification and characterization of novel mouse and human ADAM33s with potential metalloprotease activity. *Gene*, **282**, 227–36.

Zamel, N., Clean, P. A., Sandell, P. R. *et al.* (1996). Asthma on Tristan da Cunha: looking for the genetic link. The University of Toronto Genetics of Asthma Research Group. *Am. J. Respir.*, **153**, 1902–6.

Zutavern, A., Von Mutius, E., Harris, J. *et al.* (2004). The introduction of solids in relation to asthma and eczema. *Arch. Dis. Child.*, **89**, 303–8.

27

The developmental environment: influences on subsequent cognitive function and behaviour

Jason Landon, Michael Davison and Bernhard H. Breier

University of Auckland

Introduction

The concept of the developmental origins of adult disease was initially based on epidemiological observations relating evidence of a constrained fetal environment to a greater risk of metabolic and cardiovascular disorders in adult life. It was later recognised that those at greatest risk also have an increased propensity to developing obesity in childhood and during adult life (Barker and Osmond 1988, Hales and Barker 1992, Gluckman and Hanson 2004). The interest in the later effects of early environmental events has since been generalised to include possible prenatal effects on offspring behaviour and cognition. In this chapter, we review the existing human and animal literature on the early-life influences on offspring cognitive function and behaviour.

Human studies

Recently, interest has grown in the possibility of a relation between birthweight and subsequent cognitive function. Early research focused on comparisons between individuals of low birthweight (LBW) or small for gestational age (SGA) and those with normal birthweights (e.g., Ounsted et al. 1983, Pharoah et al. 1994, Strauss 2000). These studies showed that LBW and SGA individuals had an increased incidence of neurological deficits and/or poorer

cognitive skills throughout childhood. Subsequent research has examined whether this relationship persists across the normal range of birthweights (e.g. Sorenson et al. 1997, Matte et al. 2001, Richards et al. 2001, 2002, Shenkin et al. 2001, Jefferis et al. 2002). The consensus from this research is that the relationship does hold across the range of normal birthweights, but that the effect is small. However, the postnatal environment has a comparatively very large influence on cognitive function. For example, social class explains much more of the variation in cognition than does birthweight. In a longitudinal study, Jefferis et al. (2002) showed that birthweight accounted for 0.5 to 1.5% of the variation in cognition, whereas social class accounted for 2.9 to 12.5%. This was found despite the common practice of using a relatively crude surrogate (in this case, father's occupation) as the measure of social class.

Studies in which multiple measures of cognitive function were obtained throughout the life span (Richards et al. 2001, 2002) have shown that the positive association between birthweight and cognition dissipates over time, and is no longer present at age 26. In contrast, height remained positively correlated with cognition at all ages. Richards et al. therefore concluded that birthweight and postnatal growth were independently associated with cognition. Converging evidence has been provided by several independent studies. Martyn et al. (1996) showed that impaired fetal growth was not associated with poorer

Developmental Origins of Health and Disease, ed. Peter Gluckman and Mark Hanson. Published by Cambridge University Press.
© P. D. Gluckman and M. A. Hanson 2006.

cognitive performance in adulthood. In another study, Gale *et al.* (2004) investigated the relation between brain growth (measured by head circumference) both pre- and postnatally and cognitive function at age 9. In contrast to the other studies, Gale *et al.* showed a clear association between postnatal head growth and IQ at age 9, but no relation between birthweight and cognitive function at that age. The authors acknowledged that the absence of the latter relation was probably due to the comparatively smaller size of their study. However, Gale *et al.* felt able to conclude that 'brain growth during infancy is more important than growth during fetal life in determining cognitive function'.

Several studies have shown links between LBW or nutritional inadequacy during gestation and a range of behavioural problems in later life (e.g. Breslau *et al.* 1988, Breslau 1995, Neugebauer *et al.* 1999). Other studies have suggested links between birthweights in the normal range and various psychological disorders in adult life, although any conclusions drawn on the basis of these studies are very tenuous. Nonetheless, size at birth has been shown to increase risk of later schizophrenia (Wahlbeck *et al.* 2001). Wahlbeck *et al.* showed that small infants (low birthweight, shortness at birth, *or* low placental weight) who are born to lean mothers and become thin in childhood are at increased risk of developing schizophrenia. Leanness during childhood was an independent additive risk factor to being small at birth. The study showed that the association was not due to shorter gestation, thus suggesting that a reduced rate of fetal growth was causal, possibly due to prenatal undernutrition. This notion is supported by evidence showing an almost threefold increase in the risk of schizophrenia spectrum disorders in individuals conceived during the Dutch famine of 1945 (Hoek *et al.* 1998). Another recent study (Brown *et al.* 2004) has shown a dramatic increase in the risk of schizophrenia following prenatal exposure to influenza. When influenza exposure was in the first trimester, there was a sevenfold increase in the risk of schizophrenia; this dropped to a threefold risk when a broader period ('early to mid pregnancy') was used.

It remains the case, however, that the results in this area of research are mixed (e.g. Mednick *et al.* 1988, Bagalkote *et al.* 2001).

Thompson *et al.* (2001) found that the odds ratios for depression among men, but not women, rose incrementally with decreasing birthweight. However, Gale and Martyn (2004) found that women whose birthweights were less than 3 kg had an increased risk of depression when compared with women whose birthweights were over 3.5 kg. They found no effect in the normal range with men, but that LBW (less than 2.5 kg) men were more likely to report a history of depression at age 26. These discrepant results highlight the problems in interpreting these studies. Attempts are frequently made to account for numerous potential confounding variables, but essentially the task is impossible. Moreover, in all cases, the reported effects are small, and in many they apparently do not persist through the life span.

The human data, although equivocal, lend support to the notion that prenatal nutrition may affect the behaviour and cognition of offspring. They highlight the importance of establishing the nature of these potential effects, and how postnatal events may convolve with them. Small effects of birthweight on childhood cognitive performance have been repeatedly shown in human epidemiological studies; however, the effect reduces with time, presumably in response to the overwhelming effects of the postnatal environment.

Animal studies

Animal models are an ideal means of examining closely the fundamental behavioural and biological principles involved. To a large extent both pre- and postnatal environmental events can be controlled in animals. Interpretation of human epidemiological data is always clouded by their inherent nature, in particular the lack of accurate accounts of (and adequate ways of measuring) pre- and postnatal environments, and by the use of crude surrogates for behavioural measures of fundamental importance.

Thus, when testing basic principles, animal studies offer many obvious advantages.

The majority of existing animal studies have focused on the variation of nutrition during gestation, usually protein malnutrition, or overall plane of nutrition. A number of animal studies have shown that undernutrition or malnutrition prior to birth results in reduced brain size and brain-cell numbers at birth. The prevailing view has been that there is a permanent change in neuronal number throughout life. It has since been shown that many of the more dramatic anatomical alterations are reversible, but also that some of the more subtle neuronal changes are less easily reversed (see Strupp and Levitsky 1995, Morgane *et al.* 2002). However, a fundamental question remains – what effects, if any, do these changes have on an animal's ability to adapt to its environment?

Several studies have attempted to address this question, utilising an array of methodologies. Procedures such as the Morris water maze have been used to examine spatial learning, and tests such as the elevated T- and plus-mazes have been used to measure anxiety. Some studies have examined social behaviours, and a few have used variations on operant approaches to analyse behaviour. Galler and her colleagues have reported a series of studies in which they have examined the behaviour of the offspring of protein-malnourished rat dams. This model remains the most extensively investigated in the literature. In addition to behavioural studies, Galler and colleagues have provided detailed accounts of the effects on brain development, in particular on hippocampal formation, of this nutritional variation (e.g. Morgane *et al.* 2002, Mokler *et al.* 2003). The effects observed in the hippocampus promoted investigations of spatial learning using the Morris water maze (Tonkiss *et al.* 1994), and of working memory using rewarded alternation tasks (Tonkiss and Galler 1990) as hippocampal lesions have long been associated with impaired performance in such spatial tasks. However, despite this known association, neither study found any effect of prenatal protein malnutrition. A subsequent study using the Morris water maze (Tonkiss *et al.* 1997) did show a very small deficit in spatial learning. Although significant, the observed effect was so small that its functional relevance must be questionable. In addition, the mothers in this study also had prenatal saline injections. Thus, the differences could plausibly have been due to the additional, though moderate, stress of handling and injections. In yet another study (Tonkiss and Galler 1990) they found no effect of prenatal protein malnutrition on 'working memory' performance in a rewarded alternation task using a T-maze.

An operant version of the rewarded alternation task did reveal some interesting differences in the performances of the two groups. The task consisted of an observing response phase in which one of two levers was randomly presented. Following a predetermined number of responses being emitted, the lever was retracted and 5, 10, 15 or 30 seconds later both levers were presented (choice phase). Responses to the lever not presented in the observing phase were rewarded. As task difficulty was increased by reducing the number of observing responses, performance of the prenatally malnourished rats became rather better than that of the controls. Given the hippocampal differences noted in this model, this result was in direct contrast to the research hypothesis that prenatal protein malnourishment might disrupt memory performance. The authors suggested that the animals may have undergone a 'release from proactive interference' (Tonkiss and Galler 1990). However, this was not obviously reconcilable with their T-maze results. This result has not yet been investigated empirically, despite the existence of a relatively sophisticated literature on proactive interference in memory tasks.

In another study using a relatively basic operant approach, Tonkiss *et al.* (1990) showed that prenatal protein malnutrition affected acquisition on a differential reinforcement of low rates of responding (DRL) schedule. Acquisition was measured by mean percentage efficiency (rewards/responses $\times$ 100). The procedure is relatively unusual, as animals must emit responses at a sufficiently low rate (that is, 'inhibit' responding) to earn food rewards. Hippocampal lesions have been shown to impair performance and acquisition in this task (e.g. Gray and McNaughton 1983). It is important to note that the differences were not evident early in testing, but mean efficiencies of offspring of malnourished and control dams began to diverge between the ninth and seventeenth days of training. The differences thereafter were consistent and durable. This result highlights the importance of temporally extended analyses of behaviour, as more subtle or slower-developing differences can be missed using brief methods such as the Morris water maze. Given the differences that emerged, it was surprising to note that there were no differences between the groups' abilities to time accurately. This highlights the fact that differences may well be evident only given very specific environmental conditions, and that test construction and data analysis must be sufficiently sophisticated and varied to detect meaningful differences.

Galler and colleagues also showed that prenatal protein malnutrition impaired learning the avoidance response on the elevated T-maze (Almeida et al. 1996a). The procedure involves repeated trials in which a rat is placed either on the open arm or in the enclosed arm of an elevated T-maze. 'Learned' fear is measured by the latency to exit the enclosed arm (avoidance), and 'innate' fear is measured by the latency to escape the open arm. Prenatally undernourished rats showed little or no learning of the avoidance response – latencies did not progressively increase across trials as they did for the control rats. In contrast, there were no between-group differences in escape latencies (the time taken to leave an elevated open arm). Elevated-T-maze performance is purported to measure anxiety, and the impaired learning of the escape response is suggestive of reduced anxiety. It remains that the failure to learn this avoidance task could more parsimoniously be interpreted as exactly that, a deficiency in learning. The aversive nature of the open elevated arms was shown by the similar escape latencies between the two groups. The behavioural differences caused by prenatal nutrition were specific to the learning of the avoidance response. In a second study, Almeida et al. (1996b) showed that prenatal protein malnutrition resulted in increased exploration of the open arms of an elevated plus-maze. Again, this result is suggestive of reduced anxiety, or perhaps increased impulsiveness or risk taking.

More complex behavioural patterns such as depression, anxiety and schizophrenia are inherently difficult to examine in animals, perhaps impossible without substantial anthropomorphism. Nonetheless, a recent paper has leant support to the notion that prenatal exposure to influenza induces marked behavioural changes in offspring. Shi et al. (2003) showed that respiratory infection of pregnant mice resulted in offspring exhibiting deficits in prepulse inhibition in the acoustic startle response and significant changes in open-field and social-interaction tests. The authors suggested that these alterations reflected 'hyperanxiety' in novel or stressful situations. Infected offspring also showed strikingly abnormal responses to psychomimetic and antipsychotic drugs, suggesting alterations in dopaminergic and glutamatergic systems consistent with recent theories of schizophrenia.

Other researchers have investigated the effects of stress during gestation on offspring behaviour. Prenatally stressed offspring do not differ from controls in the acquisition phase of a generic Morris water-maze task. However, they seem to spend more time searching for the platform in its previous location during a reversal task (Szuran et al. 1994, Hayashi et al. 1998). A further study (Weller et al. 1988) showed that both acute and repeated gestational stress affected performance in an operant discrimination task. As with the water-maze procedures, there were no differences in acquisition or discrimination. However, prenatally stressed rats again performed more poorly in the reversal phase. Taken together, these studies suggest that the behaviour of prenatally stressed rats might be less flexible in response to environmental changes – that is, they show a reduced ability to 'unlearn'. However, several factors limit any conclusions that can be made: first, subsequent reversals were not conducted, leaving it possible that the differences might have 'washed out' and thus been functionally irrelevant; second, and relatedly, Weller et al. arranged an extinction phase and found no between-group differences, adding support to the notion that these differences on initial reversal might have been transient.

Galler and colleagues have also shown decreased social behaviours (Almeida *et al.* 1996c), and increased time taken for rat pups to approach their nest bedding (Tonkiss *et al.* 1996), following prenatal protein malnutrition. A recent study in sheep has shown that ewe–lamb 'bonding' behaviours were affected by a 35% reduction in ewe nutritional intake during gestation (Dwyer *et al.* 2003). Specifically, ewes with reduced nutrition during gestation spent less time licking their lambs after delivery, and were rated as more aggressive towards their lambs. Lamb behaviours seemed unaffected, although lambs from undernourished ewes were slower to stand, and suckled less.

The importance of early environmental interactions with respect to the epigenomic state of certain genes, and the development of neuronal systems that regulate endocrine and behavioural responses to stress, has been clearly established by Meaney and his colleagues (e.g. Francis *et al.* 1999, Meaney 2001, Menard *et al.* 2004, Weaver *et al.* 2004). Meaney and colleagues have shown that variations in maternal care in the rat influence the development of behavioural and endocrine responses to stress in offspring. Increased pup licking and grooming, and arched-back nursing, permanently alters development of the hypothalamic–pituitary–adrenal (HPA) responses to stress such that offspring of dams exhibiting high levels of these behaviours, *and* pups cross-fostered onto these dams, are less fearful as adults and show decreased HPA responses to stress. In turn, the epigenetic basis of this has been identified (see Chapter 5) (Weaver *et al.* 2004).

Recent research has also examined the effects of earlylife stress on neurogenesis. King *et al.* (2004) examined the effects of prenatal protein malnutrition and acute postnatal stress on genesis of granule cells in the hippocampal fascia. Animals were tested on postnatal days 7 and 30. Independent effects of prenatal protein malnourishment were evident at each age. Fewer cells were generated at day 7, and more at day 30. Interestingly, only control rats showed a decrease in the number of generated

cells following acute stress. Coe *et al.* (2003), using rhesus monkeys, showed that prenatal stress, both in early and late pregnancy, reduced hippocampal volume and inhibited neurogenesis in the dentate gyrus. Moreover, there was an associated increase in pituitary–adrenal activity (higher cortisol levels after a dexamethasone suppression test), and lower levels of exploratory behaviour, indicating altered emotionality. Finally, using rats, Mirescu *et al.* (2004) showed that maternal deprivation affected the regulation of adult neurogenesis in the hippocampus. Specifically, reduced cell proliferation in the dentate gyrus was evident in adult rats that were maternally separated as pups. Consistent with King *et al.* (2004) there was no normal stress-induced suppression of cell proliferation and neurogenesis despite normal activation of the HPA axis. The authors concluded that 'early adverse experience inhibits structural plasticity via hypersensitivity to glucocorticoids and diminishes the ability of the hippocampus to stress in adulthood' (Mirescu *et al.* 2004).

These relatively recent developments highlight growing understanding of the ongoing effects of early-life experiences on the developing organism. They also highlight the need to better understand the complex and dynamic gene–environment interactions in early life, and indeed across generations (Oyama *et al.* 2001). This is an avenue of research that warrants much further attention in animal models of altered prenatal nutrition, and demands an integration of a wide range of existing research into a coherent approach.

The extant research suggests differences in the effects of a range of early-life events on subsequent behaviour. To date, the behavioural outcomes of a model of overall nutritional restriction (e.g. Woodall *et al.* 1996a, 1996b, Vickers *et al.* 2000, 2001) have not been investigated extensively. However, Vickers *et al.* (2003) showed the early development of hyperphagia, and a reduction in locomotor activity in an open-field test, using this model. The interpretation and generalisability of these results remain somewhat ambiguous, but they support the fundamental principle that behaviours (eating and locomotion) that are critical in the development of metabolic disorders can be affected by prenatal nutrition. Whether these results imply that animals that were nutritionally restricted during gestation will show a reduction in the amount of work they will do in order to gain a bout of running, and/or an increased preference for eating over running, is yet to be determined.

Conclusions and future directions

The evidence reviewed here suggests that various prenatal events do have effects on the behaviour and cognition of offspring. The data, however, are not strong: behavioural research in this and other biomedical areas has often taken the form of ad-hoc additions to more biological investigations. The primary consideration appears to be to minimise the time needed to undertake the behavioural investigation, or to utilise generic procedures to investigate poorly understood and very complex multifaceted behaviours such as mood or anxiety. Moreover, although many studies show differences, in general they have no obvious external validity. Lack of external validity is, of course, a common criticism of any laboratory investigations of behaviour; it is particularly relevant, however, in biomedical research. Perhaps more important is that studies of this type commonly investigate behaviour over a very small time-window. Thus differences that emerge more gradually through an animal's interaction with its environment are missed. Some such interactions may well attenuate behavioural differences that result from gestational differences; but other interactions may well amplify the results of gestational abnormalities. The latter, of course, are likely to be the processes that cause problems for humans. Thus our thesis is that these more gradual, developing, longer-term differences in behaviour are where more focus should now be placed. The nature of their development, and environmental and other factors that influence the course of their development and persistence, are an area that has been neglected – as have possible environmental manipulations that can ameliorate a developing behavioural

problem, perhaps through to old age. Indeed, the human epidemiological data have shown that differences are not evident at all points in development, so clearly organism–environment interactions are critical in the development and alleviation of behavioural problems. In a very real sense, once we have an effective model, we must be highly sensitive to the animal or human that does *not* show the expected deficit, and ask why this may be so.

Clearly, what is required is the full utilisation of a sophisticated science of behaviour integrated with the existing sophisticated science of biology. An equality of sophistication has not yet been achieved. The plausible alternative to current practice is the use of quantitative behaviour analysis. This has been suggested by many researchers, but to date no serious attempt has been made to integrate these sciences. It seems clear to us that both sciences would benefit hugely from a transfer of knowledge.

A theoretical framework for future investigations of the interplay between behaviour, physiology and neuroendocrinology already exists. However, procedures in current use do not lend themselves to long-term behavioural measurement. The integration of serious attempts to investigate behaviour and gradually introduce greater levels of external validity will be a substantial, and necessary, step in the development of this area of research. Well-established and validated procedures are available that provide an ideal means to investigate the effects in behaviour and cognition of prenatal nutritional variations (e.g. Davison and Baum 2000, Landon and Davison 2001). Other examples of precise quantitative procedures already available are: operant choice procedures, for which an effective quantification has been available for 35 years; signal-detection and conditional-discrimination procedures for the study of discrimination and memory, for which quantification has been available for even longer; and a series of procedures in behavioural economics.

We strongly recommend these procedures, for they will provide the necessary accuracy and replicability of measures essential for discovering how environmental factors during early life affect subsequent behaviour – and, equally, many other similar research questions. The general approach is flexible, and novel tests can be constructed to investigate how animals adapt to environmental change, or to constant conditions that vary in terms of the availability of food or other goods. It is quite possible that when confronted with some conditions, perhaps similar to those signalled by reduced nutrition during gestation, offspring will show quite different and perhaps locally more adaptive patterns of behaviour. The use of food as a reward for behaviour also provides the ideal scenario to quantify preferences for food types, and what animals will do to defend a certain food intake, or distribution of diet (see e.g. Hursh 1984, Davison and McCarthy 1988). We can also investigate how this changes throughout the life span and affects the development of metabolic disorders. Exercise, via running wheels or treadmills, can be investigated in isolation, as a leisure activity, and as an activity with a 'cost', and in the context of other behavioural alternatives that will result in food reward.

In conclusion, a substantial body of research, both human and animal, has suggested strongly that early-life experiences can have significant later effects on the behavioural and cognitive development of offspring. However, there has been little agreement across experimental reports on the nature and size of the differences, and rather little consistency between the results. The current literature is limited in that the experimental procedures used have little overlap, and do not rest on any of the highly quantified behavioural measures that are readily available. The most compelling evidence remains in the epidemiological studies, and, as is well known, they are fraught with complications. Some excellent research has been reported in areas such as prenatal effects on later neurogenesis, and the effects of maternal care. However, as yet there has been little correlation with functionally relevant behavioural measures. It is also the case that in many cases the behavioural and cognitive effects are much more subtle than some of the anatomical changes evident, and are likely to be dependent on ongoing gene–environment interactions. We would predict that these effects will be even more subtle when a concerted effort is made to examine more com-

plex behaviours. A more sophisticated understanding of the complex nature of ongoing interactions between the developing organism and its environment (e.g., Oyama *et al.* 2001) would aid in understanding the long-term effects of very-early-life events.

ACKNOWLEDGMENTS

Our work is supported by the National Research Centre for Growth and Development (JL, MD and BHB), and the Health Research Council of New Zealand (BHB).

REFERENCES

Almeida, S. S., Tonkiss, J. and Galler, J. R. (1996a). Prenatal protein malnutrition affects avoidance but not escape behavior in the elevated T-maze test. *Physiol. Behav.*, **60**, 191–5.

(1996b). Prenatal protein malnutrition affects exploratory behaviour of female rats in the elevated plus-maze test. *Physiol. Behav.*, **60**, 675–80.

(1996c). Prenatal protein malnutrition affects the social interactions of juvenile rats. *Physiol. Behav.*, **60**, 197–201.

Bagalkote, H., Pang, D. and Jones, P. B. (2001). Maternal influenza and schizophrenia. *Int. J. Ment. Health*, **29**, 3–21.

Barker, D. J. P. and Osmond, C. (1988). Low birthweight and hypertension. *BMJ*, **297**, 134–5.

Breslau, N. (1995). Psychiatric sequelae of low birthweight. *Epidemiol. Rev.*, **17**, 96–106.

Breslau, N., Klein, N. and Allen, L. (1988). Very low birthweight: behavioural sequelae at nine years of age. *J. Am. Acad. Child Adolesc. Psychiatry*, **27**, 605–12.

Brown, A. S., Begg, M. S., Gravenstein, S. *et al.* (2004). Serologic evidence of prenatal influenza in the etiology of schizophrenia. *Arch. Gen. Psychiatry*, **61**, 774–80.

Coe, C. L., Kramer, M., Czéh, B. *et al.* (2003). Prenatal stress diminishes neurogenesis in the dentate gyrus of juvenile rhesus monkeys. *Biol. Psychiatry*, **54**, 1025–34.

Davison, M. and Baum, W. M. (2000). Choice in a variable environment: Every reinforcer counts. *J. Exp. Anal. Behav.*, **74**, 1–24.

Davison, M. and McCarthy, D. (1988). *The Matching Law: a Research Review*. Hillsdale, NJ: Erlbaum.

Dwyer, C. M., Lawrence, A. B., Bishop, S. C. and Lewis, M. (2003). Ewe–lamb bonding behaviours are affected by maternal undernutrition in pregnancy. *J. Nutr.*, **89**, 123–36.

Francis, D., Diorio, J., Liu, D. and Meaney, M. J. (1999). Non-genomic transmission across generations of maternal behavior and stress responses in the rat. *Science*, **286**, 1155–8.

Gale, C. R. and Martyn, C. N. (2004). Birthweight and later risk of depression in a national birth cohort. *Br. J. Psychiatry*, **184**, 28–33.

Gale, C. R., O'Callaghan, F. J., Godfrey, K. M., Law, C. M. and Martyn, C. N. (2004). Critical periods of brain growth and cognitive function in children. *Brain*, **127**, 321–9.

Gluckman, P. D. and Hanson, M. A. (2004). Living with the past: evolution, development, and patterns of disease. *Science*, **305**, 1733–6.

Gray, J. A. and McNaughton, N. (1983). Comparison between the behavioural effects of septal and hippocampal lesions: a review. *Neurosci. Biobehav. Rev.*, **7**, 119–88.

Hales, C. N. and Barker, D. J. P. (1992). Type 2 (non insulin dependent) diabetes mellitus: the thrifty phenotype hypothesis. *Diabetologia*, **35**, 595–601.

Hayashi, A., Nagaoka, M., Yamada, K., Ichitani, Y., Miake, Y. and Okado, N. (1998). Maternal stress induces synaptic loss and developmental disabilities of offspring. *Int. J. Dev. Neurosc.*, **16**, 209–16.

Hoek, H. W., Brown, A. S. and Susser, E. (1998). The Dutch famine and schizophrenia spectrum disorders. *Soc. Psychiatry Psychiatr. Epidemiol.*, **33**, 373–9.

Hursh, S. R. (1984). Behavioral economics. *J. Exp. Anal. Behav.*, **42**, 435–52.

Jefferis, B. J. M. H., Power, C. and Hertzman, C. (2002). Birthweight, childhood socioeconomic environment, and cognitive development in the 1958 British birth cohort study. *BMJ*, **325**, 305–11.

King, R. S., Debassion. W. A., Kemper, T. L. *et al.* (2004). Effects of prenatal protein malnutrition and acute postnatal stress on granule cell genesis in the fascia dentate of neonatal and juvenile rats. *Dev. Brain Res.*, **150**, 9–15.

Landon, J. and Davison, M. (2001). Reinforcer-ratio variation and its effect on rate of adaptation. *J. Exp. Anal. Behav.*, **75**, 207–34.

Martyn, C. N., Gale, C. R., Sayer, A. A. and Fall, C. (1996). Growth in utero and cognitive function in adult life: follow up study of people born between 1920 and 1943. *BMJ*, **312**, 1393–6.

Matte, T. D., Bresnahan, M., Begge, M. D. and Susser, E. (2001). Influence of variation in birthweight within normal range and within sibships on IQ at age 7 years: cohort study. *BMJ*, **323**, 310–14.

Meaney, M. J. (2001). Maternal care, gene expression, and the transmission of individual differences in stress reactivity across generations. *Annu. Rev. Neurosci.*, **24**, 1161–92.

Mednick, S. A., Machon, R. A., Huttenen, M. O. and Bonett, D. (1988). Adult schizophrenia following prenatal exposure to an influenza epidemic. *Arch. Gen. Psychiatry*, **45**, 189–92.

Menard, J. L., Champagne, D. L., Meaney, M. J. P. (2004). Variations of maternal care differentially influence 'fear' reactivity and regional patterns of cFOS immunoreactivity in response to the shock-probe burying test. *Neuroscience*, **129**, 297–308.

Mirescu, C., Peters, J. D. and Gould, E. (2004). Early life experience alters response of adult neurogenesis to stress. *Nat. Neurosci.*, **7**, 841–6.

Mokler, D. J., Galler, J. R. and Morgane, P. J. (2003). Modulation of 5-HT release in the hippocampus of 30-day-old rats exposed in-utero to protein malnutrition. *Dev. Brain Res.*, **142**, 203–8.

Morgane, P. J., Mokler, D. J. and Galler, J. R. (2002). Effects of prenatal protein malnutrition on hippocampal formation. *Neurosci. Biobehav. Rev.*, **26**, 471–83.

Neugebauer, R., Hoek, H. W. and Susser, E. (1999). Prenatal exposure to wartime famine and development of antisocial personality disorder in early adulthood. *JAMA*, **282**, 455–62.

Ounsted, M. K., Moar, V. A. and Scott, A. (1983). Small-for-dates babies at the age of four years: health, handicap, and developmental status. *Early Hum. Dev.*, **8**, 243–58.

Oyama, S., Griffiths, P. E. and Gray, R. D., eds. (2001). *Cycles of Contingency: Developmental systems and Evolution*. Cambridge, MA: MIT Press.

Pharoah, P. O., Stevenson, C. J., Cooke, R. W. and Stevenson, R. C. (1994). Clinical and sub-clinical deficits at 8 years in a geographically defined cohort of low birthweight infants. *Arch. Dis. Child.*, **70**, 264–70.

Richards M., Hardy, R., Kuh, D. and Wadsworth, M. E. J. (2001). Birthweight, and cognitive function in the British 1946 birth cohort: longitudinal population based study. *BMJ*, **322**, 199–203.

(2002). Birthweight, postnatal growth and cognitive function in a national UK birth cohort. *Int. J. Epidemiol.*, **31**, 342–8.

Shenkin, S.D, Starr, J. M., Rush, M. A., Whalley, L. J. and Deary, I. J. (2001). birthweight and cognitive function at age 11 years: the Scottish Mental Survey 1932. *Arch. Dis. Child.*, **85**, 189–97.

Shi, L., Fatemi, S. H., Sidwell, R. W. and Patterson, P. H. (2003). Maternal influenza causes marked behavioral and pharmacological changes in the offspring. *J. Neurosci.*, **23**, 297–302.

Sorenson, H. T., Sabroe, S., Olsen, J., Rothman, K. J., Gillman, M. W. and Fischer, P. (1997). Birthweight and cognitive function in young adult life: historical cohort study. *BMJ*, **315**, 401–3.

Strauss, R. S. (2000). Adult functional outcome of those born small for gestation age: twenty-six-year follow-up of the 1970 British birth cohort. *JAMA*, **283**, 625–32.

Strupp. B. J. and Levitsky, D. A. (1995). Enduring cognitive effects of early malnutrition: a theoretical reappraisal. *J. Nutr.*, **125**, 2221–32S.

Szuran, T., Zimmerman, E. and Welzl, H. (1994). Water maze performance and hippocampal weight of prenatally stressed rats. *Behav. Brain Res.*, **65**, 153–5.

Thompson, C., Syddall, H., Rosin, I., Osmond, C. and Barker, D. J. P. (2001). Birthweight and the risk of depressive disorder in later life. *Br. J. Psychiatry*, **179**, 450–5.

Tonkiss, J. and Galler, J. R. (1990). Prenatal protein malnutrition and working memory performance in adult rats. *Behav. Brain Res.*, **40**, 95–107.

Tonkiss, J., Galler, J. R., Formica, R. N., Shukitt-Hale, B. and Timm, R. R. (1990). Fetal protein malnutrition impairs acquisition of a DRL task in adult rats. *Physiol. Behav.*, **48**, 73–7.

Tonkiss, J., Shultz, P. and Galler, J. R. (1994). An analysis of spatial navigation in prenatally protein malnourished rats. *Physiol. Behav.*, **55**, 217–24.

Tonkiss, J., Harrison, R. H. and Galler, J. R. (1996). Differential effects of prenatal protein malnutrition and prenatal cocaine on a test of homing behavior in rat pups. *Physiol. Behav.*, **60**, 1013–18.

Tonkiss, J., Shultz, P. L., Shumsky, J. S. and Galler, J. R. (1997). Development of spatial navigation following prenatal cocaine and malnutrition in rats: lack of additive effects. *Neurotoxicol. Teratol.*, **19**, 363–72.

Vickers, M. H., Breier, B. H., Cutfield, W. S., Hofman, P. L. and Gluckman, P. D. (2000). Fetal origins of hyperphagia, obesity, and hypertension and postnatal amplification by hypercaloric nutrition. *Am. J. Physiol. Endocrinol. Metab.*, **279**, E83–7.

Vickers, M. H., Reddy, S., Ikenasio, B. A. and Breier, B. H. (2001). Dysregulation of the adipoinsular axis: a mechanism for the pathogenesis of hyperleptinemia and adipogenic diabetes induced by fetal programming. *J. Endocrinol.*, **170**, 323–32.

Vickers, M. H., Breier, B. H., McCarthy, D. and Gluckman, P. D. (2003). Sedentary behavior during postnatal life is determined by the prenatal environment and exacerbated by postnatal hypercaloric nutrition. *Am. J. Physiol. Regul. Integr. Comp. Physiol.*, **285**, R271–3.

Wahlbeck, K., Forsen, T., Osmond, C., Barker, D. J. P. and Eriksson, J. G. (2001). Association of schizophrenia with low maternal body mass index, small size at birth, and thinness during childhood. *Arch. Gen. Psychiatry*, **58**, 48–52.

Weaver, I. C. G., Cervoni, N., Champagne, F. A. *et al.* (2004). Epigenetic programming by maternal behavior. *Nat. Neurosci.*, **7**, 847–54.

Weller, A., Glaubman, H., Yehuda, S., Caspy, T. and Ben-Uria, Y. (1988). Acute and repeated gestational stress affect offspring learning and activity in rats. *Physiol. Behav.*, **43**, 139–43.

Woodall, S. M., Breier, B. H., Johnston, B. M. and Gluckman, P. D. (1996a). A model of intrauterine growth retardation caused by chronic maternal undernutrition in the rat: effects on the somatotrophic axis and postnatal growth. *J. Endocrinol.*, **150**, 231–42.

Woodall, S. M., Johnston, B. M., Breier, B. H. and Gluckman, P. D. (1996b). Chronic maternal undernutrition in the rat leads to delayed postnatal growth and elevated blood pressure in offspring. *Pediatr. Res.*, **40**, 438–43.

28

The developmental environment and the origins of neurological disorders

Sandra Rees,[1] Richard Harding[2] and Terrie Inder[3]

[1]University of Melbourne
[2]Monash University
[3]Murdoch Children's Research Institute

Introduction

There is now compelling evidence that many neurological disorders which become apparent after birth have their origins during fetal life. For example, epidemiological studies have shown that cerebral palsy, a heterogeneous group of non-progressive motor impairment disorders, most frequently results from prenatal rather than perinatal or postnatal causes (Nelson and Ellenberg 1986). Minimal cerebral brain dysfunction, typified by children having general reading, writing and cognitive problems, is often associated with intrauterine growth restriction (IUGR), suggesting that the neurological problems have their origins in utero. Schizophrenia, one of the most debilitating of mental disorders, affecting about 1% of the population, cannot be accounted for entirely by genetic inheritance. On the basis of histological and neurochemical observations it has been proposed that prenatal insults result in a vulnerability of the developing brain, predisposing an individual with risk factors (seen as genetic inheritance) to develop the symptoms of schizophrenia in the teenage or young adult years (Akil and Weinberger 2000). Other disorders such as epilepsy and autism are also thought to result in part from neurodevelopmental deficits. Thus there is growing evidence that abnormal development of the brain during gestation contributes to many neurological disorders which manifest in later life.

Over the last few decades there have been major advances in our understanding of the intricate sequence of events that results in the formation of the entire nervous system from a specialised sheet of cells on the dorsal surface of the embryo. At 3–4 weeks after conception, this sheet rolls into a tube (neural tube) and the formation of neurons begins. The process reaches its peak between 10 and 18 weeks of gestation, when cells are being produced at a rate of approximately 250 000 per minute. The mature brain contains about 100 billion neurons and at least twice this number of neuroglial cells which play a vital role in brain function. Once formed, neurons migrate to their appropriate sites in the developing brain and then grow processes, axons and dendrites and make specific synaptic connections. Synaptogenesis begins prenatally and continues for several months after birth, during which time environmental factors can influence the pruning and fine-tuning of these connections into their mature form. During this period axons are myelinated and hence become more rapidly conducting. Different regions of the brain form at different times, with the brainstem forming early, the cerebral hemispheres later and the cerebellum last. Thus the timing of gestational insults, and their severity and form, are likely to be important factors in determining the type of brain injury, the extent to which it will affect the function of the individual after birth and the expression of particular neurological disorders.

Developmental Origins of Health and Disease, ed. Peter Gluckman and Mark Hanson. Published by Cambridge University Press.
© P. D. Gluckman and M. A. Hanson 2006.

Factors which can affect the normal development of the brain

Cerebral hypoxia

The fetus is totally dependent on the placenta and umbilical cord for an adequate supply of oxygen and nutrients during pregnancy. Interruption to this supply could be sudden (acute), such as in umbilical cord occlusion, or of a more long-lasting (chronic) form, often due to impaired placental function resulting from maternal hypertension, maternal tobacco smoking, partial placental detachment, placental villus oedema, or damage to uterine arteries (Naeye *et al.* 1989). A critical factor affecting the fetal brain in such adverse intrauterine conditions is likely to be a reduced delivery of oxygen, which has the potential to injure neurons. This can occur as a result of (a) a reduced oxygen content of fetal blood (hypoxia), and/or (b) a reduction (or a lack of an increase) in fetal cerebral perfusion in the presence of hypoxia. It is also likely that in chronic placental dysfunction reduced nutrient supply to the fetus (e.g. glucose, amino acids, micronutrients) and an altered endocrine status could adversely affect brain development.

Hypoxia–ischaemia, which is considered to be the major cause of perinatal brain injury (Volpe 2001), leads to different neuropathologies in premature and term infants. In term infants neuronal injury predominates; neurons of the CA1 region of the hippocampus, the deeper layers of the cerebral cortex and cerebellar Purkinje cells are the most frequently injured (Rivkin 1997, Volpe 2001). Neuronal necrosis is most prominent in the border zones between the end fields of the major arteries and in the depths of the sulci, reflecting the greater effect of hypoxia–ischaemia in these regions. In contrast, in premature infants oligodendroglial/white-matter damage is the major injury. This distinctive lesion, referred to as periventricular leukomalacia (PVL), includes cystic infarcts adjacent to the lateral ventricles and gliosis extending more diffusely throughout the cerebral white matter (Banker and Larroche 1962). Magnetic-resonance imaging studies have demonstrated that the diffuse component is very common in premature infants, while focal necrosis now occurs rarely in only about 5% of infants (Inder *et al.* 2003). It is increasingly recognised that there is also primary or secondary injury to cortical or deep grey matter, including the cerebral cortex (Inder *et al.* 1999), hippocampus (Isaacs *et al.* 2000) and cerebellum (Allin *et al.* 2001). PVL is associated with cerebral palsy especially in premature infants (Kuban and Leviton 1994).

In relation to neuronal injury the principal pathways leading to cell death after hypoxia–ischaemia are initiated by energy depletion followed by (a) activation of glutamate receptors; (b) accumulation of cytosolic calcium; (c) activation of a variety of calcium-mediated deleterious events including generation of reactive oxygen species (ROS) such as superoxide anion, hydroxyl radicals and nitric oxide derivatives (reviewed by Volpe 2001). ROS interact with the lipid components of cellular membranes, initiating lipid peroxidation resulting in the breakdown of lipid constituents into highly reactive by-products including lipid aldehydes such as hydroxynonenal and malondialdehyde. These reactive aldehydes then bind to and modify protein, creating protein adducts. Nitrosative stress results from nitric oxide (NO) released from reactive microglia reacting with superoxide anions to form peroxynitrite, which targets tyrosine residues of proteins to form nitrotyrosine residues. Both of these processes are highly damaging to cell membranes. These events can result in mitochondrial disruption and immediate or delayed cell death, with the cascade of damaging events unfolding over hours to days after the primary insult (see Johnston *et al.* 2000). Immature oligodendrocytes appear to be particularly vulnerable to free-radical damage (Back *et al.* 1998, Fern and Moller 2000). Although the underlying mechanisms have not yet been definitively established, there is an association between high levels of lipid peroxidation products, such as 8-isoprostane, in the cerebrospinal fluid and white-matter injury in preterm infants (Inder *et al.* 2002).

Infection/inflammation

Recent clinical studies have indicated that maternal or intrauterine infection/inflammation might also play a critical role in perinatal brain damage. There are significant associations between maternal infection, preterm birth, neonatal brain damage and increased levels of proinflammatory cytokines in the amniotic fluid (Yoon *et al.* 1995), umbilical cord (Yoon *et al.* 1996) and brain (Deguchi *et al.* 1996). Brain damage resulting from infection can lead to long-term developmental disabilities including cerebral palsy (Dammann and Leviton 1997). Most commonly, invading microorganisms are thought to gain access to the amniotic cavity and the fetus by ascending from the vagina and cervix (Romero *et al.* 2003). Here they induce the innate immune response and cause inflammation of the chorioamniotic membranes and the production of proinflammatory cytokines. The cytokines and/or other inflammatory mediators then gain access to the fetus via swallowed amniotic fluid or fetal lungs, eyes or nasal membranes. It has been suggested that these agents increase the permeability of the blood–brain barrier with enhanced leukocyte infiltration of the brain mediated by brain chemokines. Brain microglia and astrocytes will be stimulated to up-regulate the production of cytokines, and brain injury will ensue. In human pregnancies in which intrauterine inflammation is accompanied by fetal asphyxia there appears to be a dramatic increase in the risk of cerebral palsy (Nelson and Grether 1998). It should also be noted that hypoxia–ischaemia often involves inflammatory pathways (Rothwell and Strijbos 1995), and that inflammation can interrupt haemodynamic stability. Thus there are likely to be synergistic pathways between hypoxia and infection/inflammation which will potentiate the development of brain damage.

It is also possible that infections could impair oxygen delivery to the fetal brain via effects on gas exchange in the placenta, fetal blood volume, the oxygen content of fetal blood, or fetal cerebral vascular resistance. It is likely, however, that effects will differ between acute and chronic infections. There is some evidence from preterm births that chronic placental infection may alter placental vascular structure but does not impair fetal oxygenation (Salafia *et al.* 1995); in contrast, acute infection may adversely affect placental function (Garnier *et al.* 2001, Dalitz *et al.* 2003).

Premature birth

Advances in perinatal care have led to a significant improvement in the survival of very premature (<30 weeks gestational age) infants. However, up to 10% of these infants will later develop spastic motor deficits (Holling and Leviton 1999) and another 25–50% will suffer developmental or behavioural disabilities with considerable educational, economic and social implications (Hack and Fanaroff 1999, Volpe 2001). As indicated above, the most common cerebral neuropathology observed in premature infants is white-matter damage, although there is recent evidence of injury to cerebral grey matter. Intrauterine infection and associated inflammation is the only pathological process which has so far been causally linked to premature birth. There are many potential contributors to the disabilities observed following preterm birth, including the severity of the illness, malnutrition and the nature of therapeutic regimes.

Experimental animal models

Despite promising advances in the field of neuroprotection, the development of specific neuroprotective strategies for perinatal brain damage remains limited by the current lack of understanding of the cerebral pathologies and their causative pathways. Important insights into the nature of cerebral injury in the premature infant have been made with human autopsy studies (Banker and Larroche 1962, Haynes *et al.* 2003). However, with the markedly improved survival of the premature infant over the last decade, autopsy material has become increasingly difficult to obtain and is limited by reflecting the neuropathologies associated only with the most severely ill infants.

Advances in imaging techniques (Inder *et al.* 2003) are helping to define brain injury, but animal models still provide an essential approach to elucidating the causative mechanisms underlying the vulnerability of the developing brain to changes in its environment. These models have enabled us to determine the effects of a specific insult delivered at a specific stage of brain development on the structure and function of the brain. By comparing these outcomes with the neuropathologies in human neurological disorders we can provide some insight into their possible causes.

The most frequently used model of hypoxemia–ischaemia is the one developed in the neonatal rat involving unilateral carotid artery ligation and exposure to low oxygen levels (Rice *et al.* 1981). This results in damage to the white matter, but the paucity of white matter in rodents does not allow for a close replication of the human lesion; nor does the protocol result in neurological deficits. It has, however, been valuable in providing an understanding of mechanisms involved in hypoxic–ischaemic damage. Other models include the administration of excitatory amino acid receptor agonists in rats (McDonald *et al.* 1988, Follett *et al.* 2000) and hypoxic protocols in neonatal pigs (Foster *et al.* 2001).

Fewer studies have examined the influence of intrauterine factors on the fetal brain. Although we are not yet fully aware of all the forms of compromise which might affect a fetus, our approach, and that of other laboratories (e.g. Bocking *et al.* 1988, Williams *et al.* 1992, Penning *et al.* 1994, Mallard *et al.* 2003, Baud *et al.* 2004, Derrick *et al.* 2004, Yan *et al.* 2004), has been to develop animal models of acute and chronic insults which mimic conditions commonly thought to occur during pregnancy. Over the last two decades we (and others) have used ovine models to examine the effects of a reduction in the supply of oxygen and nutrients to the fetus: (a) for 12 hours, near mid gestation (Rees *et al.* 1997, 1999); (b) brief single (Duncan *et al.* 2004a) or repeated umbilical-cord occlusions in late gestation (Loeliger *et al.* 2003), or longer occlusions (25 minutes) (Mallard *et al.* 2003); (c) chronic placental insufficiency (20–30 days) in late gestation

(Duncan *et al.* 2004b); and (d) maternal carunclectomy, which reduces the available sites for placentation, resulting in growth-restricted fetuses that are chronically hypoxaemic, hypoglycaemic and have an altered endocrine balance (Rees *et al.* 1988). Sheep have an advantage over smaller species in that vascular catheters can be chronically implanted to allow for blood sampling and controlled alterations in the intrauterine environment. Furthermore they have a long gestation (term ∼147 days) making it possible to study responses to insults over an extended period of brain development within the intrauterine environment. They also have a large volume of white matter in which the neuropathologies that develop more closely resemble human neuropathologies than do those in rodents. We have also used a guinea pig model of chronic placental insufficiency induced by uterine artery ligation during the second half of gestation (term ∼67 days) (Mallard *et al.* 1999).

Studies have focused on (a) the hippocampus, a region involved with learning and memory; (b) the cerebellum and striatum, which are essential for coordination and strategies involved in the execution of movement; (c) the cerebral cortex (particularly the motor cortex), which is involved in the initiation of movement; (d) the cerebral white matter, which contains axon tracts connecting the cortex with other parts of the brain; and (e) the retina in the eye.

These studies have allowed us to reach the following generalisations:

Acute insults in early gestation, resulting in a rapid drop in oxygen delivery to the brain at a time when neurogenesis and neural migration are at their peak, can result in the death of neurons, including Purkinje cells in the cerebellum, pyramidal cells in the hippocampus and cortical neurons (Rees *et al.* 1999), and a slowing of neural migration, at least in the hippocampus (Rees *et al.* 1997). The growth of neural processes is significantly retarded in the long term if the neurons are particularly immature at the time of the insult (as in the cerebellum) but will recover, after an initial delay, if process outgrowth is well established at the time of the insult (as in the hippocampus). Acute insults can also cause damage to the white matter resulting in diffuse injury and cystic lesions in the periventricular area, neuropathologies resembling those consistently observed in cerebral palsy. Significantly, in our studies, lesions occurred most prominently in fetuses from multiple pregnancies, a risk factor for cerebral palsy. Fetal hypotension was not a necessary accompaniment to the development of such lesions (Rees *et al.* 1997).

Acute insults (umbilical cord occlusion) in late gestation result in neuronal death in the cerebral cortex and striatum (Rees *et al.* 1999), whereas hippocampal and cerebellar neurons do not appear to be affected at the gross level. The white matter is damaged, but less extensively than when insults are delivered earlier in gestation (albeit in our experimental protocol the earlier insult was more prolonged). These observations support the finding that white-matter injury is more commonly seen in preterm than term infants; this appears to be due to the vulnerability of immature oligodendrocytes to hypoxaemia (Back *et al.* 1998).

Chronic insults (placental insufficiency) result in outcomes which differ from acute insults in several respects. Sheep fetuses compromised throughout gestation (Rees *et al.* 1988), or guinea pig fetuses compromised for the second half of gestation (Nitsos and Rees 1990, Mallard *et al.* 1999), are growth-restricted. The brain, although relatively spared in relation to other organs, is reduced in weight. There is no overt white-matter damage, although axonal myelination is reduced in the central nervous system (Nitsos and Rees 1990); this could indicate a reduction in the number of myelinating glia and a restricted capacity of those which form to generate myelin. Thinner myelin sheaths affect axonal conduction velocity, which could contribute to altered neural function in growth-restricted individuals.

Following these chronic insults the growth of neural processes and synaptogenesis is compromised

globally in the brain at term in the sheep (Rees *et al.* 1988, Rees and Harding, 1988) and guinea pig (Mallard *et al.* 1999, Dieni and Rees 2005), and this persists into young adulthood at least in some regions of the brain (Rehn *et al.* 2004). Neurons generally seem to survive chronic mild intrauterine compromise, but some populations are affected; reduced cell numbers could relate to a direct effect of hypoxia on neurogenesis or alternatively to cell death of postmitotic cells. For example, in sheep after 20 days of chronic placental insufficiency in late gestation, retinal dopaminergic amacrine cells (interneurons), which are involved in contrast sensitivity, are reduced in number but other classes of amacrine cells are not affected (Duncan *et al.* 2004b). The loss of even small numbers of specific classes of cells could significantly affect particular neural functions.

Support for the early-neurodevelopmental hypothesis of schizophrenia

In the guinea pig model, we have observed enlargement of the lateral ventricles most likely resulting from reduced growth of neural processes and reduced neuronal numbers in some brain regions (Mallard *et al.* 1999). Ventriculomegaly is one of the most consistent findings in the brains of patients with schizophrenia (Johnstone *et al.* 1976, Hopkins and Lewis 2000). Our study demonstrates experimentally for the first time that such alterations can originate from an insult in utero (Mallard *et al.* 1999) and persist into adolescence (Rehn *et al.* 2004) (Plate 4). We have also demonstrated reduced brain weight, reduced basal ganglia volume, the absence of astrogliosis and sensorimotor gating deficits (discussed below) at adolescence, paralleling the situation in some patients with schizophrenia (Rehn *et al.* 2004). Although no animal model of a complex human disorder is ever likely to emulate deficits in all aspects of structure and function observed in patients with a neuropsychiatric illness, our findings support the early-neurodevelopmental hypothesis of schizophrenia. A strength of this model is that it mimics a condition which could occur in human pregnancy, albeit at the more severe end of the spectrum of prenatal conditions. Other models in neonatal animals, such as N-methyl-D-aspartate receptor blockade (Harris *et al.* 2003), lesioning of hippocampal pathways (Lipska *et al.* 1995) and depletion of dopamine, support the neurodevelopmental hypothesis but do not replicate specific perinatal events.

How might prenatal brain damage occur in compromised fetuses?

The causes of the various forms of damage described above are likely to include many factors such as reduced oxygen availability and, in chronic insults, fetal malnutrition and altered endocrine states. Altered growth factor levels and cytokines are also likely to play a part. For example, we have shown that the neurotrophin brain-derived neurotrophic factor (BDNF) is significantly reduced in chronic placental insufficiency in the fetal hippocampus (Dieni and Rees 2005). In all regions of the brain that we have examined there are high numbers of glutamatergic synapses. We know that there is increased neuronal release, and reduced uptake of glutamate by glia, in hypoxic conditions. Excess glutamate will facilitate Ca^{2+} entry into cells via activation of NMDA receptors; this will result in the formation of reactive oxidative and nitrosative species, the peroxidation of membranes and mitochondrial disruption. Neuronal cell death will ensue if Ca^{2+} influx is high.

We have recently shown, in the fetus, that the level of glutamate efflux in the white matter positively correlates with the degree of damage to the white matter (Loeliger *et al.* 2003). Elevated glutamate levels could lead to injury by activating receptors on oligodendrocytes, or possibly on the myelin sheath itself, causing a toxic influx of Ca^{2+}. Oligodendrocytes express AMPA receptors from 63 days of gestation in fetal sheep (Furuta and Martin 1999), and it is known that activation of AMPA receptors is involved in mediating hypoxic–ischaemic injury to oligodendrocytes, at least in the developing rat brain (Follett *et al.* 2000).

White-matter damage could also occur as a result of reverse operation of the Na^+/Ca^{2+} exchanger in axons (Stys *et al.* 1991). Energy depletion causes failure of Na^+, K^+-ATPase, which allows an unopposed inward leakage of Na^+, and membrane depolarisation acts to drive the Na^+/Ca^{2+} exchanger in the Ca^{2+} import mode, leading to intracellular Ca^{2+} overload. Excess Ca^{2+} is expected to disrupt mitochondrial function, leading to axonal damage (Stys *et al.* 1991). If the insult is less severe, a sublethal influx of Ca^{2+} could significantly retard the growth of axons.

Models of infection/inflammation

Models that have been used to explore the effects of intrauterine infection include live inoculation of *E. coli* in rabbits (Yoon *et al.* 1997a, 1997b, Debillon *et al.* 2000) and fetal exposure to the endotoxin lipopolysaccharide (LPS), a component of gram negative bacteria, in sheep (Duncan *et al.* 2002, Mallard *et al.* 2003) and in rats (Cai *et al.* 2000, Bell and Hallenbeck 2002). LPS binds to the CD14 receptor on the membrane of myeloid cells and, in concert with Toll-like receptors (TLRs) including TLR4, activates a transmembrane signalling pathway (Beutler and Poltorak 2000) (Fig. 28.1). This pathway involves the activation of the transcription factor nuclear factor κB (NFκB), which is normally present in the cell cytoplasm forming an inactive complex with an inhibitor, IFκB. Following cellular activation, IFκB is degraded by cytoplasmic proteases and releases NFκB, which is translocated to the nucleus where it regulates transcription of several genes including the pro-inflammatory cytokines, interleukin 1β(IL1β), IL6 and tumour necrosis factor (TNFα). The role of NFκB in neuronal survival in vivo is controversial, with studies supporting both neurodestructive and neuroprotective roles (Mattson and Camandola 2001). It has been suggested that activation of NFκB in neurons may protect them against degeneration whereas activation in microglia promotes neuronal degeneration via cytokine production (Mattson and Camandola 2001).

In our sheep model, bolus injections of LPS administered to the fetus over five days at 0.7 of gestation resulted in brain injury within 10 days of the first exposure (Duncan *et al.* 2002). Repeated doses of endotoxin were used because fetal inflammation associated with maternal infection is likely to be chronic in nature (Romero *et al.* 2003). The injury ranged from focal cystic infarction in the peri-ventricular region to diffuse damage, characterised by reactive gliosis, in the surrounding and subcor-tical white matter (Plate 5); the pattern of injury was similar to that described in the premature infant. Blood flow was not significantly altered in the fetal ovine brain during LPS exposure but there was significant hypoxaemia due to reduced umbilical–placental blood flow, and oxygen delivery was reduced by 30–40% in the fetal brain, including the white matter (Dalitz *et al.* 2003).

The role played by hypoxia in this paradigm is still uncertain (Fig. 28.1). We know that when LPS is administered to the fetus either via constant infu-sion (Duncan *et al.* 2004c) or intra-amniotically (Nitsos *et al.* 2004), fetal hypoxaemia does not ensue and the resultant brain damage is not as signif-icant as when hypoxia is present. From previous studies we know that predominantly hypoxic insults (without fetal hypotension) (Rees *et al.* 1997) also cause white-matter damage, but that it is not as reproducible or generally as severe as that resulting from LPS exposure. Thus it appears that there are synergistic pathways between hypoxia and inflam-mation which potentiate the evolution of brain damage. In accordance with this notion, LPS has been shown to sensitise the immature rat brain to hypoxic–ischaemic injury (Eklind *et al.* 2001). Clearly the aetiology of the fetal brain damage in inflammation is multifactorial and is likely to include an increase in circulating cytokine levels; we have already shown that TNFα and IL6 levels (Duncan *et al.* 2002) increase within six hours of LPS exposure. It has been proposed that circulat-ing cytokines might act on cerebral endothelial cells or perivascular cells to up-regulate prostaglandin synthesis resulting in increased blood–brain barrier permeability (Yan *et al.* 2004); cytotoxic and pro-inflammatory substances could then pass into the brain.

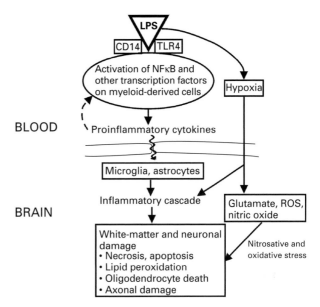

Figure 28.1 Possible activation of the inflammatory cascade by endotoxin (lipopolysaccharide, LPS). LPS binds to its receptor CD14 and in concert with Toll-like receptor 4 (TLR4) activates the NFκB signalling pathway in myeloid-derived cells. Proinflammatory and other proteins are transcribed; they affect the permeability of the blood–brain barrier, perhaps via the up-regulation of prostaglandins, and allow the entry of proinflammatory substances and circulating leukocytes into the brain. Here there is activation of microglia and astrocytes to up-regulate cytokine production; this ultimately leads to white-matter and neuronal damage. If hypoxia is also involved, excess extracellular glutamate will result in nitrosative and oxidative stress, exacerbating neuronal and axonal damage.

Model of premature birth

Although the use of nonhuman primate models for the study of neurological diseases is not always feasi-ble there is an enhanced likelihood that such models will more closely resemble the sequence of human cerebral development than other species, and that they will sustain similar brain damage. We know from the studies of Myers and colleagues (Myers 1977) in term monkeys that various regimens of total and partial asphyxia result in clinical and patho-logical findings which are similar to those in the human infant. We have recently had the opportunity to study a model of premature delivery which has

been developed for the evaluation of bronchopulmonary dysplasia (Dieni *et al.* 2004). These prematurely born primates, which are delivered at the
equivalent human age of 26–28 weeks, differ from
the human preterm infant in that delivery is elec-
tive in nature, without infection or prenatal compromise such as growth restriction. However, the model
is also uniquely similar to that of the human infant in
that the mothers receive antenatal steroids and the
infants are cared for in a neonatal intensive care unit
with very similar interventions to those received by
the human premature infant.

We have shown that the baboon brain displays
strong structural similarities to the human brain with
regards to its sequence of maturation of white and
grey matter, including gyral formation, myelination
and cortical laminar development (Dieni *et al.* 2004).
Our initial histopathological data suggest that the
prematurely born baboon sustains cerebral injury
similar to that observed in the prematurely born
human, particularly white-matter injury and gliosis, haemorrhage (Plate 6) and less frequently hippocampal sclerosis. Thus we believe that this model
has the potential to assist in shedding light on the
nature of cerebral injury in the prematurely delivered
human. We are now in a position to evaluate whether
the pattern of cerebral injury varies in relation to specific ventilatory regimens employed during neonatal
intensive care. Apart from the major neuropathologies, it is also likely that the extremely immature
infant is at risk of more subtle alterations in cerebral
structure and development, and this could account
for the behavioural and functional disabilities. MRI
studies of these prematurely delivered baboon brains
after 2–4 weeks in intensive care are helping us to
identify differences in the growth of specific areas
of grey and white matter under different respiratory
regimens.

Altered brain function in prenatally compromised offspring

Evidence of changes in the structure of the brain
are informative but they need to be supported by

studies of brain function in compromised individuals in order to obtain a clearer picture of how altering
the normal course of brain development can affect
function, particularly in the long term. We know
that babies of low or very low birthweight (VLBW),
many of whom are also growth-restricted, are at
risk for long-term auditory and visual impairment
including sensorineural hearing loss and deficits in
visual acuity, colour vision and contrast sensitivity
(Dowdeswell *et al.* 1995). In order to develop treatment strategies it is important to know whether
the deficits relate to adverse pre-, peri- or postnatal events, particularly in the light of the increasing
survival rate of VLBW infants.

In the guinea pig model of chronic placental insufficiency resulting in IUGR, we have shown that
there are long-term alterations in retinal function as
detected by measuring the electroretinogram (ERG)
in young adults (Bui *et al.* 2002). We have detected
changes in the ERG in IUGR animals, indicative
of subtle changes to photoreceptors and amacrine
cells. Such effects could contribute to the visual
impairment reported in VLBW infants. In the same
animal model we have tested the auditory system by
giving an acoustic stimulus and recording the auditory brainstem response. We have identified subtle
differences in neural conduction in auditory pathways in the prenatally compromised young adult
animals compared to controls (Rehn *et al.* 2002).
This might reflect alterations in the degree of myelination of auditory brainstem pathways or changes
in synaptic efficacy. These changes might underlie
hearing loss and speech perception abilities in VLBW
and/or growth-restricted children (Anagnostakis
et al. 1982).

Furthermore, in the prenatally compromised
guinea pig we have demonstrated a reduction in
prepulse inhibition (PPI) of the startle response
(Rehn *et al.* 2004), a behavioural paradigm which
is thought to indicate the ability of the central nervous system to filter out extraneous stimuli. PPI is
reduced in patients with schizophrenia and in some
other psychiatric disorders. Thus this result indicates
that adverse prenatal conditions lead to long-term
alterations in function which resemble alterations

in patients with schizophrenia, and hence adds further support to the early-neurodevelopmental hypothesis of schizophrenia. Recently in a rabbit model of acute placental insufficiency near term, abnormalities in motor control and hypertonia were demonstrated in neonatal offspring (Derrick *et al.* 2004). This is the first model of antenatal hypoxia–ischaemia to result in motor deficits and in neuropathology which has some parallels with deficits seen in cerebral palsy.

Possibilities for therapeutic intervention

In order to be able to provide timely therapeutic intervention for infants at risk of brain damage we need to be able to detect when an insult has occurred. This can be challenging as it has been reported that it is possible for placental and fetal brain injury to occur without significant medical problems being evident during gestation (Grafe 1994). Advanced neuroimaging is now providing the opportunity to identify and then monitor the evolution of brain injury in compromised fetuses and neonates. Another approach is to identify reliable markers of brain damage in the blood of newborns (Leviton and Dammann 2002). The presence of proteins such as S100B (from astrocytes) or neuron-specific enolase (from neurons) is considered evidence that these cells have been damaged and the proteins released into the blood through increased permeability of the blood–brain barrier.

From clinical observations and animal experimentation (Johnston *et al.* 2000) we now know that the cascade of damaging events to the brain can unfold over several days; this suggests that the window of opportunity for intervention is longer than previously envisaged. In animal models attempts have been made to inhibit the hypoxic–ischaemic cascade at almost every level, for example with N-methyl-D-aspartate (NMDA, glutamate) receptor blockade; the use of nitric oxide synthetase inhibitors; blockade of apoptosis by inhibition of caspases; blocking the up-regulation of free radical formation (reviewed by Volpe 2001). Other approaches include the application of growth factors in utero (Johnston *et al.* 1996) and the prevention of energy depletion via mild hypothermia after birth (Williams *et al.* 1997, Gluckman *et al.* 2005). Many of these approaches have been effective to varying degrees in animals but, with the exception of hypothermia, they have been less successful or have had untoward side effects in humans (Volpe 2001).

There might be an opportunity to improve the neuronal environment immediately after birth in neonates at risk, thus enhancing the growth of axons and dendrites, and synaptogenesis and myelination of axons. We know that these events are all manipulable in the period of neonatal plasticity in the months after birth. As described above, BDNF levels are decreased in chronic placental insufficiency and the growth of processes is reduced. Increasing the levels of growth factors or other molecules immediately after birth, ideally by systemic injection of small molecule mimetics of neurotrophins or growth factors which can cross the blood–brain barrier, might be successful in restoring appropriate brain development. To date, however, there are no accepted effective treatments to prevent or ameliorate human perinatal brain injury, and it remains one of the greatest challenges in perinatal medicine today.

Concluding remarks

Growing evidence supports the notion that an adverse intrauterine environment can contribute to many of the neurological disorders which manifest after birth. The timing and severity of prenatal insults are critical in determining the outcome in terms of the severity of the damage and the regions of the brain affected. In animal models it has been demonstrated that relatively brief (acute) periods of hypoxaemic compromise to the fetus can have significant effects on the fetal brain, for example death of susceptible neuronal populations (cerebellum, hippocampus, cortex) and cerebral white-matter damage. These effects appear to be more profound in mid than late gestation. Chronic mild placental insufficiency, which includes hypoxia, malnutrition and an altered endocrine status, can result in long-term deficits in neural connectivity as well as affecting postnatal function, for example the auditory and visual systems. Perinatal infection is now considered to be an important factor in causing brain damage, particularly in preterm infants; there are likely to be synergistic pathways between hypoxia and inflammation which potentiate the evolution of brain damage. By comparing findings in animal models with altered pathology and function in neurological disorders we are beginning to define the types of insult that could underlie some of the neurological disorders thought to have a prenatal origin. This will allow us to devise strategies to intervene and reduce the burden of perinatal brain injury, which is likely to increase with the increasing survival rates of preterm infants. Creating the most ideal extrauterine environment for preterm infants will also be essential if we are to facilitate appropriate neural development postnatally.

REFERENCES

Akil, M. and Weinberger, D. (2000). Neuropathology and the neurodevelopmental model. In *The Neuropathology of Schizophrenia: Progress and Interepretation* (ed. P. J. Harrison and G. W. Roberts). Oxford: Oxford University Press, pp. 189–212.

Allin, M., Matsumoto, H., Santhouse, A. M. *et al.* (2001). Cognitive and motor function and the size of the cerebellum in adolescents born very pre-term. *Brain*, **124**, 60–6.

Anagnostakis, D., Petmezakis, J., Papazissis, G., Messaritakis, J. and Matsaniotis, N. (1982). Hearing loss in low-birth-weight infants. *Am. J. Dis. Child.*, **136**, 602–4.

Back, S. A., Gan, X., Rosenberg, P. and Volpe, J. (1998). Maturation-dependent vulnerability of oligodendrocytes to oxidative stress-induced death caused by glutathione depletion. *J. Neurosci.*, **18**, 6241–53.

Banker, B. Q. and Larroche, J. C. (1962). Periventricular leukomalacia of infancy: a form of neonatal anoxic encephalopathy. *Arch. Neurol.*, **7**, 386–410.

Baud, O., Daire, J.-L., Dalmaz, Y. *et al.* (2004). Gestational hypoxia induces white matter damage in neonatal rats: a new model of periventricular leukomalacia. *Brain Pathol.*, **14**, 1–10.

Bell, M. J. and Hallenbeck, J. M. (2002). Effects of intrauterine inflammation on developing rat brain. *J. Neurosci. Res.*, **70**, 570–9.

Beutler, B. and Poltorak, A. (2000). Positional cloning of Lps, and the general role of toll-like receptors in the innate immune response. *Eur. Cytokine Netw.*, **11**, 143–52.

Bocking, A. D., Gagnon, R., White, S. E., Homan, J., Milne, K. M. and Richardson, B. S. (1988). Circulatory responses to prolonged hypoxemia in fetal sheep. *Am. J. Obstet. Gynecol.*, **159**, 1418–24.

Bui, B. V., Rees, S. M., Loeliger, M. *et al.* (2002). Altered retinal function and structure after chronic placental insufficiency. *Invest. Ophthalmol. Vis. Sci.*, **43**, 805–12.

Cai, Z., Pan, Z., Pang, Y., Evans, O. and Rhodes, P. (2000). Cytokine induction in fetal rat brains and brain injury in neonatal rats after maternal lipopolysaccharide administration. *Pediatr. Res.*, **47**, 64–72.

Dalitz, P., Harding, R., Rees, S. M. and Cock, M. L. (2003). Prolonged reductions in placental blood flow and cerebral oxygen delivery in preterm fetal sheep exposed to endotoxin: possible factors in white matter injury after acute infection. *J. Soc. Gynecol. Investig.*, **10**, 283–90.

Dammann, O. and Leviton, A. (1997). Maternal intrauterine infection, cytokines, and brain damage in the preterm newborn. *Pediatr. Res.*, **42**, 1–8.

Debillon, T., Gras-Leguen, C., Verielle, V. *et al.* (2000). Intrauterine infection induces programmed cell death in rabbit periventricular white matter. *Pediatr. Res.*, **47**, 736–42.

Deguchi, K., Mizuguchi, M. and Takashima, S. (1996). Immunohistochemical expression of tumor necrosis factor alpha in neonatal leukomalacia. *Pediatr. Neurol.*, **14**, 13–16.

Derrick, M., Luo, N. L., Bregman, J. C. *et al.* (2004). Preterm fetal hypoxia–ischemia causes hypertonia and motor deficits in the neonatal rabbit: a model for human cerebral palsy? *J. Neurosci.*, **24**, 24–34.

Dieni, S. and Rees, S. (2005). BDNF and TrkB protein expression is altered in the fetal hippocampus but not cerebellum after chronic prenatal compromise. *Exp. Neurol.*, **192**, 265–73.

Dieni, S., Inder, T., Yoder, B. *et al.* (2004). The pattern of cerebral injury in a primate model of preterm birth and neonatal intensive care. *J. Neuropathol. Exp. Neurol.*, **63**, 1297–309.

Dowdeswell, H. J., Slater, A. M., Broomhall, J. and Tripp, J. (1995). Visual deficits in children born at less than 32 weeks' gestation with and without major ocular pathology and cerebral damage. *Br. J. Ophthalmol.*, **79**, 447–52.

Duncan, J. R., Cock, M. L., Scheerlinck, J. P. *et al.* (2002). White matter injury after repeated endotoxin exposure in the preterm ovine fetus. *Pediatr. Res.*, **52**, 941–9.

Duncan, J. R., Camm, E., Loeliger, M., Cock, M. L., Harding, R. and Rees, S. M. (2004a). Effects of umbilical cord occlusion in late gestation on the ovine fetal brain and retina. *J. Soc. Gynecol. Investig.*, **11**, 369–76.

Duncan, J. R., Cock, M. L., Loeliger, M., Louey, S., Harding, R. and Rees, S. M. (2004b). Effects of exposure to chronic placental insufficiency on the postnatal brain and retina in sheep. *J. Neuropathol. Exp. Neurol.*, **63**, 1131–43.

Duncan, J. R., Cock, M. L., Suzuki, K., Rees, S. M. and Harding, R. (2004c). Brain injury in the ovine fetal brain following continuous infusion of endotoxin. Pediatric Academic Societies abstract. San Francisco, USA.

Eklind, S., Mallard, C., Leverin, A. *et al.* (2001). Bacterial endotoxin sensitizes the immature brain to hypoxic-ischaemic injury. *Eur. J. Neurosci.*, **13**, 1101–6.

Fern, R. and Moller, T. (2000). Rapid ischemic cell death in immature oligodendrocytes: a fatal glutamate release feedback loop. *J. Neurosci.*, **20**, 34–42.

Follett, P. L., Rosenberg, P. A., Volpe, J. J. and Jensen, F. E. (2000). NBQX attenuates excitotoxic injury in developing white matter. *J. Neurosci.*, **20**, 9235–41.

Foster, K. A., Colditz, P. B., Lingwood, B. E., Burke, C., Dunster, K. R. and Roberts, M. S. (2001). An improved survival model of hypoxia/ischemia in the piglet suitable for neuroprotection studies. *Brain Res.*, **919**, 122–31.

Furuta, A. and Martin, L. J. (1999). Laminar segregation of the cortical plate during corticogenesis is accompanied by changes in glutamate receptor expression. *J. Neurobiol.*, **39**, 67–80.

Garnier, Y., Coumans, A., Berger, R., Jensen, A. and Hasaart, T. H. (2001). Endotoxemia severely affects circulation during normoxia and asphyxia in immature fetal sheep. *J. Soc. Gynecol. Investig.*, **8**, 134–42.

Gluckman, P. D., Wyatt, J. S., Azzopardi, D. *et al.* (2005). Selective head cooling with mild systemic hypothermia after neonatal encephalopathy: multicentre randomised trial. *Lancet*, **365**, 663–70.

Grafe, M. R. (1994). The correlation of prenatal brain damage with placental pathology. *J. Neuropathol. Exp. Neurol.*, **53**, 407–15.

Hack, M. and Fanaroff, A. A. (1999). Outcomes of children of extremely low birthweight and gestational age in the 1990s. *Early Hum. Dev.*, **53**, 193–218.

Harris, L. W., Sharp, T., Gartlon, J., Jones, D. N. C. and Harrison, P. J. (2003). Long term behavioural, molecular and morphological effects of neonatal NMDA receptor antagonism. *Eur. J. Neurosci.*, **18**, 1706–10.

Haynes, R. L., Folkerth, R. D., Keefe, R. *et al.* (2003). Nitrosative and oxidative injury to premyelinating oligodendrocytes in periventricular leukomalacia. *J. Neuropathol. Exp. Neurol.*, **62**, 441–50.

Holling, E. E. and Leviton, A. (1999). Characteristics of cranial ultrasound white-matter echolucencies that predict disability: a review. *Dev. Med. Child Neurol.*, **41**, 136–9.

Hopkins, R. and Lewis, S. (2000). Structural imaging findings and macroscopic pathology. In *The Neuropathology of Schizophrenia: Progress and Interpretation* (ed. P. J. Harrison and G. W. Roberts). Oxford: Oxford University Press, pp. 5–56.

Inder, T. E., Huppi, P. S., Warfield, S. *et al.* (1999). Periventricular white matter injury in the premature infant is followed by reduced cerebral cortical gray matter volume at term. *Ann. Neurol.*, **46**, 755–60.

Inder, T. E., Mocatta, T. J., Darlow, B., Spencer, C., Volpe, J. J. and Winterbourn, C. (2002). Elevated free radical products in the cerebrospinal fluid of VLBW infants with cerebral white matter injury. *Pediatr. Res.*, **52**, 213–18.

Inder, T. E., Anderson, N. J., Spencer, C., Wells, S. and Volpe, J. J. (2003). White matter injury in the premature infant: a comparison between serial cranial sonographic and MR findings at term. *Am. J. Neuroradiol.*, **24**, 805–9.

Isaacs, E. B., Lucas, A., Chong, W. K. *et al.* (2000). Hippocampal volume and everyday memory in children of very low birth weight. *Pediatr. Res.*, **47**, 713–20.

Johnston, B. M., Mallard, E. C., Williams, C. and Gluckman, P. (1996). Insulin-like growth factor-1 is a potent neuronal rescue agent after hypoxic–ischemic injury in fetal lambs. *J. Clin. Invest.*, **97**, 300–8.

Johnston, M. V., Trescher, W. H., Ishida, A. and Nakajima, W. (2000). Novel treatments after experimental brain injury. *Semin. Neonatol.*, **5**, 75–86.

Johnstone, E. C., Crow, T. J., Frith, C., Husband, J. and Kreel, L. (1976). Cerebral ventricular size and cognitive impairment in chronic schizophrenia. *Lancet*, **2**, 924–6.

Kuban, K. C. and Leviton, A. (1994). Cerebral palsy. *N. Engl. J. Med.*, **330**, 188–95.

Leviton, A. and Dammann, O. (2002). Brain damage markers in children: neurobiological and clinical aspects. *Acta Pediatr.*, **91**, 9–13.

Lipska, B. K., Swerdlow, N. R. Geyer, M., Jaskiw, G., Braff, D. and Weinberger, D. (1995). Neonatal excitotoxic hippocampal damage in rats causes post-pubertal changes in prepulse inhibition of startle and its disruption by apomorphine. *Psychopharmacology (Berl.)*, **122**, 35–43.

Loeliger, M., Watson, C. S., Reynolds, J. D. *et al.* (2003). Extracellular glutamate levels and neuropathology in cerebral white matter following repeated umbilical cord occlusion in the near term fetal sheep. *Neuroscience*, **116**, 705–14.

Mallard, C., Welin, A. K., Peebles, D., Hagberg, H. and Kjellmer, I. (2003). White matter injury following systemic endotoxemia or asphyxia in the fetal sheep. *Neurochem. Res.*, **28**, 215–23.

Mallard, E. C., Rehn, A., Rees, S., Tolcos, M. and Copolov, D. (1999). Ventriculomegaly and reduced hippocampal volume following intrauterine growth-restriction: implications for the aetiology of schizophrenia. *Schizophr. Res.*, **40**, 11–21.

Mattson, M. P. and Camandola, S. (2001). NF-kappaB in neuronal plasticity and neurodegenerative disorders. *J. Clin. Invest.*, **107**, 247–54.

McDonald, J. W., Silverstein, F. S. and Johnston, M. (1988). Neurotoxicity of N-methyl-D-aspartate is markedly enhanced in developing rat central nervous system. *Brain Res.*, **459**, 200–3.

Myers, R. E. (1977). Experimental models of perinatal brain damage: relevance to human pathology. In *Intrauterine Asphyxia and the Developing Fetal Brain* (ed. L. Gluck). Chicago, IL: Year Book, pp. 37–97.

Naeye, R. L., Peters, E. C., Bartholomew, M. and Landis, J. (1989). Origins of cerebral palsy. *Am. J. Dis. Child.*, **143**, 1154–61.

Nelson, K. B. and Ellenberg, J. H. (1986). Antecedents of cerebral palsy: multivariate analysis of risk. *N. Engl. J. Med.*, **315**, 81–6.

Nelson, K. B. and Grether, J. K. (1998). Potentially asphyxiating conditions and spastic cerebral palsy in infants of normal birth weight. *Am. J. Obstet. Gynecol.*, **179**, 507–13.

Nitsos, I. and Rees, S. (1990). The effects of intrauterine growth retardation on the development of neuroglia in fetal guinea pigs: an immunohistochemical and an ultrastructural study. *Int. J. Dev. Neurosci.*, **8**, 233–44.

Nitsos, I., Moss, T. J. M., Kramer, B. W. *et al.* (2004). Fetal and Neonatal Physiological Society abstract, Italy.

Penning, D. H., Grafe, M. R., Hammond, R., Matsuda, Y., Patrick, J. and Richardson, B. (1994). Neuropathology of the near-term and midgestation ovine fetal brain after sustained in utero hypoxemia. *Am. J. Obstet. Gynecol.*, **170**, 1425–32.

Rees, S. and Harding, R. (1988). The effects of intrauterine growth retardation on the development of the Purkinje cell dendritic tree in the cerebellar cortex of fetal sheep: a note on the ontogeny of the Purkinje cell. *Int. J. Dev. Neurosci.*, **6**, 461–9.

Rees, S., Bocking, A. and Harding, R. (1988). Structure of fetal sheep brain in experimental growth retardation. *J. Dev. Physiol.*, **10**, 211–24.

Rees, S., Stringer, M., Just, Y., Hooper, S. B. and Harding, R. (1997). The vulnerability of the fetal sheep brain to hypoxemia at mid-gestation. *Dev. Brain Res.*, **103**, 103–18.

Rees, S., Breen, S., Loeliger, M., McCrabb, G. and Harding, R. (1999). Hypoxemia near mid-gestation has long-term effects on fetal brain development. *J. Neuropathol. Exp. Neurol.*, **58**, 932–45.

Rehn, A. E., Loeliger, M., Hardie, N. A., Rees, S. M., Dieni, S. and Shepherd, R. K. (2002). Chronic placental insufficiency has long-term effects on auditory function in the guinea pig. *Hear. Res.*, **166**, 159–65.

Rehn, A. E., Van den Buuse, M., Copolov, D., Briscoe, T., Lambert, G. and Rees, S. (2004). An animal model of chronic placental insufficiency: relevance to neurodevelopmental disorders including schizophrenia. *Neuroscience*, **129**, 381–91.

Rice, J. E. III, Vannucci, R. C. and Brierley, J. B. (1981). The influence of immaturity on hypoxic–ischemic brain damage in the rat. *Ann. Neurol.*, **9**, 131–41.

Rivkin, M. (1997). Hypoxic–ischemic brain injury in the term newborn: neuropathology, clinical aspects, and neuroimaging. *Clin. Perinatol.*, **24**, 607–25.

Romero, R., Chaiworapongsa, T. and Espinoza, J. (2003). Micronutrients and intrauterine infection, preterm birth and the fetal inflammatory response syndrome. *J. Nutr.*, **133**, 1668–73S.

Rothwell, N. J. and Strijbos, P. J. (1995). Cytokines in neurodegeneration and repair. *Int. J. Dev. Neurosci.*, **13**, 179–85.

Salafia, C. M., Minior, V. K., Lopez-Zeno, J. A., Whittington, S. S., Pezzullo, J. C. and Vintzileos, A. M. (1995). Relationship between placental histologic features and umbilical cord blood gases in preterm gestations. *Am. J. Obstet. Gynecol.*, **173**, 1058–64.

Stys, P. K., Waxman, S. G. and Ransom, B. R. (1991). Reverse operation of the $Na^{(+)}$–Ca^{2+} exchanger mediates Ca^{2+} influx during anoxia in mammalian CNS white matter. *Ann. NY Acad. Sci.*, **639**, 328–32.

Volpe, J. J. (2001). *Neurology of the Newborn*, 4th edn. Philadelphia, PA: Saunders.

Williams, C., Gunn, A. J., Mallard, C. and Gluckman, P. (1992). Outcome after ischaemia in the developing sheep brain: an electroencephalographic and histological study. *Ann. Neurol.*, **31**, 14–21.

Williams, G., Dardzinsky, B., Buckalew, A. and Smith, M. (1997). Modest hypothermia preserves cerebral energy metabolism during hypoxia–ischemia and correlates with brain damage: a 31P nuclear magnetic resonance study in unanesthetized neonatal rats. *Pediatr. Res.*, **42**, 700–8.

Yan, E., Castillo-Melendez, M., Nicholls, T., Hirst, J. and Walker, D. (2004). Cerebrovascular responses in the fetal sheep brain to low-dose endotoxin. *Pediatr. Res.*, **55**, 855–63.

Yoon, B. H., Romero, R., Kim, C. *et al.* (1995). Amniotic fluid interleukin-6: a sensitive test for antenatal diagnosis of acute inflammatory lesions of preterm placenta and prediction of perinatal morbidity. *Am. J. Obstet. Gynecol.*, **172**, 960–70.

Yoon, B. H., Romero, R., Yang, S. H. *et al.* (1996). Interleukin-6 concentrations in umbilical cord plasma are elevated in neonates with white matter lesions associated with periventricular leukomalacia. *Am. J. Obstet. Gynecol.*, **174**, 1433–40.

Yoon, B. H., Jun, J. K., Romero, R. *et al.* (1997a). Amniotic fluid inflammatory cytokines (interleukin-6, interleukin-1beta, and tumor necrosis factor-alpha), neonatal brain white matter lesions, and cerebral palsy. *Am. J. Obstet. Gynecol.*, **177**, 19–26.

Yoon, B. H., Kim, C. J., Romero, R. *et al.* (1997b). Experimentally induced intrauterine infection causes fetal brain white matter lesions in rabbits. *Am. J. Obstet. Gynecol.*, **177**, 797–802.

29

The developmental environment: clinical perspectives on effects on the musculoskeletal system

Cyrus Cooper, Avan Aihie Sayer and Elaine Margaret Dennison

University of Southampton

Introduction

The ability to move, the protection of vital organs and stable support for the body are the principal roles of the musculoskeletal system (muscle, bone and cartilage) (Simkin 1994). This system accounts for a large proportion of the body mass; for example, the muscle mass of a healthy adult 70-kg individual is about 20 kg (Kreisberg *et al.* 1970). The musculoskeletal system develops embryonically from the mesodermal layer, differentiating into dermatomes containing skeletal and muscle cell precursors in the first trimester. At this stage the embryo is only a few millimetres long. The growing fetus usually obtains nourishment at the expense of the mother, who tends to suffer in periods of adversity, but placental size and unrestricted blood flow through placental vessels to and from the fetus are important for optimal growth, especially during the last trimester. Fetal nutrition and the uterine environment are likely to play a part in the transcription of the genomic blueprint acquired at conception into the phenotypic newborn. Some of these developmental adaptations are now known to have long-term effects on the later risk of osteoporosis, sarcopenia and osteoarthritis. During early childhood, growth is rapid and there are windows of opportunity for environmental or lifestyle factors to have long-term effects, especially on the skeleton.

Puberty, which occurs much earlier in girls, brings growth to an end and its timing will have long-term consequences for adult stature. Women are on average physically disadvantaged compared to men throughout adult life because they have smaller skeletons and about 30% less absolute strength. They have an even poorer strength-for-weight ratio due to their extra body fat. Lower levels of physical activity which are encouraged socially, at least in the developed Western countries, compound their inevitable disadvantage.

Human ageing is accompanied by marked changes in the quantity and composition of all three musculoskeletal components. These changes underlie the enormous public health problem attributable to muscle weakness and musculoskeletal disorders in later life. It has been estimated that around 40% of adult women suffer from musculoskeletal pain (Badley and Tennant 1992). The prevalence increases markedly with age, so that at age 75–84 years some 20% of women report current back pain. The age-related losses of bone and muscle which lead to osteoporotic fracture (the most common musculoskeletal disorder in Western populations), are major contributors to this morbidity, and even mortality. It is estimated that around 40% of all white women and 13% of white men in the United States aged 50 years will experience a clinically apparent fragility fracture during their lifetime (Cooper and Melton 1996), as a result of age-related bone loss. Women are at greater risk not only because of their smaller skeletons, but also due to their dependence

Developmental Origins of Health and Disease, ed. Peter Gluckman and Mark Hanson. Published by Cambridge University Press.

on the protective effect of oestrogen, which is lost at menopause.

In this chapter we shall review the normal patterns of bone and muscle growth, the relevance of these physiological measures to later disease, and the growing body of evidence from epidemiological and mechanistic studies that environmental influences during intrauterine and early postnatal life might lead to reduced bone mass and muscle strength in late adulthood, with a consequent increase in the risk of osteoporotic fracture.

Normal skeletal growth

Peak bone mass

At any age, the size and quality of an individual's skeleton reflect everything that has happened from intrauterine life through the years of growth into young adulthood. The skeleton grows as the body grows, in length, breadth, mass and volumetric density. For men and women of normal body weight, total skeletal mass peaks a few years after fusion of the long bone epiphyses. The exact age at which bone mineral accumulation reaches a plateau varies with skeletal region and with how bone mass is measured. Areal density, the most commonly used measurement with dual-energy X-ray absorptiometry (DXA), peaks earliest (prior to age 20 years) at the proximal femur, while total skeletal mass peaks six to ten years later (Matkovic *et al.* 1994). However, total skeletal mass does not reflect the considerable heterogeneity in mineral accrual at other skeletal sites. Thus the skull continues to increase in bone mass throughout life; certain regions such as the femoral shaft and vertebral bodies continue to increase in diameter in late adulthood.

The importance of peak bone mass for bone strength during later life was initially suggested by cross-sectional observations that the dispersion of bone mass does not widen with age (Newton-John and Morgan 1970). This led to the proposition that bone mass tracks throughout life and that an individual at the high end of the population distribution at age 30 years is likely to remain at that end at age 70 years. Recent longitudinal studies have confirmed this tracking, at least across the pubertal growth spurt (Ferrari *et al.* 1998).

Bone growth in utero

The fetal skeleton develops in two distinct components, intramembranous (the skull and facial bones) and endochondral (the remainder of the skeleton) ossification. Intramembranous ossification begins with a layer or membrane of mesenchymal cells which becomes highly vascular; the mesenchymal cells then differentiate into isolated osteoblasts, which begin to secrete osteoid. The osteoid matrix is mineralised at the end of the embryonic period to form bony spicules which are precursors of the lamellae of the Haversian systems. There is no cartilage model preceding ossification in this type of bone development.

Endochondral ossification is responsible for the formation of the bones which are the main sites of fragility fracture in later life. This form of ossification depends on a pre-existing cartilaginous model that undergoes invasion by osteoblasts and is only subsequently mineralised. The development of this cartilage model can be seen by five weeks gestation with the migration and condensation of mesenchymal cells in areas destined to form the bone (DeLise *et al.* 2000). These pre-cartilagenous anlagen reflect the shape, size, position and number of skeletal elements which will be present in the mature skeleton. There is then an ordered differentiation of mesenchymal stem cells into chondrocyte precursors, proliferative chondrocytes, prehypertrophic chondrocytes and hypertrophic chondrocytes. During these stages of differentiation there is expansion of the bony template and production of an extracellular matrix rich in cytokines which facilitate vascular invasion and mineralisation. The major regulator of the proliferation of chondrocytes is parathyroid hormone-related protein (PTHrP) (Karaplis *et al.* 1994), which is secreted by the perichondral cells; other proliferative stimuli include cytokines of the GH/IGF axis (Bhaumick and Bala 1991). 1,25 $(OH)_2$

vitamin D_3 (Sylvia *et al.* 2001) and tri-iodothyronine (Quarto *et al.* 1997) are stimuli for the differentiation of the chondrocytes through different stages. Once the cartilage model has been formed, vascular growth factors embedded in the matrix are released by chondrocyte metalloproteinases. This stimulates angiogenesis and, under the influence of Cbfa1 (Ducy 2000), osteoblasts from the perichondrium invade and lay down matrix which is then mineralised.

During the period of a normal human pregnancy the fetus accumulates approximately 30 g of calcium, the majority of which is accrued during the third trimester (Widdowson *et al.* 1988). To supply this demand, there is a requirement for (1) an adequate maternal supply of calcium to the placenta and (2) increased placental calcium transfer to maintain a higher fetal serum calcium concentration than in the mother (Schauberger and Pitkin 1979). This maternofetal gradient emerges as early as 20 weeks of gestation (Forestier *et al.* 1987). There is increased calcium absorption from the gut and also bone resorption to meet this demand. A rise in maternal serum PTHrP and 1,25 $(OH)_2$ vitamin D_3 (Ardawi *et al.* 1997) is thought to drive the maternal supply of calcium to the fetus. Net resorption of the maternal skeleton, liberating calcium, starts early in gestation (Purdie *et al.* 1988), at a time when the fetal demand is small, and this contributes to maternal calciuria during pregnancy (Gambacciani *et al.* 1995). During the last trimester, maternal bone formation increases to balance bone resorption (Black *et al.* 2000). However, there is an overall decrease in the maternal bone mass of up to 10% during pregnancy (Gambacciani *et al.* 1995). Active calcium transfer across the placenta takes place in the cytotrophoblasts and involves storage of calcium by calcium-binding proteins in the cytoplasm and in the endoplasmic reticulum (Hosking 1996). Whilst in the mother 1,25 $(OH)_2$ vitamin D_3 is the principal stimulus for calcium absorption, the mid portion of PTHrP is essential at the placenta for the maintenance of the maternofetal gradient (Kovacs *et al.* 1996). Secretion of PTHrP by the fetal parathyroid glands also enhances fetal renal calcium reabsorption. The rate of maternofetal calcium transfer increases dramatically after 24 weeks, such that around two-thirds of total body calcium, phosphorous and magnesium are accumulated in a healthy term human fetus during this period. Factors which increase placental calcium transport capacity as gestation proceeds are only partly genetically controlled, and are achieved through regulatory hormones including 1,25 $(OH)_2$ vitamin D_3, parathyroid hormone, PTHrP and calcitonin. As the majority of fetal bone is gained during the last trimester, one of the major variables affecting bone mass at birth is gestational age. Other factors known to influence neonatal bone mineral content (BMC) include environmental variables such as season of birth and maternal lifestyle. Newborn total-body bone mineral content has been demonstrated to be lower among winter births than among infants born during the summer (Namgung *et al.* 1998). This observation is concordant with lower cord serum 25 $(OH)_2$ vitamin D concentrations observed during winter months, consequent upon maternal vitamin D deficiency. Other postulated contributors to impaired bone mineral acquisition during intrauterine life include maternal smoking, alcohol consumption, caffeine intake and diabetes mellitus (Specker *et al.* 2001).

Bone mineral accrual in infancy and early childhood

During infancy, average whole-body BMC increases by 389%, and total-body bone mineral density (BMD) increases by 157% (Koo *et al.* 1998). Weight and length are strong predictors of areal BMC and BMD during infancy (Li *et al.* 1989). However, because no studies of volumetric BMD have been done during the first year of life, it is not clear whether true volumetric density changes during this period. Gilsanz and colleagues (1991) found no significant differences in true volumetric density of the lumbar spine, measured using computed tomography, between male or female, black or white children aged greater than 2 years.

Developmental origins of osteoporosis and fracture

Epidemiological studies of coronary heart disease performed over a decade ago demonstrated strong geographic associations between death rate from the disorder in 1968–78 and infant mortality in 1901–10 (Barker 1995a). Subsequent research, based on individuals whose birth records had been preserved for seven decades, revealed that men and women who were undernourished during intrauterine life, and therefore had low birthweight or were thin at birth, had an increased risk for coronary heart disease, hypertension, non-insulin dependent diabetes and hypercholesterolaemia (Barker 1995b). These associations are explained by a phenomenon known as programming (Lucas 1991); this term describes persisting changes in structure and function caused by environmental stimuli acting at critical periods during early development. During embryonic life, the basic form of the human baby is laid down in miniature. However, the body does not increase greatly in size until the fetal period, when a rapid growth phase commences which continues until after birth. The main feature of fetal growth is cell division. Different tissues of the body grow during periods of rapid cell division, so-called 'critical' periods (McCance and Widdowson 1974). Their timing differs for different tissues; for example, the kidney has one in the weeks immediately before birth, while the long bones accelerate their rate of growth during the second trimester of gestation. The main adaptive response to a lack of nutrients and oxygen during this period of growth is to slow the rate of cell division, especially in tissues which are undergoing critical periods at the time. This reduction in cell division is either direct or mediated through altered concentrations of growth factors or hormones (in particular insulin, growth hormone and cortisol).

It is not in question that the human skeleton can be programmed by undernutrition. Rickets has served as a long-standing example of undernutrition at a critical stage of early life, leading to persisting changes in structure. What is new is the realisation that some of the body's 'memories' of early undernutrition become translated into pathology and thereby determine disease in later life. Evidence has now accumulated that such intrauterine programming contributes to the risk of osteoporosis in later life.

Evidence that the risk of osteoporosis might be modified by environmental influences during early life stems from four groups of studies: (a) bone mineral measurements undertaken in cohorts of adults whose detailed birth and/or childhood records have been preserved; (b) detailed physiological studies exploring the relationship between candidate endocrine systems which might be programmed (GH/IGF1, hypothalamic–pituitary–adrenal, gonadal steroid) and age-related bone loss; (c) studies characterising the nutrition, body build and lifestyle of pregnant women and relating these to the bone mass of their newborn offspring; and (d) studies relating childhood growth rates to the later risk of hip fracture.

Epidemiological studies

The first epidemiological evidence that osteoporosis risk might be programmed came from a study of 153 women born in Bath, UK, during 1968–69 who were traced and studied at age 21 years (Cooper *et al.* 1995). Data on childhood growth were obtained from linked birth and school health records. There were statistically significant ($p < 0.05$) associations between weight at one year and bone mineral content, but not density, at the lumbar spine and femoral neck; these relationships were independent of adult weight and body mass index. The data suggested a discordance between the processes which govern skeletal growth and those which influence mineralisation. They also provided direct evidence that the trajectory of bone growth might be modified in utero, an assertion previously only supported by inference from measurements of body height. The association between weight in infancy and adult bone mass was replicated in a second cohort study of 238 men and 201 women aged 60–75 years, who were born and still lived in Hertfordshire (Cooper *et al.* 1997). In this study, there were highly significant relationships

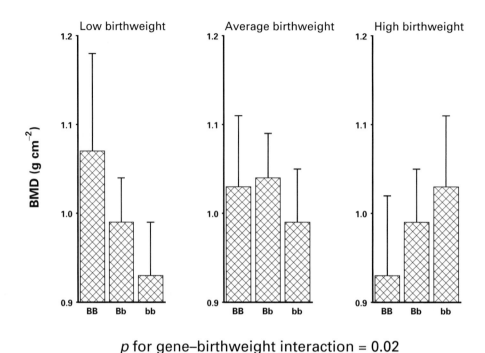

p for gene–birthweight interaction = 0.02

Figure 29.1 Relation between *VDR* genotype (BB, Bb, bb), birthweight and lumbar spine BMD among 165 men and 126 women resident in Hertfordshire. Data derived from Dennison *et al.* (2001).

between weight at 1 year and adult bone area at the spine and hip ($p < 0.005$); the relationships with BMC at these two sites were weaker but remained statistically significant ($p < 0.02$). They also remained after adjustment for known genetic markers of osteoporosis risk, such as polymorphisms in the gene for the vitamin D receptor (VDR) (Keen *et al.* 1997), and after adjustment for lifestyle characteristics in adulthood which might have influenced bone mass (physical activity, dietary calcium intake, cigarette smoking and alcohol consumption). More detailed analyses of the interactions between polymorphism in the *VDR* gene, birthweight and bone mineral density have recently been published from the same cohort study (Dennison *et al.* 2001). In the cohort as a whole, there were no significant associations between either birthweight or *VDR* genotype and bone mineral density. However, the relationship between lumbar spine BMD and *VDR* genotype varied according to birthweight (Fig. 29.1). Among individuals in the lowest

third of birthweight, spine BMD was higher ($p = 0.01$) among individuals of genotype 'BB' after adjustment for age, sex and weight at baseline. In contrast, spine BMD was reduced ($p = 0.04$) in individuals of the same genotype who were in the highest third of the birthweight distribution. A statistically significant ($p = 0.02$) interaction was also found between *VDR* genotype and birthweight as determinants of BMD. These results suggest that genetic influences on adult bone size and mineral density may be modified by undernutrition in utero. Subsequent studies from the United States, Australia and Scandinavia have replicated these relationships between weight in infancy and adult bone mass.

Physiological studies

To explore further the potential role of hypothalamic–pituitary function and its relevance to the pathogenesis of osteoporosis, profiles of circulating

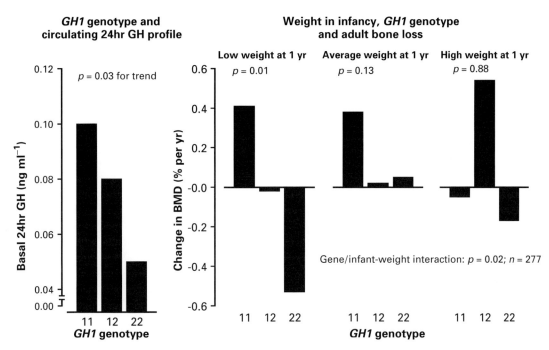

Figure 29.2 *GH1* genotype, 24-hour GH concentration, weight in infancy and adult bone loss: Hertfordshire cohort study. Data derived from Dennison *et al.* (2004).

growth hormone (GH) and cortisol were compared with bone density among groups of men and women whose birth records had been preserved. These studies revealed that birthweight and weight in infancy were predictors of basal levels of GH and cortisol during late adult life (Fall *et al.* 1998, Phillips *et al.* 1998, Dennison *et al.* 1999). The levels of these two skeletally active hormones were also found to be determinants of prospectively determined rate of bone loss. The data are compatible with the hypothesis that environmental stressors during intrauterine or early postnatal life alter the sensitivity of the growth plate to GH and cortisol. The consequence of such endocrine programming would be to reduce peak skeletal size, perhaps also to reduce mineralisation, and to predispose to an accelerated rate of bone loss during later life (Fall *et al.* 1998, Phillips *et al.* 1998, Dennison *et al.* 1999). Recent studies suggest that interactions between the genome and early environment might establish basal levels of

circulating GH, and thereby contribute to accelerated bone loss (Dennison *et al.* 2004). A single nucleotide polymorphism has been discovered at locus GH1-A5157G in the promoter region of the human growth hormone (*GH1*) gene. This is associated with significantly lower basal GH concentration, lower baseline BMD and accelerated bone loss (Fig. 29.2). As with polymorphism in the gene for the vitamin D receptor, a significant ($p = 0.02$) interaction was observed between weight at one year, allelic variation at this site and rate of bone loss.

Maternal nutrition, lifestyle and neonatal bone mineral

The third piece of epidemiological evidence that osteoporosis might arise in part through developmental maladaptation stems from investigation of a series of mothers through pregnancy; maternal anthropometric and lifestyle characteristics were

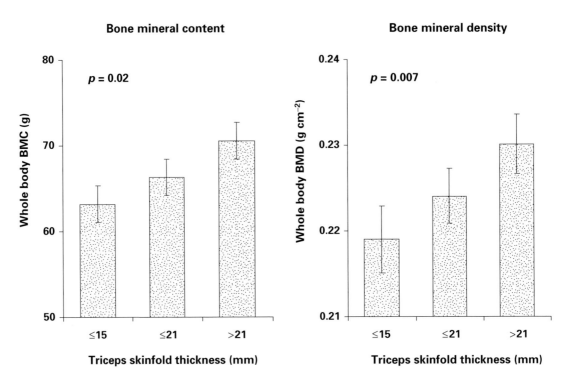

Figure 29.3 Maternal triceps skinfold thickness in early pregnancy and neonatal bone mineral among 144 term neonates. Data derived from Godfrey *et al.* (2001).

related to the bone mineral of their newborn offspring (Godfrey *et al.* 2001). After adjusting for sex and gestational age, neonatal bone mass was strongly positively associated with birthweight, birth length and placental weight. Other determinants included maternal and paternal birthweight, and maternal triceps skinfold thickness at 28 weeks (Fig. 29.3). Maternal smoking, and maternal energy intake at 18 weeks gestation, were negatively associated with neonatal BMC at both the spine and whole body (Fig. 29.4). The independent effects of maternal and paternal birthweight on fetal skeletal development support the notion that paternal influences, for example through the imprinting of growth-promoting genes such as IGF2, contribute strongly to the establishment of the early skeletal growth trajectory, while maternal nutrition and body build modify

fetal nutrient supply and subsequent bone accretion, predominantly through influences on placentation.

In the most recent data from mother/offspring cohorts, body composition has been assessed by DXA in 216 children at age 9 years (Harvey *et al.* 2004). They and their parents had previously been included in a population-based study of maternal nutrition and fetal growth. The nutrition, body build and lifestyle of the mothers had been characterised during early and late pregnancy, and samples of umbilical venous blood had been obtained at birth. Reduced maternal height, lower pre-conceptional maternal weight, reduced maternal fat stores during late pregnancy, a history of maternal smoking and lower maternal social class were all associated with reduced whole-body BMC of the child at age 9 years. Lower ionised calcium concentration in umbilical

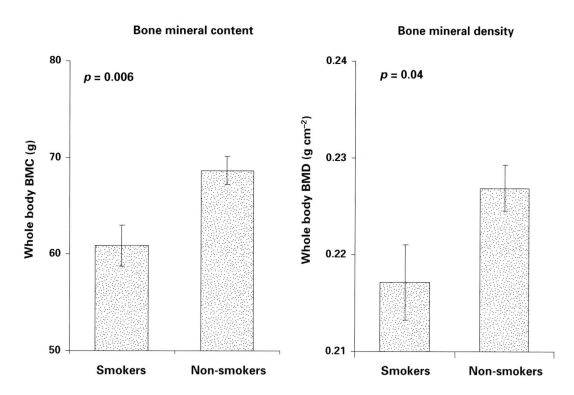

Figure 29.4 Maternal smoking during pregnancy and neonatal bone mineral among 144 term neonates. Data derived from Godfrey *et al.* (2001).

venous serum also predicted reduced childhood bone mass ($r = 0.19$, $p = 0.02$); this association appeared to mediate the effect of maternal fat stores, smoking and socioeconomic status on the bone mass of the children at age 9 years. Around 25% of the mothers had suboptimal vitamin D status as assessed by serum 25-hydroxyvitamin D concentration. The children born to these mothers had significantly ($p < 0.01$) reduced whole-body bone mineral content at age 9 years. This deficit in skeletal growth remained significant even after adjustment for childhood weight and bone area (Harvey *et al.* 2004). These data suggest that the placental capacity to maintain the maternofetal calcium gradient is important in optimising the trajectory of postnatal skeletal growth.

Childhood growth and hip fracture

Most evidence relating the intrauterine environment to later osteoporosis stems from studies utilising non-invasive assessment of bone mineral. The clinically important consequence of reduced bone mass is fracture, and data are now available which directly link growth rates in childhood with the risk of later hip fracture (Cooper *et al.* 2001). Studies of a unique Finnish cohort in whom birth and childhood growth data were linked to later hospital discharge records for hip fracture, have permitted follow-up of around 7000 men and women who were born in Helsinki University Central Hospital during 1924–33. Body size at birth was recorded and an average of 10 measurements were obtained of height and weight

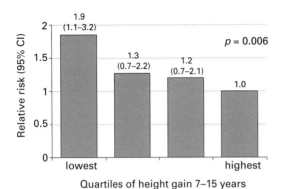

Figure 29.5 Rate of childhood height gain between age 7 and 15 years, and later risk of hip fracture among 3639 men and 3447 women born in Helsinki University Central Hospital between 1924 and 1933. Data derived from Cooper *et al.* (2001).

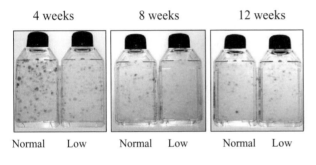

Figure 29.6 Capacity to form alkaline phosphatase-positive colony-forming units in an animal model of skeletal programming. From Oreffo *et al.* (2003).

throughout childhood. Hip-fracture incidence was assessed in this cohort using the Finnish hospital discharge registration system. After adjustment for age and sex, there were two major determinants of hip-fracture risk: tall maternal height ($p < 0.001$), and low rate of childhood growth (height, $p = 0.006$; weight, $p = 0.01$) (Fig. 29.5). The effects of maternal height and childhood growth rate were statistically independent of each other, and remained after adjusting for socioeconomic status. More important, hip-fracture risk was also elevated ($p = 0.05$) among babies born short. These data are compatible with endocrine programming influencing the risk of hip fracture. In addition, the observation that fracture subjects were shorter at birth, but of average height by age 7 years, suggests that hip-fracture risk might be particularly elevated among children in whom growth of the skeletal envelope is forced ahead of the capacity to mineralise, a phenomenon which is accelerated during pubertal growth.

Developmental plasticity and osteoporosis

Numerous animal experiments have shown that hormones, undernutrition and other influences that affect development during sensitive periods of early life permanently programme the structure and physiology of the body's tissues and systems. A remarkable example is the effect of temperature on the sex of reptiles (Barker 1998). If the eggs of an American alligator are incubated at 30 °C, all the offspring are female. If incubated at 33 °C, all the offspring are male. At temperatures between 30 and 33 °C, there are varying proportions of females and males. It is believed that the fundamental sex is female, and a transcription factor is required to divert growth along a male pathway. Instead of the transcription factor being controlled genetically by a sex chromosome, it depends on the environment, specifically temperature.

Organ systems in the body are most susceptible to developmental programming during periods when they are growing rapidly. During the first two months of life, the embryonic period, there is extensive differentiation of progenitor cells, without rapid cell replication. Thereafter, in the fetal period, the highest growth rates are observed. Growth slows in late gestation and continues to slow in childhood. The high growth rates of the fetus compared with the child are mostly the result of cell replication; the proportion of cells which are dividing becomes progressively less as the fetus becomes older. Slowing of growth is a major adaptation to undernutrition. Experiments on rats, mice, sheep and pigs have demonstrated that protein or calorie restriction of the mother during pregnancy and lactation is associated with smaller offspring (Chow and Lee 1964, McCance and Widdowson 1974, Smart *et al.* 1987, Barker 1998). In general, the earlier in life that undernutrition occurs, the more likely it is to have permanent effects on

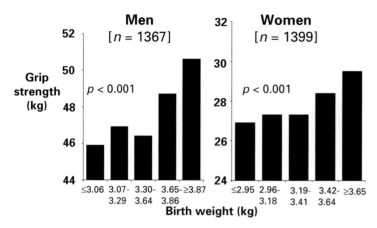

Figure 29.7 Grip strength at 53 years according to birthweight in the National Survey of Health and Development 1946 birth cohort. From Kuh *et al.* (2002).

body size (McCance and Widdowson 1962). Early in embryonic life, growth is regulated by the supply of nutrients and oxygen. At some point shortly after birth, growth begins to track. In humans, tracking is demonstrated by the way in which infants grow along centile curves. Once tracking is established, it is no longer possible to make animals grow faster by offering them unlimited food. The rate of growth has become set, homeostatically controlled by feedback systems. After a period of undernutrition, they will regain their expected size. This contrasts with the effects of undernutrition during intrauterine life, in which skeletal development is slowed and the peak skeletal proportions attained following the completion of linear growth are reduced.

There are three cellular mechanisms for the induction of programming. First, the nutrient environment may permanently alter gene expression; one example of this is permanent change in the activity of metabolic enzymes such as HMG-CoA reductase (Brown *et al.* 1990). Second, early nutrition may permanently reduce cell numbers. The small but normally proportioned rat produced by undernutrition before weaning has been shown to have fewer cells in its organs and tissues (McLeod *et al.* 1972). Growth-retarded human babies have reduced numbers of cells in their pancreas, which may limit insulin secretion (Snoeck *et al.* 1990), and reduced size of their airways, which may limit respiratory function

(Matsui *et al.* 1989). Third, certain clones of cells may be altered by environmental adversity during development; for example, an altered balance of the Th1 and Th2 lymphocyte subtypes might predispose to atopic disease in later life (Godfrey *et al.* 1994). Evidence from the human studies outlined above suggests that skeletal development might be programmed as a consequence of the first two of these mechanisms.

Animal models for the developmental origins of osteoporosis replicate the observations made in humans. In the first such model, the feeding of a low-protein diet to pregnant rats produced offspring that exhibited a reduction in bone area and BMC, with altered growth-plate morphology in adulthood (Mehta *et al.* 2002). Maternal protein restriction also down-regulated the proliferation and differentiation of bone-marrow stromal cells (Fig. 29.6) (Oreffo *et al.* 2003), as assessed by fibroblast colony formation at four and eight weeks.

Sarcopenia

Sarcopenia is defined as the loss of muscle mass and strength with ageing. The relationship between birthweight and muscle strength in later life, first described in the Hertfordshire Ageing Study (Aihie Sayer *et al.* 1998) has been replicated using a

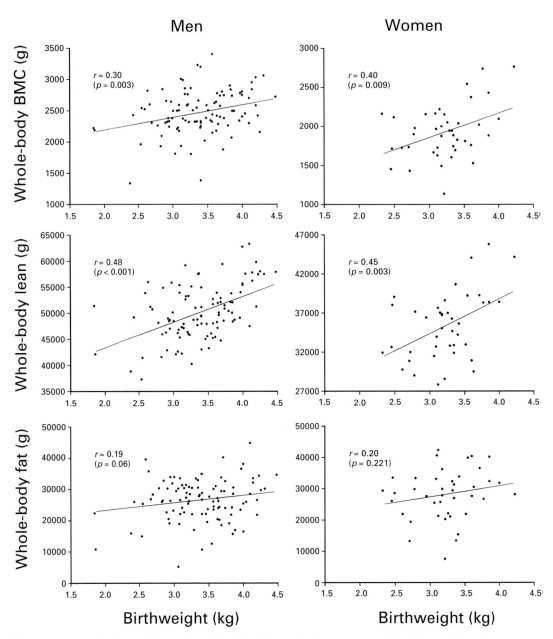

Figure 29.8 Relationship between birthweight and whole-body bone mineral content assessed by dual-energy X-ray absorptiometry (DXA) among 143 men and women aged 70–75 years born in Sheffield, UK. From Gale *et al.* (2001).

prospective national birth cohort of 1367 men and 1399 women, aged 53 years (Fig. 29.7) (Kuh *et al.* 2002). This study was also able to investigate the effect of childhood growth on adult muscle function, and demonstrated that there was no interaction between birthweight and later body size. A potential underlying mechanism is that birthweight is related to the number of muscle fibres that are established in an individual at birth, and that even in middle age compensating hypertrophy may be inadequate.

The relationship between birthweight and muscle strength may reflect a common genetic mechanism, but this has been little explored. One study investigated the role of polymorphism in the *IGF2* gene (Aihie Sayer *et al.* 2002). The product of this gene, insulin-like growth factor 2, is central to fetal growth and has a proliferative action in adult muscle. However, the study showed that birthweight and polymorphism of the *IGF2* gene had independent effects on grip strength in men, suggesting that this polymorphism did not explain the observed association between early growth and grip.

Adult muscle mass, as estimated by urinary creatinine excretion, is also related to early size independent of adult size (Phillips 1995). A study of men and women aged 50 years showed that muscle mass was predicted by low birthweight and small head circumference, but not by thinness at birth. A study of adult body composition in 143 people aged 65–75 years using whole-body DXA confirmed that low birthweight was associated with significantly lower adult lean mass in both men and women. About 25% of the variation in whole-body lean mass was explained by birthweight. There was no significant relationship with fat mass, but low birthweight was related to lower bone mass (Fig. 29.8) (Gale *et al.* 2001). This suggests that allocation of cells to different body compartments (muscle, bone and fat) during critical periods of development may be influenced by early growth and nutrition.

Conclusions

Several modifiable factors influence the growing musculoskeletal system and permit it to achieve

its full genetic potential. These may act during intrauterine or early postnatal life, in childhood, or in adolescence. While many important research questions need to be addressed in this area, concerted action in health policy should be directed at: (1) optimising maternal nutrition and intrauterine growth; (2) improving the calcium intake and general nutritional levels of all children; (3) increasing the general exercise level of prepubertal and pubertal children; (4) ensuring adequate vitamin D status, not just during infancy but throughout the period of growth. Further research into the interaction between the genome and early environmental risk factors for osteoporotic fracture is urgently required, in order that environmental modification can be targeted to those at the greatest risk. Finally, intervention studies exploring the role of maternal lifestyle and nutrition on bone mineral accrual will provide much-needed evidence on this approach to the reduction in fracture risk of future generations.

ACKNOWLEDGMENTS

We are grateful to the Medical Research Council, the Wellcome Trust, the Arthritis Research Campaign, the National Osteoporosis Society and the British Heart Foundation for support of our research programme into the developmental origins of osteoporotic fracture. The manuscript was prepared by Gill Strange.

REFERENCES

Aihie Sayer, A., Cooper, C., Evans, J. R. *et al.* (1998). Are rates of ageing determined *in utero*? *Age Ageing*, **27**, 579–83.

Aihie Sayer, A., Syddall, H., O'Dell, S. D. *et al.* (2002). Polymorphism of the IGF-2 gene, birthweight and grip strength in adult men. *Age Ageing*, **31**, 468–70.

Ardawi, M. S. M., Nasrat, H. A. N. and BA'Aqueel, H. S. (1997). Calcium-regulating hormones and parathyroid hormone-related peptide in normal human pregnancy and postpartum: a longitudinal study. *Eur. J. Endocrinol.*, **137**, 402–9.

Badley, E. M. and Tennant, A. (1992). The changing profile of joint troubles with age: findings from a postal survey of the population. *Ann. Rheum. Dis.*, **51**, 366–71.

Barker, D. J. P. (1995a). Fetal origins of coronary heart disease. *BMJ*, **311**, 171–4.

Barker, D. J. P. (1995b). The fetal origins of adult disease. *Proc. R. Soc. Lond. B*, **262**, 37–43.

(1998). Programming the baby. In *Mothers, Babies and Health in Later Life* (ed. D. J. P. Barker). Edinburgh: Churchill Livingstone, pp. 13–41.

Bhaumick, B. and Bala, R. M. (1991). Differential effects of insulin-like growth factors I and II on growth, differentiation and glucoregulation in differentiating chondrocyte cells in culture. *Acta Endocrinol. (Copenh.)*, **125**, 201–11.

Black, A. J., Topping, J., Durham, B., Farquharson, R. G. and Fraser, W. D. (2000). A detailed assessment of alterations in bone turnover, calcium homeostasis, and bone density in normal pregnancy. *J. Bone Miner. Res.*, **15**, 557–63.

Brown, S. A., Rogers, L. K., Dunn, J. K., Gotto, A. M. and Patsch, W. (1990). Development of cholesterol homeostatic memory in the rat is influenced by maternal diets. *Metabolism*, **39**, 468–73.

Chow, B. F. and Lee, C. J. (1964). Effect of dietary restriction of pregnant rats on body weight gain of the offspring. *J. Nutr.*, **82**, 10–18.

Cooper, C. and Melton, L. J. (1996). Magnitude and impact of osteoporosis and fractures. In *Osteoporosis* (ed. R. Marcus, D. Feldman and J. Kelsey). San Diego, CA: Academic Press, pp. 419–34.

Cooper, C., Cawley, M. I. D., Bhalla, A. *et al.* (1995). Childhood growth, physical activity and peak bone mass in women. *J. Bone Miner. Res.*, **10**, 940–7.

Cooper, C., Fall, C., Egger, P., Hobbs, R., Eastell, R. and Barker, D. (1997). Growth in infancy and bone mass in later life. *Ann. Rheum. Dis.*, **56**, 17–21.

Cooper, C., Eriksson, J. G., Forsén, T., Osmond, C., Tuomilehto, J. and Barker, D. J. P. (2001). Maternal height, childhood growth and risk of hip fracture in later life: a longitudinal study. *Osteoporos. Int.*, **12**, 623–9.

DeLise, A. M., Fischer, L. and Tuan, R. S. (2000). Cellular interactions and signaling in cartilage development. *Osteoarthritis Cartilage*, **8**, 309–34.

Dennison, E., Hindmarsh, P., Fall, C. *et al.* (1999). Profiles of endogenous circulating cortisol and bone mineral density in healthy elderly men. *J. Clin. Endocrinol. Metab.*, **84**, 3058–63.

Dennison, E. M., Arden, N. K., Keen, R. W. *et al.* (2001). Birthweight, vitamin D receptor genotype and the programming of osteoporosis. *Paediatr. Perinat. Epidemiol.*, **15**, 211–19.

Dennison, E. M., Syddall, H. E., Rodriguez, S., Voropanov, A., Day, I. N. M., Cooper, C., and the Southampton Genetic Epidemiology Research Group (2004). Polymorphism in the growth hormone gene, weight in infancy, and adult bone mass. *J. Clin. Endocrinol. Metab.*, **89**, 4898–903.

Ducy, P. (2000). Cbfa1: a molecular switch in osteoblast biology. *Dev. Dyn.*, **219**, 461–71.

Fall, C., Hindmarsh, P., Dennison, E., Kellingray, S., Barker, D. and Cooper, C. (1998). Programming of growth hormone secretion and bone mineral density in elderly men: an hypothesis. *J. Clin. Endocrinol. Metab.*, **83**, 135–9.

Ferrari, S., Rizzoli, R., Slosman, D. and Bonjour, J. P. (1998). Familial resemblance for bone mineral mass is expressed before puberty. *J. Clin. Endocrinol. Metab.*, **83**, 358–61.

Forestier, F., Daffos, F., Rainaut, M., Bruneau, M. and Trivin, F. (1987). Blood chemistry of normal human fetuses at midtrimester of pregnancy. *Pediatr. Res.*, **21**, 579–83.

Gale, C. R., Martyn C. N., Kellingray, S., Eastell, R. and Cooper, C. (2001). Intrauterine programming of adult body composition. *J. Clin. Endocrinol. Metab.*, **86**, 267–72.

Gambacciani, M., Spinetti, A., Gallo, R., Cappagli, B., Teti, G. C. and Facchini, V. (1995). Ultrasonographic bone characteristics during normal pregnancy: longitudinal and cross-sectional evaluation. *Am. J. Obstet. Gynecol.*, **173**, 890–3.

Gilsanz, V., Roe, T. F., Mora, S., Costin, G. and Goodman, W. G. (1991). Changes in vertebral bone density in black girls and white girls during childhood and puberty. *N. Engl. J. Med.*, **325**, 1597–600.

Godfrey, K., Walker-Bone, K., Robinson, S. *et al.* (2001). Neonatal bone mass: influence of parental birthweight, maternal smoking, body composition, and activity during pregnancy. *J. Bone Miner. Res.*, **16**, 1694–703.

Godfrey, K. M., Barker, D. J. P. and Osmond, C. (1994). Disproportionate fetal growth and raised IGE concentration in adult life. *Clin. Exp. Allergy*, **24**, 641–8.

Harvey, N. C. W., Javaid, M. K., Taylor, P. *et al.* (2004). Umbilical cord calcium and maternal vitamin D status predict different lumbar spine bone parameters in the offspring at 9 years. *J. Bone. Miner. Res.*, **19**, 1032.

Hosking, D. J. (1996). Calcium homeostasis in pregnancy. *Clin. Endocrinol. (Oxf.)*, **45**, 1–6.

Karaplis, A. C., Luz, A., Glowacki, J. *et al.* (1994). Lethal skeletal dysplasia from targeted disruption of the parathyroid hormone-related peptide gene. *Genes Dev.*, **8**, 277–89.

Keen, R., Egger, P., Fall, C. *et al.* (1997). Polymorphisms of the vitamin D receptor, infant growth and adult bone mass. *Calcif. Tissue Int.*, **60**, 233–5.

Koo, W. W. K., Bush, A. J., Walters, J. and Carlson, S. E. (1998). Postnatal development of bone mineral status during infancy. *J. Am. Coll. Nutr.*, **17**, 65–70.

Kovacs, C. S., Lanske, B., Hunzelman, J. L., Guo, J., Karaplis, A. C. and Kronenberg, H. M. (1996). Parathyroid hormone-related peptide (PTHrP) regulates fetal–placental calcium transport through a receptor distinct from the PTH/PTHrP receptor. *Proc. Natl. Acad. Sci. USA*, **93**, 15233–8.

Kreisberg, R. A., Bowdoin, B. and Meador, C. K. (1970). Measurement of muscle mass in humans by isotopic dilution of creatine 14C. *J. Appl. Physiol.*, **28**, 264–7.

Kuh, D., Bassey, E. J., Hardy, R., Aihie Sayer, A., Wadsworth, M. and Cooper, C. (2002). Birthweight, childhood size and muscle strength in adult life: evidence from a birth cohort study. *Am. J. Epidemiol.*, **156**, 627–33.

Li, J. Y., Specker, B. L., Ho, M. L. and Tsang, R. C. (1989). Bone mineral content in black and white children 1–6 years of age. *Am. J. Dis. Child.*, **143**, 1346–9.

Lucas, A. (1991). Programming by early nutrition in man. In *The Childhood Environment and Adult Disease* (ed. G. R. Bock and J. Whelan). New York, NY: Wiley, pp. 38–55.

Matkovic, V., Jelic, T., Wardlaw, G. M. *et al.* (1994). Timing of peak bone mass in Caucasian females and its implication for the prevention of osteoporosis. *J. Clin. Invest.*, **93**, 799–808.

Matsui, R., Thurlbeck, W. M., Fujita, Y., Yu, S. Y. and Kida, K. (1989). Connective tissue, mechanical, and morphometric changes in the lungs of weanling rats fed a low protein diet. *Pediatr. Pulmonol.*, **7**, 159–66.

McCance, R. A. and Widdowson, E. M. (1962). Nutrition and growth. *Proc. R. Soc. Lond. B*, **156**, 326–37.

(1974). The determinants of growth and form. *Proc. R. Soc. Lond. B*, **185**, 1–17.

McLeod, K. I., Goldrick, R. B. and Whyte, H. M. (1972). The effect of maternal malnutrition on the progeny in the rat: studies on growth, body composition and organ cellularity in first and second generation progeny. *Aust. J. Exp. Biol. Med. Sci.*, **50**, 435–46.

Mehta, G., Roach, H. I., Langley-Evans, S. *et al.* (2002). Intrauterine exposure to a maternal low protein diet reduces adult bone mass and alters growth plate morphology in rats. *Calcif. Tissue Int.*, **71**, 493–8.

Namgung, R., Tsang, R. C., Lee, C., Han, D. G., Ho, M. L. and Sierra, R. I. (1998). Low total body bone mineral content and high bone resorption in Korean winter-born versus summer-born newborn infants. *J. Pediatr.*, **132**, 421–5.

Newton-John, H. F. and Morgan, B. D. (1970). The loss of bone with age, osteoporosis and fractures. *Clin. Orthop. Relat. Res.*, **71**, 229–52.

Oreffo, R. O. C., Lashbrooke, B., Roach, H. I., Clarke, N. M. P. and Cooper, C. (2003). Maternal protein deficiency affects mesenchymal stem cell activity in the developing offspring. *Bone*, **33**, 100–7.

Phillips, D. I. W. (1995). Relation of fetal growth to adult muscle mass and glucose tolerance. *Diabetic Med.*, **12**, 686–90.

Phillips, D. I. W., Barker, D. J. P., Fall, C. H. D. *et al.* (1998). Elevated plasma cortisol concentrations: a link between low birthweight and the insulin resistance syndrome? *J. Clin. Endocrinol. Metab.*, **83**, 757–60.

Purdie, D. W., Aaron, J. E. and Selby, P. L. (1988). Bone histology and mineral homeostasis in human pregnancy. *Br. J. Obstet. Gynaecol.*, **95**, 849–54.

Quarto, R., Campanile, G., Cancedda, R. and Dozin, B. (1997). Modulation of commitment, proliferation, and differentiation of chondrogenic cells in defined culture medium. *Endocrinology*, **138**, 4966–76.

Schauberger, C. W. and Pitkin, R. M. (1979). Maternal–perinatal calcium relationships. *Obstet. Gynecol.*, **53**, 74–6.

Simkin, P. A. (1994). The musculoskeletal system. In *Rheumatology*, (ed. J. H. Klippel and P. A., Dieppe). London: Mosby, pp. 1.2.1–1.2.10.

Smart, J. L., Massey, R. F., Nash, S. C. and Tonkiss, J. (1987). Effects of early life undernutrition in artificially reared rats: subsequent body and organ growth. *Br. J. Nutr.*, **58**, 245–55.

Snoeck, A., Remacle, C., Reusens, B. and Hoet, J. J. (1990). Effect of a low protein diet during pregnancy on the fetal rat endocrine pancreas. *Biol. Neonate*, **57**, 107–18.

Specker, B. L., Namgung, R. and Tsang, R. C. (2001). Bone mineral acquisition *in utero*, during infancy, and throughout childhood. In *Osteoporosis*, 2nd edn (ed. R. Marcus, D. Feldman and J. Kelsey). New York, NY: Academic Press, vol. 1, pp. 599–620.

Sylvia, V. L., Del Toro, F., Hardin, R. R., Dean, D. D., Boyan, B. D. and Schwartz, Z. (2001). Characterization of PGE(2) receptors (EP) and their role as mediators of 1alpha,25-(OH)(2)D(3) effects on growth zone chondrocytes. *J. Steroid Biochem. Mol. Biol.*, **78**, 261–74.

Widdowson, E. M., Southgate, D. A. T. and Hey, E. (1988). Fetal growth and body composition. In *Perinatal Nutrition* (ed. B. S. Landblad). New York, NY: Academic Press, pp. 3–14.

30

The developmental environment: experimental perspectives on skeletal development

Richard O. C. Oreffo and Helmtrud I. Roach

University of Southampton

Introduction

Osteoporosis is a multifactorial skeletal disorder characterised by low bone mass and microarchitectural deterioration of bony tissue, with a consequent increase in the risk of fracture (Jordan and Cooper 2002). The bone mass of an individual in later life depends upon the peak obtained during skeletal growth, and the subsequent rate of bone loss. Preventive strategies against osteoporotic fracture may be aimed at either increasing the peak bone mass attained or reducing the rates of bone loss. As shown in the previous chapter, epidemiological studies have indicated that poor growth during fetal life, infancy and childhood is associated with decreased bone mass in adulthood and an increased risk of fracture (Cooper *et al.* 1995, 1997, Fall *et al.* 1998). These relationships appear to be mediated through the programming of metabolic and endocrine systems governing bone growth, by environmental influences acting during critical periods of intrauterine or early postnatal development (Barker 1995, 2000, Barker and Martyn 1997, Godfrey and Barker 2001). In particular, maternal nutrition appears to be important in determining skeletal size at maturity. However, to date, there is little understanding of the cellular and molecular mechanisms whereby environmental modulation in utero could lead to an altered skeletal development among the offspring. This review will examine the benefits and information gained from animal models of intrauterine programming (maternal dietary modulation) with respect to the skeletal development of the young offspring, peak bone mass and bone quality of aged offspring, and will correlate to other animal studies undertaken ex utero and, as appropriate, to the human scenario.

The link between nutrition and bone development

Over the last 40 years, animal studies have proved informative of the role of nutrition in skeletal development. Seminal studies from Widdowson and McCance (1963) used a rat model and demonstrated that programming of growth may arise through nutritional modulation during critical windows of early life. They found that rats undernourished early on in bone development (3–6 weeks after birth) lost weight compared to control groups, permanently remaining smaller, even after resumption of a normal diet. In contrast, rats undernourished later on in bone development (9–12 weeks after birth) initially lost weight but regained their normal growth trajectory on resumption of a normal diet with 'catch-up growth' whereby their weight gain actually exceeded that of the control group. A further example of nutritional influences on bone development is rickets, where incomplete mineralisation of the organic bone matrix arises as a consequence of poor

Developmental Origins of Health and Disease, ed. Peter Gluckman and Mark Hanson. Published by Cambridge University Press.
© P. D. Gluckman and M. A. Hanson 2006.

childhood nutrition. Hence the postnatal influence of nutrition on bone development is well established, but much less is known about the long-term effects of prenatal maternal nutrition on bone development of the offspring.

Programming and skeletal development and function

In this chapter we shall summarise what is known to date about the consequences of a maternal nutritional challenge on the skeletal development of the offspring. The following parameters of bone development and structure have been studied so far: (1) the characteristics of bone-marrow stromal cells in young and skeletally mature rats; (2) the growth-plate structure at skeletal maturity and old age and (3) bone area, bone mineral content and bone mineral density in aged offspring.

The Langley-Evans model of fetal protein insufficiency

The best-characterised animal model for studying the effects of maternal nutritional deficiencies on the development of the offspring is the low-protein rat model developed by Langley-Evans (Langley and Jackson 1994). In essence, pregnant rats are either fed a diet containing 180 g casein per kg (control diet) or 90 g casein per kg (low-protein diet), balanced in energy content through the addition of carbohydrates. Throughout the studies, animals have free access to water and food at all times. After birth, the litters are culled to a maximum of eight pups per litter, and dams are fed the control diet, as are the pups after weaning. Thus any differences in bone development observed in the pups in later life could be attributed directly to protein insufficiency in utero. The feeding of a low-protein diet to pregnant rats produces offspring that exhibit growth retardation in late pregnancy. Pups from dams on a low-protein diet subsequently develop functional changes in adulthood, including hypertension, progressive deterioration of renal function, cardiovascu-

lar disease, impaired immune responses and altered life spans (Langley-Evans et al. 1996, 1999a, 1999b, Langley-Evans 1999, Aihie Sayer et al. 2001).

Effects of maternal protein deficiency on rat bone-marrow stromal cells

Bone formation and bone growth in the developing offspring depends on differentiation of bone-marrow mesenchymal stem cells into cells of the osteogenic lineage (Triffitt and Oreffo 1998, Bianco et al. 2001). Hence any effects on bone quality are likely to be a consequence of the regulation of osteoblast/mesenchymal stem-cell activity. It is likely, therefore, that alterations in the regulation of mesenchymal stem cell and osteoblastic activity are important candidate mechanisms for the programming of the skeletal growth trajectory by dietary protein restriction during intrauterine life. Using the Langley-Evans model of protein insufficiency, Oreffo and coworkers (2003) examined the cellular mechanisms involved in the programming of bone development, specifically whether colony formation (colony-forming unit–fibroblastic, CFU-F), proliferation and differentiation of bone-marrow stromal cells from offspring of female rats maintained on normal (18% casein) or low (9% casein) protein was altered, and whether their responses to growth hormone (GH), 1,25 $(OH)_2$ vitamin D_3 and IGF1 differed. Total CFU-F numbers, indicative of the colony-forming efficiency of the mesenchymal stem cells and proliferation potential of these cells, was found to be reduced by approximately 40% in cultures from offspring whose mothers were fed a low-protein diet compared to the normal-protein group at eight weeks (Fig. 30.1). However, no difference in total CFU-F was observed at 12 weeks between normal and low-protein group cultures. In contrast, at 16 weeks, a significant increase of 111% in total CFU-F number in the low-protein group compared to cultures from the control-group offspring was recorded.

Similar results were observed following examination of alkaline phosphatase-positive CFU-F number, indicative of osteogenic potential and

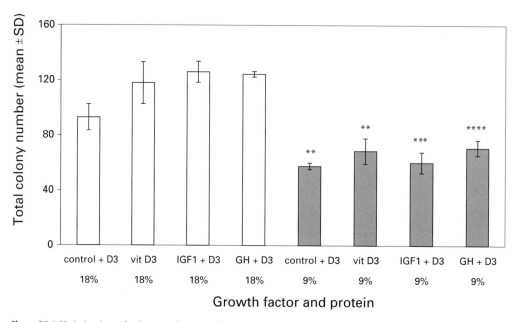

Figure 30.1 Variation in total colony number in rat bone-marrow cultures from offspring of mothers maintained on a control (18% casein) or low-protein (9% casein) diet. Significance levels refer to comparison of counterpart 18% and 9% protein group results analysed using Bonferroni multiple group analysis. ** $p < 0.01$, *** $p < 0.001$, **** $p < 0.0001$.

differentiation. At eight weeks, a significant reduction (approximately 90%) in alkaline phosphatase-positive CFU-F number was observed in cultures from the low-protein group compared to counterpart normal-protein cultures. At 12 weeks no significant differences between the groups were observed, while at 16 weeks, as observed for total CFU-F number, cultures from the low-protein group had significantly increased alkaline phosphatase-positive CFU-F numbers compared to normal-protein cultures. Interestingly, the addition of osteogenic growth factors, GH, 1,25 (OH)$_2$ vitamin D$_3$ and IGF1, under the conditions examined, was insufficient to overcome or reverse the effects of maternal dietary manipulation. The findings of altered CFU-F colony formation and alkaline phosphatase activity suggest an association between maternal diet in pregnancy and bone growth in the young offspring as assessed by parameters of osteoblast proliferation, with normal proliferation and differentiation of mesenchymal stem cells and subsequent skeletal maturity delayed as a consequence of maternal protein restriction during early life.

It is known that in rats puberty is reached at 9 weeks and skeletal maturity is attained at 13 weeks (Hughes and Tanner 1970). In skeletally mature offspring (12–16 weeks of age) whose mothers were fed a normal-protein diet, the reduction in CFU-F colony number and alkaline phosphatase-specific activity reflects reduced osteoblast activity as skeletal growth maturity is reached. In contrast, in offspring from mothers on a low-protein diet the reduced osteoblast activity/skeletal development at 8 weeks during peak skeletal growth, and the significantly increased osteoblast activity at 12 and 16 weeks, may be attributable to intrauterine programming, with subsequent 'catch-up' skeletal growth occurring at 12 and 16 weeks. These studies on bone-marrow stromal activity are limited by the absence of information from later time-points (greater than 20 weeks) that would indicate if the 'catch-up' in skeletal growth in the low-protein offspring is followed by a degree of growth overshoot.

Catch-up growth has previously been observed in malnourished rats. Studies by Reichling and German (2000) found that rats fed a low-protein diet from weaning (22 days) grew for longer periods, a finding replicated in a previous study looking at craniofacial development in rats (Miller and German 1999), which found that protein malnutrition affected growth trajectory, with animals growing for a significantly longer period of time. Both of these studies add support to the theory that maternal protein restriction may delay skeletal maturity.

The data from these animal studies are particularly intriguing when extrapolated to data from human studies such as the Finnish cohort (Cooper et al. 2001) and the Saskatchewan bone mineral accrual study (Bailey et al. 1999), in that maturational delay may increase the risk of hip fracture through altered accrual of bone density and disproportionate bone growth. Furthermore, a number of studies have shown that human intrauterine growth-retarded babies are capable of demonstrating a 'catch-up' of growth for various anthropometric parameters (Villar et al. 1982, 1984). Furthermore, Walther et al. (1981) found that infants malnourished in utero had a significant retardation in skeletal maturity at birth, when compared to infants in the control group. However, at 2.5–3.5 years of age, the average skeletal maturity of the intrauterine malnourished children approached that of controls, demonstrating 'catch-up' in skeletal growth during infancy.

Studies from Rizzoli's group (Bourrin et al. 2000a, 2000b, Ammann et al. 2000) have shown that dietary protein deprivation in adult rats results in decreased bone mineral mass as well as in thinning of cortical and trabecular bone leading to decreased bone strength. The same group (Bourrin et al. 2000b) found adult rats maintained on a restricted-protein diet (2.5% casein) had reduced plasma osteocalcin, IGF1, periosteal bone formation and mineral apposition rates, indicating decreased osteoblast recruitment and activity as a result of direct dietary manipulation in those animals. Thus these results, in combination with the studies from the maternal nutrition challenge studies, indicate that changes in osteoblast activity are, at least in part, a consequence of maternal dietary protein restriction and that, in turn, osteoblast activity will affect subsequent bone development of offspring.

Effects of maternal protein deficiency on growth-plate structure

Bone development and in particular the longitudinal growth of long bones depends on a functional growth plate with precise coordination, both temporally and spatially, of a multitude of processes. As is well known, overall skeletal growth is regulated systemically by growth hormone with important contributions from glucocorticoids and thyroid hormone (Siebler et al. 2001). At the growth plate, the effects of all three factors converge via locally acting IGF1, which binds to IGF1 receptors on chondrocytes, stimulating proliferation. Since the 'programming' by fetal protein insufficiency is thought to occur via the growth hormone neuroendocrine axis, any changes could potentially affect growth-plate structure and function, possibly mediated via the local availability of IGF1. However, IGF1 mainly influences cell proliferation, which is not the only aspect contributing to bone growth. In fact, the main parameters contributing to linear growth are matrix synthesis and cellular enlargement during hypertrophy (Hunziker and Schenk 1989, Breur et al. 1991, Kuhn et al. 1996, Farnum et al. 2002). For example, in the proximal tibial growth plate of a 4-week-old rat, which is in its pubertal growth spurt, only 9% of growth is contributed by proliferation, whereas 32% is due to matrix synthesis and 59% due to chondrocyte enlargement (Wilsman et al. 1996). Thus, to understand possible effects of 'programming' on the growth plate, an understanding of the regulation of longitudinal growth that occurs at the growth plate is critical.

Morphologically distinct zones, termed 'reserve' (or 'resting'), 'proliferative' and 'hypertrophic' zones, correspond to stages in chondrocyte differentiation. Reserve chondrocytes are committed progenitor cells that, upon receival of the IGF1 stimulus, start to proliferate, forming columns of flattened cells. In the lower proliferative/upper hypertrophic zone, a number of changes take place, including loss of proliferation and a considerable increase in cell volume, as chondrocytes differentiate into hypertrophic cells. Other accompanying changes include increased expression of alkaline phosphatase, type X collagen and vascular endothelial growth factor. Regulatory genes, such as Indian hedgehog (Kronenberg and Chung 2001), bone morphogenetic protein-6 (Grimsrud *et al.* 1999) and *RUNX2* are up-regulated as cells enter hypertrophy. Chondrocyte proliferation is maintained via the Indian hedgehog/PTHrP feedback loop and any interference with this loop results in stunted patterns of bone pattern. Finally, in the lower hypertrophic zone, calcification of the matrix is initiated (Anderson 1995) and chondrocytes undergo programmed cell death (Horton *et al.* 1998, Roach and Clarke 2000, Roach *et al.* 2004).

The role of fetal programming in modulation of these complex interactions is unclear, with only limited preliminary data available. However, the data available are suggestive of a possible interaction. In larger mammals (rabbit upwards), the growth plates close at skeletal maturity and longitudinal growth ceases. However, smaller mammals (rats, mice) maintain a growth plate into old age (Roach *et al.* 2003a). Upon examination of the growth plates of 8-week-old rats derived from mothers maintained on a low-protein diet or control diet (Langley-Evans model), the height of the growth plates from rats from the low-protein group was considerably greater than the growth-plate height from control rats. (Plate 7).

This finding was contrary to expectations, since the prediction had been that reduced IGF1 levels would slow down growth, which would be reflected in a decreased height of the growth plates. In rapidly growing animals, the height and morphology of the growth plates have a direct positive relationship to the rate of longitudinal growth. Thus the greater the height of the growth plate, the greater the rate of bone growth. Examination of anthropometric measurements between the two groups regarding tibial or femoral length, width, cortical width or trabecular bone volume showed no evidence of increased growth rates in pups from mothers on a low-protein diet. However, the relationship between growth-plate height and rate of longitudinal growth depends on the age of the animal. In young rats, the *rate* of growth increases between 1 and 5 weeks, then declines until skeletal maturity, which is achieved by 11.5–13 weeks (Kember 1973, Hunziker and Schenk 1989). Bones will continue to grow, albeit at a reduced rate, until about 26 weeks of age, after which growth virtually ceases in rats. Hence, after 5 weeks, the rate of growth starts to decline and the height of the growth plate progressively decreases (Roach *et al.* 2003a). During this time the height of the growth plate is inversely related to maturation, i.e. the greater the height, the lower the skeletal maturity. The growth plates of the low-protein pups had been examined at 8 weeks, a time when the rate of growth was in decline, and thus the increased height probably reflected a lesser degree of skeletal maturity.

After about 26 weeks of age, rats have virtually ceased to grow and growth-plate heights no longer change. However, changes take place within the growth-plate structure with increasing age, as described in detail by Roach *et al.* (2003a). The growth plates become increasingly irregular due to a combination of events. In some parts of the growth plates, chondrocyte death leads to large acellular areas, in other parts the 'core' cartilage is resorbed and replaced by bone, while in some regions direct bone formation by former growth-plate chondrocytes is observed.

To investigate whether the changes in growth-plate height that were observed in the offspring of the low-protein group at skeletal maturity persisted until old age, rats were maintained for over a year. Sixteen male offspring, closely matched for age, were selected for histological analyses of the proximal tibial growth plates. To take account of the above-mentioned irregularities in cartilage resorption and acellularity, several measures of the heights of the growth plates were taken and adjusted for these irregularities. Seventy measurements of growth-plate width were available from the seven animals in the control group and 90 from the nine animals in the low-protein group. Mehta and coworkers (2002) found that the height of the growth plates was significantly greater in rats that were protein-undernourished in utero (control mean 170 μm, 95% CI 20 μm; low-protein mean 220 μm, 95% CI 30 μm). These differences were highly statistically significant ($p < 0.001$) when analysed using a non-paired t-test and remained after Bonferroni correction for multiple testing. In the random effects model, which took account of gender, weight and effects within and between mothers, the trend towards higher growth plates in the offspring of dams fed a low-protein diet persisted, but became non-significant. These findings indicate that the height of the growth plate had been greater in this group at the time-point when longitudinal bone growth had ceased and suggest that the cessation of growth *at an earlier age* in the protein-undernourished rats.

The observed changes in the height and the nature of the growth cartilage may be secondary to other metabolic effects of developmental undernutrition. Nwagwu *et al.* (2000) recently demonstrated that the kidneys of rats exposed to a similar degree of intrauterine protein restriction were structurally different and lost function more rapidly than those of control animals. Although in the studies from Mehta *et al.* (2002) reliable causes of death were not established for most of the rats whose bones were analysed histologically, renal disease was a common finding at post mortem of the larger group of animals. Renal osteodystrophy is associated with disordered bone remodelling due to disruption of the complex interactions between parathyroid hormone, vitamin D_3 and local growth factors. Cobo *et al.* (1999) have also found increased growth-plate height, and irregularity at the growth cartilage–metaphyseal junction, in young rats with experimental renal failure. Therefore, although the animals used in this study were much older and there was unlikely to be any renal compromise during active skeletal growth, it is possible that an increased incidence of renal dysfunction in the aged rats caused changes in growth-plate morphology in late adulthood. In a parallel study, catabolic as well as anabolic phases of osteodystro-

phy could be demonstrated within the cortical bone in a subgroup of the aged rats (Roach *et al.* 2003b), but this was not correlated with maternal protein insufficiency. A further possibility is that intrauterine protein restriction may have programmed the function of the vitamin D system, resulting in rachitic effects on skeletal growth and the appearance of the growth plate. Investigation of these hypotheses was not examined in the studies from Mehta and coworkers (2002) due to the lack of data concerning renal function and vitamin D status in these animals.

An alternative interpretation is that the findings represent direct programming of bone growth. This explanation would be consistent with the observations made in human studies, where relationships between weight in infancy and adult bone mass are independent of renal function (Cooper *et al.* 1997). This interpretation is also supported by studies of the proliferation of growth-plate chondrocytes. During normal ageing, the proliferative rate of growth-plate chondrocytes diminishes with each successive cell cycle. Glucocorticoid administration to the growth plates suppresses proliferation of these chondrocytes (Baron *et al.* 1994), and thus the progenitor cells in the affected growth plate had undergone fewer cell divisions than those of the control growth plate. After glucocorticoid removal, these cells were able to proliferate faster and thus return to the original growth trajectory. Thus, growth-plate senescence may not be a function of time per se, but of the cumulative number of divisions the stem cell has undergone. Programming of growth trajectory may therefore occur at the level of chondrocyte cell number and division potential. Such a mechanism, although speculative, is consistent with the results of the study of Baron and coworkers (1994), and with the findings from Mehta *et al.* (2002) presented here. Interestingly, the young offspring of rats fed low-protein diets in pregnancy exhibit hypersensitivity to glucocorticoids in liver and brain, which appears to be mediated by increased glucocorticoid receptor numbers and expression (Langley-Evans *et al.* 1996). In conclusion, the increased height and irregularity of the growth plates from maternally undernourished rats may represent programming of chondrocyte function.

Maternal protein deficiencies and adult bone mass

The Langley-Evans rat model has also been used to evaluate bone mineral using dual-energy X-ray absorptiometry (DXA) (Mehta *et al.* 2002). Whole-body bone mineral content (BMC), area and areal bone mineral density (BMD) (g cm^{-2}) were evaluated in 54 aged offspring (23 from maternal low-protein and 31 from control dams). Measurements were also obtained of whole-body lean and fat mass. There was a statistically significant difference in the mean whole-body area (low-protein 53.6 cm^2, control 58.1 cm^2); this difference ($p = 0.01$) in a random effects model allowed for gender, body weight, and animal and mother interrelationships. Thus the mean bone area of adult offspring born to dams fed low-protein diets was around 10% lower than that of the offspring born to dams fed a control diet during gestation. A similar magnitude of difference was observed for whole BMC (low-protein 8.29 g, control 9.01 g), but the variance in BMC measurements was greater and the difference between the two groups just failed to reach statistical significance ($p = 0.06$) in the random effects model. There was no comparable difference between the groups in whole-body BMD ($p = 0.88$). There was a significant positive association ($p < 0.001$) between whole body-fat mass and whole-body BMC, and when examined in a multivariant model the adjustment for differences in fat mass was able to eliminate the significant effect of maternal diet on the BMC of the offspring. No such effect was observed for whole-body lean mass. The difference between the two groups in bone area remained after adjusting for both lean and fat mass. These results suggest that maternal protein deficiencies result in a reduction in bone area and BMC, but not BMD, among the aged offspring. Thus bone size, rather than volumetric bone density, is the principal outcome modified by maternal protein restriction. These results thus mirror the results of epidemiological studies among

the human population, as discussed in the previous chapter.

Summary and future perspectives

In conclusion, a low-protein diet in utero is associated with reduced bone mineral content and changes in the appearance of the epiphyseal growth plates in aged rats. This is consistent with an overall reduction in mineralised bone, as indicated by the lower bone area of low-protein-exposed rats. The profound effects on skeletal architecture, growth and bone size are mirrored by changes in mesenchymal stem-cell activity, which is also subject to maturational delay as a consequence of maternal protein restriction during early life. Studies to date therefore suggest that abnormalities of skeletal development are initiated in early life, possibly through a combination of elevated glucocorticoid activity and impaired IGF1 activity, which together would favour a down-regulation of bone deposition. Thus, it is possible that changes in skeletal growth and structure following poor nutrition in pregnancy may act as a precursor for reduced bone mass in later life and, potentially, osteoporotic fracture in humans, although caution must be applied before extrapolation of these animal findings to human populations.

There is no doubt that rat and mouse models of maternal protein insufficiency provide useful models to study programming in utero. However, we are still at an early stage in defining how such insufficiency affects bone development and bone quality in the offspring. The rat model will permit more detailed experimental investigations than would be possible in human subjects, although, like all animal models, the rat model has a number of caveats that should be borne in mind. In particular it must be stressed that (1) bone development differs from humans in that a growth plate persists until old age (2) rodents do not have Harversian systems and (3) rodents do not remodel bone in the same manner as larger animals. Notwithstanding these limitations, further research into the mechanisms of programming of bone growth may increase our understanding of the factors influencing bone development as well as adult bone structure and peak bone mass. To achieve this it will be necessary not only to examine changes in anthropometric and gross skeletal structure and growth-plate function, but also to harness currently available molecular and biochemical approaches, including gene array and proteomics, to gain a molecular and proteomic fingerprint of cells from offspring whose mothers have been nutritionally challenged. Elucidation of the mechanisms of skeletal programming and the implications therein for improving nutrition in pregnancy offers significant clinical implications in reducing the burden of osteoporosis and improving the quality of life for all those affected by this debilitating disease.

REFERENCES

Aihie Sayer, A., Dunn, R., Langley-Evans, S. and Cooper, C. (2001). Prenatal exposure to a maternal low protein diet shortens life span in rats. *Gerontology*, **47**, 9–14.

Ammann, P., Bourrin, S., Bonjour, J. P., Meyer, J. M. and Rizzoli, R. (2000). Protein undernutrition-induced bone loss is associated with decreased IGF-I levels and estrogen deficiency. *J. Bone Miner. Res.*, **15**, 683–90.

Anderson, H. C. (1995). Molecular biology of matrix vesicles. *Clin. Orthop.*, **314**, 266–80.

Bailey, D. A., McKay, H. A., Mirwald, R. L., Crocker, P. R. and Faulkner, R. A. (1999). A six-year longitudinal study of the relationship of physical activity to bone mineral accrual in growing children: the University of Saskatchewan bone mineral accrual study. *J. Bone Miner. Res.*, **14**, 1672–9.

Barker, D. J. P. (1995). Intrauterine programming of adult disease. *Mol. Med. Today*, **1**, 418–23.

Barker, D. J. P. (2000). In utero programming of cardiovascular disease. *Theriogenology*, **53**, 555–74.

Barker, D. J. P. and Martyn, C. N. (1997). The fetal origins of hypertension. *Adv. Nephrol. Necker Hosp.*, **26**, 65–72.

Baron, J., Klein, K. O., Colli, M. J. et al. (1994). Catch-up growth after glucocorticoid excess: a mechanism intrinsic to the growth plate. *Endocrinology*, **135**, 1367–71.

Bianco, P., Riminucci, M., Gronthos, S. and Robey, P. G. (2001). Bone marrow stromal stem cells: nature, biology, and potential applications. *Stem Cells*, **19**, 180–92.

Bourrin, S., Toromanoff, A., Ammann, P., Bonjour, J. P. and Rizzoli, R. (2000a). Dietary protein deficiency induces osteoporosis in aged male rats. *J. Bone Miner. Res.*, **15**, 1555–63.

Bourrin, S., Ammann, P., Bonjour, J. P. and Rizzoli, R. (2000b). Dietary protein restriction lowers plasma insulin-like growth factor I (IGF-I), impairs cortical bone formation, and induces osteoblastic resistance to IGF-I in adult female rats. *Endocrinology*, **141**, 3149–55.

Breur, G. J., Vanenkevort, B. A., Farnum, C. E. and Wilsman, N. J. (1991). Linear relationship between the volume of hypertrophic chondrocytes and the rate of longitudinal bone growth in growth plates. *J. Orthop. Res.*, **9**, 348–59.

Cobo, A., Lopez, J. M., Carbajo, E. et al. (1999). Growth plate cartilage formation and resorption are differentially depressed in growth retarded uremic rats. *J. Am. Soc. Nephrol.*, **10**, 971–9.

Cooper, C., Cawley, M., Bhalla, A. et al. (1995). Childhood growth, physical activity, and peak bone mass in women. *J. Bone Miner. Res.*, **10**, 940–7.

Cooper, C., Fall, C., Egger, P., Hobbs, R., Eastell, R. and Barker, D. (1997). Growth in infancy and bone mass in later life. *Ann. Rheum. Dis.*, **56**, 17–21.

Cooper, C., Eriksson, J. G., Forsen, T., Osmond, C., Tuomilehto, J. and Barker, D. J. P. (2001). Maternal height, childhood growth and risk of hip fracture in later life: a longitudinal study. *Osteoporos. Int.*, **12**, 623–9.

Fall, C., Hindmarsh, P., Dennison, E., Kellingray, S., Barker, D. and, Cooper, C. (1998). Programming of growth hormone secretion and bone mineral density in elderly men: a hypothesis. *J. Clin. Endocrinol. Metab.*, **83**, 135–9.

Farnum, C. E., Lee, R., O'Hara, K. and Urban, J. P. (2002). Volume increase in growth plate chondrocytes during hypertrophy: the contribution of organic osmolytes. *Bone*, **30**, 574–81.

Godfrey, K. M. and Barker, D. J. P. (2001). Fetal programming and adult health. *Public Health Nutr.*, **4**, 611–24.

Grimsrud C. D., Romano, P. R., D'Souza, M. et al. (1999). BMP-6 is an autocrine stimulator of chondrocyte differentiation. *J. Bone Miner. Res.*, **14**, 475–82.

Horton, W. E., Feng, L. and Adams, C. (1998). Chondrocyte apoptosis in development, aging and disease. *Matrix Biol.*, **17**, 107–15.

Hughes, P. C. and Tanner, J. M. (1970). The assessment of skeletal maturity in the growing rat. *J. Anat.*, **106**, 371–402.

Hunziker, E. B. and Schenk, R. K. (1989). Physiological mechanisms adopted by chondrocytes in regulating longitudinal bone growth in rats. *J. Physiol.*, **414**, 55–71.

Jordan, K. M. and Cooper, C. (2002). Epidemiology of osteoporosis. *Best Pract. Res. Clin. Rheumatol.*, **16**, 795–806.

Kember, N. F. (1973). Aspects of the maturation process in growth cartilage in the rat tibia. *Clin. Orthop.*, **95**, 288–94.

Kronenberg, H. M. and Chung, U. (2001). The parathyroid hormone-related protein and Indian hedgehog feedback loop in the growth plate. *Novartis. Found. Symp.*, **232**, 144–52.

Kuhn, J. L., DeLacey, J. H. and Leenellett, E. E. (1996). Relationship between bone growth rate and hypertrophic chondrocyte volume in New Zealand white rabbits of varying ages. *J. Orthop. Res.*, **14**, 706–11.

Langley, S. C. and Jackson, A. A. (1994). Increased systolic blood pressure in adult rats induced by fetal exposure to maternal low-protein diets. *Clin. Sci.*, **86**, 217–22.

Langley-Evans, S. C. (1999). Fetal origins of adult disease. *Br. J. Nutr.*, **81**, 5–6.

Langley-Evans, S. C., Gardner, D. S. and Jackson, A. A. (1996). Maternal protein restriction influences the programming of the rat hypothalamic–pituitary–adrenal axis. *J. Nutr.*, **126**, 1578–85.

Langley-Evans, S. C., Welham, S. J. and Jackson, A. A. (1999a). Fetal exposure to a maternal low protein diet impairs nephrogenesis and promotes hypertension in the rat. *Life Sci.*, **64**, 965–74.

Langley-Evans, S. C., Sherman, R. C., Welham, S. J., Nwagwu, M. O., Gardner, D. S. and Jackson, A. A. (1999b). Intrauterine programming of hypertension: the role of the reninangiotensin system. *Biochem. Soc. Trans.*, **27**, 88–93.

Mehta, G., Roach, H. I., Langley-Evans, S. *et al.* (2002). Intrauterine exposure to a maternal low protein diet reduces adult bone mass and alters growth plate morphology in rats. *Calcif. Tissue Int.*, **71**, 493–8.

Miller, J. P. and German, R. Z. (1999). Protein malnutrition affects the growth trajectories of the craniofacial skeleton in rats. *J. Nutr.*, **129**, 2061–9.

Nwagwu, M. O., Cook, A. and Langley-Evans, S. C. (2000). Evidence of progressive deterioration of renal function in rats exposed to a maternal low-protein diet in utero. *Br. J. Nutr.*, **83**, 79–85.

Oreffo, R. O. C., Lashbrooke, B., Roach, H. I., Clarke, N. M. P. and Cooper, C. (2003). Maternal protein deficiency affects mesenchymal stem cell activity in the developing offspring. *Bone*, **33**, 100–7.

Reichling, T. D. and German, R. Z. (2000). Bones, muscles and visceral organs of protein-malnourished rats (*Rattus norvegicus*) grow more slowly but for longer durations to reach normal final size. *J. Nutr.*, **130**, 2326–32.

Roach, H. I. and Clarke, N. M. P. (2000). Programmed cell death of chondrocytes in vivo: apoptosis, dark chondrocytes, and cell paralysis. In *Chemistry and Biology of Mineralized Tissues: Proceedings of the Sixth International Conference* (ed. M. Goldberg, A. Boskey and C. Robinson). Rosemont, IL, American Academy of Orthopedic Surgeons, pp. 325–30.

Roach, H. I., Mehta, G., Oreffo, R. O., Clarke, N. M. and Cooper, C. (2003a). Temporal analysis of rat growth plates: cessation of growth with age despite presence of a physis. *J. Histochem. Cytochem.*, **51**, 373–83.

Roach, H. I., Clarke, N. M., Langley-Evans, S. and Cooper, C. (2003b). Catabolic and anabolic phases of osteodystrophy in aged rats. *J. Bone Miner. Metab.*, **21**, 299–306.

Roach, H. I., Aigner, T. and Kouri, J. B. (2004). Chondroptosis: a variant of apoptotic cell death in chondrocytes? *Apoptosis*, **9**, 265–77.

Siebler, T., Robson, H., Shalet, S. M. and Williams, G. R. (2001). Glucocorticoids, thyroid hormone and growth hormone interactions: implications for the growth plate. *Horm. Res.*, **56** (Suppl 1), 7–12.

Triffitt, J. T. and Oreffo, R. O. C. (1998). The osteoblast lineage In *Molecular and Cellular Biology of Bone* (ed. M. Zaidi) Advances in Organ Biology, vol. 5B. Stamford, CT: JAI Press. pp. 429–51.

Villar, J., Belizan, J. M., Spalding, J. and Klein, R. E. (1982). Postnatal growth of intrauterine growth retarded infants. *Early Hum. Dev.*, **6**, 265–71.

Villar, J., Smeriglio, V., Martorell, R., Brown, C. H. and Klein, R. E. (1984). Heterogeneous growth and mental development of intrauterine growth-retarded infants during the first 3 years of life. *Pediatrics*, **74**, 783–91.

Walther, F. J., Ramaekers, L. H. and van Engelshoven J. M. (1981). Skeletal maturity at birth and at the age of 3 years of infants malnourished in utero. *Early Hum. Dev.*, **5**, 139–43.

Widdowson, E. M. and McCance, R. A. (1963). The effect of finite periods of undernutrition at different ages on the composition and subsequent development of the rat. *Proc. R. Soc. Lond. B*, **158**, 329–42.

Wilsman, N. J., Farnum, C. E., Green, E. M., Lieferman, E. M. and Clayton, M. K. (1996). Cell cycle analysis of proliferating zone chondrocytes in growth plates elongating at different rates. *J. Orthop. Res.*, **14**, 562–72.

31

The developmental environment and the early origins of cancer

Anders Ekbom

Karolinska University Hospital

Introduction

The hypothesis that the intrauterine environment is of importance to the aetiology of certain forms of cancer is not new. Studies of children exposed in utero to radiation in Japan at the end of the Second World War indicate a special vulnerability during the perinatal period for future cancer risks (Kato *et al.* 1989). Although the increased risk was most pronounced for haematopoietic cancers, an excess number of breast cancers has also been demonstrated. Similarly, strong associations have been shown between exposure to diethylstilbestrol (DES) given to expectant mothers during pregnancy and vaginal adenocarcinoma in young women (Greenwald *et al.* 1971). These two examples are of major importance as they show that there is a window of vulnerability already 'open' in utero.

Although the findings mentioned above prove that there are biological pathways which can act in a cancerogenic process at an early stage in life, the two exposures (DES and radiation on a level with Hiroshima and Nagasaki) are extremely rare. However, in the case of haematopoietic cancers, especially leukaemia in childhood, studies have shown that chromosomal translocations are already present at birth in children that later will manifest with leukaemia (Hjalgrim *et al.* 2002), indicating that factors other than those mentioned above are of importance in utero. However, in order to study other cancers that will occur in adult life, researchers are facing a formidable challenge. What sort of exposures are we interested in? How can these be assessed, especially if the time lag between exposure and the outcome can exceed 50 years? Focus has to a great extent been on hormonal exposures, especially oestrogens, due to the fact that during pregnancy the concentration of oestrogens is 10 times higher in female fetuses and 100 times higher in male fetuses than it will be later in life (Genuth 1983). However, even if data from different observational studies during recent years are strongly suggestive of an association, the underlying mechanisms seem to be more complex than originally perceived.

The aim of this review is to assess what is known up to now about intrauterine exposures and cancer in adult life with special emphasis on cancers of the breast, testis and prostate.

Breast cancer

Breast cancer is the most common cancer form among women in the westernised world. In the United States, more than 10% of all women will have a diagnosis of breast cancer. There is a genetic component, and known hereditary factors can so far explain approximately 5% of all cases in younger women. Reproductive patterns influence the risk to some extent, young age at first full-term pregnancy

Developmental Origins of Health and Disease, ed. Peter Gluckman and Mark Hanson. Published by Cambridge University Press.

as well as multiple pregnancies being protective factors (Adami *et al.* 1995). Other environmental factors must therefore be of importance, as studies on immigrants from low-risk areas (such as Japan) to high-risk areas (such as the United States) show that the third generation has incidence rates very similar to those in the total US population (Haenszel and Kurihara 1968).

The incidence of breast cancer is increasing in the westernised world. Although mammographic screening and changes in reproductive patterns, such as fewer children and an increase in age at first birth, can partly explain this increase, there are reasons to believe that we are facing a 'real' increase in the incidence. The underlying reasons for this remain unknown, and different hypotheses have been put forward with regards to diet, physical exercise, etc. None of these hypotheses can, however, convincingly explain the changes in incidence over time. The hypothesis put forward by Dimitrios Trichopoulos (1990) was therefore seductive when he proposed that breast cancer might originate in utero. He pointed out that oestrogens are important components in breast cancer carcinogenesis, that oestrogen concentrations are increased during pregnancy, and that the concentration differs between individuals and populations. The hypothesis was supported by a number of observations. In animal models, a diet high in n-6 polyunsaturated fatty acids during pregnancy affects the risk of breast cancer in the offspring (Hilakivi-Clarke *et al.* 1997). Familial risk of breast cancer among first-degree relatives is higher when the sister rather than the mother is affected (Eby *et al.* 1994), which is not in line with the common conception of familial inheritance, but can be explained by similarities in the intrauterine milieu of the sisters. A further indication is the seasonality with regard to month of birth and the risk of breast cancer (Yuen *et al.* 1994).

In order to test the hypothesis of an association between intrauterine exposures and the risk of cancer in adults, one has to rely on indirect measures which act as proxies for endogenous or exogenous exposures known to affect pregnancy, hormonally or by other means. Proxy variables which have

been used are birth and placental weight, height, gestational age, age and parity of the mother, preeclampsia, smoking, twinning, and jaundice in the newborn.

Birthweight has been the most common proxy variable used to assess the impact of intrauterine exposures on the risk of breast cancer. Birthweight is associated with levels of different pregnancy hormones including oestrogen (Kaijser *et al.* 2000), which was initially the hormone implicated in the hypothesis of intrauterine exposures and breast cancer. There have been quite a few studies which have assessed the association between breast cancer risk and birthweight (Ekbom *et al.* 1992, 1997, Michels *et al.* 1996, Sanderson *et al.* 1996, 2002, Innes *et al.* 2000, Titus-Ernstoff *et al.* 2002, Vatten *et al.* 2002, Ahlgren *et al.* 2003, McCormack *et al.* 2003, Mellemkjaer *et al.* 2003). The results of different studies are given in Table 31.1. There seems to be a consistent pattern that the risk of breast cancer increases with increasing birthweight. However, in some studies this pattern is only evident for premenopausal cancers, and in others for postmenopausal cancer. In some, no adjustments have been made for other known risk factors such as reproductive factors. There are also differences in how the birthweight was assessed. In some studies self-reported birthweight was used, in others birthweight was assessed through interviews with the mother or, especially in the Scandinavian studies, through data from archives or registries. Studies that rely on information from mothers face the problems of selection, as early death of the mother could be associated with lifestyle factors which would affect the birthweight of the offspring. However, although there are some inconsistencies in the results of different studies, the results clearly indicate that there is an association between increasing birthweight and the risk of breast cancer, with a clear tendency to a graded ('dose-dependent') effect.

Maternal age has been implicated as a risk factor for breast cancer in some studies (Ekbom *et al.* 1997, Innes *et al.* 2000), but these findings are not consistent as there are reports of no such association in other studies (Sanderson *et al.* 1996). **Parity**, on the other hand, does not appear to affect the risk

Table 31.1 Published studies on birthweight and subsequent risk of breast cancer.

Study	Type of study	Number of breast cancers	Age restrictions	Type of information	Association with birthweight	Pre- or post-menopause
Ekbom *et al.* 1992	Case–control	458	–	Birth records	+	Pre and post
Michels *et al.* 1996	Case–control	582	–	Interview mother	+	Pre and post
Sanderson *et al.* 1996	Case–control	746	< 46 years	Interview	+	Pre
Sanderson *et al.* 1996	Case–control	401	50–64	Interview	0	Post
Ekbom *et al.* 1997	Case–control	1068	–	Birth records	0	Pre and post
Innes *et al.* 2000	Case–control	484	< 38 years	Birth records	+	Pre
Sanderson *et al.* 2002	Case–control	288	< 46 years	Interview mother	0	Pre
Titus-Ernstoff *et al.* 2002	Case–control	1716	≥ 50 years	Interview	+	Post
Vatten *et al.* 2002	Case–control	373	–	Birth records	+	Pre and post
Ahlgren *et al.* 2003	Cohort	2334	–	Registry	+	Pre and post
McCormack *et al.* 2003	Cohort	359	–	Birth records	+	Pre and post
Mellemkjaer *et al.* 2003	Case–control	881	< 40 years	Birth records	+	Pre

of breast cancer in the offspring. Previous reports of an association between pregnancy hormone levels and age of the mother have not been substantiated in a recently published study (Kaijser *et al.* 2002), and there is no underlying biological rationale. The association between an increase in the age of the mother and breast cancer risk can therefore probably be explained by confounding factors: fertility patterns in the mother and daughter will be similar, not due to genetics but due to social influences. As an increased age at first birth is associated with an excess risk of breast cancer, a spurious association can therefore emerge.

Pre-eclampsia is associated with a dysfunctional placenta and will lead to decreased levels of many pregnancy hormones, for instance oestrogens (Garoff and Seppala 1976, Long *et al.* 1979). A protective effect in the offspring against breast cancer following a history of pre-eclampsia in the mother during pregnancy is therefore of particular interest (Ekbom *et al.* 1992, 1997). These findings indicate that placental function is of importance for a future risk of breast cancer in the offspring. Confounding by changes in the reproductive patterns in the offspring does not seem to be the underlying reason, as follow-up studies of offspring born to pre-eclamptic mothers do not show any differences in age at menarche and other characteristics with an impact

on breast cancer, such as adult height (Ros *et al.* 2001).

Twin pregnancies are characterised by high levels of placental hormones and it has also been reported that oestrogen levels are higher in dizygotic than in monozygotic twin pregnancies (Kappel *et al.* 1985). Therefore, if endogenous hormone levels in utero are of importance for developing cancer later in life, twins would run a higher risk, than singletons. However, cohort studies on twins have failed to reveal any significant increase in risk, although a study based on the Swedish Twin Registry found a substantially higher incidence of breast cancer in dizygotic same-sexed female twins in the age range 20–29 but not thereafter (Braun *et al.* 1995). However, the duration of gestation in twin pregnancy is, on average, substantially shorter than for singleton pregnancy (Nylander 1983). Thus, twins will be exposed to the hormonal environment in utero for a shorter time and the cumulative exposure will be lower than for singletons. Therefore, if gestational age is taken into account, it may well be that twins in fact have a substantially increased risk. Moreover, in a Swedish study on breast cancer in same-sexed twins, the mean birthweight and ponderal index were higher among cases compared to their co-twin, and the risk of breast cancer increased with increasing birthweight with a gradient that was greater in twins than in singletons (Hubinette *et al.* 2001). Similarly, in a study of opposite-sexed twins, the gradient with birthweight was extremely steep. There was a 12-fold increased risk among twins from an opposite-sexed pair with a birthweight over 3000 g compared to one with a birthweight less than 2000 g (Kaijser *et al.* 2001). This indicates that interaction may well be present, with androgens from the opposite-sexed twin enhancing the exposures in utero.

Gestational age. As mentioned previously, the cumulative exposure in utero will be dependent on gestational length. Low birthweight is dependent not only on the growth velocity in utero but also on the gestational duration. Unfortunately, data are scarce with regards to gestational age in the studies published so far on birthweight and the risk of breast cancer. Another group of women of interest are those born severely premature, i.e. before the 33rd week of gestation. Some of these women produce extreme levels of endogenous oestrogens during the first months of life, probably due to an immature ovarian feedback system that leads to oestradiol-producing ovarian cysts (Sedin *et al.* 1985). These women seem to have an excess risk of breast cancer (Ekbom *et al.* 2000a, Kaijser *et al.* 2003a), which indicates that it is the exposures not only in utero but also during the period around birth which could be of importance for the risk of breast cancer.

DES. As mentioned previously, the finding of a causal association between exposure to DES in utero and the risk of vaginal cancer in young women (Greenwald *et al.* 1971) is one of the cornerstones of the hypothesis of intrauterine exposures and the risk of adult cancers (see also Chapter 7). It is therefore of particular interest to assess to what extent exposure to DES in utero will impact the risk of breast cancer. Data are scarce but in the largest study so far close to 5000 women were followed up from the 1950s and 1960s and compared to unexposed siblings; there was a significant twofold excess risk for breast cancer after the age of 40 and a 40% non-significant increased risk overall (Palmer *et al.* 2002). Although not conclusive, these results further implicate the intrauterine environment for breast cancer

and also hint that specific hormonal exposures are of importance.

Smoking during pregnancy will affect placental function substantially. Besides reduced birthweight there will be decreased levels of placental hormones such as oestrogen (Kaijser *et al.* 2000). However, smoking in the mother has so far not been associated with the offspring's risk for breast cancer (Okasha *et al.* 2003). This suggests that oestrogen is not the only hormonal mechanism in operation.

Neonatal jaundice has been shown to be associated with an increased risk of breast cancer (Ekbom *et al.* 1997). Neonatal jaundice is characterised by high levels of oestrogen and other hormones in the newborn, possibly due to an impaired metabolism of maternal or endogenous hormones (Robine *et al.* 1988). As for extreme prematurity, this is of particular interest as it shows that early exposures are not necessarily confined to the prenatal period.

Perinatal determinants for breast size. There is good empirical evidence linking mammary-gland mass to risk of breast cancer. It is known that women with high-density mammograms (75% or more of the total breast with dense mammographic appearance) have a fourfold risk compared to low-density mammograms (25% or less of the total breast area with dense mammographic appearance) (Byrne *et al.* 2001). Women with small breasts who have undergone augmentation mammoplasty, who could serve as a proxy for low mammary-gland mass, have a reduced risk of breast cancer (Brinton *et al.* 2000). Likewise, women who have undergone surgical reduction of their breasts also have a reduced breast-cancer risk (Brinton *et al.* 2001). Mammary-gland mass, which is likely to reflect the total number of mammary cells and be correlated to mammary cells at risk of transformation, can also explain several of the descriptive aspects of breast-cancer epidemiology, for instance differences in incidence between Asian and Caucasian women (Trichopoulos and Lipman 1992). Another interesting observation is that breast cancer is more common in the left, larger, breast than in the right breast (Ekbom *et al.* 1994). This difference in size is probably due to differences in blood supply. The haemodynamic asymmetry starts at birth when the ductus arteriosus is closed; up to that time, the blood distribution to the two breasts is similar (Garson *et al.* 1990). There is, however, no difference in incidence among women younger than 45 years, which strongly indicates that exposures early in life, i.e. in utero, are of major importance, as this is the only time period where no asymmetry is present in the blood supply.

There is only one study that has studied mammographic patterns and breast size and associations with birth characteristics. There was a very strong association between high placental weight, as well as birthweight and length, and the risk of high-density patterns (Ekbom *et al.* 1995). The increase in breast-cancer incidence may therefore, at least partly, be explained by the better nutritional status of pregnant women in the twentieth than in the eighteenth century, resulting in more cells at risk for malignant transformation. This model would also explain results from immigration studies and the emerging breast-cancer epidemic in Asia among young women, possibly due to a better nutritional status in utero.

Testicular cancer

Testicular cancer, a relatively uncommon malignancy, shows one of the most pronounced increases in relative terms in the westernised world. The annual increase varies between 2.3% and 5.2% in different populations. Also, there is a wide variation in incidence between adjacent populations, e.g. a tenfold difference between Denmark and Lithuania, and twofold between Denmark and Sweden (Adami *et al.* 1994). Analyses of the temporal trends in incidence have revealed strong birth-cohort phenomena, i.e. year of birth is more important to the risk than age. This phenomenon is seen in all countries around the Baltic Sea. However, in Denmark, Norway, and Sweden, no increase was seen for birth cohort for the years after the Second World War, nor was there a tendency towards a decrease (Moller 1989, Bergstrom *et al.* 1996). Similar observations have been reported from British Columbia (Coleman

et al. 1993). In contrast, Finland, former East Germany and Poland show a continuous increase, including among the birth-cohorts born during the Second World War (Bergstrom *et al.* 1996).

A pronounced birth-cohort effect, as well as results from immigration studies, where origin of birth regardless of duration of stay in a high-incidence area is the determinant for cancer risk (Ekbom *et al.* 2003), suggests that factors early in life, probably in utero, are major determinants for the risk of testicular cancer. This hypothesis is further strengthened by the fact that the only established risk factor for testicular cancer is cryptorchidism, i.e. an undescended testicle, which is already present at birth (Schottenfeld *et al.* 1980). Cryptorchidism as such is probably not a risk factor, but indicates shared factors in the intrauterine environment that affect the risk of cryptorchidism as well as testicular cancer. This hypothesis is further strengthened by the fact that men with unilateral cryptorchidism are at an increased risk for testicular cancer in the contralateral testicle (Pinczowski *et al.* 1991).

There are two major histopathological types of testicular cancer, seminomas and non-seminomas, which differ with regards to mean age at diagnosis and age-specific incidence peak: both are lower for non-seminomas than for seminomas. The annual incidence of the two forms is strongly correlated (Levi *et al.* 1990) and common or similar aetiological factors are therefore likely, especially as mixed forms of the two types are quite frequent. The increased risk associated with cryptorchidism and a birth-cohort phenomenon are present for both forms (Wanderas *et al.* 1995). Irrespective of type, testicular cancer is believed to originate from germ cells present early in life. It has been proposed that the temporal trends in the incidence of testicular cancer could be a result of increased exposure to oestrogens in utero caused by changes in dietary habits or exposures to environmental oestrogen-like chemicals (Sharpe and Skakkebaek 1993). It has also been proposed, and also seems likely, that testicular cancer, cryptorchidism, other urogenital malformations such as hypospadias, and the reported decrease in sperm counts, could be the result of a common syndrome

(Boisen *et al.* 2001). Further credance for such a hypothesis is lent by the fact that there is evidence that patients with testicular cancer are subfertile at the time of diagnosis. A decreased fecundity was evident among testicular cancer cases some years before diagnosis in a Norwegian study (Fossa and Kravdal 2000). A cohort study from Denmark with 30 000 men who received semen analysis due to fertility problems found an increased risk for testicular cancer present after 15 years of follow-up (Jacobsen *et al.* 2000). Finally, a recent study from Sweden was able to demonstrate that fathering dizygotic twins occurred less than expected among males who later would be diagnosed with testicular cancer, irrespective of duration of follow-up (Richiardi *et al.* 2004a). Making the assumption that twinning rate is a better marker for fertility, these results are in line with the hypothesis of a common syndrome including testicular cancer and poor sperm quality.

It is therefore not surprising that there has been a lot of focus on birth characteristics and the risk of testicular cancer. Short gestational age and both low and high birthweight have been implicated repeatedly as risk factors (Henderson *et al.* 1979, Depue *et al.* 1983, Brown *et al.* 1986, Moss *et al.* 1986, Pearce *et al.* 1987, Swerdlow *et al.* 1987, Haughey *et al.* 1989, Prener *et al.* 1992, Akre *et al.* 1996, Wanderas *et al.* 1998, Richiardi *et al.* 2002). Moreover, as for breast cancer, neonatal jaundice has been found to be associated with a twofold or larger excess risk in studies from Norway (Wanderas *et al.* 1998) and Sweden (Akre *et al.* 1996). Birth order is another proxy that has been investigated repeatedly. It has been shown that birth order and sibship size affect testicular cancer risk independently of each other (Richiardi *et al.* 2004b).

Smoking during pregnancy, as mentioned previously, will affect the intrauterine hormonal milieu substantially. It is therefore of interest that the differences in incidence of testicular cancer in different populations over time have a very good correlation with the frequency of female smokers 20–30 years prior to the testicular cancer incidence measurement (Pettersson *et al.* 2004). It has also been shown that male offspring of female victims of lung cancer have a significant excess risk of testicular cancer (Kaijser *et al.* 2003b). This may suggest that a hormonal disturbance from smoking during the intrauterine period can affect the risk.

Prostate cancer

As for breast cancer, the incidence of prostate cancer is increasing in many countries and ethnic groups, most markedly in North America and northern Europe. Better detection can explain part of the increased incidence but, as for breast cancer, not the entire increase (Potosky *et al.* 1990). The only known risk factor besides age is ethnicity. African-Americans have a substantially higher incidence and mortality in all age groups than other ethnic groups in the United States (Parkin *et al.* 1992). As for breast cancer, the intrauterine period has been proposed to be of aetiological importance (Ross and Henderson 1994). Animal studies have shown that exposure to oestrogen during the neonatal period causes permanent disturbance in the adult prostate including epithelial dysplasia. The underlying reason for this has been postulated to be up-regulation of the oestrogen receptor expression (Prins and Birch 1997).

However, in contrast to breast cancer, there is a fairly limited number of studies that have assessed a potential association between birth characteristics and risk of prostate cancer. In the first study of this kind, a small Swedish cohort study of 366 men with known birthweight collected from midwives' charts, who were followed up for the occurrence of cancer, 21 cases of prostate cancer were subsequently identified. There was a sixfold increase in the risk of prostate cancer among men with the highest decentile of birthweight compared to men with the lowest (Tibblin *et al.* 1995). In a subsequent case–control study of 250 cases, a weak association between an increased risk of prostate cancer and high birthweight and placental weight could be demonstrated (Ekbom *et al.* 1996a). However, in a large study consisting of 844 cases of prostate cancer, no such association could be found (Ekbom *et al.* 2000b). However, as for breast cancer, a history of pre-eclampsia in the mother was associated with a protective effect (Ekbom *et al.* 2000a) and there were indications that gestational age was inversely associated with risk of prostate cancer (Ekbom *et al.* 2000b). There were also hints that neonatal jaundice was associated with an excess risk, but low statistical power prevented any firm conclusions (Ekbom *et al.* 2000b).

In an American study on health professionals there were 1375 cases of prostate cancer, and 545 of these had information on birthweight. The authors failed to show any significant association between birth characteristics and prostate cancer (Platz *et al.* 1998). Similarly, in a recent American study of 192 men with early onset of prostate cancer, no association could be found with birthweight (Boland *et al.* 2003). Thus, even if it is tempting to draw a parallel in the aetiology between prostate and breast cancer, so far the data with regards to prostate cancer are inconsistent. If the perinatal period is of importance, birthweight does not seem to be a good marker for potential aetiological factors.

Underlying mechanisms

In Table 31.2, different features of breast, testis, and prostate cancer are summarised. It is obvious that in the case of testicular cancer, and to a lesser extent breast cancer, there is a time-window in utero or perinatally that has an impact on the risk of cancer. One should, however, be somewhat more cautious before one infers such an association for prostate cancer. There are also some common features such as neonatal jaundice, high and low birthweight, gestational age and pre-eclampsia that have an effect on the future risk of cancer. Initially, it was generally assumed that the underlying mechanism was hormonal, and a special focus was on oestrogens. However, androgens have also been implicated, especially in the case of prostate cancer – where the incidence among African-Americans gives some hints that oestrogens cannot, at least exclusively, be responsible. The lack of any association with smoking in the mother further discred-

Table 31.2 Associations of different perinatal characteristics with cancer of testis, breast, and prostate.

Cancer form	High birth-weight	Low birth-weight	pre-eclampsia	Jaundice	Smoking in the mother
Testis	+	+	−	+	+
Breast	+	(+)	+	+	0
Prostate	(+)	−	(+)	(+)	−

its oestrogens for at least breast cancer. In other words, we have presently very little knowledge of what kind of exposure should be assessed in future studies in order to enhance our understanding of the underlying biological mechanisms. However, there are a number of mechanisms, not necessarily mutually exclusive, which could explain the association between adult cancer and pre- or perinatal factors.

(1) Placental hormones acting as growth factors will affect the number of stem cells and thereby the size of the organ and the number of cells at risk later in life. Breast cancer is probably the best example of a cancer form where such an underlying mechanism is probable.

(2) Hormones acting as growth factors will induce cell proliferation. Increased cell division may increase the risk of malignant transformation by increasing the risk for genetic errors. Increased levels of pregnancy hormones will then provide a 'fertile soil' either through a first 'hit' in the process towards a malignant transformation or through up-regulation of different hormone receptors. The latter has been proposed in animal models for prostate cancer.

(3) Oestrogens or other hormones or their metabolites may be directly genotoxic (Service 1998), and different enzymes have been linked to increased risk of breast cancer. The substantially increased risk especially for premenopausal breast cancer in women born extremely preterm and twins born at full term could be the result of direct genotoxic effects.

The implication that the early prenatal and perinatal periods are the window of opportunity for the risk of developing cancer as an adult does not mean that exposures later in life are of no importance. Variation in endogenous hormone levels over time and between populations can probably explain only some of the temporal trends and geographical differences (Henderson *et al.* 1997). One should therefore be somewhat sceptical when the changes in incidence of testicular cancer, for instance, are proposed to be the result of decreasing maternal age at first full-term pregnancy. Exogenous oestrogen-like substances have also been proposed to be of major importance, especially for testicular cancer but also for prostate and breast cancer (Sharpe 1995). With the exception of smoking, the scientific community has so far failed to identify a causal relationship with any other external exposure which has a hormonal effect. This includes antiandrogenic compounds such as pp'DDE, where ecological data from Scandinavia argue against such an association, at least for testicular cancer (Ekbom *et al.* 1996b). However, it is fair to say that the last ten years have given us new insights into the importance of the early period of life as a potential window of opportunity. What we now need is a better understanding of the underlying mechanisms, in order to enhance our understanding of the associations documented between different markers for exposures early in life and the risk of adult cancer.

REFERENCES

Adami, H. O., Bergstrom, R., Mohner, M. *et al.* (1994). Testicular cancer in nine northern European countries. *Int. J. Cancer*, **59**, 33–8.

Adami, H. O., Persson, I., Ekbom, A. *et al.* (1995). The aetiology and pathogenesis of human breast cancer. *Mutat. Res.*, **333**, 29–35.

Ahlgren, M., Sorensen, T., Wohlfahrt, J. *et al.* (2003). birthweight and risk of breast cancer in a cohort of 106,504 women. *Int. J. Cancer*, **107**, 997–1000.

Akre, O., Ekbom, A., Hsieh, C. C., Trichopoulos, D. and Adami, H. O. (1996). Testicular nonseminoma and seminoma in relation to perinatal characteristics. *J. Natl. Cancer. Inst.*, **88**, 883–9.

Bergstrom, R., Adami, H. O., Mohner, M. *et al.* (1996). Increase in testicular cancer incidence in six European countries: a birth cohort phenomenon. *J. Natl. Cancer. Inst.*, **88**, 727–33.

Boisen, K. A., Main, K. M., Rajpert-De Meyts, E. and Skakkebaek, N. E. (2001). Are male reproductive disorders a common entity? The testicular dysgenesis syndrome. *Ann. NY Acad. Sci.*, **948**, 90–9.

Boland, L. L., Mink, P. J., Bushhouse, S. A. and Folsom, A. R. (2003). Weight and length at birth and risk of early-onset prostate cancer (United States). *Cancer Causes Control*, **14**, 335–8.

Braun, M. M., Ahlbom, A., Floderus, B., Brinton, L. A. and Hoover, R. N. (1995). Effect of twinship on incidence of cancer of the testis, breast, and other sites (Sweden). *Cancer Causes Control*, **6**, 519–24.

Brinton, L. A., Lubin, J. H., Burich, M. C. *et al.* (2000). Breast cancer following augmentation mammoplasty (United States). *Cancer Causes Control*, **11**, 819–27.

Brinton, L. A., Persson, I., Boice, J. D., McLaughlin, J. K. and Fraumeni, J. F. (2001). Breast cancer risk in relation to amount of tissue removed during breast reduction operations in Sweden. *Cancer*, **91**, 478–83.

Brown, L. M. Pottern, L. M. and Hoover, R. N. (1986). Prenatal and perinatal risk factors for testicular cancer. *Cancer Res.*, **46**, 4812–16.

Byrne, C., Schairer, C., Brinton, L. A. (2001). Effects of mammographic density and benign breast disease on breast cancer risk (United States). *Cancer Causes Control*, **12**, 103–10.

Depue, R. H., Pike, M. C. and Henderson, B. E. (1983). Estrogen exposure during gestation and risk of testicular cancer. *J. Natl. Cancer Inst.*, **71**, 1151–5.

Eby, N., Chang-Claude, J. and Bishop, D. T. (1994). Familial risk and genetic susceptibility for breast cancer. *Cancer Causes Control*, **5**, 458–70.

Ekbom, A., Trichopoulos, D., Adami, H. O., Hsieh, C. C. and Lan, S. J. (1992). Evidence of prenatal influences on breast cancer risk. *Lancet*, **340**, 1015–18.

Ekbom, A., Adami, H. O., Trichopoulos, D. (1994). Epidemiologic correlates of breast cancer laterality (Sweden). *Cancer Causes Control*, **5**, 510–16.

Ekbom, A., Thurfjell, E., Hsieh, C. C., Trichopoulos, D. and Adami, H. O. (1995). Perinatal characteristics and adult mammographic patterns. *Int. J. Cancer*, **61**, 177–80.

Ekbom, A., Hsieh, C. C., Lipworth, L. *et al.* (1996a). Perinatal characteristics in relation to incidence of and mortality from prostate cancer. *BMJ*, **313**, 337–41.

Ekbom, A., Wicklund-Glynn, A. and Adami, H. O. (1996b). DDT and testicular cancer. *Lancet*, **347**, 553–4.

Ekbom, A., Hsieh, C. C., Lipworth, L., Adami, H. O. and Trichopoulos, D. (1997). Intrauterine environment and breast cancer risk in women: a population-based study. *J. Natl. Cancer Inst.*, **89**, 71–6.

Ekbom, A., Erlandsson, G., Hsieh, C. *et al.* (2000a). Risk of breast cancer in prematurely born women. *J. Natl. Cancer Inst.*, **92**, 840–1.

Ekbom, A., Wuu, J., Adami, H. O. *et al.* (2000b). Duration of gestation and prostate cancer risk in offspring. *Cancer Epidemiol. Biomarkers Prev.*, **9**, 221–3.

Ekbom, A., Richiardi, L., Akre, O., Montgomery, S. M. and Sparen, P. (2003). Age at immigration and duration of stay in relation to risk for testicular cancer among Finnish immigrants in Sweden. *J. Natl. Cancer Inst.*, **95**, 1238–40.

Fossa, S. D. and Kravdal, O. (2000). Fertility in Norwegian testicular cancer patients. *Br. J. Cancer*, **82**, 737–41.

Garoff, L. and Seppala, M. (1976). Toxemia of pregnancy: assessment of fetal distress by urinary estriol and circulating human placental lactogen and alpha-fetoprotein levels. *Am. J. Obstet. Gynecol.*, **126**, 1027–33.

Garson, A., Bricker, J. T. and McNamara, D. G., eds. (1990). *The Science and Practice of Pediatric Cardiology*. Philadelphia, PA: Lea and Febiger.

Genuth, S. M. (1983). The reproductive glands. In *Physiology* (ed. M. N. Levy). St Louis, MO: Mosby, pp. 1069–115.

Greenwald, P., Barlow, J. J., Nasca, P. C. and Burnett, W. S. (1971). Vaginal cancer after maternal treatment with synthetic oestrogen. *N. Engl. J. Med.*, **285**, 390–2.

Haenszel, W. and Kurihara, M. (1968). Studies of Japanese migrants. I. Mortality from cancer and other diseases among Japanese in the United States. *J. Natl. Cancer Inst.*, **40**, 43–68.

Haughey, B. P., Graham, S., Brasure, J. *et al.* (1989). The epidemiology of testicular cancer in upstate New York. *Am. J. Epidemiol.*, **130**, 25–36.

Henderson, B. E., Benton, B., Jing, J., Yu, M.C. and Pike, M. C. (1979). Risk factors for cancer of the testis in young men. *Int. J. Cancer*, **23**, 598–602.

Henderson, B. E., Ross, R. K., Yu, M. C. and Bernstein, L. (1997). An explanation for the increasing incidence of testis cancer: decreasing age at first full-term pregnancy. *J. Natl. Cancer Inst.*, **89**, 818–20.

Hilakivi-Clarke, L., Clarke, R., Onojafe, I. *et al.* (1997). A maternal diet high in n-6 polyunsaturated fats alters mammary gland development, puberty onset, and breast cancer risk among female rat offspring. *Proc. Natl. Acad. Sci. USA*, **94**, 9372–7.

Hjalgrim, L. L., Madsen, H. O., Melbye, M. *et al.* (2002). Presence of clone-specific markers at birth in children with acute lymphoblastic leukaemia. *Br. J. Cancer*, **87**, 994–9.

Hubinette, A., Cnattingius, S., Ekbom, A. *et al.* (2001). Birthweight, early environment, and genetics: a study of twins discordant for acute myocardial infarction. *Lancet*, **357**, 1997–2001.

Innes, K., Byers, T. and Schymura, M. *et al.* (2000). Birth characteristics and subsequent risk for breast cancer in very young women. *Am. J. Epidemiol.*, **152**, 1121–8.

Jacobsen, R., Bostofte, E., Engholm, G. *et al.* (2000). Risk of testicular cancer in men with abnormal semen characteristics: cohort study. *BMJ*, **321**, 789–92.

Kaijser, M., Granath, F., Jacobsen, G., Cnattingius, S. and Ekbom, A. (2000). Maternal pregnancy estriol levels in relation to anamnestic and fetal anthropometric data. *Epidemiology*, **11**, 315–19.

Kaijser, M., Lichtenstein, P., Granath, F. *et al.* (2001). in utero exposures and breast cancer: a study of opposite-sexed twins. *J. Natl. Cancer Inst.*, **93**, 60–2.

Kaijser, M., Jacobsen, G., Granath, F., Cnattingius, S. and Ekbom, A. (2002). Maternal age, anthropometrics and pregnancy oestriol. *Paediatr. Perinat. Epidemiol.*, **16**, 149–53.

Kaijser, M., Akre, O., Cnattingius, S. and Ekbom, A. (2003a). Preterm birth, birthweight, and subsequent risk of female breast cancer. *Br. J. Cancer*, **89**, 1664–6.

(2003b). Maternal lung cancer and testicular cancer risk in the offspring. *Cancer Epidemiol. Biomarkers Prev.*, **12**, 643–6.

Kappel, B., Hansen, K., Moller, J. and Faaborg-Andersen, J. (1985). Human placental lactogen and dU-oestrogen levels in normal twin pregnancies. *Acta Genet. Med. Gemellol. (Roma)*, **34**, 59–65.

Kato, H., Yoshimoto, Y. and Schull, W. J. (1989). Risk of cancer among children exposed to atomic bomb radiation in utero: a review. *IARC Sci. Publ.*, **96**, 365–74.

Levi, F., Te, V. C. and La Vecchia, C. (1990). Testicular cancer trends in the Canton of Vaud, Switzerland, 1974–1987. *Br. J. Cancer*, **62**, 871–3.

Long, P. A., Abell, D. A. and Beischer, N. A. (1979). Fetal growth and placental function assessed by urinary estriol excretion before the onset of pre-eclampsia. *Am. J. Obstet. Gynecol.*, **135**, 344–7.

McCormack, V. A., dos Santos Silva, I., De Stavola, B. L. *et al.* (2003). Fetal growth and subsequent risk of breast cancer: results from long term follow up of Swedish cohort. *BMJ*, **326**, 248.

Mellemkjaer, L., Olsen, M. L., Sorensen, H. T. *et al.* (2003). Birth-weight and risk of early-onset breast cancer (Denmark). *Cancer Causes Control*, **14**, 61–4.

Michels, K. B., Trichopoulos, D., Robins, J. M. *et al.* (1996). Birthweight as a risk factor for breast cancer. *Lancet*, **348**, 1542–6.

Moller, H. (1989). Decreased testicular cancer risk in men born in wartime. *J. Natl. Cancer Inst.*, **81**, 1668–9.

Moss, A. R., Osmond, D., Bacchetti, P., Torti, F. M. and Gurgin, V. *et al.* (1986). Hormonal risk factors in testicular cancer: a case-control study. *Am. J. Epidemiol*, **124**, 39–52.

Nylander, P. P. S. (1983). The phenomenon of twinning. In *Obstetrical Epidemiology* (ed. A. M. Thomson). London: Academic Press, pp. 143–65.

Okasha, M., McCarron, P., Gunnell, D. and Davey Smith, G. (2003). Exposures in childhood, adolescence and early adulthood and breast cancer risk: a systematic review of the literature. *Breast Cancer Res. Treat.*, **78**, 223–76.

Palmer, J. R., Hatch, E. E., Rosenberg, C. L. *et al.* (2002). Risk of breast cancer in women exposed to diethylstilbestrol in utero: preliminary results (United States). *Cancer Causes Control*, **13**, 753–8.

Parkin, D. M., Muir, C. S. and Whelan, S. L. (1992). *Cancer Incidence in Five Continents*, vol 6. Lyon: IARC.

Pearce, N., Sheppard, R. A., Howard, J. K., Fraser, J. and Lilley, B. M. (1987). Time trends and occupational differences in cancer of the testis in New Zealand. *Cancer*, **59**, 1677–82.

Pettersson, A., Kaijser, M., Richiardi L. *et al.* (2004). Women smoking and testicular cancer: one epidemic causing another? *Int. J. Cancer*, **109**, 941–4.

Pinczowski, D., McLaughlin, J. K., Lackgren, G., Adami, H. O. and Persson, I. (1991). Occurrence of testicular cancer in patients operated on for cryptorchidism and inguinal hernia. *J. Urol.*, **146**, 1291–4.

Platz, E. A., Giovannucci, E., Rimm, E. B. *et al.* (1998). Retrospective analysis of birthweight and prostate cancer in the Health Professionals Follow-up Study. *Am. J. Epidemiol.*, **147**, 1140–4.

Potosky, A. L., Kessler, L., Gridley, G., Brown, C. C. and Horm, J. W. (1990). Rise in prostatic cancer incidence associated with increased use of transurethral resection. *J. Natl. Cancer Inst.*, **82**, 1624–8.

Prener, A., Hsieh, C. C., Engholm, G., Trichopoulos, D. and Jensen, O. M. (1992). Birth order and risk of testicular cancer. *Cancer Causes Control.*, **3**, 265–72.

Prins, G. S. and Birch, L. (1997). Neonatal oestrogen exposure up-regulates oestrogen receptor expression in the developing and adult rat prostate lobes. *Endocrinology*, **138**, 1801–9.

Richiardi, L., Akre, O., Bellocco, R. and Ekbom, A. (2002). Perinatal determinants of germ-cell testicular cancer in relation to histological subtypes. *Br. J. Cancer*, **87**, 545–50.

Richiardi, L., Akre, O., Montgomery, S. M. *et al.* (2004a). Fecundity and twinning rates as measures of fertility before diagnosis of germ-cell testicular cancer. *J. Natl. Cancer Inst.*, **96**, 145–7.

Richiardi, L., Akre, O., Lambe, M. *et al.* (2004b). Birth order, sibship size, and risk for germ-cell testicular cancer. *Epidemiology*, **15**, 323–9.

Robine, N., Relier, J. P. and Le Bars, S. (1988). Urocytogram, an index of maturity in premature infants. *Biol. Neonate*, **54**, 93–9.

Ros, H. S., Lichtenstein, P., Exbom, A. and Cnattingius, S. (2001). Tall or short? Twenty years after pre-eclampsia exposure *in utero*: comparisons of final height, body mass index, waist-to-hip ratio, and age at menarche among women, exposed and unexposed to pre-eclampsia during fetal life. *Pediatr. Res.*, **49**, 763–9.

Ross, R. K. and Henderson, B. E. (1994). Do diet and androgens alter prostate cancer risk via a common etiologic pathway? *J. Natl. Cancer Inst.*, **86**, 252–4.

Sanderson, M., Williams, M. A., Malone, K. E. *et al.* (1996). Perinatal factors and risk of breast cancer. *Epidemiology*, **7**, 34–7.

Sanderson, M., Shu, X. O., Jin, F. *et al.* (2002). Weight at birth and adolescence and premenopausal breast cancer risk in a low-risk population. *Br. J. Cancer*, **86**, 84–8.

Schottenfeld, D., Warshauer, M. E., Sherlock, S. *et al.* (1980). The epidemiology of testicular cancer in young adults. *Am. J. Epidemiol.*, **112**, 232–46.

Sedin, G., Bergquist, C. and Lindgern, P. G. *et al.* (1985). Ovarian hyperstimulation syndrome in preterm infants. *Pediatr. Res.*, **19**, 548–52.

Service, R. F. (1998). New role for oestrogen in cancer? *Science*, **279**, 1631–3.

Sharpe, R. M. (1995). Reproductive biology: another DDT connection. *Nature*, **375**, 538–9.

Sharpe, R. M. and Skakkebaek, N. E. (1993). Are oestrogens involved in falling sperm counts and disorders of the male reproductive tract? *Lancet*, **341**, 1392–5.

Swerdlow, A. J., Huttly, S. R. and Smith, P. G. *et al.* (1987). Prenatal and familial associations of testicular cancer. *Br. J. Cancer*, **55**, 571–7.

Tibblin, G., Eriksson, M., Cnattingius, S. and Ekbom, A. (1995). High birthweight as a predictor of prostate cancer risk. *Epidemiology*, **6**, 423–4.

Titus-Ernstoff, L., Egan, K. M., Newcomb, P. A. *et al.* (2002). Early life factors in relation to breast cancer risk in postmenopausal women. *Cancer Epidemiol. Biomarkers Prev.*, **11**, 207–10.

Trichopoulos, D. (1990). Is breast cancer initiated in utero? *Epidemiology*, **1**, 95–6.

Trichopoulos, D. and Lipman, R. D. (1992). Mammary gland mass and breast cancer risk. *Epidemiology*, **3**, 523–6.

Wanderas, E. H., Tretli, S. and Fossa, S. D. (1995). Trends in incidence of testicular cancer in Norway 1955–1992. *Eur. J. Cancer*, **31A**, 2044–8.

Wanderas, E. H., Grotmol, T., Fossa, S. D. and Tretli, S. (1998). Maternal health and pre- and perinatal characteristics in the etiology of testicular cancer: a prospective population- and register-based study on Norwegian males born between 1967 and 1995. *Cancer Causes Control*, **9**, 475–86.

Vatten, L. J., Maehle, B. O., Lund Nilsen, T. I. *et al.* (2002). birthweight as a predictor of breast cancer: a case–control study in Norway. *Br. J. Cancer*, **86**, 89–91.

Yuen, J., Ekbom, A., Trichopoulos, D., Hsieh, C. C. and Adami, H. O. (1994). Season of birth and breast cancer risk in Sweden. *Br. J. Cancer*, **70**, 564–8.

32

The developmental environment: implications for ageing and life span

Thomas B. L. Kirkwood

University of Newcastle

Introduction

The ageing process is generally taken to refer to the final stages of an organism's life cycle, 'ageing' often being defined as a progressive, generalised impairment of function resulting in an increasing risk of frailty, disability, disease, and eventually death. Although ageing is thus distanced from the developmental processes of early life, a continuum of cellular and molecular processes connects the beginning and end of life, and recent advances in research on ageing have highlighted the life-course nature of the factors that influence ageing and longevity. In particular, it is now widely accepted that events occurring early in life can have important impacts on the outcomes of the ageing process, influencing both health in old age and the length of life itself.

Three principal kinds of mechanism can be distinguished that connect development with ageing. First, the ageing process is driven by the lifelong accumulation of cellular and molecular damage, arising from processes such as oxidative damage and errors in macromolecule synthesis and processing. These errors begin to accumulate from a very early stage of development, so stresses in early life that increase rates of damage, even transiently, can have long-term consequences. Second, as we shall see below, the cellular maintenance and repair processes that influence damage accumulation appear to be influenced in some circumstances by environmental factors,

such as nutrition. Therefore, variations in the developmental environment can affect the efficiency of repair, which in turn can affect ageing and life span. Third, although the developmental process is under close genetic control, so that organisms generally follow a highly reproducible path from egg to adult, there is growing evidence that developmental variations arising purely by chance can have significant effects on how the individual organism experiences the end stages of the ageing process, even though these variations have little visible effect during earlier life.

This chapter considers current understanding of the factors governing ageing and longevity and of how these are linked to development.

What causes ageing?

A common misconception about the ageing process is that organisms such as humans are programmed to die, perhaps because this is necessary to get rid of older generations and make space for the new. The fallacies in this view have been thoroughly described (Kirkwood and Cremer 1982) and will be summarised only briefly here. The main objection is that there is little evidence that ageing serves as a major contributor to mortality in natural populations (Medawar 1952), which means that ageing apparently does not serve the role suggested for it.

Developmental Origins of Health and Disease, ed. Peter Gluckman and Mark Hanson. Published by Cambridge University Press.
© P. D. Gluckman and M. A. Hanson 2006.

The theory also embodies the questionable supposition that selection for advantage at the species level will be more effective than selection among individuals for the advantages of a longer life. Ageing is clearly a disadvantage to the individual, so any mutation that inactivated any hypothetical 'ageing genes' would confer a fitness advantage, and therefore the non-ageing mutation should spread through the population unless countered by selection at the species or group level. Conditions under which 'group selection' can work successfully are highly restrictive (Maynard Smith 1976), especially when there is selection in the opposite direction acting at the level of the individual. Briefly, it is necessary that the population be divided among fairly isolated groups, and that the introduction of a non-ageing genotype into a group should rapidly lead to the group's extinction. The latter condition is necessary to provide the selection between groups that might, in principle, counter the tendency for selection at the level of individuals to favour the spread of non-ageing mutants. It is unlikely that these conditions will be met with sufficient generality to explain the evolution of ageing.

If ageing is not actively programmed, how can it be accounted for in terms of natural selection? The key comes from looking more closely at the observation that ageing makes negligible contribution to mortality in wild populations of animals. For example, 90% of wild mice are dead by age 10 months, although the same animals might live for three years if protected (Austad 1997). This has an important bearing on how far the mouse genome should invest in mechanisms for the long-term maintenance and repair of its somatic cells. If 90% of wild mice are dead by 10 months, any investment in maintenance to keep the body in good condition much beyond this point can benefit at most 10% of the population. This immediately suggests that there will be little evolutionary advantage in building long-term survival capacity into a mouse. The argument is further strengthened when we observe that nearly all of the survival mechanisms required by the mouse to combat intrinsic deterioration (DNA damage, protein oxidation, etc.) require metabolic resources. Metabolic resources are

scarce, as is evidenced by the fact that the major cause of mortality for wild mice is cold, due to insufficient energy to maintain body temperature (Berry and Bronson 1992). From a Darwinian point of view, the mouse will benefit more from investing any spare resource into thermogenesis or reproduction than into better DNA repair capacity than it needs.

This concept, with its explicit focus on evolution of optimal levels of cell maintenance, is termed the disposable soma theory (Kirkwood 1977, 1997). In essence, the investments in durability and maintenance of somatic (non-reproductive) tissues are predicted to be sufficient to keep the body in good repair through the normal expectation of life in the wild environment, with some measure of reserve capacity. Thus, it makes sense that mice (with 90% mortality by 10 months) have intrinsic life spans of around three years, while humans (who probably experienced something like 90% mortality by age 50 in our ancestral environment) have intrinsic life spans limited to about 100 years. The distinction between somatic and reproductive tissues is important because the reproductive cell lineage, or germ line, must be maintained at a level that preserves viability across the generations, whereas the soma needs only to support the survival of a single generation. As far as is known, all species that have a clear distinction between soma and germ line undergo somatic senescence, while animals that do not show senescence, such as the freshwater hydra (Martinez 1997), have germ cells distributed throughout their body.

The disposable soma theory leads to a number of clear predictions about the nature of the underlying mechanisms that lead to age-related frailty, disability and disease. In essence, ageing is neither more nor less than the progressive accumulation through life of a variety of random molecular defects that build up within cells and tissues. These defects start to arise very early in life, probably in utero, but in the early years both the fraction of affected cells and the average burden of damage per affected cell are low. But over time the faults increase, resulting eventually in age-related functional impairment of tissues and organs.

This view also helps us examine the sometimes controversial relationship between 'normal ageing' and age-related disease. At one extreme, the term 'normal ageing' is reserved for individuals in whom identifiable pathology is absent. An obvious difficulty that arises, however, when any attempt is made to draw a line between normal ageing and age-related disease is that as a cohort ages, the fraction of individuals who can be said to be ageing 'normally' declines to very low levels. Whether the word 'normal' can usefully be applied to such an atypical subset is debatable. The majority of chronic degenerative conditions, such as dementia, osteoporosis and osteoarthritis, involve the progressive accumulation of specific types of cellular and molecular lesions. Since the ageing process, as we have seen, is likely to be caused by the general accumulation of such lesions, there may be much greater overlap between the causative pathways leading to normal ageing and age-related diseases than has hitherto been recognised. In the case of Alzheimer's disease, most people above age 70 have extensive cortical amyloid plaques and neurofibrillary tangles (the so-called 'hallmarks' of classic Alzheimer's disease) even though they may show no evidence of major cognitive decline (Esiri *et al.* 2001). Osteoporosis provides another interesting example, since progressive bone loss from the late 20s onwards is the norm. Whether an individual reaches a critically low bone density, making him or her highly susceptible to fracture, is governed by how much bone mass they had to start with and by their individual rate of bone loss. The process that leads eventually to osteoporosis is thus entirely 'normal', but what distinguishes whether or not this process results in an overtly pathological outcome is a range of moderating factors, including developmental factors.

In terms of underlying cellular and molecular mechanisms, ageing is highly complex, involving multiple mechanisms at different levels. Much recent evidence suggests that an important theme linking several different kinds of damage is the action of reactive oxygen species (ROS; also known as 'free radicals') which are produced as by-products of the body's essential use of oxygen to produce cellular energy (Martin *et al.* 1996, von Zglinicki *et al.* 2000). Of particular significance are the contributions of ROS-induced damage to cellular DNA through (1) damage to the chromosomal DNA of the cell nucleus resulting in impaired gene function, (2) damage to telomeres – the protective DNA structures that appear to 'cap' the ends of chromosomes (analogous to the plastic tips of shoelaces), and (3) damage to the DNA that exists within the cell's energy-generating organelles, the mitochondria, resulting in impaired energy production.

Damage to DNA is particularly likely to play a role in the lifelong accumulation of molecular damage within cells, since it can readily result in permanent alteration of the cell's DNA sequence. Cells are subject to mutation all the time, both through errors that may become fixed when cells divide and as a result of ROS-induced damage which can occur at any time. Numerous studies have reported age-related increases in somatic mutation and other forms of DNA damage, suggesting that an important determinant of the rate of ageing at the cellular and molecular level is the capacity for DNA repair (Promislow 1994, Bürkle *et al.* 2002).

The role of damage to telomeres has received much attention in ageing research. In many human somatic tissues a decline in cellular division capacity with age appears to be linked to the fact that the telomeres, which protect the ends of chromosomes, get progressively shorter as cells divide (Kim *et al.* 2002). This is due to the absence of the enzyme telomerase, which is normally expressed only in germ cells (in testis and ovary) and in certain adult stem cells. Some have suggested that in dividing somatic cells telomeres act as an intrinsic 'division counter', perhaps to protect us against runaway cell division as happens in cancer but causing ageing as the price for this protection (Campisi 1997). Erosion of telomere length below a critical length appears to trigger activation of cell cycle checkpoints resulting in permanent arrest of the cell division process. While the loss of telomeric DNA is often attributed mainly to the so-called 'end replication' problem – the inability of the normal DNA copying machinery to copy right to the very end of the strand in the absence of telomerase – it has been found that stress, especially oxidative stress, has an even bigger effect on the rate of telomere erosion (von Zglinicki 2002). Telomere shortening is greatly accelerated (or slowed) in cells with increased (or reduced) levels of stress. The clinical relevance of understanding telomere maintenance and its interaction with stress is considerable. A growing body of evidence suggests that telomere length is linked with ageing and mortality (e.g. Cawthon *et al.* 2003). Not only do telomeres shorten with normal ageing in several tissues (e.g. lymphocytes, vascular endothelial cells, kidney, liver), but also their reduction is more marked in certain disease states. For example, there appears to be a 100-fold higher incidence of vascular dementia in people with prematurely short telomeres (von Zglinicki *et al.* 2000).

An important connection between oxidative stress and ageing is suggested by the accumulation of mitochondrial DNA (mtDNA) deletions and point mutations with age (Wallace 1992). Mitochondria are intracellular organelles, each carrying its own small DNA genome, which are responsible for generating cellular energy. As a by-product of energy generation, mitochondria are also the major source of ROS within the cell, and they are therefore both responsible for, and a major target of, oxidative stress. Any age-related increase in mutation of mtDNA is likely to contribute to a progressive decline in the cell and tissue capacity for energy production. Age-related increases in frequency of cytochrome c oxidase (COX)-deficient cells have been reported in human muscle (Müller-Höcker 1989, Müller-Höcker *et al.* 1993, Brierley *et al.* 1998) and brain (Cottrell *et al.* 2000), associated with increased frequency of mutated mtDNA. Until recently, the evidence for age-related accumulation of mtDNA mutations came mainly from tissues such as brain and muscle where cell division in the adult, if it occurs at all, is rare. This led to the idea that accumulation of mtDNA mutation was driven mainly by the dynamics of mitochondrial multiplication and turnover within non-dividing cells (Kowald and Kirkwood 2000). However, recent work has revealed a strongly age-dependent accumulation of mtDNA mutations in human gut epithelium, which has the highest cell division rate of any tissue in the body (Taylor *et al.* 2003). Thus it appears that mtDNA mutation accumulation may be a widespread phenomenon.

What controls life span?

From an evolutionary and ecological perspective, the level of extrinsic mortality experienced by a population in the wild is clearly the principal driver in the evolution of longevity. If the level of extrinsic mortality is high, the average survival period is short and there is little selection for a high level of maintenance. Any spare resources should go instead towards reproduction. Consequently, the organism is not long-lived even in a protected environment. Conversely, if the level of extrinsic mortality is low, selection is likely to direct a higher investment in building and maintaining a durable soma. Studies comparing the biochemistry of cellular repair among long- and short-lived species bear this prediction out. Cells from long-lived organisms exhibit greater capacity to repair molecular damage and withstand biochemical stresses than cells from short-lived species (Kapahi *et al.* 1999, Ogburn *et al.* 2001). In terms of DNA repair capacity, a key player in the immediate cellular response to DNA damage is the enzyme poly(ADP-ribose) polymerase 1 (PARP1). Grube and Bürkle (1992) discovered a strong, positive correlation of PARP1 activity with the species' life span, cells from long-lived species having higher levels of PARP1 activity than cells from short-lived species. In a similar vein, it was found that human centenarians, who have often maintained remarkably good general health, have a significantly greater poly(ADP-ribosyl)ation capacity than the general population (Muiras *et al.* 1998). Numerous opportunities exist to test the evolutionary prediction that in safe environments (those with low extrinsic mortality) ageing will evolve to be retarded, whereas ageing should evolve to be more rapid in hazardous environments. Field observations comparing a mainland population of opossums, subject to significant predation by mammals, with an island population not subject to mammalian predation, found the predicted slower ageing in the island population (Austad 1993).

What is interesting from the perspective of how longevity is controlled is to understand how these ecologically driven effects are mediated at the level of cellular and molecular mechanisms. The disposable soma theory predicts that the proportional effort devoted to cellular maintenance and repair processes will vary directly with longevity. For instance, the long-lived rodent species *Peromyscus leucopus* exhibits lower generation of reactive oxygen species (ROS), higher cellular concentrations of some antioxidant enzymes, and overall lower levels of protein oxidative damage than the shorter-lived species *Mus musculus* (Sohal *et al.* 1993). A direct relation between species longevity and rate of mitochondrial ROS production in captive mammals has also been found (Ku *et al.* 1993; Barja and Herrero 2000), as has a similar relationship between mammals and similar-sized but much longer-lived birds (Herrero and Barja 1999). Markers of glycoxidation, the non-enzymatic modification of reducing sugars, are also found to accumulate more slowly in long-lived, as opposed to short-lived, mammals (Sell *et al.* 1996).

Of particular significance in terms of metabolic factors influencing ageing rates has been the discovery that insulin signalling pathways appear to have effects on ageing that may be strongly conserved across the species range (Gems and Partridge 2001). Insulin signalling regulates responses to varying nutrient levels, and so the discovery of the major role for these pathways in ageing fits well with the central concept of the disposable soma theory, namely that ageing results from, and is controlled by, the metabolic allocation of the organism's metabolic resources to maintenance and repair.

One of the clearest examples of how metabolic signalling affects ageing and longevity comes from a study on genes of the insulin signalling pathway in the nematode *Caenorhabditis elegans* (Murphy *et al.* 2003). When threatened with overcrowding, which the larval worm detects by the increasing concentration of a pheromone, it diverts its development from the normal succession of larval moults into a long-lived dispersal form called the dauer larva

(Larsen *et al.* 1995). Dauers show increased resistance to stress and can survive very much longer than the normal form, reverting to complete their development should more favorable conditions be detected. An insulin/IGF1-like gene, *daf-2*, heads the gene regulatory pathway that controls the switch into the dauer form, and mutations in *daf-2* produce animals that develop into adults with substantially increased life spans (Kenyon *et al.* 1993). In common with other members of the evolutionarily conserved insulin/IGF1 signalling pathway, *daf-2* also regulates lipid metabolism and reproduction. The *daf-2* gene product exerts its effects by influencing 'downstream' gene expression, in particular via the actions of another gene belonging to the dauer-formation gene family, *daf-16*, which it inhibits (Kimura *et al.* 1997). It was shown by Murphy *et al.* (2003) that more than 300 genes appeared to have their expression levels altered by *daf-16* regulation. These genes turned out to be a heterogeneous group in which three major categories could be discerned. The first category comprised a variety of stress-response genes, including antioxidant enzymes. A second group of genes encoded antimicrobial proteins, important for survival in this organism because its death is commonly caused by proliferation of bacteria in the gut. A third group included genes involved in protein turnover, which is an important cellular maintenance system. Thus the metabolic regulation of the rate of ageing in *C. elegans* is mediated through genetic effects on a diverse array of survival mechanisms, exactly as the disposable soma theory predicted.

Plasticity of ageing processes

The example of *C. elegans* just considered shows how life span may be regulated by environmental factors such as crowding. This introduces an important principle, directly compatible with the underlying hypothesis of the disposable soma theory, that the optimal allocation of resources between growth, maintenance and reproduction may exhibit an evolved plasticity that allows the individual to respond to varying circumstances. In addition to the dauer larva of *C. elegans*, a much-studied phenomenon is that of life-span extension through dietary restriction in rodents.

It has long been known that life span in laboratory rodents is extended by restricting their food intake, with typical increases of 20–30% in both mean and maximum life span (McCay *et al.* 1935, Weindruch and Walford 1988). Long-term calorie restriction results in a small, lean animal, with impaired fertility, but which is otherwise healthy and active. Recent interest has focused on identifying the physiological mechanisms that maintain the animal in what appears to be a youthful state. Almost without exception somatic maintenance functions are up-regulated (Holehan and Merry 1986, Masoro 1993; Yu 1994, Merry 1995).

At first sight, it seems paradoxical that an organism with less energy available can up-regulate physiological processes, which must have an associated metabolic cost. This requires that metabolic savings be made elsewhere. The most obvious saving is in reproductive effort. Not only is reproduction costly in direct physiological terms, but behaviours associated with reproduction can also be expensive. Rodents typically invest a large fraction of their energy budget in reproduction. Calorie restriction results in animals that are mostly infertile, although there is some variation depending on the sex, the degree of restriction and the age at which restriction is first applied (Weindruch and Walford 1988). For example, in mice, calorie restriction by 40% arrests follicular cycles in females (Nelson *et al.* 1985), whereas in female rats subjected to the same level of restriction, some reproductive activity continues (McShane and Wise 1996). Puberty in female rodents is delayed and reproductive senescence occurs later (Merry and Holehan 1979; Nelson *et al.* 1985). On re-feeding, female rodents previously kept on restricted diets are able to reproduce at much later ages than fully fed controls (see Holehan and Merry 1986).

Posing the evolutionary question of why a calorie-restricted organism should retard ageing helps to throw light on the physiological basis of this phenomenon. Harrison and Archer (1988) suggested that the primary role of calorie restriction is to postpone reproductive senescence. If a famine lasts longer than the normal reproductive lifespan of the animal, any female that delays reproductive senescence and is able to breed after the famine has passed will experience a selective advantage. A more explicit hypothesis was proposed by Holliday (1989), based on the disposable soma theory of ageing. This proposed that during periods of famine the animal might improve its Darwinian fitness by temporarily shifting resources away from reproduction and towards increased somatic maintenance. The potential benefit is that the animal gains an increased chance of survival with a reduced intrinsic rate of senescence, thereby permitting reproductive value to be preserved for when the famine is over. Shanley and Kirkwood (2000) explored these ideas in a quantitative life-history analysis, based on extensive physiological data, and confirmed that the evolutionary hypothesis would work, provided certain plausible conditions were fulfilled, the main requirements being (1) that survival of juveniles is reduced during periods of famine, and (2) that the organism needs to pay an energetic 'overhead' before any litter of offspring can be produced.

A further instance of plasticity of ageing processes is seen in social insects, such as ants and bees, where queens are generally long-lived and workers have life spans which can vary among the castes. In the case of the honeybee (*Apis mellifera*), the worker caste possesses a capacity for regulation of ageing in which the same genotype may, depending upon its environment, end up in either of two temporal groups that differ dramatically with respect to life span as well as physiological profiles related to somatic maintenance (Omholt *et al.* in press). In summer, worker bees need to forage, and as foraging is risky, they do not normally live long (Visscher and Dukas 1997). In this case there is likely to be selection against investing resources to increase the potential life span of the workers. This is supported by the fact that honeybee foragers do not eat and process pollen themselves but are fed proteinaceous jelly on a regular basis by the hive bees in accordance with their foraging activity level (Riessberger and Crailsheim 1997 Hrassnigg and Crailsheim 1998). Furthermore, turning off vitellogenin synthesis in the forager (Pinto *et al.* 2000), and reprogramming its hypopharyngeal glands to synthesise honey-processing enzymes at low rates (Bozic and Woodring 2000), is likely to be a means to optimise the allocation of the colony's protein budget, as this will prevent build-up of a vitellogenin store that will be lost when the forager perishes in the field (Amdam and Omholt 2002; Amdam *et al.* 2003). In winter, on the other hand, when there is no risky foraging and the colony has to survive for several months before it can resume reproduction, there is likely to be a selection pressure to allocate enough resources to keep the workers alive for a long time. This is clearly supported by the observed accumulation of vitellogenin and the maintenance of a high haemocyte load in the long-lived caste of overwintering hive bees (Fluri *et al.* 1977).

The possibility that adaptive plasticity of ageing and life span occurs also in humans has been raised by the discovery that the fetal nutritional environment can affect the risk of developing age-related diseases in the adult (O'Brien *et al.* 1999, Barker *et al.* 2002, Gluckman and Hanson 2004a, 2004b, Bateson *et al.* 2004). Whether these effects are mediated by adaptive plasticity affecting the allocation of metabolic resources to somatic maintenance remains to be discovered.

Developmental origins of life-span variability

Life span varies greatly within populations. In free-living, outbred populations this variation is usually attributed to the combined effects of individual genetic and environmental factors and to causes such as infection, accident, starvation, predation and cold. However, even when a population comprises genetically uniform individuals, reared in a constant environment, and protected from extrinsic mortality, the individuals display very different life spans (Finch and Kirkwood 2000, Kirkwood and Finch 2002). Although some of this non-genetic, non-environmental variation can be attributed to the

stochastic nature of the intrinsic mechanisms of cell and molecular ageing, there is growing evidence that some of it may also be due to the effects of intrinsic chance on developmental processes.

The overall process of morphogenesis is remarkably reliable. Nevertheless, small early perturbations can result in large effects, and there is evidence of significant organ size variations among genetically identical organisms (Finch and Kirkwood 2000), or even between the two sides of a single individual (known as 'fluctuating asymmetry'; Moller and Swaddle 1997). In addition to variations in the endpoints of development, such as adult organ size, there can be significant variations in the timing of key developmental events, such as puberty (vom Saal *et al.* 1990). In keeping with our understanding of the evolution of ageing reviewed earlier, we can see that any source of developmental variation that has little effect on the fitness of young organisms but that contributes to the pathophysiology of ageing, will largely escape the attentions of natural selection. The cumulative effects of intrinsic variations at the cell level during development are seen in the variability of organ size and cell number when morphogenesis is complete. In genetically identical individuals, such as inbred mice or monozygotic human twins, the variation in organ size can be large (Finch and Kirkwood 2000). For example, the size of the ovary in newborn mice of the same strain may vary three fold (Jones and Krohn 1961, Gosden *et al.* 1982), and there can be differences of 10–20% in the sizes of the hippocampi in human twin pairs (Plassman *et al.* 1997). These variations affect the size of the respective organ's 'reserve capacity', which in turn can affect the time taken for its function to become terminally compromised by the accumulation of cellular and molecular damage.

REFERENCES

Amdam, G. V. and Omholt, S. W. (2002). The regulatory anatomy of honeybee lifespan. *J. Theor. Biol.*, **216**, 209–28.
Amdam, G. V., Norberg, K., Hagen, A. and Omholt, S. W. (2003). Social exploitation of vitellogenin. *Proc. Natl. Acad. Sci. USA*, **100**, 1799–802.

Austad, S. N. (1993). Retarded senescence in an insular population of opossums. *J. Zool.*, **229**, 695–708.

(1997). Comparative aging and life histories in mammals. *Exp. Gerontol.*, **32**, 23–38.

Barja, G. and Herrero, A. (2000). Oxidative damage to mitochondrial DNA is inversely related to maximum life span in the heart and brain of mammals. *FASEB J.*, **14**, 312–18.

Barker, D. J. P., Eriksson, J. G., Forsen, T. and Osmond, C. (2002). Fetal origins of adult disease: strength of effects and biological basis. *Int. J. Epidemiol.*, **31**, 1235–9.

Bateson, P., Barker, D., Clutton-Brock, T. *et al.* (2004). Developmental plasticity and human health. *Nature*, **430**, 419–21.

Berry, R. J. and Bronson, F. H. (1992). Life history and bioeconomy of the house mouse. *Biol. Rev. Camb. Philos. Soc.*, **67**, 519–50.

Bozic, J. and Woodring, J. (2000). Variation in JH synthesis rate in mature honeybees and its possible role in reprogramming of hypopharyngeal gland function. *Pflügers Arch.*, **439**, R163–4.

Brierley, E. J., Johnson, M. A., Lightowlers, R. N., James, O. F. W. and Turnbull, D. M. (1998). Role of mitochondrial DNA mutations in human aging: implications for the central nervous system and muscle. *Ann. Neurol.*, **43**, 217–23.

Bürkle, A., Beneke, S., Brabeck, C. *et al.* (2002). Poly(ADP-ribose) polymerase-1, DNA repair and mammalian longevity. *Exp. Gerontol.*, **37**, 1203–5.

Campisi, J. (1997). Aging and cancer: the double-edged sword of replicative senescence. *J. Am. Geriatr. Soc.*, **45**, 482–8.

Cawthon, R. M., Smith, K. R., O'Brien, E., Sivatchenko, A. and Kerber, R. A. (2003). Association between telomere length in blood and mortality in people aged 60 years or older. *Lancet*, **361**, 393–5.

Cottrell, D. A., Blakely, E. L., Johnson, M. A., Ince, P. G., Borthwick, G. M. and Turnbull, D. M. (2000). Cytochrome c oxidase deficient cells accumulate in the hippocampus and choroid plexus with age. *Neurobiol. Aging*, **22**, 265–72.

Esiri, M. M., Matthews, F., Brayne, C. *et al.* (2001). Pathological correlates of late-onset dementia in a multicentre, community-based population in England and Wales. *Lancet*, **357**, 169–75.

Finch, C. E. and Kirkwood, T. B. L. (2000). *Chance, Development, and Aging*. New York, NY: Oxford University Press.

Fluri, P., Wille, H., Gerig, L. and Lüscher, M. (1977). Juvenile hormone, vitellogenin and haemocyte composition in winter worker honeybees (*Apis mellifera*). *Experientia*, **33**, 1240–1.

Gems, D. and Partridge, L. (2001). Insulin/IGF signalling and ageing: seeing the bigger picture. *Curr. Opin. Genet. Dev.*, **11**, 287–92.

Gluckman, P. D. and Hanson, M. A. (2004a). The developmental origins of the metabolic syndrome. *Trends Endocrinol. Metab.*, **15**, 183–7.

(2004b). Living with the past: evolution, development, and patterns of disease. *Science*, **305**, 1733–6.

Gosden, R. G., Laing, S. C., Felicio, L. S., Nelson, J. F. and Finch, C. E. (1982). Imminent oocyte exhaustion and reduced follicular recruitment mark the transition to acyclicity in aging C57BL/6J mice. *Biol. Reprod.*, **28**, 255–60.

Grube, K. and Bürkle, A. (1992). Poly(ADP-ribose) polymerase activity in mononuclear leukocytes of 13 mammalian species correlates with species-specific life span. *Proc. Natl. Acad. Sci. USA*, **89**, 11759–63.

Harrison, D. E. and J. R. Archer. (1988). Natural selection for extended longevity from food restriction. *Growth Dev. Aging*, **52**, 65.

Herrero, A. and Barja, G. (1999). 8-oxo-deoxyguanosine levels in heart and brain mitochondrial and nuclear DNA of two mammals and three birds in relation to their different rates of aging. *Aging Clin. Exp. Res.*, **11**, 294–300.

Holehan, A. M. and B. J. Merry. (1986). The experimental manipulation of aging by diet. *Biol. Rev. Camb. Philos. Soc.*, **61**, 329–68.

Holliday, R. (1989). Food, reproduction and longevity: is the extended lifespan of calorie-restricted animals an evolutionary adaptation? *Bioessays*, **10**, 125–7.

Hrassnigg, N. and Crailsheim, K. (1998). The influence of brood on the pollen consumption of worker bees (*Apis mellifera* L.). *J. Insect Physiol.*, **44**, 393–404.

Jones, E. C. and Krohn, P. L. (1961). The relationships between age, numbers of oocytes, and fertility in virgin and multiparous mice. *J. Endocrinol.*, **21**, 469–96.

Kapahi, P., Boulton, M. E. and Kirkwood, T. B. L. (1999). Positive correlation between mammalian life span and cellular resistance to stress. *Free Radic. Biol. Med.*, **26**, 495–500.

Kenyon, C., Chang, J., Gensch, E., Rudner, A. and Tabtiang, R. (1993). A *C. elegans* mutant that lives twice as long as wild-type. *Nature*, **366**, 461–4.

Kim, S., Kaminker, P. and Campisi, J. (2002). Telomeres, aging and cancer: in search of a happy ending. *Oncogene*, **21**, 503–11.

Kimura, K. D., Tissenbaum, H. A., Liu, Y. X. and Ruvkun, G. (1997). *daf-2*, an insulin receptor-like gene that regulates longevity and diapause in *Caenorhabditis elegans*. *Science*, **277**, 942–6.

Kirkwood, T. B. L. (1977). Evolution of ageing. *Nature*, **270**, 301–4.

(1997). The origins of human ageing. *Phil. Trans. R. Soc. Lond. B*, **352**, 1765–72.

Kirkwood, T. B. L. and Cremer, T. (1982). Cytogerontology since 1881: a reappraisal of August Weismann and a review of modern progress. *Hum. Genet.*, **60**, 101–21.

Kirkwood, T. B. L. and Finch, C. E. (2002). The old worm turns more slowly. *Nature*, **419**, 794–5.

Kowald, A. and Kirkwood, T. B. L. (2000). Accumulation of defective mitochondria through delayed degradation of damaged organelles and its possible role in the ageing of post-mitotic and dividing cells. *J. Theor. Biol.*, **202**, 145–60.

Ku, H.-H., Brunk, U. T. and Sohal, R. S. (1993). Relationship between mitochondrial superoxide and hydrogen peroxide production and longevity of mammalian species. *Free Radic. Biol. Med.*, **15**, 621–7.

Larsen, P. L., Albert, P. and Riddle, D. L. (1995). Genes that regulate both development and longevity in *Caenorhabditis elegans*. *Genetics*, **139**, 1567–83.

Martin, G. M., Austad, S. N. and Johnson, T. E. (1996). Genetic analysis of ageing: role of oxidative damage and environmental stresses. *Nat. Genet.*, **13**, 25–34.

Martinez, D. E. (1997). Mortality patterns suggest lack of senescence in hydra. *Exp. Gerontol.*, **33**, 217–25.

Masoro, E. J. (1993). Dietary restriction and aging. *J. Am. Geriatr. Soc.*, **41**, 994–9.

Maynard Smith, J. (1976). Group selection. *Q. Rev. Biol.*, **1**, 277–83.

McCay, C. M., Crowell, M. F. and Maynard, L. A. (1935). The effect of retarded growth upon the length of the life span and upon the ultimate body size. *J. Nutr.*, **10**, 63–79.

McShane, T. M. and Wise, P. M. (1996). Life-long moderate caloric restriction prolongs reproductive life span in rats without interrupting estrous cyclicity: effects on the gonadotropin-releasing hormone luteinizing hormone axis. *Biol. Reprod.*, **54**, 70–5.

Medawar, P. B. (1952). *An Unsolved Problem of Biology*. London: Lewis.

Merry, B. J. (1995). Effect of dietary restriction on aging: an update. *Rev. Clin. Gerontol.*, **5**, 247–58.

Merry, B. J. and Holehan, A. M. (1979). Onset of puberty and duration of fertility in rats fed a restricted diet. *J. Reprod. Fertil.*, **57**, 253–9.

Moller, A. P. and Swaddle, J. P. (1997). *Asymmetry, Developmental Stability, and Evolution*. Oxford: Oxford University Press.

Muiras, M.-L., Müller, M., Schächter, F. and Bürkle, A. (1998). Increased poly(ADP-ribose) polymerase activity in lymphoblastoid cell lines from centenarians. *J. Mol. Med.*, **76**, 346–54.

Müller-Höcker, J. (1989). Cytochrome-c-oxidase deficient cardiomyocytes in the human heart: an age-related phenomenon. A histochemical ultracytochemical study. *Am. J. Pathol.*, **134**, 1167–73.

Müller-Höcker, J., Seibel, P., Schneiderbanger, K. and Kadenbach, B. (1993). Different *in situ* hybridization patterns of mitochondrial DNA in cytochrome c oxidase-deficient extraocular muscle fibres in the elderly. *Virchows Arch. A*, **422**, 7–15.

Murphy, C. T., McCarroll, S. A., Bargmann, C. I. *et al.* (2003). Genes that act downstream of DAF-16 to influence the lifespan of *Caenorhabditis elegans*. *Nature*, **424**, 277–84.

Nelson, J. F., Gosden, R. G. and Felicio, L. S.. (1985). Effect of calorie-restriction on estrous cyclicity and follicular reserves in aging C57BL6J mice. *Biol. Reprod.*, **32**, 515–22.

O'Brien, P. M. S., Wheeler, T. and Barker, D. J. P. (1999). *Fetal Programming: Influences on Development and Disease in Later Life*. London: Royal College of Obstetricians and Gynaecologists.

Ogburn, C. E., Carlberg, K., Ottinger, M. A., Holmes, D. J., Martin, G. M. and Austad, S. N. (2001). Exceptional cellular resistance to oxidative damage in long-lived birds requires active gene expression. *J. Gerontol. A*, **56**, B468–74.

Omholt, S. W., Kirkwood, T. B. L. and Amdam, G. V. (in press). Evolutionary regulation of aging: lessons from the honeybee. *Exp. Gerontal.*

Pinto, L. Z., Bitondi, M. M. G. and Simões, Z. L. P. (2000). Inhibition of vitellogenin synthesis in *Apis mellifera* workers by a juvenile hormone analogue, pyriproxyfen. *J. Insect Physiol.*, **46**, 153–60.

Plassman, B. L., Welsh-Bohmer, K. A., Bigler, E. D. *et al.* (1997). Apolipoprotein E4 allele and hippocampal volume in twins with normal cognition. *Neurology*, **48**, 985–9.

Promislow, D. E. L. (1994). DNA-repair and the evolution of longevity: a critical analysis. *J. Theor. Biol.*, **170**, 291–300.

Riessberger, U. and Crailsheim, K. (1997). Short-term effect of different weather conditions upon the behaviour of forager and nurse honey bees (*Apis mellifera carnica* Pollmann). *Apidologie*, **28**, 411–26.

Sell, D. R., Lane, M. A., Johnson, W. A. *et al.* (1996). Longevity and the genetic determination of collagen glycoxidation kinetics in mammalian senescence. *Proc. Natl. Acad. Sci. USA*, **93**, 485–90.

Shanley, D. P. and Kirkwood, T. B. L. (2000). Calorie restriction and aging: a life history analysis. *Evolution*, **54**, 740–50.

Sohal, R. S., Ku, H.-H. and Agarwal, S. (1993). Biochemical correlates of longevity in two closely-related rodent species. *Biochem. Biophys. Res. Comm.*, **196**, 7–11.

Taylor, R. W., Barron, M. J., Borthwick, G. M. *et al.* (2003). Mitochondrial DNA mutations in human colonic crypt stem cells. *J. Clin. Invest.*, **112**, 1351–60.

Visscher, P. K. and Dukas, R. (1997). Survivorship of foraging honey bees. *Insectes Soc.*, **44**, 1–5.

Vom Saal, F. S., Quadagno, D. M., Even, M. D., Keisler, L. W., Keisler, D. H. and Khan, S. (1990). Paradoxical effects of maternal stress on fetal steroids and postnatal reproductive traits in female mice from different intrauterine positions. *Biol. Reprod.*, **43**, 751–61.

von Zglinicki, T. (2002), Oxidative stress shortens telomeres. *Trends Biochem. Sci.*, **27**, 339–44.

von Zglinicki, T., Serra, V., Lorenz, M. *et al.* (2000). Short telomeres in patients with vascular dementia: an indicator of low antioxidative capacity and a possible prognostic factor? *Lab. Invest.*, **80**, 1739–47.

Wallace, D. C. (1992). Mitochondrial genetics: a paradigm for aging and degenerative diseases? *Science*, **256**, 628–32.

Weindruch, R. and Walford, R. L. (1988). *The Retardation of Aging and Disease by Dietary Restriction.* Springfield, IL: Charles C. Thomas.

Yu, B. P. (1994). How diet influences the aging process of the rat. *Proc. Soc. Exp. Biol. Med.*, **205**, 97–105.

33

Developmental origins of health and disease: implications for primary intervention for cardiovascular and metabolic disease

Terrence Forrester

University of the West Indies

Introduction

The impact of the environment on our lives over the aeons has been a dominant force helping to shape our genome, and within it the encrypted forms and functions that characterise our species. Throughout most of our evolutionary history, the environment has posed its nutritional challenges within the rubric of malnutrition and infection, and the drive to establish and retain food security has so dominated our activities over these millennia that survival advantage has accrued to thrifty genomes and thrifty 'phenomes' (Neel 1999, Hales and Barker 2001). That we should now be threatened by agricultural surplus is perhaps poetic justice. Regardless, in establishing our mastery over nature, and extracting three square meals per day, every day, as well as essentially relieving ourselves of the requirement for muscular work to secure food or defend life, we have fallen prey to the asynchronous kinetics of biological adaptation and environmental change (Gluckman and Hanson 2004). We have simply not had enough evolutionary time to adapt successfully to the increasing availability of food and reduction in physical activity required for daily life that have taken place at an increasingly rapid pace over the past 300 years.

The invention of agriculture some 10 000 years ago enabled the emergence of modern civilisations by ensuring surplus, fostering labour specialisation and thus the eventual rise of the capitalist approach to economic growth (Diamond 1998). Consistent food supply for populations enabled escape from malnutrition and infection. With the advent of the industrial revolution approximately 300 years ago, the more recent uptake of technology into food production has resulted in an abundance of dietary animal products and carbohydrates, especially simple sugars, as well as oils and fats, changes that are associated with increased energy density of our diets. The simultaneous uptake of technology into production processes has displaced human physical activity from economic activity while the incorporation of technology into the domestic environment has reduced energy expenditure even further. Essentially unrestricted access to calories and reduced physical activity have combined to create a positive energy balance at the individual level, manifested as increasing adiposity (Francois and James 1994).

Adiposity is captured by a summary anthropometric measure, the body mass index (BMI) which is highly correlated with percentage of fat within any one population. However, the intercept of the curves relating percentage of fat and BMI varies across populations. For example, among Nigerian men a BMI of 25 kg m^{-2} represents a fat level of 16%, among Jamaican men of African origin, 21.5%, while among African-American men it corresponds to over 25% fat (Luke *et al.* 1997).

Developmental Origins of Health and Disease, ed. Peter Gluckman and Mark Hanson. Published by Cambridge University Press.

Nevertheless, despite its limitations, BMI remains the best available summary measure of adiposity for the purpose of global estimates and comparisons (Norgan 1994).

Obesity: marker and mediator of the metabolic syndrome?

Controversy exists around the question, whether adipose tissue is a proxy for metabolic and physiological changes which accompany chronic energy surplus or whether, rather, adipose tissue lies directly on the causal pathway to cardiovascular disease. Were the storage of the energy surplus in the body to be in an inert form, then perhaps the main challenges resulting from obesity might have been mechanical. However, if adipose tissue is a functional entity involved in the pathogenesis of disease, then mechanical problems would be accompanied by cardiovascular pathology. In this chapter the position taken is that whether proxy or causal agent, adiposity is associated with the emergence of a cluster of cardiovascular diseases – hypertension, diabetes, and atherosclerotic vascular disease. The pattern of depot storage which results in a high BMI ($>25 \, \mathrm{kg \, m^{-2}}$) and central adiposity, captured as waist circumference or waist/hip ratio, is that which is most closely related to the risk of the metabolic syndrome and its sequelae.

Hypertension and diabetes are cardiovascular diseases in their own right, and are simultaneously risk factors for atherosclerotic vascular disease. The coexistence of several potent risk factors for atherosclerotic disease, obesity (especially central obesity), insulin resistance, hypertension and dyslipidaemia (low HDL and hypertriglyceridaemia) is referred to as the metabolic syndrome. An efficient way, therefore, to examine the cardiovascular diseases related to the interaction of the environment and our underlying genetic and non-genetic, programmed susceptibilities is to focus on the metabolic syndrome. This series of interrelated metabolic and physiological disturbances constitute a risk slate for atherosclerosis and lie at the base of the current epidemics of chronic cardiovascular disease.

Pathophysiology of the metabolic syndrome

Adipose tissue produces adipocytokines which participate in the pathogenetic pathways leading to the metabolic syndrome. These include tumour necrosis factor alpha (TNFα), interleukin 6 (IL6), plasminogen activator inhibitor type 1, adiponectin, angiotensinogen/angiotensin II, and resistin (Shirai 2004).

Adipocytokines exert influence on the metabolism of both carbohydrates and lipids (Shirai 2004). Adipose tissue releases TNFα which induces insulin resistance at the level of muscle and liver. It is also one of the inflammatory stimuli which stimulates the production of adhesion molecules in endothelium, and so promotes monocyte adherence and the downstream actions leading to atherogenesis. IL6 also induces insulin resistance. It is atherogenic insofar as it also promotes release of adhesion molecules by the endothelium, fibrinogen from the liver and procoagulant behaviour by platelets. Resistin causes insulin resistance and glucose intolerance. Adiponectin, on the other hand, also an adipocytokine released from adipose tissue, stimulates insulin sensitivity. This cytokine also reduces adhesion of monocytes to endothelial cells.

There is also a family of nuclear receptors which are activated by circulating lipids, and in turn modulate both lipid and carbohydrate metabolism. They are released in proportion to circulating lipids, and the mass of adipose tissue is related to the concentrations and flux of lipids through the circulation. Circulating lipids elicit the expression of a family of nuclear receptors, peroxisome proliferator-activated receptors (PPARs), which modulate both lipid and glucose metabolism (Evans *et al.* 2004). PPARs function as lipid sensors and modulate metabolism by controlling networks of genes. PPARα and PPARγ are found in liver and adipose tissue while PPARδ is expressed in all tissues of the body, albeit at lower levels. PPARγ is induced during adipocyte differentiation and acts to increase triglyceride content of tissues, thus lowering circulating fatty acids and triglycerides, and so improving insulin sensitivity. PPARα is expressed mainly in liver and heart muscle and controls fatty acid oxidation. PPARα is induced by circulating fatty acids and stimulates hepatic fatty acid oxidation, leading to the production of ketone bodies which are used as fuel in overnight or prolonged fasts. PPARδ opposes the lipid storage activities of PPARγ by promoting fatty acid oxidation and adaptive thermogenesis.

Obesity is also associated with altered hypothalamopituitary (HPA) activity. The direction of the sometimes subtle relationships is not known with certainty. Current hypotheses assume that the relationship starts with repeated/chronic stress, activation of the HPA and the sympathetic nervous system (SNS) axes, and that insulin resistance, lipid abnormalities and central storage of fat emerge as consequences (Bjorntorp and Rosmond 2000). Regardless of the direction of the causal vectors, central adiposity is associated with abnormalities of HPA and SNS function, and these neurohumoral abnormalities can explain some of the changes in lipid and carbohydrate metabolism seen in the metabolic syndrome. These are basically insulin resistance and raised blood pressure (Bjorntorp 1992).

The mechanisms underpinning the dyslipidaemia associated with the metabolic syndrome are incompletely understood. HDL concentrations are low, and triglyceride concentrations are high, both changes constituting an increased risk of atherosclerotic vascular disease. Hypertriglyceridaemia might be related to differential tissue sensitivity to the inhibitory effects of insulin on lipolysis versus glucose disposal (Hales and Ozanne 2003a, 2003b).

Hypertension is an integral part of the metabolic syndrome. The mechanisms underlying the elevation of blood pressure are multiple and include HPA axis hyperactivity. Circulating cortisol levels are higher and/or the circadian rhythm is flattened, glucocortioid receptor concentrations in vascular tissue are higher (Langley-Evans 2001, Bertram and Hanson 2002). Cortisol acts directly on vascular smooth muscle and increases its sensitivity to vasoconstrictor stimuli by enhancing accumulation of calcium and its availability to the contractile machinery. Cortisol also modulates the renin angiotensin aldosterone system (RAAS). Receptors for angiotensin II are expressed in greater concentration in vascular tissue and kidney, resulting in increased sensitivity to circulating angiotensin II, which causes vasoconstriction. Up-regulation of the renin–angiotensin–aldosteron system also promotes renal salt retention.

Susceptibility to the metabolic syndrome: developmental contributions

A genetic susceptibility to cardiovascular disease appears to exist. Hypertension, diabetes and dyslipidaemia are all regarded as polygenic disorders with genetic contributions of up to a third. However, no clear delineation of the putative influential genes is yet available. Obesity itself appears to be a prime driver or co-traveller of the epidemics of the metabolic syndrome in all populations studied. The consistency of these relationships raises a fundamental biological question: why are common risk factors common? Perhaps the most attractive hypothesis addressing this question is the common-disease/common-variant (CVCD) hypothesis (Doris 2002). If we use hypertension as an example (though it would be equally applicable to each component of the metabolic syndrome), then the CVCD hypothesis would propose the following line of thought. Hypertension is a common disorder. 'Common' implies that the disorder is prevalent within populations, and that it is widespread across populations, globally. High prevalence and widespread distribution could arise if susceptibility alleles for hypertension were prevalent in the founding population of modern human beings and became distributed globally with human dispersal. The information available to date from genetic studies in hypertension suggests that it is a polygenic disorder with small contributions from multiple genes, although no gene on this putative panel has yet been identified with confidence.

Equally, there is a growing literature on a less obviously genetic modulation of cardiovascular disease risk arising out of early-life environments. Thus, accumulating evidence describes a relationship between maternal nutrition before and during pregnancy, fetal growth, postnatal catch-up growth and risk of cardiovascular disease in later life (Osmond and Barker 2000, Barker *et al*. 2002). Epigenetic effects have been proposed as underlying these relationships, both from mother to child and across wider familial and intergenerational distances (Drake and Walker 2004). Methylation of DNA and acetylation of nuclear histones are detailed mechanisms proposed to explain the modulation of gene expression by environmental factors. The epigenetic changes affect the pattern of ontogeny, fetal growth, metabolic and physiological set-points and response characteristics in the offspring. Thus, the quality of the ovum, maternal weight for height, body composition, and dietary intake in pregnancy all combine to provide changing environments which influence gene expression and thus set the parameters within which fetal development takes place.

In a teleological context, these epigenetically elicited alterations in capabilities and capacities of the newborn enable the developing fetus to 'forecast' the extrauterine environment and to establish a range of attributes best suited to traversing the environment 'envisioned' (Gluckman and Hanson 2004). Any mismatch therefore between postnatal environmental demands and metabolic and physiological capabilities and capacities will determine whether an individual will have his or her capacities exceeded, with consequent risk of disease (Hales and Barker 2001).

The hypothesis of the early-life origins of cardiovascular disease rests on the demonstration of a consistent relationship between maternal nutrition, and/or size and proportions of the offspring at birth, and risk of the metabolic syndrome, and posits a process whereby the programming of fetal metabolism and physiology has carry-over effects into postnatal life which increase the risk of developing cardiovascular diseases in adulthood (Barker 1998). Size and proportions at birth are direct results of the

cadence and rate of fetal growth. Fetal growth itself is largely regulated by placentally mediated nutrient flow, which is in turn determined by maternal body mass and composition, as well as by the pattern of dietary intake during pregnancy. Fetal undernutrition results in catabolism and growth faltering if the catabolism is prolonged. The timing of undernutrition determines which organs are primarily affected. Specific impairment occurs in those organs most rapidly developing at the time of insult, and the adaptation to the intrauterine insult secures a redistribution of blood flow from organs in less critical stages of development, or lower down on a teleological priority listing, to organs higher up the priority scale in order to salvage vital organs such as the brain at the expense of abdominal organs and skeletal muscle.

Fetal undernutrition occurs in a setting of maternal undernutrition and is associated with the programming of fetal metabolic and physiological competences (Lucas 1991). Maternal undernutrition is associated with up-regulation of the maternal HPA axis, leading to increased cortisol production (Benediktsson *et al*. 1993, Lindsay *et al*. 1996, Seckl 1998). Access of maternal cortisol to the fetus is simultaneously enhanced by changes in placental cortisol receptors (11β hydroxysteroid dehydrogenase 2), which are down-regulated, thereby increasing entry of glucocorticoids into the fetal circulation. In addition, fetal HPA axis sensitivity is centrally enhanced. Increased fetal exposure to cortisol causes accelerated ontogeny through the process of accelerated differentiation (Fowden *et al*. 1998). This results, for example, in a reduced number of nephrons at birth, a reduced pancreatic β-cell mass and shifts in the balance of hepatic enzymes that affect carbohydrate metabolism, promoting gluconeogenesis at the expense of glycogenesis (Brenner and Chertow 1994, Langley-Evans *et al*. 1999, Ozanne 1999, Ozanne and Hales 1999, Wintour *et al*. 2003, McMullen *et al*. 2004).

Programming of obesity

A large number of studies from both developed and developing countries have shown that the metabolic syndrome is associated with low birthweight and thinness at birth (Law *et al.* 1992).

The propensity to develop obesity, as well as to deposit fat centrally, leading to or associated with the development of syndrome X, appears to be modulated in association with size and proportions at birth and/or maternal undernutrition (Law *et al.* 1992, Martorell *et al.* 2001). There is also evidence that the pattern of BMI change in early infancy predicts later obesity (Rolland-Cachera *et al.* 1984). For example, the age at which BMI rebounds from its first minimum after birth is predictive of later obesity and diabetes (Rolland-Cachera *et al.* 1984). Early age of adiposity rebound is associated with risk of diabetes in later life (Eriksson *et al.* 2003).

Programming of renal body-fluid blood pressure control

Maternal (rat) undernutrition in pregnancy is associated with smaller kidney size, altered shape, a reduction in nephron number and earlier progression to renal failure (Langley and Jackson 1994). Analogously, post-mortem studies in humans show that intrauterine growth retardation is also associated with reduced nephron number. The limitation in nephron number is thought to enhance blood pressure sensitivity to salt intake and might be the basis of the Guyton renal body-fluid mechanism which dominates long-term salt and water and blood pressure control (Brenner and Chertow 1994). This is an intuitively attractive hypothesis which claims that reduced nephron number effectively resets the pressure natriuresis curve rightward when the individual is exposed to salt intakes typically encountered in the Western lifestyle (Dodic *et al.* 1998, Nwagau *et al.* 2000). Chronic exposure to these high salt intakes in individuals with reduced nephron number would produce permanent changes in nephron structure and function, further nephron loss and eventually hypertension. Thus maternal undernutrition would programme hypertension risk through renal capacities of the offspring.

Programming of the pancreas

Similarly, the ontogeny of the pancreas is altered in the context of maternal undernutrition (Petrik *et al.* 1999, Hill and Duville 2000). The temporal pattern of pancreatic cell apoptosis is altered such that there is a net reduction in the number of β cells available to the individual in adult life. Such a diminution in pancreatic reserve is thought to result in pancreatic exhaustion and a fall in insulin secretion after a period of sustained exposure of the β cells to demands for elevated insulin secretion when insulin resistance is present. When compensatory insulin secretion falls away, diabetes emerges (Hales and Ozanne 2003b).

Programming of the liver

Lastly, undernutrition in utero also alters the ontogeny of the liver such that the balance of periportal and perivenous cells is altered, and the expression of enzymes influencing glucose storage as glycogen versus hepatic glucose production changes (Ozanne 1999, Ozanne and Hales 1999). The combination of a relative insensitivity of adipose tissue inhibition of lipolysis by circulating insulin while hepatic glucose production goes unchecked results in a diabetes-like profile of glucose and fatty acid metabolism (Hales and Ozanne 2003b).

In summary, therefore, maternal size before and during pregnancy and her dietary intakes during these periods are directly related to fetal growth, birthweight, and proportions of the newborn. Smaller size at birth is related to higher blood pressure and risk of hypertension, and this increase in risk is probably mediated through programmed susceptibility to adiposity and its physiological effects and, less well demonstrated, programming of blood pressure sensitivity to salt intake. An interlocking cascade of other metabolic and physiological mechanisms produces insulin resistance and impaired glucose tolerance, hypertriglyceridaemia, low HDL, and together with raised blood pressure constitute the metabolic syndrome.

Clinical syndromes

Hypertension, insulin resistance, diabetes and dys-lipidaemia are all risk factors for poor vascular out-comes, including atherosclerotic vascular disease, congestive heart failure and stroke. Atheroscler-otic vascular disease in coronary vessels (ischaemic heart disease) and peripheral arteries (peripheral vascular disease), are the macrovascular complica-tions that attend diabetes, dyslipidaemia and hyper-tension. Large-vessel ischaemic stroke also arises as an atherosclerotic outcome within this context. Congestive heart failure complicates hypertension, and coronary disease can also contribute to this outcome.

Hypertension

While obesity, salt intake, alcohol intake, physical inactivity and psychosocial stress in humans are recognised risk factors for hypertension, fetal pro-gramming is increasingly recognised as an inde-pendent risk factor. The gestational influences (above) comprising maternal pre-pregnancy nutri-tional plane, coupled with her dietary intake and weight gain in pregnancy, combine to present a metabolic and physiological context for fetal devel-opment. Maternal undernutrition at any of these stages, especially if associated with impaired fetal growth, is strongly associated with raised blood pres-sure in childhood and risk of hypertension in adult life (Law and Shiell 1996). Prevalence of hyperten-sion is also related to adiposity, and it is not cur-rently settled whether fetal programming also affects blood pressure through the programming of adipos-ity (Huxley *et al.* 2000).

Diabetes

Type 2 diabetes is strongly related to adiposity, especially central adiposity, and physical inactivity (Knowler *et al.* 1993, Haffner 1998, Newsome *et al.* 2003). There is also growing evidence that insulin resistance and emergence of diabetes is related to

pregnancy programming (Hales and Ozanne 2003b). Gross phenotypes of the epigenetic and metabolic programming which manifest as insulin resistance and diabetes include birthweight and ponderal index, lower birthweight and thinness at birth being predictive, especially within an adult context of obesity.

Dyslipidaemia

Likewise, obesity and dietary intake of saturated fats and cholesterol are the largest determinants of high serum cholesterol in humans. There is some evi-dence also to implicate in utero events with the subsequent development of dyslipidaemia (Barker 1995). The interaction of such programmed suscep-tibility with acquired and/or programmed obesity triggers clinically relevant hypercholesterolaemia and triglyceridaemia.

Primary prevention

Hypertension and diabetes have well-recognised natural histories and complication profiles (Amer-ican Heart Association 2003). Although improved treatment and control have reduced the incidence of stroke and metabolic deaths from diabetes, death from coronary disease has emerged as the number-one vascular outcome of the metabolic syndrome. Risk of atherosclerotic vascular disease, whether coronary syndromes, peripheral vascular disease or stroke, is amplified by cigarette smoking, dietary patterns which emphasise saturated fats and low intake of fruit and vegetables, and physical inac-tivity. The clinical management of these syndromes is the domain of numerous excellent textbooks of medicine and systematic reviews in the peer-reviewed literature. These aspects of management will not be covered here. Rather, emphasis will be placed on a broader approach to the amelioration and eventual reversal of the epidemics.

In this regard the primary prevention of obe-sity and comorbidities is paramount. Prevention is simple in principle, but successful population-level outcomes have proven elusive in practice (World Health Organization 2000, 2003, Murray *et al.* 2003). Consequently, the field is replete with considerable angst, public policy initiatives, international and national programmes, and community and individual effort to reverse obesity and prevent its emergence. Yet, at least at the reductionist level, the strategic objectives are clear.

The chief aim is to avoid prolonged periods of positive energy balance. This implies a combination of reduction in energy intake and an increase of physical activity. Energy intake is subtly raised and physical activity reduced in most individuals who become obese. The mean rate of rise of body weight at the population level is usually small, of the order of a kilogram per annum, implying modest daily energy surplus.

The pathways leading to increased energy intake are a combination of the consumption of energy-dense foods, large portion sizes, and highly effective marketing of foods. Foods are made energy-dense through use of simple sugars, oils and fats, during both processing and cooking (Hu and Willett 2002, World Health Organization 2003). It is easier to accumulate excess calories on exposure to energy-dense foods, since satiety is primarily related to stomach volume as opposed to caloric intake.

The decision-making space within which people in countries from lower-middle to high income make choices about food and physical activity is not neutral (Handy *et al.* 2002, Frumkin 2002, World Health Organization 2003). The variety, availability, price, convenience, marketing thrust and cultural norms are some of the inputs into the current patterns of food consumption where animal products, cereal-based products, salt, oils, fats and simple sugars are emphasised, and fruit and vegetable intake not. The obvious implication is that eliciting changes in the pattern of food consumption as a public health measure to reduce the incidence of obesity and its comorbidities will require changes in this decision-making environment to support the desired changes.

Similarly, the primary aim for physical activity is to raise both physical activity and physical fitness. It is important to point out that the considerations here are primarily applicable to those groups whose daily physical activity has fallen and who are not malnourished. Hence, they not applicable to subsistence farmers in resource-poor settings even though their relatives on migration to the built city experience a surge in weight. Thus, in low-income countries with the twin burdens of infection/malnutrition and emerging cardiovascular disease epidemics in subpopulations, initiatives have to be appropriately targeted.

Physical activity is constrained by our physical environments as well as by the uptake of labour-saving technologies (Handy *et al.* 2002, Frumkin 2002). Workplace design and work process design inhibit physical activity. Likewise the design of housing, communities and cities, policies for automobiles and public transport all conspire to limit physical activity.

An effective response will require a mix of national and international policy changes that need to be adopted in order to put human development at the centre of policy right alongside profit (Forrester 2003). Health is a critical component of human development, and nutrition is central to the capture and retention of good health. At individual levels, decision making and behaviour change can and should take place despite operating in a non-ideal environment. Thus strategies to alter the mix and quantity of foods eaten, as well as methods of food preparation, need to be designed and tested for population uptake and impact. Similarly, environment-specific strategies to elicit increases in physical activity and physical fitness need to be identified at individual level.

Disease management

Hypertension

The commonest cardiovascular disease related to obesity is eminently treatable even if not curable. The strategies include universal prescription of dietary and activity lifestyle changes to foster weight reduction, dietary sodium reduction, optimising alcohol intake, and increase of other mineral and vitamin micronutrients that play a role in blood pressure regulation, e.g. potassium and calcium.

Treatment and control with pharmaceuticals is paramount to success in reducing organ damage, whether brain (stroke), kidney (renal failure), heart (cardiac failure and coronary disease) or other important vascular bed (peripheral vascular disease). We possess an enviable armamentarium of effective drugs with a minimal side-effects profile. However, we have been manifestly unsuccessful in (a) identifying most of the individuals who should be treated, (b) enrolling these into treatment groups and (c) eliciting adherence. Thus control rates vary between <10% in European countries, 17% in Canada and 29% in the United States – countries where drug prices are not an issue – and, paradoxically, 20–30% in low-middle-income countries such as Barbados and Jamaica, where cost is a significant barrier to coverage (Freeman *et al.* 1996). Clearly there is scope for improvement here.

Diabetes

Diabetes, while a disease in its own right, is important for the burden of disease because it is such a potent risk factor for atherosclerotic vascular disease. Individuals die more from cardiovascular complications than from diabetes per se. Management of diabetes is therefore aimed at two levels. First, maintaining tight metabolic control in order to minimise risk of microvascular complications as well as metabolic complications (nonketotic or ketoacidotic coma etc.). Increasingly, however, it is believed that diabetes should be treated as a prevascular syndrome and thus treated as for secondary prevention of a vascular event with aspirin, statin, ace inhibitor, hypertensive agent, as well as with the currently emphasised hypoglycaemic agent. Lifestyle change aimed at meal planning, weight reduction if possible, increase of physical fitness and avoidance of tobacco are cornerstones of the approach to improve insulin action and thus return the disordered glucose and lipid metabolism to normal.

Atherosclerotic vascular disease

Established coronary disease is treated on its merits and is outside the scope of this chapter (but see Chapter 22). High-quality curative medical and surgical procedures with well-established cost-benefit and cost-effectiveness information exist and are in clinical use (Braunwald 1997).

Conclusions

Chronic cardiovascular disease arising in transitional and high-income countries comes about in the setting of obesity. Obesity is associated with the metabolic syndrome, which is a constellation of risk factors for atherosclerotic vascular disease while at the same time constituting a cluster of subsidiary diseases in themselves (hypertension, diabetes, hypercholesterolaemia) with their own burden of pathological sequelae. The global challenges are to prevent the emergence of obesity and comorbidities in epidemic proportions in low-income countries now treading the path to economic prosperity, and simultaneously to reverse the epidemic in low-middle middle- and high-income countries. An alternative route to economic development must be found that does not include consumption patterns and environmental changes which promote obesogenic behaviours and tobacco use. Where the full epidemic flourishes primary prevention should be targeted at unaffected individuals, e.g. children and young adults who are not yet overweight or obese. Novel approaches to secondary prevention within the context of our existing hostile environments need to be identified in order to reverse obesity and ameliorate its impact. Additionally, full use of existing knowledge should be made and come to be reflected in improvements in detection, treatment and control. Lastly, primary prevention could conceivably extend to optimisation of newborn physiology for the current calorie-replete, indolent postnatal environment (World Health Organization 2002). While conceptually feasible and aimed at optimising fetal development to entrain metabolic and physiologic capability to safely traverse our modern environments without incurring the burden of disease, such interventions have not yet been identified – but they are among our highest priorities.

REFERENCES

American Heart Association (2003). *Hypertension Primer: the Essentials of High Blood Pressure*, 3rd edn. Baltimore, MD: Lippincott Williams and Wilkins.

Barker, D. J. P. (1995). Fetal origins of coronary heart disease. *BMJ*, **311**, 51–7.

(1998). *Mothers, Babies and Health in Later Life*, London: Churchill Livingstone.

Barker, D. J. P., Eriksson, J. G., Forsen, T. and Osmond, C. (2002). Fetal origins of adult disease: strength of effects and biological basis. *Int. J. Epidemiol.*, **31**, 1235–9.

Benediktsson, R., Lindsay, R. M., Noble, J., Seckl, J. R. and Edwards, C. R. (1993). Glucocorticoid exposure in utero: a new model for adult hypertension. *Lancet*, **41**, 339–41.

Bertram, C. E. and Hanson, M. A. (2002). Prenatal programming of postnatal endocrine glucocorticoids. *Reproduction*, **124**, 459–67.

Bjorntorp, P. (1992). Abdominal obesity and the metabolic syndrome. *Ann. Med.*, **24**, 465–8.

Bjorntorp, P. and Rosmond, R. (2000). The metabolic syndrome: a neuroendocrine disorder? *Br. J. Nutr.*, **83** (Suppl. 1), S49–57.

Braunwald, E. (1997). *Heart Disease: a Texbook of Cardiovascular Medicine*, 5th edn. Philadelphia, PA: Saunders.

Brenner, B. M. and Chertow, G. M. (1994). Congenital oligonephropathy and the etiology of adult hypertension and progressive injury. *Am. J. Kidney Dis.*, **23**, 171–5.

Diamond, J. (1998). *Guns, Germs and Steel: a Short History of Everybody for the Last 13,000 Years*. London: Vintage.

Dodic, M., May, C. N., Wintour, E. M. and Coughlan, J. P. (1998). An early prenatal exposure to excess glucocorticoid leads to hypertensive offspring in sheep. *Clin. Sci.*, **94**, 149–55.

Doris, P. A. (2002). Hypertension genetics, single nucleotide polymorphisms, and the common disease:common variant hypothesis. *Hypertension*, **39**, 323–33.

Drake, A. J. and Walker, B. R. (2004). The intergenerational effects of fetal programming: non-genomic mechanisms for the inheritance of low birth weight and cardiovascular risk. *J. Epidemiol.*, **180**, 1–16.

Eriksson, J. G., Forsen, T., Tuomelhito, J., Osmond, C. and Barker, D. J. P. (2003). Early adiposity rebound in childhood and risk of type 2 diabetes in adult life. *Diabetologia*, **46**, 190–4.

Evans, R. M., Barish, G. D. and Wang, Y. (2004). PPARS and the complex journey to obesity. *Nat. Med.*, **10**, 1–7.

Forrester, T. E. (2003). Research into policy: hypertension and diabetes mellitus in the Caribbean. *West Indian Med. J.*, **52**, 164–9.

Fowden, A. L., Li, J. and Forhead, A. J. (1998). Glucocorticoids and the preparation for life after birth: are there long term consequences of the life insurance? *Proc. Nutr. Soc.*, **57**, 113–22.

Francois, P. J. and James, W. P. T. (1994). An assessment of nutritional factors affecting the BMI of a population. *Eur. J. Clin. Nutr.*, **48** (Suppl. 3) S90–7.

Freeman, V., Fraser, H., Forrester, T. E. *et al.* (1996). A comparative study of hypertension prevalence, awareness, treatment and control rates in St. Lucia, Jamaica and Barbados. *J. Hypertens.*, **14**, 495–502.

Frumkin, H. (2002). Urban sprawl and public health. *Public Health Rep.*, **117**, 201–17.

Gluckman, P. D. and Hanson, M. A. (2004). The developmental origins of the metabolic syndrome. *Trends Endocrinol. Metab.*, **15**, 183–7.

Haffner, S. M. (1998). Epidemiology of type 2 diabetes: risk factors. *Diabetes Care*, **21** (Suppl. 3) C3–6.

Hales, C. N. and Barker, D. J. P. (2001). The thrifty phenotype hypothesis. *Br. Med. Bull.*, **60**, 5–20.

Hales, C. N. and Ozanne, S. E. (2003a). The dangerous road of catch-up growth. *J. Physiol.*, **547**, 5–10.

(2003b). For debate: fetal and early postnatal growth restriction lead to diabetes, the metabolic syndrome and renal failure. *Diabetologia*, **46**, 1013–19.

Handy, S. C., Boarnet, M. G., Ewing, R. and Killingsworth, R. E. (2002). How the built environment affects physical activity: views from urban planning. *Am. J. Prev. Med.*, **23**, 64–73.

Hill, D. J. and Duville, B. (2000). Pancreatic development and adult diabetes. *Pediatr. Res.*, **48**, 269–74.

Hu, F. B. and Wilett, W. C. (2002). Optimal diets for prevention of coronary heart disease. *JAMA*, **288**, 2569–78.

Huxley, R. R., Shiell, A. W. and Law, C. M. (2000). The role of size at birth and postnatal catch-up growth in determining systolic blood pressure: a systematic review of the literature. *J. Hypertens.*, **18**, 815–31.

Knowler, W. C., Saad, M. F., Pettitt, D. J., Nelson, R. G. and Bennett, P. H. (1993). Determinants of Diabetes mellitus in Pima Indians. *Diabetes Care*, **16**, 216–27.

Langley, S. C. and Jackson, A. A. (1994). Increased systolic pressure in adult rats induced by fetal exposure to maternal low protein diets. *Clin. Sci.*, **86**, 217–22.

Langley-Evans, S. C. (2001). Fetal programming of cardiovascular function through exposure to maternal undernutrition. *Proc. Nutr. Soc.*, **60**, 505–13.

Langley-Evans, S. C., Sherman, R. C., Welham, S. J., Nwagwu, M. O., Gardner, D. S. and Jackson, A. A. (1999). Intrauterine programming of hypertension: the role of the renin angiotensin system. *Biochem. Soc. Trans.*, **27**, 88–93.

Law, C. M. and Shiell, A. W. (1996). Is blood pressure inversely related to birth weight? The strength of evidence from a systematic review of the literature. *J. Hypertens.*, **14**, 935–41.

Law, C. M., Barker, D. J. P., Osmond, C., Fall, C. H. and Simmonds, S. J. (1992). Early growth and abdominal fatness in adult life. *J. Epidemiol. Comm. Health*, **46**, 184–6.

Lindsay, R. S., Lindsay, R. M., Waddell, B. J. and Seckl, J. R. (1996). Programming of glucose tolerance in the rat: role of placental 11 beta-hydroxysteroid dehydrogenase. *Diabetologia*, **39**, 1299–305.

Lucas, A. (1991). The childhood environment and adult disease. In *Programming by Early Nutrition in Man* (ed. G. R. Bock. and J. Whelan). Chichester: Wiley, pp. 38–55.

Luke, A., Durazo-Arvisu, R., Rotimi, C. *et al.* (1997). Relation between body mass index and body fat in black population samples from Nigeria, Jamaica and the United States. *Am. J. Epidemiol.*, **145**, 620–8.

Martorell, R., Stein, A. D. and Schroeder, D. G. (2001). Early nutrition and later adiposity. *J. Nutr.*, **13**, 874–80s.

McMullen, S., Gardner, D. S. and Langley-Evans, S. C. (2004). Prenatal programming of angiotensin 11 type 2 receptor expression in the rat. *Br. J. Nutr.*, **91**, 133–40.

Murray, C. J., Lauer, J. A., Hutubessy, R. C. *et al.* (2003). Effectiveness and costs of interventions to lower blood pressure and cholesterol: a global and regional analysis on reduction of cardiovascular-disease risk. *Lancet*, **361**, 717–25.

Neel, J. V. (1999). The thrifty genotype in 1998. *Nutr. Rev.*, **57**, 52–9.

Newsome, C. A., Shiell, A. W., Fall, C. H., Phillips, D. I., Shier, R. and Law, C. M. (2003). Is birth weight related to later glucose and insulin metabolism? A systematic review. *Diabet. Med.*, **20**, 339–48.

Norgan, N. G. (1994). Population differences in body composition in relation to body mass index. *Eur. J. Clin. Nutr.*, **48** (Suppl. 3), S10–27.

Nwagau, M. D., Cook, A. and Langley-Evans, S. C. (2000). Evidence of progressive deterioration of renal function in rats exposed to a maternal low protein diet in utero. *Br. J. Nutr.*, **83**, 79–85.

Osmond, C. and Barker, D. J. P. (2000). Fetal, infant and childhood growth are predictors of coronary heart disease, diabetes, and hypertension in adult men and women. *Environ. Health Perspect.*, **108** (Suppl. 3), 545–53.

Ozanne, S. E. (1999). Programming of hepatic and peripheral insulin sensitivity by maternal protein restriction. *Biochem. Soc. Trans.*, **27**, 94–7.

Ozanne, S. E. and Hales, C. N. (1999). The long term consequences of intrauterine protein malnutriton for glucose metabolism. *Proc. Nutr. Soc.*, **58**, 615–19.

Petrik, J., Reusens, B., Arany, E. *et al.* (1999). A low protein diet alters the balance of islet cell replication and apoptosis in the fetal and neonatal rat and is associated with a reduced pancreatic expression of insulin-like growth factor 11. *Endocrinology*, **140**, 4861–73.

Rolland-Cachera, M. F., Deheeger, M., Bellisle, F., Sempe, M., Guillaud-Bataille, M. and Patois, E. (1984). Adiposity rebound in children: a simple marker for predicting obesity. *Am. J. Clin. Nutr.*, **39**, 129–35.

Seckl, J. R. (1998). Physiological programming of the fetus. *Clin. Perinatol.*, **25**, 939–62.

Shirai, K. (2004). Obesity as the core of the metabolic syndrome and the management of coronary disease. *Curr. Med. Res. Opin.*, **20**, 295–304.

Wintour, E. M., Moritz, K. M., Johnson, K., Ricardo, S., Samuel, C. S. and Dodic, M. (2003). Reduced nephron number in adult sheep hypertensive as a result of prenatal glucocorticoid treatment. *J. Physiol.*, **549**, 929–35.

World Health Organization (2000). *Obesity: Preventing and Managing the Global Epidemic*. WHO Technical Report Series, 894. Geneva: World Health Organization.

  (2002). *Programming of Chronic Disease by Impaired Fetal Nutrition: Evidence and Implications for Policy and Intervention Strategies*. WHO/NHD/02.3; WHO/NPH/02.1. Geneva: World Health Organization.

  (2003). *Diet, Nutrition and Prevention of Chronic Diseases: Report of the Joint WHO/FAO Expert Consultation. WHO Technical Report Series, 916*. Geneva: World Health Organization.

34

Developmental origins of health and disease: public-health perspectives

Catherine Law[1] and Janis Baird[2]

[1]University College London
[2]University of Southampton

Introduction

The World Health Organization (WHO) describes public health as a social and political concept. It is based in 'a comprehensive understanding of the ways in which lifestyles and living conditions determine health status, and a recognition of the need to mobilise resources and make sound investments in policies, programmes and services which create, maintain and protect health by supporting healthy lifestyles and creating supportive environments for health' (World Health Organization 1998). From this, it follows that a public-health perspective on developmental origins of health and disease is focused on effecting change rather than dissection of the aetiology. Nonetheless, understanding of the mechanisms that underlie relationships between early life and adult disease would be helpful, though arguably not essential, in developing policies or programmes to improve public health.

The preceding chapters have illustrated the complexity of the human as a biological organism. In the biomedical science base the determinants of adult health include concepts such as gene expression, modulation of physiological systems and evolutionary pressures such as predictive adaptive responses (Hanson *et al.* 2004). Figure 34.1 shows a public-health view of the determinants of health. In this, the biological characteristics of individuals are central,

but they are influenced by and interact with layers of influence deriving from their lifestyles, their social and community networks and the services (public and private) that they need or can access. All of these may be influenced by general economic, cultural and environmental conditions. Studying these complex interactions as they relate to early life and adult disease is a huge potential area of research that might yield great dividends for public health. Yet the evidence base here is small and, despite pockets of excellence, social and public health science are yet to be fully engaged in the research agenda of developmental origins of health and disease.

Figure 34.1 illustrates two important tensions in developing the evidence base and in using it to promote public health. First, the effect of public health interventions applied at an individual level (sometimes called 'downstream' interventions), for example health education or food supplementation, are relatively easily studied, albeit the effects may rely on complex biological mechanisms. However, effective 'downstream' interventions cannot be successfully implemented if other so-called 'upstream' influences are unfavourable. For example, health education can reduce maternal smoking in pregnancy but is ineffective in women whose social and community networks ('upstream' influences) reinforce smoking habits (Independent Inquiry into Inequalities in Health 1998). Second, public health interventions focused on the outer layers of the

Developmental Origins of Health and Disease, ed. Peter Gluckman and Mark Hanson. Published by Cambridge University Press.
© P. D. Gluckman and M. A. Hanson 2006.

determinants of health, for example through improving education or reducing unemployment, may have profound effects on societies and individuals but are nearly always applied in a context in which other change is occurring, thus challenging the scientific concepts of controlled experiments.

This chapter will examine evidence on the developmental origins of health and disease, as it applies to public health, under three headings. The first will describe the nature of the evidence base and the challenges of using it for public health action. The second will discuss approaches to applying the evidence base, particularly for developing public policy. The third will set out some of the issues that need to be addressed in developing interventions. Though each of the sections will draw on a wide range of evidence, the illustrations will be focused on early growth and cardiovascular risks as this is one of the areas in developmental origins of health and disease where most evidence in humans exists.

The nature of the evidence

The scientific evidence on developmental origins of health and disease derives from a range of disciplines in basic, clinical and public health sciences. Put at their simplest, the arguments for public health action are sequenced as follows: observational evidence in humans shows associations between events in early life and adult disease or its risk factors, which are not (fully) explained by confounders in adult life; experiments in animal models and basic science provide evidence that these associations might be causal; these and other experiments in animal models suggest that early interventions might lead to reduction in adult disease; limited intervention studies in humans suggest that early intervention can lead to long-term change (though not always in the expected direction); therefore public health interventions should be developed and tested. Consideration of the types of evidence that are used to support each thread of this argument reveal some of the areas for differential interpretation and inform the strong debates which charac-

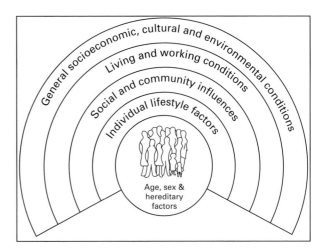

Figure 34.1 The determinants of health. From Dahlgren and Whitehead (1991).

terise this field of inquiry (Susser and Levin 1999, Kramer 2000, Marmot 2001, Robinson 2001, Barker 2002, Singhal and Lucas 2004).

The early studies of the Hertfordshire and Sheffield cohorts (Barker *et al.* 1989, Hales *et al.* 1991, Fall *et al.* 1992, 1995, Martyn *et al.* 1996), referred to extensively in earlier chapters, were the first of a series of cohort studies from different groups around the world that used historical records to associate some aspect of early life with the chronic degenerative diseases of adulthood or their risk factors (Stein *et al.* 1996, Forsen *et al.* 1997, Leon *et al.* 1998, Mi *et al.* 2000). Others used existing or regenerated cohort studies to test the hypotheses being generated (Rich-Edwards *et al.* 1995, Curhan *et al.* 1996, Gunnell *et al.* 1998, De Stavola *et al.* 2000, Parsons *et al.* 2001). Cohort studies are the gold standard in observational study design for assessing such associations. However, they are difficult, time-consuming and expensive to carry out and, as with all observational studies, suffer from a number of susceptibilities to bias. One difficulty in studying the developmental origins of health and disease is the very long latent period between exposure (some aspect of early life) and the effect of interest, cardiovascular death for example, which makes loss to follow-up a particularly likely source of bias. Fortunately a number of cohort studies derive from record linkage (Leon *et al.* 1998, Eriksson *et al.* 2001), in which loss to follow-up is usually much less. For the outcomes where more than a few studies have assessed its association with the same exposure, the findings are reasonably consistent. For example, most studies have found an inverse association of birthweight with ischaemic heart disease (Osmond *et al.* 1993, Frankel *et al.* 1996, Martyn *et al.* 1996, Leon *et al.* 1998, Eriksson *et al.* 1999, Forsen *et al.* 1999). However, for many important adult disease outcomes, particularly cancers and chronic disabling conditions which rarely cause death directly, such as depression, there is little published information. Thus, even if we accept that the associations shown in cohort studies are unbiased, they are still limited in scope.

The second challenge of the cohort studies is that the early 'exposure' information is often just an indicator of early life, rather than the putative causal agent. The most widely cited example is birthweight, which is a summary measure of growth over a specified period reflecting length, body mass and head size, which in turn reflects skeletal and muscle growth, fat mass and organ size. If information on gestational age is not available, then birthweight also reflects the duration of time a fetus spends in utero. Thus the demonstration of a consistent association between, for example, reduced birthweight and an increased risk of death from ischaemic heart disease (Osmond *et al.* 1993, Frankel *et al.* 1996, Martyn *et al.* 1996, Leon *et al.* 1998, Eriksson *et al.* 1999, Forsen *et al.* 1999) does not necessarily mean that raising mean birthweight will lead to reduction in the rate of ischaemic heart disease in that generation, a point that will be returned to later. Furthermore, in utero exposures may be associated with change in adult disease risk with little alteration of fetal growth. For instance, in the Dutch 'hunger winter', exposure to famine in different stages of pregnancy was associated with altered glucose tolerance in mid adult life, without substantial changes in birthweight (Ravelli *et al.* 1998).

Much of the work in animal models has been developed to explain the biological mechanisms that underlie the relationships between indicators such as birthweight and risk factors such as blood pressure or glucose tolerance. The contribution of such work to our understanding of human biology is evident in earlier chapters. But can this work be used to improve human health – that is, as an agent for change? As with all debates on the applicability of animal evidence to human health, the choice of animal model is important. For example, much of the animal kingdom experiences multiple pregnancies. This is a particular challenge in understanding the mechanisms that underlie the observed epidemiological associations between early life and adult disease, most of which have been studied in singletons. However, knowledge of these mechanisms might assist in developing specific and targeted interventions. For example, numerous studies have shown that the manipulation of the diets of pregnant animals results in both short- and long-term physiological changes to the offspring (Harding 2001, Langley-Evans *et al.* 2003). This suggests mechanisms through which early life could influence later health, and points to the potential for development of a dietary intervention during pregnancy. Yet some argue that these models have limited applicability to intervening in human health (Croce 1999). Many of the experimental manipulations are extreme, and young animals appear to be almost infinitely capable of change in relation to early stimuli (Hanson *et al.* 2004). Furthermore, experimental research paradigms tend to be based on the study of specific systems or exposures, whereas individuals within populations experience clusters of exposures and frequently suffer from co-morbidity. For example, pregnant women suffering from undernutrition in rural sub-Saharan Africa are also more likely to bear a high burden of infection, and their impoverished status renders them at high risk of domestic abuse and violence, all risk factors for impaired fetal growth (Podja and Kelly 2000). In these circumstances, arguments for public health interventions may be made more on the basis of human rights than scientific knowledge, though the latter might enhance the capacity of interventions to be effective.

Because of the Hippocratic imperative to 'at least, do no harm' (Jones 1923), some have argued that causality must be established before experimental interventions in humans are justified (Kramer 2000). However, it is difficult to see how causality will be established, given the challenges to the available methodology in both animal and human research outlined above. Furthermore, one classical method of assessing the likelihood of an exposure causing a change in an outcome is to assess research evidence against a set of criteria developed by Bradford Hill (1965). One important criterion is that the research evidence shows that experimental manipulation of the exposure leads to change in the outcome. This reveals a catch-22 situation – intervention in humans cannot be justified until causality is proven but causality cannot be proven until evidence from interventions in humans is provided. Thus, we may never have the ideal combination of evidence to inform public health policy.

Applying the evidence to public health

Research into the developmental origins of health and disease is the domain of the specialist, often working on specific physiological or other systems, or for particular mechanisms or exposures. This reflects the pattern of research more generally and is necessary, given the sophistication of research methods and the complex subject under study. However, public health policy makers are forced to be generalists. They have to base policy on an overview, both of the population at a point in time and on the life courses of the individuals within it. They are also risk-averse, so the possibility of doing harm, or of being seen to do harm by doing nothing, is preoccupying. In addition, at a political level, there is a preference for short-term outcomes consistent with demonstration of achievement within the timescales of a political career.

Many governments and non-governmental organisations now espouse the need for evidence-based policy, though some have argued that policy can, at best, only be informed by, and not be based on, evidence (Black 2001). By analogy with clinical trials and complex healthcare interventions, public policy

interventions should be preceded by a careful assessment of the evidence base, including explicit consideration of any harm or disbenefits that might occur (Campbell *et al.* 2000). In developmental origins of health and disease, such collations of evidence are rare, though some have been commissioned by policy-making organisations (World Health Organization 2001, Delisle 2002). More formal systematic reviews or meta-analyses have been carried out, but these have been to investigate aetiology or to estimate effect sizes, and have been in relation to specific exposures and outcomes (Huxley *et al.* 2000, 2002, Lawlor *et al.* 2002, Owen *et al.* 2003a, 2003b). Some sections of the scientific community have worked together to develop the evidence base across disciplines (Hanson *et al.* 2004) but much has also developed in relative isolation. Thus the science base on which public health policy could be developed is dissipated.

In addition, we know that there are many gaps in our knowledge. For example, a recent systematic review aimed to describe the patterns of infant growth associated with adult health and disease, as a prelude to informing policy in developed countries. Adult disease outcomes were chosen to include those diseases which result in the highest burden to the population. The Global Burden of Disease Study has estimated these by calculating, for different groups of countries, the disability-adjusted life years (DALYs) lost as a consequence of various diseases or risks (Murray and Lopez 1997). Table 34.1 sets out the 12 conditions that, between them, constitute the top 10 causes of DALYs lost for men and for women. The number beside each condition shows the number of papers which describe the association of each condition with infant growth (Baird *et al.* 2005). These numbers are based on a rigorous search of a number of literature databases and result from screening over 70 000 abstracts (J. Baird and D. J. Fisher, unpublished data). Only ischaemic heart disease and type 2 diabetes have sufficient numbers of studies to be able to make general (rather than study-specific) comments on the associations observed. Furthermore, this literature is dependent on three cohort

Table 34.1 Papers reporting the association of infant growth or size with disease or conditions of adulthood.

	Number of papers	Reference
Ischaemic heart disease	5	Fall *et al.* 1995
		Eriksson *et al.* 2001
		Forsen *et al.* 2004
		Syddall *et al.* 2005
		Barker *et al.* 2005
Cerebrovascular disease	1	Martyn *et al.* 1996
Major depression	1	Thompson *et al.* 2001
Lung cancer	1	Syddall *et al.* 2005
Road traffic accidents	0	
Alcohol use	0	
Dementia	1	Syddall *et al.* 2005
Osteoarthritis	1	Aihie Sayer *et al.* 2003
Chronic obstructive pulmonary disease	1	Syddall *et al.* 2005
Self-injury	1	Barker *et al.* 1995
Breast cancer	1	De Stavola *et al.* 2004
Type 2 diabetes	3	Hales *et al.* 1991
		Eriksson *et al.* 2003
		Bhargava *et al.* 2004

Total number of papers is 13.

* Based on Global Burden of Disease Study (Murray and Lopez 1997).

studies, two British (MRC National Survey of Health and Development 1946 and Hertfordshire; (Barker *et al.* 1995, 2005, Hales *et al.* 1991, Fall *et al.* 1995, Martyn *et al.* 1996, Thompson *et al.* 2001, Aihie Sayer *et al.* 2003, De Stavola *et al.* 2004, Syddall *et al.* 2005) and one Finnish (Helsinki; Eriksson *et al.* 2001, 2003, Forsen *et al.* 2004) with few studies from developing countries (Bhargava *et al.* 2004).

Understanding the context in which research studies were undertaken is critical for using the results in developing public health policy. The importance of using research in developmental origins of health and disease, most of which has been carried out in developed countries, for resource-poor countries is discussed fully elsewhere (Chapter 35). Context also has a dimension in time. Much of the epidemio-

logical research refers to historical cohort studies, conducted on people born decades ago. Their lives would have been different in many ways from those of today's infants. Relative to those born in developed countries now, they would, for example, have been born into larger families, to mothers who were thinner and had lower educational attainment and relative income. They would have been more likely to have been breast-fed but to have had a higher burden of infection. Similarly, current trends suggest that we will have to re-interpret evidence for today's children and for the generation of children soon to be born. For example, some historical cohort studies have indicated that the combination of small size at birth, together with poor growth in infancy and accelerated growth in the remainder of childhood, is associated with increased risk of ischaemic heart disease and type 2 diabetes (Eriksson *et al.* 2001, 2002, Bhargava *et al.* 2004). This raises concern that the increased survival of growth-retarded babies, together with the rising prevalence of childhood obesity, may greatly increase the risk of cardiovascular disease in this group of babies when they grow up (Singhal and Lucas 2004).

In much of the application of research to public health policy, the views of parents and children are not considered, despite this right being enshrined in the UN Convention on the Rights of the Child (United Nations 1999). In a recent study, a systematic review of lay perspectives on infant growth was combined with focus groups seeking views on the importance of early growth for later health. Parents and health professionals saw growth as an indicator of (early) health, and not as important in its own right. On direct questioning, there was little support for intervening to alter infant growth in the absence of pathologically abnormal patterns (Lucas *et al.* 2004). Children themselves seem unlikely to regard childhood as a training ground for a particular type of adult life required to meet public-health mortality targets, though they deserve to be asked if this is true (Law 2002). The falls in rates of immunisation against measles, mumps and rubella as a result of parental uncertainty about the safety of the triple vaccine is demonstration, if it were needed, that parents' views cannot be forced to coincide with those of public health experts (Kmietowicz 2002).

Related to these views is policymakers' understandable preference for short-term 'payback'. This relates not just to political expediency but also to commonly expressed time preferences in the population (Trostel and Taylor 2001), and the need to be cost-effective. Thus, when choosing a policy intervention to reduce ischaemic heart disease, pressures to achieve mortality targets in the foreseeable future will tend to favour measures which target older adults, for example by encouraging smoking cessation. Prevention of adult disease by the promotion of maternal and child health is more likely to be politically possible if it is aligned to wider strategies which emphasise the importance of early life for other reasons (Independent Inquiry into Inequalities in Health 1998, Department of Health 2003).

Thus, applying evidence of the developmental origins of health and disease to public health relies on balances: whether to act for the short term or for the long; the likelihood of benefit compared to harm; and political strength from knowledge versus uncertainties due to the absence of evidence. The final section of this chapter will discuss an area for which the evidence is most limited – that of public health interventions.

Public health interventions

Because the determinants of health cover a broad range (Fig. 34.1), so must public health interventions. They can range from brief interventions applied at the level of an individual to complex national or international public policy. Ideally, all policy would be based on research of effectiveness, yet, as noted earlier, current methods for determining effectiveness are limited and relate mainly to interventions delivered at the level of individuals. There is an urgent need to develop the methods and means for evaluating public health interventions. Until this occurs, policymakers will be caught between having to implement public health interventions which are not known to be effective (and which may do harm) or using lack of evidence as a reason for inaction. In the meantime, the potential for improving public health is lost.

Clinical studies afford a rare opportunity to collect information on interventions through experimental or quasi-experimental designs. For example, Lucas and colleagues carried out a randomised controlled trial of breast milk versus different types of infant formula in a selected sample of preterm infants whose mothers had chosen not to provide their own breast milk to feed their baby. At follow-up, aged 13–16 years, those who had received breast milk had systolic blood pressures that were on average around 3 mm Hg lower than those who had received infant formula (Singhal *et al.* 2001). However, there are no other trials with which to compare this result, and so it is difficult to apply this information to a normal population of term babies. A systematic review of observational studies of the association of breast-feeding with blood pressure found that individuals who had been breast-fed (most of whom would not have been premature) had, on average, systolic pressures that were around 1 mm Hg lower than those who had not been breast-fed (Owen *et al.* 2003b). This suggests that the benefits to the population from increasing rates of breast-feeding in the general population would be modest. However, these would be added to the shorter-term benefits with which breast-feeding is associated.

The arguments for whole-population (rather than targeted) approaches to prevention have been laid out by Rose (1992). Briefly, targeting those at highest risk, for example screening of older adults for individuals who have undiagnosed hypertension, can be an efficient means of focusing on those who are most likely to benefit from an intervention such as antihypertensive treatment. However, applying an appropriate public health intervention to an entire population is likely to achieve a greater reduction in adverse outcomes. This occurs because a very large number of individuals will all have reduced their risk by a small amount, but the sum reduction in risk will result in a large decrease in adverse outcomes.

Cumulative incidence of ischaemic heart disease (%)

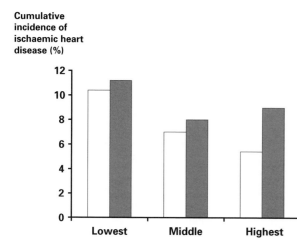

Third of BMI at 1 year

Change in BMI SDS, 3–11 years
☐ Decrease   ■ Increase

Figure 34.2 Cumulative incidence of ischaemic heart disease, according to body mass index BMI at 1 year, and change in standard deviation score for BMI between 3 and 11 years of age (3387 men born 1934–44, Helsinki, Finland)

Using the blood-pressure analogy again, it has been calculated that an intervention that reduced the mean population blood pressure by 10 mm Hg would reduce deaths related to hypertension by 30% (Rose 1985).

Targeted and whole-population approaches are not mutually exclusive and each might be used in early interventions to prevent adult disease. Leaving aside the important issue of causality (which has been discussed earlier), the effectiveness of either approach is dependent on the size of association between the exposure to be modified, such as birthweight, and the outcome, such as blood pressure. Using this example, some have argued that the size of 'effect' (the association of birthweight with blood pressure) is small (Huxley *et al.* 2002), or artificially inflated (Lucas *et al.* 1999), at least in relation to other modifiable factors such as adult lifestyle (Kramer 2000). On the other hand, the relationship may be stronger at the extremes of the population distribution for blood pressure (Curhan *et al.* 1996) or body

mass (Whincup *et al.* 1989, Leon *et al.* 1996), suggesting some merit in an intervention strategy targeted at high-risk groups. For either strategy, precise interventions have yet to be defined, with the epidemiological evidence to date limited to suggesting potential for public health improvement in general terms. For example, Fig. 34.2 shows analysis from the Helsinki cohort of men relating the cumulative incidence of ischaemic heart disease to body mass index (BMI), and changes in BMI, in early life. The increase/decrease shown in the figure refers to a change in the standard deviation score for BMI, and thus is a relative measure. If each man had been in the highest third of BMI at 1 year and had lowered his standard deviation score for BMI between 3 and 11 years, the incidence of ischaemic heart disease would have been lowered by 40%, a significant improvement in public health (Barker *et al.* 2002). However, the required changes in the population distribution both of body mass in infancy and of change in body mass between 3 and 11 years are considerable. Furthermore, it is not clear how changes of this magnitude could be effected, particularly as they imply opposite growth patterns at different ages (increase in average body mass in infancy and decrease in childhood). So, while changes in early growth have the potential to create reductions in adult disease (assuming the two are causally related), the means to achieve this potential are unclear.

Finally, basic science suggests that the greatest potential for programming of an organism occurs in very early life, suggesting that the best time for intervention might be periconceptionally or in early pregnancy. Interventions applied to one person (a mother) for the benefit of another (her baby) raise complex ethical issues which are discussed elsewhere (Chapter 36). These issues loom over public health policy. For example, it has long been feared that strategies to reduce low birthweight in some developing countries will be at the cost of a rising prevalence of obstructed labour which, in the absence of obstetric care, will be accompanied by an increase in maternal mortality (Rush 2000). In addition to the high cost of avoidable mortality, the death of a mother in a resource-poor setting has profound effects on the health and mortality of her family (Measham and Gillespie 1998). The recent publications of trials from developing countries strengthens the evidence base on which such policies may be made for short-term and long-term health (Merialdi *et al.* 2003).

Conclusion

Bismarck said that 'politics is the art of the possible'. The promotion of maternal and child health has long been seen as an unfulfilled right in many countries. The research evidence on developmental health and disease may give further impetus to improving the health of mothers, children and families – making it possible politically. It may also alert us to unintended potential consequences, both beneficial and harmful, of public health policy change.

REFERENCES

Aihie Sayer, A., Poole, J., Cox, V. *et al.* (2003). Weight from birth to 53 years: a longitudinal study of the influence on clinical hand osteoarthritis. *Arthritis Rheum*, **48**, 1030–3.

Baird, J., Lucas, P., Fisher, D., Kleijnen, J., Roberts, H. and Law, C. M. (2005). Defining optimal infant growth for lifetime health: a systematic review of lay and scientific literature. MRC Epidemiology Resource Centre, University of Southampton. www.mrc.soton.ac.uk.

Barker, D. J. P. (2002). Commentary: components in the interpretation of the high mortality in the county of Finland. *Int. J. Epidemiol.*, **31**, 309–10.

Barker, D. J. P., Winter, P. D., Osmond, C., Margetts, B. and Simmonds, S. J. (1989). Weight in infancy and death from ischaemic heart disease. *Lancet*, **2**, 577–80.

Barker, D. J. P., Osmond, C., Rodin, I., Fall, C. H. D. and Winter, P. D. (1995). Low weight gain in infancy and suicide in adult life. *BMJ*, **311**, 1203.

Barker, D. J. P., Eriksson, J. G., Forsen T. and Osmond, C. (2002). Fetal origins of adult disease: strength of effects and biological basis. *Int. J. Epidemiol.*, **31**, 1235–9.

Barker, D. J. P., Osmond, C., Forsen, T. J., Kajantie, E. and Eriksson, J. G. (2005). Trajectories of growth among children who have coronary events as adults. *N. Engl. J. Med.*, **353**, 1802–9.

Bhargava, S. K., Sachdev, H. S., Fall, C. H. *et al.* (2004). Relation of serial changes in childhood body-mass index to impaired glucose tolerance in young adulthood. *N. Engl. J. Med.*, **350**, 865–75.

Black, N. (2001). Evidence based policy: proceed with care. *BMJ*, **323**, 275–9.

Campbell, M., Fitzpatrick, R., Haines, A. *et al.* (2000). Framework for design and evaluation of complex interventions to improve health. *BMJ*, **321**, 694–6.

Croce, P. (1999). *Vivisection or Science? An Investigation into Testing Drugs and Safeguarding Health*. London: Zed Books.

Curhan, G. C., Willett, W. C., Rimm, E. B., Spiegelman, D., Ascherio, A. L. and Stampfer, M. J. (1996). Birth weight and adult hypertension, diabetes mellitus and obesity in US men. *Circulation*, **94**, 3246–50.

Dahlgren, G. and Whitehead, M. (1991). *Policies and Strategies to Promote Social Equity in Health*. Stockholm: Institute of Futures Studies.

Delisle, H. (2002). *Programming of Chronic Disease by Impaired Fetal Nutrition; Evidence and Implications for Policy and Intervention Strategies*. Geneva: World Health Organization.

Department of Health (2003). *Tackling Health Inequalities*. London: Department of Health.

De Stavola, B. L., Hardy, R., Kuh, D., dos Santos Silva, I., Wadsworth, M. and Swerdlow, A. J. (2000). Birthweight, childhood growth and risk of breast cancer in a British cohort. *Br. J. Cancer*, **83**, 964–8.

De Stavola, B. L., dos Santos Silva, I., McCormack, V., Hardy, R. J., Kuh, D. J. and Wadsworth, M. E. (2004). Childhood growth and breast cancer. *Am. J. Epidemiol.*, **159**, 671–82.

Eriksson, J. G., Forsen, T., Tuomilehto, J., Winter, P. D., Osmond, C. and Barker, D. J. P. (1999). Catch-up growth in childhood and death from coronary heart disease: longitudinal study. *BMJ*, **318**, 427–31.

Eriksson, J. G., Forsen, T., Tuomilehto, J., Osmond, C. and Barker, D. J. P. (2001). Early growth and coronary heart disease in later life: longitudinal study. *BMJ*, **322**, 949–53.

Eriksson, J. G., Forsen, T., Tuomilehto, J., Jaddoe, V. W. V., Osmond, C. and Barker, D. J. P. (2002). Effects of size at birth and childhood growth on the insulin resistance syndrome in elderly individuals. *Diabetologia*, **45**, 342–8.

Eriksson, J. G., Forsen, T., Tuomilehto, J., Osmond, C. and Barker, D. P. J. (2003). Early adiposity rebound in childhood and risk of type 2 diabetes in adult life. *Diabetologia*, **46**, 190–4.

Fall, C. H. D., Barker, D. J. P., Osmond, C., Winter, P. D., Clark, P. M. S. and Hales, C. N. (1992). Relation of infant feeding to adult serum cholesterol concentration and death from ischaemic heart disease. *BMJ*, **304**, 801–5.

Fall, C. H. D., Osmond, C., Barker, D. J. P. *et al.* (1995). Fetal and infant growth and cardiovascular risk factors in women. *BMJ*, **310**, 428–32.

Fisher, D. J., Baird, J., Lucas, P., Roberts, H., Kleijnan, J. and Law, C. M. (2004). Is infant growth related to health and well-being in adulthood? A systematic review of the evidence. Poster presented at the Society for Social Medicine 48th Annual Scientific Meeting. University of Birmingham, 15–17 September 2004.

Forsen T, Eriksson, J. G., Tuomilehto, J., Teramo, K., Osmond, C. and Barker, D. J. P. (1997). Mother's weight in pregnancy and coronary heart disease in a cohort of Finnish men: follow up study. *BMJ*, **315**, 837–40.

Forsen T, Eriksson, J. G., Tuomilehto, J., Osmond, C. and Barker, D. J. P. (1999). Growth in utero and during childhood among women who develop coronary heart disease: longitudinal study. *BMJ*, **319**, 1403–7.

Forsen, T., Osmond, C., Eriksson, J. G. and Barker, D. J. P. (2004). Growth of girls who later develop coronary heart disease. *Heart*, **90**, 20–4.

Frankel, S., Elwood, J. H., Sweetnam, P., Yarnell, J. and Davey Smith, G. (1996). Birthweight, adult risk factors and incident coronary heart disease: the Caerphilly study. *Public Health*, **110**, 139–43.

Gunnell, D. J., Davey Smith, G., Frankel, S. *et al.* (1998). Childhood leg length and adult mortality: follow up of the Carnegie (Boyd Orr) Survey of Diet and Health in Pre-war Britain. *J. Epid. Comm. Health*, **52**, 142–52.

Hales, C. N., Barker, D. J. P., Clark, P. M. S. *et al.* (1991). Fetal and infant growth and impaired glucose tolerance at age 64. *BMJ*, **303**, 1019–22.

Hanson, M., Gluckman, P., Bier, D. *et al.* (2004). Report of the 2nd World Congress on Fetal Origins of Adult Disease, Brighton, UK., June 7–10, 2003. *Pediatr. Res.*, **55**, 894–7.

Harding, J. E. (2001). The nutritional basis of the fetal origins of adult disease. *Int. J. Epidemiol.*, **30**, 15–23.

Hill, A. B. (1965). The environment and disease: association or causation? *Proc. R. Soc. Med.*, **58**, 295–300.

Huxley, R., Neil, A. and Collins, R. (2002). Unravelling the fetal origins hypothesis: is there really an inverse association between birthweight and subsequent blood pressure? *Lancet*, **360**, 659–65.

Huxley, R. R., Shiell, A. W. and Law, C. M. (2000). The role of size at birth and postnatal catch-up growth in determining systolic blood pressure: a systematic review of the literature. *J. Hypertens.*, **18**, 815–31.

Independent Inquiry into Inequalities in Health. (1998). *Report of the Independent Inquiry into Inequalities in Health*. London: Stationery Office.

Jones, W. H. S. (1923). *Hipprocrates*. Loeb Classical Libary, 147: Ancient Medicine. Cambridge, MA; Harvard University Press.

Kmietowicz, Z. (2002). Government launches intensive media campaign on MMR. *BMJ*, **324**, 383.

Kramer, M. S. (2000). Invited commentary: association between restricted fetal growth and adult chronic disease. Is it causal? Is it important? *Am. J. Epidemiol*, **152**, 605–8.

Langley-Evans, S. C., Langley-Evans, A. J. and Marchand, M. C. (2003). Nutritional programming of blood pressure and renal morphology. *Arch. Physiol. Biochem.*, **111**, 8–16.

Law, C. M. (2002). Commentary: using research evidence to promote cardiovascular health in children. *Int. J. Epidemiol.*, **31**, 1127–9.

Lawlor, D. A., Ebrahim, S. and Davey Smith, G. (2002). Is there a sex difference in the association between birth weight and systolic blood pressure in later life? Findings from a meta-regression analysis. *Am. J. Epidemiol.*, **156**, 1100–4.

Leon, D. A., Koupilova, I., Lithell, H. O. *et al.* (1996). Failure to realise growth potential in utero and adult obesity in relation to blood pressure in 50 year old Swedish men. *BMJ*, **312**, 401–6.

Leon, D. A., Lithell, H. O., Vagero, D. *et al.* (1998). Reduced fetal growth rate and increased risk of death from ischaemic heart disease: cohort study of 15,000 Swedish men and women born 1915–29. *BMJ*, **317**, 241–5.

Lucas, A., Fewtrell, M. S. and Cole, T. J. (1999). Fetal origins of adult disease: the hypothesis revisited. *BMJ*, **319**, 245–9.

Lucas, P. J., Roberts, H., Baird, J., Fisher, D. J. and Law, C. M. (2004). Who cares about growth? The views of parents and others on the importance of growth in babies. Poster presented at the Society for Social Medicine 48th Annual Scientific Meeting. University of Birmingham, 15–17 September 2004.

Marmot, M. (2001). Aetiology of coronary heart disease. *BMJ*, **323**, 1261–2.

Martyn, C. N., Barker, D. J. P. and Osmond, C. (1996). Mothers' pelvic size, fetal growth, and death from stroke and coronary heart disease in men in the UK. *Lancet*, **348**, 1264–8.

Measham, A. and Gillespie, S. (1998). *Implementation Completion Report: Second Tamil Nadu Integrated Nutrition Project*. Washington, DC: World Bank.

Merialdi, M., Carroli, G., Villar, J. *et al.* (2003). Nutritional interventions during pregnancy for the prevention or treatment of impaired fetal growth: an overview of randomized controlled trials. *J Nutr.*, **133**, 1626–31S.

Mi, J., Law, C. M., Zhang, K-L., Osmond C., Stein, C. and Barker, D. (2000). Effects of infant birthweight and maternal body mass index in pregnancy on components of the insulin resistance syndrome in China. *Ann. Int. Med.*, **132**, 253–60.

Murray, C. J. L. and Lopez, A. D. (1997). Alternative projections of mortality and disability by cause 1990–2020: Global Burden of Disease Study. *Lancet*, **349**, 1498–504.

Osmond, C., Barker, D. J. P., Winter, P. D., Fall, C. H. D. and Simmonds, S. J. (1993). Early growth and death from cardiovascular disease in women. *BMJ*, **307**, 1519–24.

Owen, C. G., Whincup, P. H., Odoki, K., Gilg, J. A. and Cook, D. G. (2003a). Birthweight and blood cholesterol level: a study of adolescents and systematic review. *Pediatrics*, **111**, 1081–9.

Owen, C. G., Whincup, P. H., Gilg, J. A. and Cook, D. G. (2003b). Effect of breast feeding in infancy on blood pressure in later life: systematic review and meta-analysis. *BMJ*, **327**, 1189–95.

Parsons, T. J., Power, C. and Manor, O. (2001). Fetal and early life growth and body mass index from birth to early adulthood in 1958 British cohort. *BMJ*, **323**, 1331–5.

Podja, J. and Kelly, L. (2000). Low birthweight: a report based on the International Low Birthweight Symposium, Dhaka, Bangladesh, June 1999. United Nations Administrative Committee on Coordination / Sub-Committee on Nutrition. Geneva; World Health Organization.

Ravelli, A. C. J., van der Meulen, J. H. P., Michels, R. P. J. *et al.* (1998). Glucose tolerance in adults after prenatal exposure to famine. *Lancet*, **351**, 173–7.

Rich-Edwards, J., Stampfer, M., Manson, J. *et al.* (1995). Birthweight, breastfeeding and the risk of coronary heart disease in the Nurses Health Study. *Am. J. Epidemiol*, **141**, S78.

Robinson, R. (2001). The fetal origins of adult disease. *BMJ*, **322**, 375–6.

Rose, G. (1985). Sick individuals and sick populations. *Int. J. Epidemiol.*, **14**, 32–8.

(1992). *The Strategy of Preventive Medicine.* Oxford: Oxford University Press.

Rush, D. (2000). Nutrition and maternal mortality in the developing world. *Am. J. Clin. Nutr.*, **72**, 212–40S.

Singhal, A. and Lucas, A. (2004). Early origins of cardiovascular disease: is there a unifying hypothesis? *Lancet*, **363**, 1642–5.

Singhal, A., Cole, T. J. and Lucas, A. (2001). Early nutrition in preterm infants and later blood pressure: two cohorts after randomised trials. *Lancet*, **357**, 413–19.

Stein, C. E., Fall, C. H. D., Kumaran, K., Osmond, C., Cox, V. and Barker, D. J. P. (1996). Fetal growth and coronary heart disease in South India. *Lancet*, **348**, 1269–73.

Susser, M. and Levin, B. (1999). Ordeals for the fetal programming hypothesis: the hypothesis largely survives one ordeal but not another. *BMJ*, **318**, 885–6.

Syddall, H. E., Aihie Sayer, A., Simmonds, S. J. *et al.* (2005). Birth weight, infant weight gain, and cause-specific mortality: the Hertfordshire Cohort Study. *Am. J. Epidemiol.*, **161**, 1074–80.

Thompson, C., Syddall, H., Rodin, I., Osmond, C. and Barker, D. J. P. (2001). Birth weight and the risk of depressive disorder in late life. *Br. J. Psychiatry*, **179**, 450–5.

Trostel, P. A. and Taylor, G. A. (2001). A theory of time preference. *Economic Inquiry* 39, 379–95.

United Nations (1999). *UN Convention on the Rights of the Child.* Geneva: United Nations.

Whincup, P. H., Cook, D. G. and Shaper, A. G. (1989). Early influences on blood pressure: a study of children aged 5–7 years. *BMJ*, **299**, 587–91.

World Health Organization (1998). *Health Promotion Glossary.* Geneva: World Health Organization.

World Health Organization. (2001). *Life Course Perspectives on Coronary Heart Disease, Stroke and Diabetes.* Geneva: WHO.

35

Developmental origins of health and disease: implications for developing countries

Caroline H. D. Fall[1] and Harshpal Singh Sachdev[2]

[1]University of Southampton
[2]Maulana Azad Medical College

Introduction

The series of epidemiological studies that set the ball rolling for DOHaD research, by linking data from old obstetric and child health records to adult outcomes, were based in (so-called) developed countries. In brief, they showed that adult cardiovascular disease, type 2 diabetes and the metabolic syndrome were increased in people who were light or thin at birth and during infancy, gained weight or body mass index (BMI) rapidly in childhood, and became overweight or obese adults (Barker 1989, Hales *et al.* 1991, Barker *et al.* 1993, Osmond *et al.* 1993, Forsen *et al.* 1997, 1999, Eriksson *et al.* 2001, 2003). The associations with accelerated childhood weight gain and adult obesity were strongest in those who were smallest at birth. These findings led to the 'fetal origins' and 'thrifty phenotype' hypotheses, which proposed that undernutrition during early development, and a mismatch between undernutrition at this time and later overnutrition and obesity, are crucial factors in the development of these adult diseases (Barker 1989, 1995, Hales and Barker 1992).

The concept that cardiovascular disease and type 2 diabetes, generally considered diseases of affluence, have their origins in transition from poverty and undernutrition offered an explanation for the epidemics of coronary heart disease that swept Europe and the USA in the mid twentieth century (Barker *et al.* 1989). These appeared first in higher socioeconomic groups (the first to experience transition) and later shifted to the less advantaged (the last to experience improvements in fetal and infant nutrition).

Potential relevance for developing countries

In simple terms, the thrifty-phenotype hypothesis predicts high rates of disease in people exposed to undernutrition in fetal life and infancy followed by adequate or excess nutrition in childhood and adult life. This describes the experience of large numbers of people in developing countries. The incidence of intrauterine growth restriction (IUGR) is high in developing countries (Fig. 35.1) (De Onis *et al.* 1998). This is attributed at least partly to poor nutrition among girls and women, resulting in maternal short stature, low body weight, and macro- and micronutrient deficiencies during pregnancy (Kramer 1987, World Health Organization 1995). Growth faltering in infancy (the first 1–2 postnatal years) is also common in developing countries, especially after the cessation of breast-feeding, because of suboptimal weaning practices and frequent infections (Shrimpton *et al.* 2001).

At the same time, economic development and improvements in agricultural production are transforming the nutritional situation for children and adults. In India, national surveys have shown a right

Developmental Origins of Health and Disease, ed. Peter Gluckman and Mark Hanson. Published by Cambridge University Press.
© P. D. Gluckman and M. A. Hanson 2006.

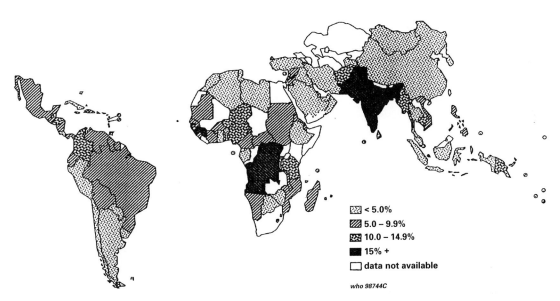

Figure 35.1 Intrauterine growth restriction in developing countries. From De Onis *et al.* (1998), with permission of Nature Publishing Group.

shift in BMI and skinfold thickness among children and adults even in poor urban and rural populations (Sachdev 2003). The proportion of children underweight-for-age below the age of 5 years fell from 78% in the late 1970s to 47% in 1998–9. Although these trends reflect an escape from hunger, with considerable benefits for health, they are all too quickly giving rise to a new concern: the emergence of obesity and obesity-related disease (James *et al.* 2001, Popkin 2004). Developing countries are reporting high rates of coronary heart disease and type 2 diabetes that have 'come out of nowhere' in one or two generations, to become leading causes of morbidity and mortality (Bulatao and Stephens 1992, Fall 2001).

These epidemics are expected to intensify. By the year 2030, the prevalence of diabetes is predicted to rise by 151% in India, 104% in China, 161% in sub-Saharan Africa, 148% in Latin America and the Caribbean and 163% in the Middle East, all far exceeding the predicted increase in established market economies (54%) (Wild *et al.* 2004). The highest number of people with diabetes will be of working age (45–64 years) unlike in developed countries, where the greatest number are in older age groups.

Data for cardiovascular disease are less complete but there is evidence of increasing hypertension, coronary heart disease and stroke in Africa, Asia and South America (Bulatao and Stephens 1992). Coronary heart disease is predicted to become the commonest cause of death in India by 2025 (Bulatao and Stephens 1992, Ghaffar *et al.* 2004).

Currently, the worst affected are the urban rich, because of a host of factors causing obesity (Ghaffar *et al.* 2004, Sachdev 2004). However, this is changing. Industrialisation is bringing urban lifestyles to rural populations. In India, there are high and rising rates of impaired glucose tolerance (IGT) in rural communities, suggesting a large reservoir of incipient diabetes (Ramachandran *et al.* 1992). Some developing countries are reporting a shift in disease towards the poorer sectors, especially in urban slums (Sawaya *et al.* 2003). It is generally agreed that the epidemics of disease have been triggered by obesity consequent upon urbanisation. However, if the thrifty-phenotype hypothesis is correct, they are also exacerbated by persisting suboptimal fetal and infant development, linked to undernutrition in mothers.

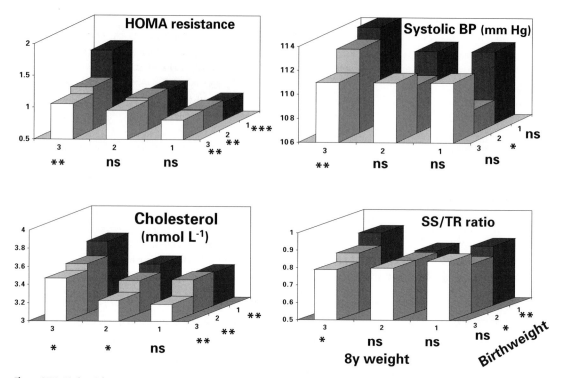

Figure 35.2 Birthweight, current (8-year) weight and cardiovascular disease risk factors among Indian children. Birthweight and 8-year weight shown in three groups, from lightest (1) to heaviest (3). Significance level for trend in each row and column (adjusted for age and sex): ns, not significant; * $p < 0.05$; ** $p < 0.01$; *** $p < 0.001$. From Bavdekar *et al.* (1999). © 1999 American Diabetes Association. Reprinted with permission.

Born small, becoming big

A study of cardiovascular disease risk factors in Indian children was the first in a developing country to examine associations between size at birth and later risk. Among 4-year-old children born in the KEM Hospital, Pune, lower birthweight was associated with higher plasma glucose concentrations after an oral glucose load (Yajnik *et al.* 1995). After adjusting for current (4-year) weight, which was strongly positively related to glucose and insulin concentrations, lower birthweight was also associated with higher insulin concentrations. When the children were examined again at 8 years, those of lower birthweight had higher LDL-cholesterol concentrations and subscapular/triceps skinfold ratios and, after adjusting for 8-year weight, higher sys-

tolic blood pressure and insulin resistance (Bavdekar *et al.* 2000). These risk factors were highest in children who were born small but became the biggest (heaviest, tallest and most adipose) at 8 years (Fig. 35.2).

Studies in other developing countries, mainly in children, have shown similar results. Blood pressure has been studied in children in Africa (Margetts *et al.* 1991, Woelk *et al.* 1998, Levitt *et al.* 1999, Law *et al.* 2000), the West Indies (Forrester *et al.* 1996), Asia (Law *et al.* 2000, Adair and Cole 2003, Cole 2004, Kumar *et al.* 2004) and South and Central America (Barros and Victora 1999, Bergel *et al.* 2000, Law *et al.* 2000) and measurements of glucose/insulin metabolism (glucose tolerance, insulin concentrations and glycosylated haemoglobin) in South Africa (Crowther *et al.* 1998) and Jamaica (Forrester *et al.*

1996, Bennett *et al.* 2002). The majority showed no direct associations between low birthweight (or other measurements at birth) and later outcomes. However, after adjusting for current weight, most showed higher blood pressure and glucose and insulin concentrations in children of lower birthweight, birth length or ponderal index. Being born small was not on its own associated with these outcomes, but 'becoming big' was strongly associated with them, and a combination of the two (small becoming big) was associated with the highest levels. Though fewer, follow-up studies in adults in South Africa (Levitt *et al.* 2000), China (Jie *et al.* 2000, Zhao *et al.* 2002) and India (Bhargava *et al.* 2004) have shown similar results.

In all of these studies, the inverse associations between disease (or risk factors) and size at birth were statistically considerably weaker than the positive associations with current size. This is true of studies in developed countries, though perhaps more marked in developing countries, especially for adults. While in Hertfordshire and Helsinki, coronary heart disease and type 2 diabetes were related to small size at birth without any adjustment for adult size, in South Africa (Levitt *et al.* 2000), China (Jie *et al.* 2000, Zhao *et al.* 2002) and India (Bhargava *et al.* 2004) associations with birth size were generally only statistically significant after adjusting for adult BMI. This suggests that being 'born small' becomes a problem only if there is also a 'becoming big' in childhood or adult life.

A clear example of the 'small becoming big' phenomenon came from a study of young adults in New Delhi, India, who were measured at birth and every six months until the age of 21 years (Bhargava *et al.* 2004). Mean birthweight was only 2.9 kg and as children a high proportion of the cohort was underweight for age (53% at the age of 2 years, using National Center for Health Statistics standards). When they were re-traced at the age of 26–32 years, over 40% were overweight (BMI > 25 kg m^{-2}) and over 10% were obese (BMI > 30 kg m^{-2}). Four per cent of the cohort already had type 2 diabetes and 15% had IGT. After adjusting for adult BMI,

plasma glucose concentrations and insulin resistance were inversely related to birthweight, and IGT and diabetes were associated with lower weight and BMI at the age of 1 year. In contrast, the *childhood* growth of those who developed IGT or diabetes was characterised by accelerated BMI gain relative to the rest of the cohort (Fig. 35.3, right-hand graph). From being below the cohort mean for BMI at 2 years they were well above the mean at 30 years, while height standard deviation (SD) scores were close to the cohort mean throughout (Fig. 35.3, left-hand graph). The highest prevalence of IGT and diabetes was in men and women who had low BMI SD scores in infancy but high SD scores at 12 years or later. An increase in BMI SD score between 2 and 12 years was a strong risk factor for adult IGT and diabetes, independently of adult BMI. It is important to point out that even at the age of 12 their mean BMI was not high by international standards. They had 'become big relative to themselves' rather than in absolute terms. We will return to this distinction later.

Born big

Hard on the heels of studies showing associations between low birthweight and adult disease came data showing an increased risk of type 2 diabetes at *both* extremes of birthweight (McCance *et al.* 1994, Rich-Edwards *et al.* 1999). The increased risk at high birthweights was in men and women whose mothers were diabetic during pregnancy. Although this mother-to-offspring transmission of diabetes probably has a genetic component, the main driver is thought to be hyperglycaemia and hyperinsulinism in the fetus of the diabetic mother (Dabelea *et al.* 2000a, 2000b), an example of 'fuel-mediated teratogenesis' (long-term functional changes in offspring of diabetic mothers exposed to altered fuels during pregnancy) as proposed by Freinkel (1980).

A recent survey among schoolchildren in Taiwan has shown a similar phenomenon. Type 2 diabetes was rare at this age (<20 per 100 000) but the risk of disease was increased at both low and

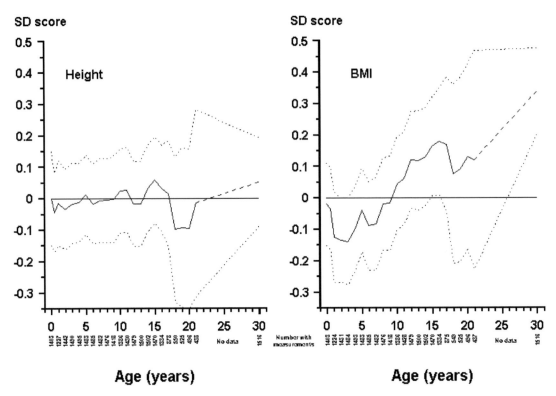

Figure 35.3 Mean sex-specific SD scores for height (left) and BMI (right) at every age from birth to 21 years, and when studied at 26–32 years, for subjects in New Delhi, India, who developed IGT or diabetes. Mean SD scores are indicated by the solid line, and 95% CIs by dotted lines. The mean SD score for the whole cohort is zero. From Bhargava *et al.* (2004). © 2004 Massachusetts Medical Society. All rights reserved. Reprinted with permission.

high birthweights (Fig. 35.4) (Wei *et al.* 2003) . The latter was explained by maternal gestational diabetes and higher current weight among these children. Maternal glucose intolerance was also suggested as an explanation for findings in men and women aged 40–60 years born in Mysore, India (Fall *et al.* 1998). Coronary heart disease was associated with smaller size at birth (Stein *et al.* 1996) but the prevalence of type 2 diabetes was increased in men and women who had a higher ponderal index at birth and heavier mothers (Fall *et al.* 1998). When they were born (1934–54), few mothers would have had gestational diabetes, but it was proposed that heavier fatter mothers had milder degrees of glucose intolerance, to account for these findings.

In a recent study of contemporary women giving birth in Mysore, the prevalence of gestational diabetes was high (6%) despite a low average maternal age and BMI (Hill *et al.* 2005). As expected, babies born to diabetic mothers were heavier (mean birthweight 3339 g) and more adipose than babies of mothers with normal glucose tolerance (2956 g). Though macrosomic they were still below the average birthweight for most developed countries, and only three out of 41 weighed >4 kg, the standard definition of macrosomia. These data suggest that gestational diabetes is common in some developing-country populations and that macrosomic effects on the fetus may be masked because of lower mean birthweight. The relationship between birthweight

Odds ratio

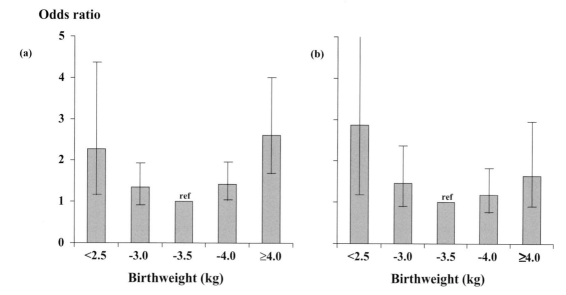

Figure 35.4 Odds ratios for type 2 diabetes among Taiwan schoolchildren according to birthweight: (a) adjusted for age and sex; (b) adjusted for the child's current BMI, socioeconomic status, family history of diabetes, and maternal gestational diabetes. From Wei *et al.* (2003). © 2003 American Diabetes Association. Reprinted with permission.

and later diabetes may vary, and may be inverse, U-shaped or positive, depending on mean birthweight, maternal size, and incidence of gestational diabetes in the population studied (Yajnik 2004a).

Even among non-diabetic mothers in Mysore there were positive associations between maternal glucose concentrations and newborn size (Fig. 35.5) (Hill *et al.* 2005). These became mainly non-significant after adjusting for maternal BMI or fat mass, which were strongly positively related to both maternal glucose and insulin concentrations and newborn size. With a secular trend of increasing body size in all populations, including pregnant women, fetuses will become exposed to more 'fuels', not only glucose, but also amino acids and lipids. These may bring about the reductions in low birthweight that are observed as populations become better nourished. However, if there is *rapid* nutritional transition, and maternal adiposity increases ahead of maternal stature and lean tissue mass, some components of fetal body composition may be enhanced by fuels linked

to maternal adiposity, while others remain growth-restricted. The 'thin–fat' Indian baby may be an example of this.

The 'thin–fat' Indian baby

The Pune Maternal Nutrition Study was a prospective population-based observational study of maternal nutrition and neonatal outcome in rural Indian women (Rao *et al.* 2001, Yajnik *et al.* 2003). The mothers were short and thin (mean pre-pregnant height and BMI 152 cm and 18.1 kg m^{-2}) and the mean full-term birthweight was only 2.7 kg. Detailed anthropometry of the newborns showed that their body composition differed from white Caucasian babies born in the UK (Fig. 35.6) (Yajnik *et al.* 2003). They were lighter by almost two standard deviations, and measures of non-fat soft tissue such as muscle (mid-upper-arm circumference) and abdominal viscera (abdominal circumference) showed a similar deficit. Measurements of truncal fat (subscapular

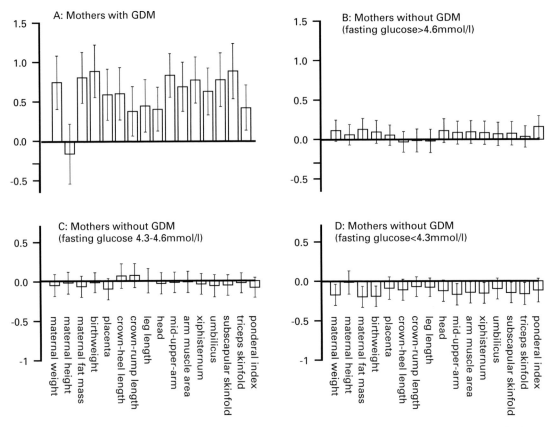

Figure 35.5 Standard deviation (SD) scores for mothers and their babies born in Mysore, South India. The mean SD score for the whole cohort is zero. (A) Mothers with gestational diabetes (GDM) and their babies; (B), (C), (D) mothers without GDM, in thirds of fasting blood glucose. Values adjusted for gestation. Error bars show 95% confidence intervals.

skinfolds), however, were relatively 'spared' (−0.5 SD). Thus, although extremely small and thin, the Indian babies were relatively adipose. A similar pattern has been confirmed in urban Indian populations (Yajnik *et al*. 2002, Krishnaveni *et al*. 2005).

The aetiology of the muscle-thin but adipose 'thin–fat' phenotype of Indian newborns is unknown. The above studies showed that disproportionate neonatal adiposity is related to greater maternal adiposity, and higher maternal glucose and insulin concentrations, but the low lean mass is unexplained. The phenotype may be 'adaptive' and carry some survival advantage; for example, in the face of a nutritional deficit, muscle growth may be sacrificed, and fat laid

down preferentially as a substrate for brain growth and/or immune function (Yajnik 2004a). Alternatively it may have a genetic basis. Its consequences for later health, if any, are also unknown; however it echoes the well-described adult Indian phenotype (lower muscle mass, higher percentage body fat, and greater tendency to central adiposity than white Caucasians) that is strongly associated with type 2 diabetes (Yajnik 2004a, 2004b). The findings highlight the fact that birthweight provides only a crude summary of fetal growth and fails to describe potentially important differences in the development of specific tissues. They also suggest that 'improvements' in maternal nutrition that simply increase maternal

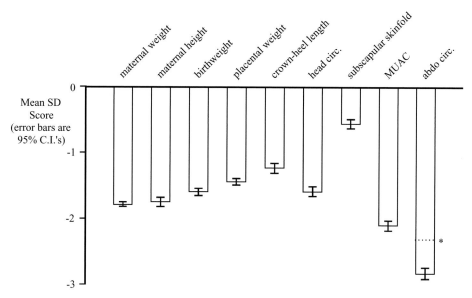

Figure 35.6 Mean SD scores for maternal pre-pregnant weight and height, and measurements of the babies, in Pune, India, compared with Southampton, UK. The Southampton mean is represented by zero. * indicates estimated SD score adjusted for difference in measurement techniques. From Yajnik *et al.* (2003), with permission of Nature Publishing Group.

adiposity, and hence insulin resistance, could exacerbate this unbalanced phenotype (Yajnik 2004a).

Weight gain in infancy

There are few cohort studies able to examine the relationship of weight gain in infancy to later risk factors and disease outcomes. In Hertfordshire, Helsinki and New Delhi (Fig. 35.3) lower weight or BMI at one year were associated with a higher risk of adult cardiovascular disease and/or type 2 diabetes (Barker 1989, Hales *et al.* 1991, Barker *et al.* 1993, Osmond *et al.* 1993, Forsen *et al.* 1997, 1999, Eriksson *et al.* 2001, 2003, Bhargava *et al.* 2004). These findings were encouraging for paediatricians in developing countries, where it is usual to encourage infant weight gain in small babies. This practice probably has significant short-term benefits, including improved immunity from infection and reduced infant mortality (Victora *et al.* 2001). Furthermore, optimising nutrition in infancy is more effective than in later

childhood for preventing stunting (Martorell *et al.* 1994, Stein *et al.* 2004). On the other hand, recent data from randomised controlled trials in UK newborns have shown associations between rapid infant weight gain and higher levels of cardiovascular risk factors during childhood (Singhal and Lucas 2004).

There are several possible explanations for the different findings in adults (Hertfordshire, Helsinki and New Delhi) and children. Cardiovascular risk factors measured in childhood may be misleading in relation to later disease risk. This seems unlikely as there is evidence that risk factors 'track' from childhood into adult life (Ronnemaa *et al.* 1991, Kelder *et al.* 2002). Patterns of infant growth, and the environmental factors that determine them, may differ for babies born today in affluent countries from those of the adult cohorts. The poor social conditions that led to infant growth faltering and high infant mortality in the past, and possibly cardiovascular disease in later life, have disappeared for most in developed countries and for many in developing countries. Infant weight gain may therefore have different long-term effects in contemporary children than in the past. Finally, there may be survival effects; metabolic characteristics that enabled small infants to survive may also increase their risk of later disease – this has also been proposed as an explanation for the association between lower birthweight and adult disease (McCance et al. 1994). Whatever the explanation, the optimal trajectory of infant weight gain for later health, among today's infants in developing countries, is not known.

The relationship, if any, between mode of feeding during infancy, and later health, is also unclear. Studies comparing people who were breast-fed or artificially fed are difficult to interpret because of confounding by socioeconomic influences on how mothers feed their babies. In developing countries there is good evidence that breast-feeding protects against infection and reduces infant mortality (Cunningham et al. 1991). In comparison, effects on adult outcomes are probably small (Owen et al. 2003, Martin et al. 2004a), although this needs further research. There is some evidence that the risk of hypertension and obesity may be reduced in adults who were breast-fed as infants (Victora et al. 2003, Swinburn et al. 2004).

Height growth in childhood

While accelerated childhood BMI gain is clearly associated with an increased risk of adult disease, the picture is less clear regarding height growth. In developed countries, short adult stature is strongly associated with an increased risk of developing cardiovascular disease, type 2 diabetes and gestational diabetes (Marmot et al. 1978, Waaler 1984, Rich-Edwards et al. 1995, Anastasiou et al. 1998). Suggested explanations are that taller people have larger coronary arteries and lean body mass, that factors associated with poor childhood growth (poor nutrition, hormonal disturbances or genetic differences) also lead to an increased risk of disease, and (reverse causality) that people with poor adult health 'shrink' faster with age. Stunting in childhood has been linked to increased adult obesity and central

obesity in developing countries (Sawaya et al. 2003), and to higher cardiovascular risk factors in childhood (Gaskin et al. 2000, Sawaya et al. 2003). On the other hand, among the 8-year-old Pune children blood pressure and insulin resistance were higher in taller children (Bavdekar et al. 2000). The Delhi study showed no relationship between height SD scores throughout childhood, or adult height, and IGT or type 2 diabetes (Bhargava et al. 2004). In developing countries, height is strongly related to socioeconomic status. For this reason alone, taller height may be associated with an increased risk of disease at the start of the transition process, but become associated with a lower risk of disease as the transition 'matures' and switches to lower socioeconomic groups.

Maternal nutrition

Newborn size increases with increasing maternal BMI and fat mass (Kramer 1987, World Health Organization 1995). The effects on fetal growth of variations in maternal diet, however, have been poorly characterised. Trials of balanced energy and protein supplements, usually started in mid to late pregnancy, have shown small but consistent increases in birthweight (around 50 g) (Kramer and Kakuma 2003). A very high calorie supplement for severely undernourished women in The Gambia increased birthweight by 136 g (and reduced stillbirths and neonatal deaths) (Ceesay et al. 1997). Trials have sometimes shown paradoxical results; for example high-density protein supplements have consistently reduced fetal growth (Rush 2001). Women in developing countries frequently have multiple micronutrient deficiencies (the so-called 'hidden hunger') which may prevent the utilisation of energy and protein for fetal growth (Ramakrishnan 2002, Fall et al. 2003). The results of single micronutrient supplements have been largely negative, perhaps unsurprisingly, because the effect of any one limiting nutrient will be constrained by deficiencies of other limiting nutrients. However, multiple micronutrient trials have also had mixed results, ranging from a large increase in birthweight (+100 g) among HIV-positive women in Tanzania to no effect among undernourished women in Nepal, Mexico and Zimbabwe (Fawzi *et al.* 1998, Christian *et al.* 2003, Fall *et al.* 2003, Ramakrishnan *et al.* 2003, Friis *et al.* 2004). Data from experimental animals suggest that the mother's pre- and peri-conceptional nutritional status influences the trajectory of fetal growth and newborn size (Robinson *et al.* 1999, Kwong *et al.* 2000), but few trials have assessed the effect on fetal growth of starting supplementation pre-conceptionally. Importantly, no trials have assessed effects of maternal supplementation on neonatal body composition.

It seems likely that dietary influences on fetal growth vary with the ethnic and geographical characteristics of populations. In Southampton, UK, mothers with high carbohydrate intakes in early pregnancy and low dairy or meat protein intakes in late pregnancy had lower-birthweight babies (Godfrey *et al.* 1996). In the Pune Maternal Nutrition Study, neonatal size was unrelated to maternal energy or protein intakes but mothers with higher intakes of green leafy vegetables, fruit and milk, and higher folate and vitamin C status had larger babies (Rao *et al.* 2001). In well-nourished US women, moderate exercise was associated with higher birthweight (Clapp 2003), while in Pune, thin mothers with a high physical workload, associated with farm labour, had smaller babies (Rao *et al.* 2003).

In addition to maternal BMI and fat mass, newborn size increases with the mother's height, head circumference and even birthweight. These associations probably have both genetic and environmental components but suggest that a female's nutrition during her physical growth in fetal life and childhood, as well as during pregnancy, influences the growth of her fetus. Further evidence of this is that maternal leg length in childhood predicts the birthweight of her children, independently of her final height (Martin *et al.* 2004b). Pregnancy during adolescence is associated with reduced fetal growth, perhaps because nutrients are preferentially diverted to maternal growth (King 2003). The term 'maternal constraint'

has been given to the poorly understood phenomenon, first described in animal cross-breeding studies, whereby fetal growth is limited if the mother is small in size (Adair and Prentice 2004). This may be important in preventing obstructed labour in small mothers. It may also explain why changes in newborn size have lagged behind the marked increases in the weight and height of children that have accompanied recent improvements in nutrition in developing countries. Mothers will probably be taller in future generations, although paradoxically the emerging problem of obesity may threaten this; accelerated weight gain after early malnutrition can lead to earlier menarche, compromising final height (Rush 2000).

Barker proposed that maternal ill health, poverty and undernutrition were important causes of impaired fetal and infant development and, in turn, adult disease (Barker 1989, 1995). If so, correlations would be expected between indices of poor maternal nutrition and cardiovascular disease and its risk factors in the offspring. The problem is that there are so far only limited data available to test this, especially in populations old enough to measure disease outcomes. Several studies in developing countries have shown that low maternal weight gain, BMI or skinfold thickness in pregnancy are associated with higher offspring blood pressure (Fig. 35.7) (Godfrey *et al.* 1994, Adair *et al.* 2001), insulin resistance (Jie *et al.* 2000) and risk of coronary heart disease (Stein *et al.* 1996). There have been few follow-up studies relating outcomes to maternal diet. In The Gambia there is an annual period of severe undernutrition during the rainy season, and being born at this time is associated with a tenfold increase in mortality from infectious disease in young adult life (Moore *et al.* 2004). Cardiovascular disease risk factors in young Gambian adults, however, were unrelated to month of birth or infant anthropometry (Moore *et al.* 2001). The authors suggested this could be because the subjects remained undernourished as adults (no 'becoming big'). In the only follow-up study so far of a randomised controlled trial of a nutritional intervention in pregnancy, blood pressure was lower in Argentinean children whose mothers were supplemented

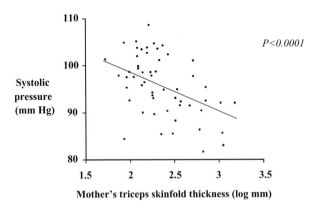

Figure 35.7 Children's systolic blood pressure (adjusted for sex and current weight) according to the mother's triceps skinfold thickness at 15 weeks of gestation. From Godfrey *et al.* (1994), by permission of the Royal College of Obstetricians and Gynaecologists.

with calcium to prevent pregnancy-induced hypertension (Belizan *et al.* 1997).

As described above (see 'Born big'), maternal overnutrition and obesity may also programme disease in the offspring. This may be a particular problem if women were undernourished in childhood; in Finland, higher maternal BMI was associated with increased mortality from cardiovascular disease in the offspring, but only if the mother was short in stature (possible evidence of childhood stunting) (Forsen *et al.* 1997). 'Optimal' maternal nutrition thus depends on what has gone before and, especially in populations undergoing nutritional transition, is likely to change with time.

Implications for further research and for public health policy

The data presented suggest that nutrition and growth during fetal life, infancy, childhood and adolescence have important effects on adult health in developing countries. 'Sufficient' energy, macronutrients and micronutrients are required for normal growth and function. However, not enough is known about the ideal balance of these at different stages of the

life cycle, in different environmental circumstances and in people whose genes have evolved in different settings. In developing countries the emphasis up to now has been on eradicating undernutrition. These efforts need to continue because, although severe protein and energy malnutrition have been reduced considerably, milder degrees persist and micronutrient deficiencies remain common. However, energy overnutrition, resulting in overweight and obesity, is emerging as a serious threat to health. Moreover, the rapidity of transition has led to the coexistence of undernutrition and overnutrition within populations and even within individuals. There is therefore a delicate balance to be achieved.

Maternal nutrition

The attractiveness of the 'fetal origins' hypothesis is that improvements in maternal nutrition could, among other (short-term) benefits, prevent common chronic diseases of adult life. This has not yet, however, been proved or disproved, nor do we know what constitutes optimal maternal nutrition for fetal development and later health. The hypothesis is sufficiently plausible, however, and of such potential importance that research in this area should be vigorously pursued. It seems imperative to study the effects of improving the diet of undernourished women, before and during pregnancy, on their own health and that of their offspring. There is good evidence that both extremes of maternal BMI are harmful. In developing-country populations, relatively small increases in maternal adiposity may have adverse effects. We suggest therefore that nutritional intervention studies in mothers should focus on diet quality and be designed to avoid increasing maternal adiposity. Birthweight is not sufficient as an outcome; studies should examine neonatal body composition and functional outcomes, and incorporate long-term follow-up.

Accelerated BMI or adiposity gain in childhood

There is good evidence that childhood obesity increases the risk of adult obesity and disease, and this has stimulated programmes in developed countries to treat obese children. However, there are problems with this approach. Current methods of treating established obesity in children, as in adults, are not very effective (Reilly and McDowell 2003, Summerbell *et al.* 2003, Swinburn *et al.* 2004). Also, this approach may not capture the majority of at-risk children in developing countries. The Delhi study showed that adults with IGT or diabetes were not overweight or obese as children; in fact they were thinner than average as young children (Bhargava *et al.* 2004). At the age of 12 years only 3% of them were overweight, and none were obese. What characterised them was a steady upward change across BMI categories from about the age of 2 years (Fig. 35.3). These data suggest that it is not obesity in absolute terms that carries long-term risk, but becoming 'obese relative to oneself', i.e. crossing from lower to higher categories of adiposity. To identify these children would require serial measurements of adiposity and suitable population-specific reference standards. International anthropometric standards are unhelpful for detecting this 'relative' overnutrition. Data from the Delhi study are currently being used to determine the feasibility of detecting upward changes in BMI in Indian children. Further research is needed, as it is not known whether this trajectory is modifiable, and, if so, whether this will be beneficial.

The emergence of obesity in developing countries certainly requires urgent action. Messages about the health risks of adult obesity and of sedentary lifestyles need to go out much more strongly. In the case of children, there is the problem that such messages would conflict with current policies, which still emphasise the prevention of childhood undernutrition. Limiting children's food intake would probably be unacceptable in developing countries. However, it is important to make parents aware of the harmful effects of obesity, inform them about healthy diets (for example upper limits of energy and fat intakes and necessary intakes of micronutrient-rich foods) and promote physical activity. National programmes that provide universal supplementary midday meals for children in many developing countries should be reviewed, possibly targeted only to the most undernourished children, and the micronutrient quality improved (Uauy and Kain 2002, Sachdev 2004).

Infancy

As described above, it is not clear whether 'catch-up' weight gain in infancy is good or bad in relation to later disease risk. Infancy may be an accessible window in which better nutrition could prevent later disease, or a time when rapid weight gain increases later risk. Data from randomised controlled trials of nutritional interventions in infancy are currently limited to special groups such as preterm babies, and there are no data from developing countries. We do not know therefore whether infant weight gain should be 'promoted', 'protected' or 'restrained'. However, because of evidence that encouraging weight gain in IUGR babies has important benefits for short-term health and survival, and may prevent stunting, we think there is insufficient evidence to alter current policies. Further research in this area is needed. Breast-feeding should be promoted for its known short-term benefits, and current data on adult outcomes do not conflict with this recommendation.

Conclusions

The DOHaD concept, that common chronic diseases of adult life are linked to nutritional experience in early life, has potentially huge implications for public health strategies in developing countries. This was recognised in the Global Strategy on Diet, Physical Activity and Health presented at the 2004 World Health Assembly, which stated for the first time that 'maternal health and nutrition before and during pregnancy, and early infant nutrition may be important in the prevention of non-communicable diseases throughout the life course' (World Health Organization 2004). Currently, however, DOHaD research poses more questions than answers, and despite the urgency created by epidemics of disease in developing countries, it is not yet possible to derive clear public health recommendations. The emergence of overnutrition and obesity complicates the issue; the answer is not simply to 'improve' (i.e. increase) birthweight. Further research into the link between maternal diet, fetal growth and both short- and long-term outcomes is a high priority. There is good evidence that accelerated BMI gain in childhood ('becoming obese relative to oneself'), at least after the period of infancy, increases the risk of adult cardiovascular disease and type 2 diabetes. More research is needed even here, however, to determine the feasibility and outcome of modifying fat gain in childhood.

REFERENCES

Adair, L. S. and Cole, T. J. (2003). Faster childhood growth increases risk of high blood pressure in adolescent boys who were thin at birth. *Hypertension*, **41**, 451–6.

Adair, L. S. and Prentice, A. M. (2004). A critical evaluation of the fetal origins hypothesis and its implications for developing countries. *J. Nutr.*, **134**, 191–3.

Adair, L. S., Kuzawa B. B. A. and Borja, J. (2001). Maternal energy stores and diet composition during pregnancy program adolescent blood pressure. *Circulation*, **104**, 1034–9.

Anastasiou, E., Alevizaki, M., Grigorakis, S. J., Philippou, G., Kyprianou, M. and Souvatzoglou, A. (1998). Decreased stature in gestational diabetes mellitus. *Diabetologia*, **41**, 997–1001.

Barker, D. J. P. (1989). Rise and fall of Western diseases. *Nature*, **338**, 371–2.

(1995). The fetal origins of coronary heart disease. *BMJ*, **311**, 171–4.

Barker, D. J. P., Osmond, C., Winter, P. D. W., Margetts, B. and Simmonds, S. J. (1989). Weight in infancy and death from ischaemic heart disease. *Lancet*, **2**, 577–80.

Barker, D. J. P., Hales, C. N., Fall, C. H. D., Osmond, C., Phipps, K. and Clark, P. M. S. (1993). Type 2 (non-insulin-dependent) diabetes mellitus, hypertension and hyperlipidaemia (syndrome X): relation to reduced fetal growth. *Diabetologia*, **36**, 62–7.

Barros, F. and Victora, C. (1999). Increased blood pressure in adolescents who were small for gestational age at birth: a cohort study in Brazil. *Int. J. Epidemiol.*, **28**, 676–81.

Bavdekar, A., Yajnik, C. S., Fall, C. H. D. *et al.* (2000). The insulin resistance syndrome (IRS) in eight-year-old Indian children: small at birth, big at 8 years or both? *Diabetes*, **48**, 2422–9.

Belizan, J. M., Villar, J., Bergel, E., del Pino, A., Di Fulvio, S. and Galliano, S. V. (1997). Long-term effect of calcium supplementation during pregnancy on the blood pressure of offspring: follow up of a randomised controlled trial. *BMJ*, **315**, 281–5.

Bennett, F., Watson-Brown, C., Thame, M. *et al.* (2002). Shortness at birth is associated with insulin resistance in pre-pubertal Jamaican children. *Eur. J. Clin. Nutr.*, **56**, 506–11.

Bergel, E., Haelterman, E., Belizan, J., Villar, J. and Carroli, G. (2000). Perinatal factors associated with blood pressure during childhood. *Am. J. Epidemiol.*, **151**, 594–601.

Bhargava, S. K., Sachdev, H. P. S., Fall, C. H. D. *et al.* (2004). Relation of serial changes in childhood body mass index to impaired glucose tolerance in young adulthood. *N. Engl. J. Med.*, **350**, 865–75.

Bulatao, R. A. and Stephens, P. W. (1992). *Global Estimates and Projections of Mortality by Cause, 1970–2015.* Working Paper Series 1007. Washington, DC: World Bank.

Ceesay, S. M., Prentice, A. M., Cole, T. J. *et al.* (1997). Effects on birth weight and perinatal mortality of maternal dietary supplements in rural Gambia: 5 year randomised controlled trial. *BMJ*, **315**, 786–90.

Christian, P., Khatry, S. K., Katz, J. *et al.* (2003). Effects of alternative maternal micronutrient supplements on low birth weight in rural Nepal: double blind randomised community trial. *BMJ*, **326**, 571–6.

Clapp, J. F. (2003). The effects of maternal exercise on fetal oxygenation and feto-placental growth. *Eur. J. Obstet. Gynecol. Reprod. Biol.*, **110** (Suppl. 1), S80–5.

Cole, T. J. (2004). Modelling postnatal exposures and their interactions with birth size. *J. Nutr.*, **134**, 201–4.

Crowther, N. J., Cameron, N., Trusler, J. and Gray, I. P. (1998). Association between poor glucose tolerance and rapid postnatal weight gain in seven year old children. *Diabetologia*, **41**, 1163–7.

Cunningham, A. S., Jelliffe, D. B. and Jelliffe, E. F. (1991). Breast-feeding and health in the 1980s: a global epidemiologic review. *J. Pediatr.*, **118**, 659–66.

Dabelea, D., Hanson, R. L., Lindsay, R. S. *et al.* (2000a). Intrauterine exposure to diabetes conveys risks for type 2 diabetes and obesity: a study of discordant sibships. *Diabetes*, **49**, 2208–11.

Dabelea, D., Knowler, W. C. and Pettitt, D. J. (2000b). Effect of diabetes in pregnancy and offspring: follow-up research in the Pima Indians. *J. Matern. Fetal Med.*, **9**, 83–8.

De Onis, M., Blossner, M. and Villar, J. (1998). Levels of intrauterine growth retardation in developing countries. *Eur. J. Clin. Nutr.*, **52**: S1, S5–15.

Eriksson, J. G., Forsen, T., Tuomilehto, H. J. and Barker, D. J. P. (2001). Early growth and coronary heart disease in later life: longitudinal study. *BMJ*, **322**, 949–53.

Eriksson J. G., Forsen, T., Tuomilehto, J., Osmond, C. and Barker, D. J. P. (2003). Early adiposity rebound in childhood and risk of type 2 diabetes in adult life. *Diabetologia*, **46**, 190–4.

Fall, C. H. D. (2001). Non-industrialised countries and affluence: relationship with type 2 diabetes. *Br. Med. Bull.*, **60**, 33–50.

Fall, C. H. D., Stein, C., Kumaran, K. *et al.* (1998). Size at birth, maternal weight, and non-insulin-dependent diabetes (NIDDM) in south Indian adults. *Diabet. Med.*, **15**, 220–7.

Fall, C. H. D., Yajnik, C. S., Rao, S., Davies, A. A., Brown, N. and Farrant, H. J. W. (2003). Micronutrients and fetal growth. *J. Nutr.*, **133**, 1747–56S.

Fawzi, W. W., Msamanga, G., Spiegelman, D. *et al.* (1998). Randomised trial of effects of vitamin A supplements on pregnancy outcomes and T cell counts in HIV-1 infected women in Tanzania. *Lancet*, **351**, 1477–82.

Forrester, T. E., Wilks, R. J., Bennett, F. I. *et al.* (1996). Fetal growth and cardiovascular risk factors in Jamaican schoolchildren. *BMJ*, **312**, 156–60.

Forsen, T., Eriksson, J. G., Tuomilehto, J., Teramo, K., Osmond, C. and Barker, D. J. P. (1997). Mother's weight in pregnancy and coronary heart disease in a cohort of Finnish men: follow up study. *BMJ*, **315**, 837–40.

Forsen, T., Eriksson, J. G., Tuomilehto, J., Osmond, C. and Barker, D. J. P. (1999). Growth in utero and during childhood among women who develop coronary heart disease: longitudinal study. *BMJ*, **319**, 1403–7.

Freinkel, N. (1980). Of pregnancy and progeny. *Diabetes*, **29**, 1023–35.

Friis, H., Gomo, E., Nyazema, N. *et al.* (2004). Effect of multimicronutrient supplementation on gestational length and birth size: a randomized, placebo-controlled, double-blind effectiveness trial in Zimbabwe. *Am. J. Clin. Nutr.*, **80**, 178–84.

Gaskin, P. S., Walker, S. P., Forrester, T. E. and Grantham-McGregor, S. M. (2000). Early linear growth retardation and later blood pressure. *Eur. J. Clin. Nutr.*, **54**, 563–7.

Ghaffar, A., Reddy, K. S. and Singhi, M. (2004). Burden of non-communicable diseases in South Asia. *BMJ*, **328**, 807–10.

Godfrey, K. M., Forrester, T., Barker, D. J. P. *et al.* (1994). Maternal nutritional status in pregnancy and blood pressure in childhood. *Br. J. Obstet. Gynaecol.*, **101**, 398–403.

Godfrey, K. M., Robinson, S., Barker, D. J. P., Osmond, C. and Cox, V. (1996). Maternal nutrition in early and late pregnancy in relation to placental and fetal growth. *BMJ*, **312**, 410–14.

Hales, C. N. and Barker, D. J. P. (1992). Type 2 (non-insulin-dependent) diabetes mellitus: the thrifty phenotype hypothesis. *Diabetologia*, **35**, 595–601.

Hales, C. N., Barker, D. J. P., Clark, P. M. S. *et al.* (1991). Fetal and infant growth and impaired glucose tolerance at age 64. *BMJ*, **303**, 1019–22.

Hill, J. C., Krishnaveni, G. V., Annamma, I., Leary, S. and Fall, C. H. D. (2005). Glucose tolerance in pregnancy in South India; relationships to neonatal anthropometry. *Acta. Obstet. Gynecol. Scand.*, **84**, 159–65.

James, W. P. T., Leach, R., Kalamara, E. and Shayeghi, M. (2001). The worldwide obesity epidemic. *Obes. Res.*, **9** (Suppl. 4), 220–33S.

Jie, M., Law, C., Zhang, K.-L., Osmond, C., Stein, C. and Barker, D. (2000). Effects of infant birthweight and maternal body mass index in pregnancy on components of the insulin resistance syndrome in China. *Ann. Intern. Med.*, **132**, 253–60.

Kelder, S. H., Osganian, S. K., Feldman, H. A. *et al.* (2002). Tracking of physical and physiological risk variables among ethnic subgroups from third to eighth grade: the Child and Adolescent Trial for Cardiovascular Health cohort study. *Prev. Med.*, **34**, 324–33.

King, J. C. (2003). The risk of maternal nutritional depletion and poor outcomes increases in early or closely spaced pregnancies. *J. Nutr.*, **133**, 1732–6S.

Kramer, M. S. (1987). Determinants of low birth weight: methodological assessment and meta-analysis. *Bull. World Health Organ.*, **65**, 663–737.

Kramer, M. S. and Kakuma, R. (2003). Energy and protein intake in pregnancy. *Cochrane Database Syst. Rev.*, **2003** (4), CD000032.

Krishnaveni, G. V., Hill, J. C., Veena, S. R. *et al.* (2005). Truncal adiposity is present at birth and in early childhood in South Indian children. *Indian Pediatrics*, **42**, 527–38.

Kumar, R., Bandyopadhyay, S., Aggarwal, A. K. and Khullar, M. (2004). Relation between birthweight and blood pressure among 7–8 year old rural children in India. *Int. J. Epidemiol.*, **33**, 87–91.

Kwong, W. Y., Wild, A. E., Roberts, P., Willis, A. C. and Fleming, T. (2000). Maternal undernutrition during the pre-implantation period of rat development causes blastocyst abnormalities and programming of postnatal hypertension. *Development*, **127**, 4195–202.

Law, C. M., Egger, P., Dada, O. *et al.* (2000). Body size at birth and blood pressure among children in developing countries. *Int. J. Epidemiol.*, **29**, 52–9.

Levitt, N. S., Steyn, K., de Wet, T. *et al.* (1999). An inverse relation between blood pressure and birth weight among 5 year old children from Soweto, South Africa. *J. Epidemiol. Community Health*, **53**, 264–8.

Levitt, N. S., Lambert, E. V., Woods, D., Hales, C. N., Andrew, R. and Seckl, J. (2000). Impaired glucose tolerance and elevated blood pressure in low birthweight non-obese young South African adults: early programming of cortisol axis. *J. Clin. Endocrinol. Metab.*, **85**, 4611–18.

Margetts, B. M., Rowland, M. G. M., Foord, F. A., Cruddas, A. M., Cole, T. J. and Barker, D. J. P. (1991). The relation of maternal weight to the blood pressures of Gambian children. *Int. J. Epidemiol.*, **20**, 938–43.

Marmot, M. G., Rose, G., Shipley, M. and Hamilton, P. S. (1978). Employment grade and coronary heart disease in British civil servants. *J. Epidemiol. Community Health*, **32**, 244–9.

Martin, R. M., Davey Smith, G., Mangtani, P., Tilling, K., Frankel, S. and Gunnell, D. (2004a). Breastfeeding and cardiovascular mortality: the Boyd Orr cohort and a systematic review with meta-analysis. *Eur. Heart J.*, **25**, 778–86.

Martin, R. M., Davey Smith, G., Frankel, S., and Gunnell, D. (2004b). Parent's growth in childhood and the birth weight of their offspring. *Epidemiology*, **15**, 308–16.

Martorell, R., Kettel Khan, L. and Schroeder, D. G. (1994). Reversibility of stunting: epidemiological findings in children from developing countries. *Eur. J. Clin. Nutr.*, **48** (Suppl. 1), S45–57.

McCance, D. R., Pettitt, D. J., Hanson, R. L., Jacobsson, L. T. H., Knowle, W. C. and Bennett, P. H. (1994). Birth weight and non-insulin dependent diabetes: thrifty genotype, thrifty phenotype, or surviving small baby genotype? *BMJ*, **308**, 942–5.

Moore, S. E., Halsall, I., Howarth, D., Poskitt, E. M. and Prentice, A. M. (2001). Glucose, insulin and lipid metabolism in rural Gambians exposed to early malnutrition. *Diabet. Med.*, **18**, 646–53.

Moore, S. E., Fulford, A. J. C., Streatfield, P. K., Persson, L. A. and Prentice, A. M. (2004). Comparative analysis of patterns of survival by season of birth in rural Bangladeshi and Gambian populations. *Int. J. Epidemiol.*, **33**, 137–43.

Osmond, C., Barker, D. J. P., Winter, P. D., Fall, C. H. D. and Simmonds, S. J. (1993). Early growth and death from cardiovascular disease in women. *BMJ*, **307**, 1519–24.

Owen, C. G., Whincup, P. H., Gilg, J. A. and Cook, D. G. (2003). Effect of breast feeding in infancy on blood pressure in later life: systematic review and meta-analysis. *BMJ*, **327**, 1189–95.

Popkin, B. M. (2004). The nutrition transition: an overview of world patterns of change. *Nutr. Rev.*, **62**, S140–3.

Ramachandran, A., Snehalatha, C., Dharmaraj, D. and Viswanathan, M. (1992). Prevalence of glucose intolerance in Asian Indians: urban–rural difference and significance of upper body adiposity. *Diabetes Care*, **15**, l348–55.

Ramakrishnan, U. (2002). Prevalence of micronutrient malnutrition worldwide. *Nutr. Rev.*, **60**, S46–52.

Ramakrishnan, U., Gonzalez-Cossio, T., Neufeld, L. M., Rivera, J. and Martorell, R. (2003). Multiple micronutrient supplementation during pregnancy does not lead to greater infant birth size than does iron-only supplementation: a randomized controlled trial in a semirural community in Mexico. *Am. J. Clin. Nutr.*, **77**, 720–5.

Rao, S., Yajnik, C. S., Kanade, A. *et al.* (2001). Maternal fat intakes and micronutrient status are related to fetal size at birth in rural India: the Pune Maternal Nutrition Study. *J. Nutr.*, **131**, 1217–24.

Rao, S., Kanade, A., Margetts, B. M. *et al.* (2003). Maternal activity in relation to birth size in rural India: the Pune Maternal Nutrition Study. *Eur. J. Clin. Nutr.*, **57**, 531–42.

Reilly, J. J. and McDowell, Z. C. (2003). Physical activity interventions in the prevention and treatment of paediatric obesity: systematic review and critical appraisal. *Proc. Nutr. Soc.*, **62**, 611–19.

Rich-Edwards, J. W., Manson, J. E., Stampfer, M. J. *et al.* (1995). Height and risk of cardiovascular disease in women. *Am. J. Epidemiol.*, **142**, 909–17.

Rich-Edwards, J. W., Colditz, G. A., Stampfer, M. J. *et al.* (1999). Birthweight and the risk of type 2 diabetes in adult women. *Ann. Int. Med.*, **130**, 278–84.

Robinson, J. J., Sinclair, K. D. and McEvoy, T. G. (1999). Nutritional effects on foetal growth. *Anim. Sci.*, **68**, 315–31.

Ronnemaa, T., Knip, M., Lautala, P. *et al.* (1991). Serum insulin and other cardiovascular risk indicators in children, adolescents and young adults. *Ann. Med.*, **23**, 67–72.

Rush, D. (2000). Nutrition and maternal mortality in the developing world. *Am. J. Clin. Nutr.*, **72** (suppl.), 212–40S.

  (2001). Maternal nutrition and perinatal survival. *Nutr. Rev.*, **59**, 315–26.

Sachdev, H. P. S. (2003). Recent transitions in the anthropometric profile of Indian children: clinical and public health implications. *NFI Bull.*, **24**, 6–8.

(2004). Nutritional transition in the backdrop of early life origins of adult diseases: a challenge for the future. *Indian J. Med. Res.*, **119**, iii–iv.

Sawaya, A. L., Martins, P., Hoffman, D. and Roberts, S. B. (2003). The link between childhood undernutrition and risk of chronic diseases in adulthood: a case study of Brazil. *Nutr. Rev.*, **61**, 168–75.

Shrimpton, R., Victora, C. G., de Onis, M., Lima, R. C., Blossner, M. and Clugston, G. (2001). Worldwide timing of growth faltering: implications for nutritional interventions. *Pediatrics*, **107**, E75.

Singhal, A. and Lucas, A. (2004). Early origins of cardiovascular disease: is there a unifying hypothesis? *Lancet*, **363**, 1642–5.

Stein, A. D., Barnhardt, H. X., Wang, M. *et al.* (2004). Comparison of linear growth patterns in the first three years of life across two generations in Guatemala. *Pediatrics*, **113**, 270–5.

Stein, C., Fall, C. H. D., Kumaran, K., Osmond, C., Cox, V. and Barker, D. J. P. (1996). Fetal growth and coronary heart disease in South India. *Lancet*, **348**, 1269–73.

Summerbell, C. D., Ashton, V., Campbell, K. J., Edmunds, L., Kelly, S. and Waters, E. (2003). Interventions for treating obesity in children. *Cochrane Database Syst. Rev.*, **2003** (3), CD001872.

Swinburn, B. A., Caterson, I., Seidell, J. C. and James, W. P. T. (2004). Diet, nutrition and the prevention of excess weight gain and obesity. *Public Health Nutr.*, **7**, 123–46.

Uauy, R. and Kain, J. (2002). The epidemiological transition: need to incorporate obesity prevention into nutrition programmes. *Public Health Nutr.*, **5**, 223–9.

Victora, C. G., Barros, F. C., Horta, B. L. and Martorell, R. (2001). Short-term benefits of catch-up growth for small-for-gestational-age infants. *Int. J. Epidemiol.*, **30**, 1325–30.

Victora, C. G., Barros, F. C., Lima, R. C., Horta, B. L. and Wells, J. (2003). Anthropometry and body composition of 18 year old men according to duration of breast feeding: birth cohort study from Brazil. *BMJ*, **327**, 901–6.

Waaler, H. T. (1984). Height, weight and mortality: the Norwegian experience. *Acta Med. Scand. Suppl.*, **679**, 1–56.

Wei, J.-N., Sung, F.-C., Li, C.-Y. *et al.* (2003). Low birthweight and high birthweight infants are both at risk to have type 2 diabetes among schoolchildren in Taiwan. *Diabetes Care*, **26**, 343–8.

Wild, S., Roglic, G., Green, A., Sicree, R. and King, H. (2004). Global prevalence of diabetes: estimates for the year 2000 and projections for 2030. *Diabetes Care*, **27**, 1047–53.

Woelk, G., Emanuel, I., Weiss, N. S. and Psaty, B. M. (1998). Birthweight and blood pressure among children in Harare, Zimbabwe. *Arch. Dis. Child. Fetal Neonatal Ed.*, **79**, F119–22.

World Health Organization (1995). Maternal anthropometry and pregnancy outcomes: a WHO collaborative study. *Bull. World Health Organ.*, **73** (suppl.).

(2004). *Global Strategy on Diet, Physical Activity and Health.* 57th World Health Assembly. www.who.int/features/2004/wha57/en, accessed 10 October 2004.

Yajnik, C. S. (2004a). Obesity epidemic in India: intrauterine origins? *Proc. Nutr. Soc.*, **63**, 1–10.

(2004b). Early life origins of insulin resistance and type 2 diabetes in India and other Asian countries. *J. Nutr.*, **134**, 205–10.

Yajnik, C. S., Fall, C. H. D., Vaidya, U. *et al.* (1995). Fetal growth and glucose and insulin metabolism in four-year old Indian children. *Diabet. Med.*, **12**, 330–6.

Yajnik, C. S., Lubree, H. G., Rege, S. S. *et al.* (2002). Adiposity and hyperinsulinaemia in Indians are present at birth. *J. Clin. Endocrinol. Metab.*, **87**, 5575–80.

Yajnik, C. S., Fall, C. H. D., Coyaji, K. J. *et al.* (2003). Neonatal anthropometry: the thin–fat Indian baby. The Pune Maternal Nutrition Study. *Int. J. Obes.*, **27**, 173–80.

Zhao, M., Shu, X. O., Jin, F. *et al.* (2002). Birthweight, childhood growth and hypertension in adulthood. *Int. J. Epidemiol.*, **31**, 1043–51.

36

Developmental origins of health and disease: ethical and social considerations

Ray Noble

University College London

Introduction

The discovery of a link between low birthweight and adult disease has opened exciting and rewarding areas of research (Nathanielsz and Thornburg 2003). The 'Barker hypothesis' of fetal programming, where fetal adaptations to nutritional deprivation increase vulnerability to disorders in later life (Barker 1998), creates the prospect of new strategies to prevent adult diseases either by changing maternal nutrition or by new therapeutic approaches to fetal growth. With the focus on possible benefits of these strategies and the prospect of breaking the cycle of poverty and disease, there has been little consideration of associated ethical and social issues.

In this chapter I will argue that, as currently presented, the concept of the fetal origin of adult disease creates a pseudo-pathological condition by regarding low birthweight, even within the normal range, as impairment. It renders pathological that which we currently regard as normal. It seeks to fix that which may be damaged later (adult disease) by altering that which is not yet broken (fetal growth and function) (Flake 2003). It establishes and fosters a simplistic creed of 'big babies good, small babies bad', and it shifts the focus away from socioeconomic influences and places the onus of responsibility on women.

Furthermore, the aim of increasing mean birthweight and employing therapeutic strategies to protect the fetus may further intensify what some already argue is an intimidating environment, challenging the autonomy and rights of pregnant women (Roth 2000). Public health strategies at the population level, or clinical approaches to individual health, should aim to be supportive and empowering rather than prescriptive and onerous. Research involving humans should proceed with caution with clearly understood objectives. It should be carried out only with informed consent of the participants and should be part of an economic and social framework supporting human rights.

Programming for disease or programming for life?

Two strands of evidence presented in this book support the programming hypothesis of adult disease. Epidemiology shows a strong link between size at birth and adult disease or outcome (Hales and Barker 2001), with experiments using animals demonstrating changes in fetal and neonatal function in response to restricted maternal nutrition (Hoet and Hanson 1999). Taken together, these studies are convincing; but we need to consider value judgments used in making the case for public health initiatives or human trials, and how this case is perceived and acted upon.

Developmental Origins of Health and Disease, ed. Peter Gluckman and Mark Hanson. Published by Cambridge University Press.
© P. D. Gluckman and M. A. Hanson 2006.

One crucial judgment is whether the effects of programming are harmful or beneficial. If programming is defined as adaptation then it is shown to exist; if it is characterised by changes in function persisting after birth then programming exists; but whether such programming *fixes* a life strategy leading to adult disease has yet to be determined. It is as likely to be a strategy for promoting health as it is a part of the process in inducing disease. There is a clear difference between changes in fetal and neonatal function and a programmed life trajectory. Changes in function may increase the risk of adult disease, but through the course of a lifetime it is one factor amongst several. Nor is it clear that fetal growth is the primary factor. On the contrary, recent studies have shown that restricted nutrition produces changes preserving rather than reducing growth (Hoet and Hanson 1999, Ravelli *et al.* 1999), and there is little to suggest that these changes should be regarded as impairments rather than strategies for survival (Hales and Ozanne 2003). Far from being malfunctions, they are part of a normal range of adaptation enhancing rather than reducing survival (Rose 1992).

Different species have growth and metabolic strategies to meet specific requirements after birth and beyond. Many studies have been carried out using sheep, a species with a much higher growth rate and a lower percentage of body fat than humans (Harding 2001). Human beings and sheep, of course, have different feeding behaviours and requirements. Human beings can alter their environment and cope with changing social and economic circumstances. Environmental, social or economic factors existing in one generation may not hold for the next even if changes in biological function are found to persist. Circumstances during pregnancy and infancy may not be those encountered when the offspring become adults. Effective health strategies would be those accounting for factors throughout life, rather than those focusing on events before or during pregnancy. A focus on the biogenic nature of risk without considering socioeconomic factors is a value judgment likely to lead to discriminative and potentially harmful strategies.

'Big babies good, small babies bad'

Programming is a powerful concept. By implying that events are predetermined, it shifts the focus of causes of adult disease to the fetus and events in utero. 'Impaired growth and development in utero' are said to be widespread in the population 'affecting many babies whose birthweights are within the normal range.'

Thus, what was formerly considered normal or 'within the normal range' becomes an impairment (Merialdi *et al.* 2003) and 'small baby' falls within the same category as genetic or congenital diseases. Other life events are viewed, not as causes, but as factors with which the 'impaired' individual is maladapted to cope. Rather than being considered a predisposing factor, 'small baby' becomes a new pathology and a primary cause of adult disease. It is a factitious pathology; yet this simplistic doctrine of 'small babies bad' leads to a prescription of maternal behaviour whilst creating pressure for clinical or nutritional intervention (Merialdi *et al.* 2003). '*Only* when the causes in early life of these human diseases are established,' a recent review concluded, 'will it be possible to devise ways for their primary prevention'(Hoet and Hanson 1999; my emphasis). Fetal programming becomes a target causal factor in primary public health, the 'risk' becomes a cause, 'small baby' becomes a benchmark for a new pathology and it lays the burden of responsibility for adult disease on young women and mothers.

The role of the mother and her relationship to the fetus

Developments in fetal assessment foster new attitudes to both mother and fetus. The emergence of fetuses as patients (if not in their own right, then at least with a quasi-independent consideration of interest) (James 1998) puts moral pressure on both clinicians and prospective mothers. Considerations of fetal wellbeing and the interests of the fetus have loaded the moral scales, with the burden falling heavily on pregnant women, and it is within this context that we must consider the impact of the concept of the developmental origin of adult disease.

These advances in fetal and neonatal medicine have been accompanied by a changing view of the status of the fetus. If a baby can survive prematurity at younger gestational ages, then there is considered to be little difference in moral status between a late-gestation fetus and a newborn baby. Indeed a fetus is referred to as 'baby' as though it had a separate existence, or at least a separate consideration from that of its mother. In the words of a leading specialist in fetal medicine 'most professionals and parents consider the fetus as a separate individual' (James 1998).

At one extreme, this changing view of the fetus is expressed in the concept of 'fetal rights', the 'right to life' and the 'right to be born'. But there has been a further extension of this notion of fetal rights, and that is the 'right to be born healthy', the right to protection from harm (Bewley 2002). To a greater or lesser measure, the fetus and mother have been ethically and legally separated and in some circumstances are considered to be in conflict. But this conflict is not between fetus and mother, but between the pregnant woman and what the fetus means to others. As the American lawyer Janet Gallagher has put it:

The fetus becomes an icon, the object of a quasi-religious cult. And the woman within whose body that new object of devotion exists drops out of sight as an individual with hopes and plans and choices. She becomes instead the environment of the fetus, 'the mother ship', or the 'uterine capsule'. (Gallagher 1995)

With the right to be born healthy comes the right to protection from harm. There is an attempt to give the fetus a separate legal status and to control the behaviour of pregnant women in the interest of the unborn child (Roth 2000). It is as if there were fetuses without women (Mahowald 1995). As the novelist Rachel Cusk describes in her book on her experiences of becoming a mother:

I am living not freely but in some curious tithe. I have surrendered my solitude and become . . . a bridge, a link, a vehicle. I read newspaper reports of women in America being prosecuted for harming their unborn foetuses and wonder how this can be; how the body can become a public space, like a telephone box, that can unlawfully vandalise itself . . . Now it is as if some spy is embedded within me . . . It is not, I feel sure, the baby who exerts this watchful pressure: it is the baby's meaning for other people, *the world's sense of ownership stating its claim.* (Cusk 2001; my emphasis)

I have argued that what was formally part of the normal distribution of birthweight becomes a new pathology, a pseudo-pathological condition because there is in fact no impairment. As a result, the mother becomes responsible not for the health of her fetus and newborn baby alone but also for the health of the future adult. To the 'right to be born healthy' is now added the 'right to be born with a healthy future'. But by this process women are responsible not only for the health of their own offspring but also for the *cost to the community* of an unhealthy future population.

Fetal protection and the challenge to the autonomy of women are expressed not only by legal constraint but also through social and moral pressure (Roth 2000). Women are caught in a pincer movement between those seeking to protect the fetus and those concerned with the social and economic cost or burden of ill health. Public health discourse portrays pregnant women as needing constant self-surveillance to protect the health of their fetuses (Petersen and Lupton 1996). Others are recruited in this surveillance as society stakes its claim to the future health of its citizens, finding expression in simplified accounts in the media such as that in *Men's Health*, where we find the following under the headline 'Dieting can harm future children':

If you want healthy kids, stop your partner dieting excessively before becoming pregnant, researchers from Southampton University claim. They discovered that even when women change their eating habits once they are pregnant, their children are more likely than average to suffer heart disease, hypertension, diabetes and strokes. (Anon 2001)

This report neither suggests how the reader should stop his partner dieting excessively nor defines what this means. But the message is clear. It calls upon *men* to exert pressure on *women* on behalf of their future offspring.

Biological and social causes of adult disease: the blame game

Creating a new pathology creates a new approach to health; and it is likely to do so at the expense of other strategies. Just as a relationship exists between birth-weight and cardiovascular disease, so a correlation exists between poverty, chronic ill health and mortality (Spencer 2000). Inequality itself increases vulnerability to chronic diseases (Townsend *et al.* 1988); people die younger in countries with the greatest income inequalities (Wilkinson 2000). There is also a correlation between poverty and low birthweight, and doubtless these factors are mutually cause and effect. The real message from the concept of developmental programming is that the environment is a key factor in the origin of disease, not solely that biogenic factors make disease inevitable. But an emphasis on fetal growth and events around pregnancy shifts the target from economic and social causes of poverty – poor housing, poor access to health care, financial stress, poor education and limited work opportunities – towards a panacea, a cure-all for cardiovascular disease (Spencer 2000). Perversely, it allows the blame for these inequalities to shift from the rich to the poor themselves for not heeding advice to follow a 'healthy lifestyle'. It leads to discriminative social and economic policies producing negative social attitudes with underprivileged groups targeted as those primarily affected, with a stereotypic assumption that poor women fail to make appropriate life decisions (Rose 1992).

Such an approach stems from two curiously contradictory assumptions:

- an overly simplistic interpretation of the significance of 'intractable' genetic and biological forces working to determine susceptibility to disease and chronic ill health;
- an ability of all those affected to make appropriate choices for their own health.

Contradictory because it places the responsibility of ill health on individuals and yet it is argued that 'biogenetic factors in and of themselves are altogether too powerful to be ignored' (Marsland 1995). Yet the choice is not to ignore them, but to understand them. Biology tells us how the body functions and what it needs to be healthy. Education becomes then the main primary health strategy, with the assumption that it is within the power of all to act on its message. But it is a false prospectus to assume that this message alone provides a solution, or that the message is without a potential to harm.

Identifying a biological cause of disease does not render a solution by itself. We need to shift the focus to incorporate and take into account the social context of behaviour and the 'intimate links which tie behaviour to social and environmental circumstances' (Spencer 2000). As a recent world report on women's health concluded, improvements in women's health require not only advances in science and health care, but also social justice for women and the removal of social and cultural barriers to equal opportunities (Fathalla 1994). This ethical and moral view has been summarised by Keith Tones thus:

> To cajole people into taking responsibility for their health, while at the same time ignoring the social and environmental circumstances which conspire to make them ill, is a fundamentally defective strategy – and unethical. (Tones 1988)

The real potential of the concept of developmental programming is that it provides a better understanding of how these circumstances conspire to make people ill. Rather than emphasising the biological over the social it should be used to better understand the importance of economic and social wellbeing, of justice and equality of opportunity.

The 'duty to be well' and the 'risky persona'

Contemporary public health strategies are generally based on the concept of an individual 'duty to be well' and the targeting of individuals or groups considered at greatest risk. This approach can be liberating for those who can make effective and appropriate lifestyle choices, but oppressive for those who are powerless to make such choices – and all the more so if the burden of responsibility falls on a particular group, as it does for women in relation to reproductive health. It is a consumerist view of autonomy, with a notion that individuals can 'buy into' a 'healthy' lifestyle, and that society, social welfare and health are simply an aggregate of individual behaviours, without regard for social, economic and cultural influences. But, as Rose has argued, society is not merely a collection of individuals but is also 'a collectivity', and the behaviour and health of its individual members are profoundly influenced by 'collective characteristics and social norms' (Rose 1992). An emphasis on the individual 'duty to be well' ignores the specific needs of groups within society and the interdependency of humans as social beings (World Health Organization 1978).

Such is the position of women as mothers, or potential mothers. Not only that they be held culpable for 'failing to protect' their own health, but also for failing to protect the health of their offspring and, in the context of the fetal origin of adult disease, for failing to protect the health of future adults. In this context women as 'healthy citizens' are viewed as a resource for the reproduction and health of other healthy citizens. They are deemed to have a 'duty to be healthy' not simply for themselves as autonomous beings, nor solely for their offspring, but for the economic wellbeing of others. This forms part of a strategy to target those at 'high risk', with a focus on those most likely to develop disease. It involves discriminating a minority of the population with special problems or 'at greatest risk' from the 'normal' majority of the population (Rose 1992).

Thus, the 'risky persona' in medicine and public health discourse tends to be stereotyped as an aspect of gender, social class, ethnicity and sexuality. As Petersen and Lupton (1996) put it 'women, the feminised gay male, non-white peoples, the poor and members of the working class have been stereotypically portrayed as more "contaminating" and therefore more culpable.' Under the seemingly good intent of public beneficence, public health discourse and public health policy can be unfairly discriminating and prejudicial. It relies on programmes of 'education' coupled with moral pressure on target or culprit groups.

Public health discourses are pursued on the premise that the concept of 'healthy lifestyle' can be understood and acted upon. In this context it might be argued that the concept of programming in response to maternal diet would provide better information for women to make appropriate choices. Yet, the plethora of conflicting dietary advice available in libraries, bookshops and magazines can create confusion rather than understanding (Cusk 2001). Furthermore, health as duty can lead to unattainable aims (Davey Smith 2001), particularly if women are not able to make effective choices for economic, social or cultural reasons. To put an onus of responsibility on women for the health of the population would be unethical; to do so without tackling the underlying causes of poverty would be immoral (Ottawa Charter 1986).

Designer diets for designer babies – human trials

Ethical research involving human participants is premised on two fundamental commitments: to improve human welfare by advancing knowledge and understanding of disease; and equally to preserve and protect the dignity and health interests of research participants. Clinical research aims to benefit individual participants and patient groups through the identification and testing of improved treatments, and to benefit society by making them widely available. The potential risk of harm to participants has led to widespread agreement that sound ethical standards must be observed in clinical research regardless of the perceived benefits (World Medical Association 1964, Nuffield Council on Bioethics 1999). The ends alone, no matter how good, are insufficient justification of the means employed if they may harm those involved. Research involving human subjects 'should be preceded by careful assessment of predictable risks and burdens in comparison with foreseeable benefits to the subjects or to others' (World Medical Association 1964: Helsinki Declaration, article 10.16) and should 'only occur if the importance of the objective outweighs the inherent risks and burdens to the subject' (Helsinki Declaration, article 10.18). Informed consent is a fundamental principle in any research involving human participants. Consent can only be informed if the potential harms and benefits are clearly understood; or where there is doubt, if the participants understand the nature of such doubt. It should be clear what the proposed research or intervention might achieve and who will be the likely beneficiaries.

Research into the early programming of chronic disease offers the prospects of novel strategies to prevent adult disease. Whilst these studies are still at an early stage, it is suggested nonetheless that 'sufficient is now known to implement policies which improve fetal growth by protecting the nutrition and growth of girls and young women' (University of Southampton 2003). However, other than involving 'public health interventions' and improving access to a balanced diet, the details of this novel strategy are unclear. In any event, it is not at all clear who the target of such dietary advice should be. Too little is known to set clear and achievable goals for projects that are truly informed and inclusive rather than presumptuous and prescriptive. Nor is it clear what the endpoint of such intervention or trials should be. If the goal is a shift in mean birthweight then it is not clear on what grounds it would be justified or by what method it could be achieved. A general improvement in economic and social wellbeing raises ethical issues only about how this is achieved. A specific target of increasing mean birthweight by nutritional or therapeutic intervention raises specific ethical issues.

In the 'Hertfordshire study' those at greatest risk of coronary heart disease were apparently men who were small at birth but who became obese as infants or adults (Fall *et al.* 1995). Thus diet and activity of infants and adults is also important, and not solely the nutrition of their mothers (Hales and Barker 1992). Yet by focusing on the concept of fetal programming it is suggested that public health interventions should be aimed at the health of mothers and the growth of girls and young women (Robinson 2001).

Understanding the relationship between diet and fetal growth may provide women with information to make balanced choices for the healthy outcomes of their pregnancies and the wellbeing of their children. It may also be possible to provide dietary supplements where this can be shown to be beneficial, particularly in the poorer regions of the world, and these strategies might be better aimed at the health of young women. Thus, recent studies suggest that small amounts of n-3 fatty acids, a constituent of fish oil, can increase birthweight by prolonging gestation or increasing fetal growth. It has been suggested that 'adequate' amounts of these fatty acids should be provided during the perinatal period (Das 2002). But such interventionist strategies can be helpful only if the evidence upon which they are based and the advice given is clear and the goals achievable. It is not at all certain that this is so (Merialdi *et al.* 2003).

It would be easy to adopt a simple notion that enhancing the diet of undernourished mothers can only be good. Improving the health of future adults by tackling the developmental origin of disease will reduce suffering, improve economic productivity, and may reduce the burden on over-stretched healthcare systems. This is a prescriptive approach: being undernourished is bad therefore giving supplements to improve diet must be good. But it can only be 'good' if we know that the risks are small in relation to the benefits.

Targeting young women: the risk of harm

An overly enthusiastic claim that sufficient is now known to promote the growth of babies in the womb by protecting the nutrition of young women is clearly wide of the mark. First, it is acknowledged that there is still 'insufficient evidence that maternal nutrition underlies cardiovascular disease in humans and insufficient data to make specific dietary recommendations to pregnant mothers' (Fall 2003). Second, inappropriate intervention with dietary supplements to young women 'may simply increase obesity and harm the fetus'. The risk of doing harm is certainly sufficient reason to be cautious. There is at least evidence from both animal and human studies to suggest that nutritional supplementation in adolescent women may reduce rather than increase fetal growth (Rush 1989, Scholl *et al.* 1990, Delisle *et al.* 2001). There may also be a risk of neonatal death (Villar *et al.* 2003).

In a recent overview of randomised controlled trials it was concluded that there is 'little evidence to support the implementation of specific nutrition public health interventions to prevent impaired growth'(Merialdi *et al.* 2003). Thus any strategy targeting specifically adolescent women in developing countries for nutritional supplementation with the aim of increasing birthweight would at best be experimental, and may do harm rather than good. Clear ethical guidelines need to be applied (World Medical Association 1964). It is unclear on what basis the participants in such a programme could give informed consent based on an understanding of the possible harms and benefits, particularly as these are still uncertain (Fall 2003).

Specific programmes to date have targeted the poor in underdeveloped countries or in poor socio-economic positions in developed countries, with the positive motive of breaking the cycle of poverty and disease. But it is unclear whether such programmes will form part of a more comprehensive approach to addressing the nature of poverty, or how such a vulnerable group would be recruited, or what economic pressure would apply to their recruitment. In undernourished communities young women may be urged to sign up to such programmes without understanding the inherent risks of 'improving' their diets to 'protect' their future offspring. There would be an additional ethical concern if health care were offered in exchange for participation. A controlled nutritional environment 'tricking' the fetus to adopt a growth strategy inappropriate for the prevailing nutritional environment as a neonate or in subsequent development may certainly be harmful. A nutritional 'fix' without tackling the underlying causes of poverty and poor nutritional choice in such circumstances would be irresponsible. Action to tackle malnutrition at one level, without clear

coordinated action at other levels (communal, social and economic) would be not only unlikely to succeed but also ethically questionable. Any action to improve the diet of young women specifically should be empowering rather than prescriptive. Action to improve the nutritional situation of young women with the aim of increasing birthweight should involve a reallocation of resources in their favour to allow them to exercise choice; furthermore, any such action should be sustainable (Jonsson 1995).

Nor is it axiomatic that nutritional supplements would be beneficial. Nutrient restriction in early pregnancy appears to produce persistent changes in function. It does so even when growth is unaffected. Changes may thus be produced by dietary supplements that make the fetus poorly adapted for the prevailing neonatal environment regardless of birthweight. This may lead to the babies becoming obese in later life, with an increased risk of associated disease. Thus dietary supplementation in such a scenario may be harmful rather than beneficial.

Conclusions: human rights and public health

The utilitarian argument for preventive medicine is that it is better to be healthy than ill or dead, and it is better that more people are healthy than ill. This may be sufficient justification for preventive medicine as a concept (Rose 1992), but it cannot alone suffice to justify the means employed in public health policy. Ethical preventive strategies are those that enhance human rights and empower citizens in attaining health objectives. A public health programme that protects and promotes human rights is better than one of equal effectiveness that burdens or restricts them (International Federation of Red Cross and Red Crescent Societies 1999).

The developmental programming concept of adult disease may improve our understanding of why some people are more susceptible to chronic conditions. It may also lead to better strategies for prevention. However, whilst chronic adult diseases may owe a great deal to events in early life, it remains the case that the causes and factors influencing the onset of such diseases are varied. Furthermore, the interplay of these factors is likely to be complex. Regarding small babies as impaired places undue pressure on pregnant women whilst setting the scene for health care or clinical intervention. For this reason, care should be taken both in presenting the concept of the developmental programming of disease and in assessing strategies designed to influence the health of young women.

REFERENCES

Anon. (2001). *Mens Health*, **7** (9).

Barker, D. J. P. (1998). In utero programming of chronic disease. *Clin. Sci.*, **95**, 115–28.

Bewley, S. (2002). Restricting the freedom of pregnant women. In *Ethical Issues in Maternal–Fetal Medicine* (ed. D. L. Dickenson). Cambridge: Cambridge University Press, pp. 131–46.

Cusk, R. (2001). *A Life's Work: on Becoming a Mother*. London: Fourth Estate.

Das, U. N. (2002). Long chain polyunsaturated fatty acids and fetal programming. Electronic letter. *BMJ*. www.bmj.com/cgi/eletters/324/7335/447.

Davey Smith, G. (2001). Reflections on the limitations to epidemiology. *J. Clin. Epidemiol.*, **54**, 325–31.

Delisle, H., Chandra-Mouli, V. and de Benoist, B. (2001). Should adolescents be specifically targeted for nutrition in developing countries? To address which problems, and how? World Health Organization. www.who.int/child-adolescent-health.

Fall, C. H. D. (2003). The fetal and early origins of adult disease. *Indian Pediatr.*, **40**, 480–502.

Fall, C. H. D., Osmond, C., Barker, D. J. P., Clark, P. M. S., Stirling, Y. and Meade, T. W. (1995). Fetal and infant growth and cardiovascular risk factors in women. *BMJ*, **310**, 428–32.

Fathalla, M. F. (1994). Women's health: an overview. *Int. J. Gynaecol. Obstet.*, **46**, 105–18.

Flake, A. W. (2003). Surgery in the human fetus: the future. *J. Physiol.*, **547**, 45–51.

Gallagher, J. (1995). Collective bad faith: 'protecting' the Fetus. In *Reproduction, Ethics, and the Law: Feminist Perspectives*. (ed. J. C. Callahan). Bloomington, IN: Indiana University Press, pp. 343–79.

Hales, C. N and Barker, D. J. P. (1992). Type 2 (non-insulin-dependent) diabetus mellitus: the thrifty phenotype hypothesis. *Diabetologia*, **35**, 595–601.

Hales, C. N. and Barker, D. J. P. (2001). The thrifty phenotype hypothesis. *Br. Med. Bull.*, **60**, 5–21.

Hales, C. N. and Ozanne, S. E. (2003). The dangerous road of catch-up growth. *J. Physiol.*, **547**, 5–10.

Harding, J. E. (2001). The nutritional basis of the fetal origin of adult disease. *Int. J. Epidemiol.*, **30**, 15–23.

Hoet, J. J. and Hanson, M. A. (1999). Intrauterine nutrition: its importance during critical periods for cardiovascular and endocrine development. *J. Physiol.*, **514**, 617–27.

International Federation of Red Cross and Red Crescent Societies (1999). The public health – human rights dialogue. In *Health and Human Rights* (ed. J. M. Mann, S. Gruskin, M. A. Grodin and G. J. Annas). New York, NY: Routledge, pp. 46–53.

James, D. (1998). Recent advances: fetal medicine. *BMJ*, **316**, 1580–3.

Jonsson, U. (1995). Ethics and child nutrition. *Food Nutr. Bull.*, **16**, 293–8.

Mahowald, M. B. (1995). As if there were fetuses without women: a remedial essay. In *Reproduction, Ethics, and the Law: Feminist Perspectives* (ed. J. C. Callahan). Bloomington, IN: Indiana University Press, pp. 199–218.

Marsland, D. (1995). *Social Misconstruction: the Neglect of Biology in Contemporary British Sociology*. Sociological Notes, **22**. London: Libertarian Alliance.

Merialdi, M., Carroli, G., Villar, J. *et al.* (2003). Nutrtitional interventions during pregnancy for the prevention or treatment of impaired fetal growth: an overview of randomized controlled trials. *J. Nutr.*, **133**, 1626–31S.

Nathanielsz, P. W. and Thornburg, K. L. (2003). Fetal programming: from gene to functional systems. An overview. *J. Physiol.*, **547**, 3–4.

Nuffield Council on Bioethics (1999). *The Ethics of Clinical Research in Developing Countries*. London: Nuffield Council.

Ottawa Charter (1986). *Ottawa Charter for Health Promotion*. Presented at the first International Conference on Health Promotion, Ottawa, 1986.

Petersen, A. and Lupton, D. (1996). *The New Public Health: Health and Self in the Age of Risk*. London: Sage.

Ravelli, A. C. J., van der Meulen, J. H. P., Osmond, C., Barker, D. J. P. and Bleker, O. (1999). Obesity at the age of 50 years in men and women exposed to famine prenatally. *Am. J. Clin. Nutr.*, **70**, 811–16.

Robinson, R. (2001). The fetal origins of adult disease. *BMJ*, **322**, 375–6.

Rose, G. (1992). *The Strategy of Preventive Medicine*. Oxford: Oxford University Press.

Roth, R. (2000). *Making Women Pay: the Hidden Costs of Fetal Rights*. New York, NY: Cornell University Press.

Rush D. (1989). Effects of changes in maternal energy and protein intake during pregnancy, with special reference to fetal growth. In *Fetal Growth* (ed. F. Sharp, R. B. Fraser and R. D. G. Milner). London: Royal College of Obstetricians and Gynaecologists, pp. 203–29.

Scholl, T. O., Hediger, M. L. and Ances, I. G. (1990). Maternal growth during pregnancy and decreased infant birth weight. *Am. J. Clin. Nutr.*, **51**, 790–3.

Spencer, N. (2000). *Poverty and Child Health*, 2nd edn. Oxford: Radcliffe Medical Press.

Tones, K. (1988). Health education and the promotion of health: seeking wisely to empower. In *Health and Empowerment: Research and Practice* (ed. S. Kendall). London: Arnold, pp. 57–88.

Townsend, P., Davidson, N. and Whitehead, M., eds. (1988). *Inequalities in Health: The Black Report and the Health Divide*. London: Penguin.

University of Southampton (2003). Centre for the Origins of Adult Disease. Press release, 5 June 2003.

Villar, J., Merialdi, M., Gulmezoglu, A. M. *et al.* (2003). Characteristics of randomized controlled trials included in systematic reviews of nutritional interventions reporting maternal morbidity, mortality, preterm delivery, intrauterine growth restriction and small for gestational age and birth weight outcomes. *J. Nutr.*, **133**, 1632–9S.

Wilkinson, R. (2000). *Mind the Gap: Heirarchies, Health and Human Evolution*. London: Weidenfeld and Nicolson.

World Health Organization (1978). *Declaration of Alma-Ata.* 'Health for All' series, no. 1. Geneva: WHO.

World Medical Association (1964). *Declaration of Helisnki: Ethical Principles for Medical Research Involving Human Subjects.* Adopted by the 18th WMA General Assembly, Helsinki, Finland, June 1964.

37

Past obstacles and future promise

D. J. P. Barker

University of Southampton

Introduction

The idea that common chronic diseases are initiated through developmental processes that begin before birth arose from geographical studies published 20 years ago (Barker and Osmond 1986). The evidence was circumstantial and the mechanisms unknown. Today even a perfunctory reading of this book would lead to the conclusion that the 'developmental origins of health and disease' now has a sound scientific basis in both human and animal studies. This being so, the need to expand research is urgent. Almost a million people in the USA died of coronary heart disease last year. One hundred and fifty million people in the world have type 2 diabetes and the epidemic is rising. Ten million Americans over the age of 50 have osteoporosis and one out of every two women over the age of 50 will have an osteoporotic fracture in their lifetime.

Differences in adult lifestyle provide only a partial explanation of why one person develops these disorders while another does not; nor does lifestyle account for the higher rates of these disorders among poorer people and ethnic minorities in Western countries. The effects of modifying adult lifestyle, when formally tested in randomised trials, have been disappointingly small (Ebrahim and Davey Smith 1997). One explanation could be that there are differences in people's vulnerability to adverse lifestyles and hence differences in the benefits of lifestyle

modification. The new 'developmental' model for chronic disease postulates that initiating events occur during early development, and that individual differences in vulnerability to lifestyle and other aspects of the environment are acquired at that time.

To elucidate this, traditional 'risk factor' epidemiology has had to acquire a developmental perspective. This review describes obstacles that have had to be overcome and some areas where progress can be expected.

Obstacles to progress

Confounding variables

The association between low birthweight and later cardiovascular disease in individuals has provided a platform for further epidemiological research. This is reviewed in more detail by Godfrey (Chapter 2). The original observations in Hertfordshire, UK, are shown in Table 37.1. Among men death rates from coronary heart disease fell with increasing birthweight and weight at 1 year (Barker et al. 1989). There were similar tends with birthweight among women (Osmond et al. 1993). An early obstacle to be overcome was the argument that people whose growth was impaired in utero and during infancy may continue to be exposed to an adverse environment in childhood and adult life, and it is this later environment that produces the effects attributed to

Developmental Origins of Health and Disease, ed. Peter Gluckman and Mark Hanson. Published by Cambridge University Press.
© P. D. Gluckman and M. A. Hanson 2006.

Table 37.1 Hazard ratios (95% confidence intervals) for death from coronary heart disease before age 65 years, according to birthweight and weight at 1 year in 10 636 men in Hertfordshire.

Weight (pounds)	Death from coronary heart disease
Birthweight	
≤ 5.5 (n = 486)	1.50 (0.98 to 2.31)
5.6–6.5 (n = 1385)	1.27 (0.89 to 1.83)
6.6–7.5 (n = 3162)	1.17 (0.84 to 1.63)
7.6–8.5 (n = 3308)	1.07 (0.77 to 1.49)
8.6–9.5 (n = 1564)	0.96 (0.66 to 1.39)
≥ 10 (n = 731)	1.00
p for trend	< 0.001
Weight at 1 year old	
≤ 18 (n = 715)	2.22 (1.33 to 3.73)
18.1–20 (n = 1806)	1.80 (1.11 to 2.93)
20.1–22 (n = 3404)	1.96 (1.23 to 3.12)
22.1–24 (n = 2824)	1.52 (0.95 to 2.45)
24.1–26 (n = 1391)	1.36 (0.82 to 2.26)
≥ 27 (n = 496)	1.00
p for trend	< 0.001

Source: Barker *et al.* (1989).

intrauterine influences. There is now strong evidence that this argument cannot be sustained (Frankel *et al.* 1996, Rich-Edwards *et al.* 1997, Leon *et al.* 1998). The associations between low birthweight and later disease have been shown to be independent of influences such as smoking habits, employment, alcohol consumption and exercise. Adult lifestyle, however, adds to the effects of early life: for example, the studies in Finland have shown that the highest incidence of coronary heart disease occurs among men who were thin at birth and had low household incomes as adults (Barker *et al.* 2001; see Eriksson, Chapter 15).

Graded associations

In the many studies which have shown associations between low birthweight and disease in later life, a consistent feature has been that the associations are graded (Hales *et al.* 1991, McCance *et al.* 1994,

Frankel *et al.* 1996, Lithell *et al.* 1996, Stein *et al.* 1996, Rich-Edwards *et al.* 1997, 1999, Leon *et al.* 1998, Eriksson *et al.* 2001). Table 37.1 shows how disease rates fall across the range of birthweight and infant weight. This suggests that what were regarded as normal variations in the delivery of nutrients to the human fetus and infant have profound implications for health in later life. This has proved a difficult concept for some clinicians, whose attention is necessarily focused on people with pathologically low birthweight.

Fetal nutrition

The different size of newborn human babies exemplifies developmental plasticity (West-Eberhard 1989). The growth of babies has to be constrained by the size of the mother, otherwise normal birth could not occur. Small women have small babies: in pregnancies after ovum donation they have small babies even if the woman donating the egg is large (Brooks *et al.* 1995). Babies may be small because their growth is constrained in this way or because they lack the nutrients for growth. As McCance (1962) wrote, 'The size attained in utero depends on the services which the mother is able to supply. These are mainly food and accommodation.' Mother's height or bony pelvic dimensions are generally not found to be important predictors of the baby's long-term health, and research into the developmental origins of disease has focused on the nutrient supply to the baby, while recognising that other influences such as hypoxia and stress also influence fetal growth. This focus on fetal nutrition was endorsed in a recent review (Harding 2001), and is reviewed in relation to fetal metabolism by Fowden *et al.* (Chapter 10).

An obstacle has been that fetal nutrition is sometimes equated with maternal nutrition. Because Western women are adequately nourished, the argument runs, Western babies must also be adequately nourished. Such a view does not take into account the long and vulnerable fetal supply line, which may limit transfer of nutrients from a well-nourished mother to her fetus. It does not give adequate consideration to the role of the placenta in this process (reviewed by Myatt and Roberts in Chapter 9). Nor does it acknowledge the sometimes competing demands of mother and fetus (Barker 1998).

Small effects

A criticism of the 'developmental origins' hypothesis is that associations between birthweight and some intermediary markers are small. For example, a 1 kg increase in birthweight is associated with around a 3 mm Hg reduction in systolic pressure (Huxley *et al.* 2000). This contrasts with the large effect of low birthweight on clinical hypertension, the risk of which doubles between people who weighed 4 kg or more at birth and those who weighed 3 kg or less (Eriksson *et al.* 2000). It suggests that lesions accompanying poor fetal growth which ultimately lead to hypertension have a small influence on blood pressure within the normal range, because counter-regulating mechanisms are able to maintain normal blood pressure levels for many years after birth. Ultimately, these mechanisms fail to maintain homeostasis, and clinical hypertension develops.

Sensitivity of the embryo

Because babies seem able to grow to reasonable size, almost irrespective of what the mother eats in late pregnancy, the view has developed that the baby in the womb is a highly successful parasite, able to take from the mother whatever it requires to satisfy its modest needs. Not until late pregnancy, when it becomes large, do its food requirements become substantial and even these, it seems, are readily satisfied at the mother's expense. Even in the wartime famine in Holland pregnant women lost weight but their babies continued to grow (Ravelli *et al.* 1998). Thus, it has been suggested, the baby in the womb is protected, buffered from the world by the mother's body, a shield pierced only by poisons or infections. Alone in its padded cell it lives out its genetic potential to emerge, preordained and bespoke.

Such a comfortable picture is far from the true one. It resonates with the position on child growth adopted by the hereditarians a century ago. The children of the poor were stunted and thin, they maintained, because they came from genetically inferior stock. Therefore there was no compelling reason to improve their nutrition and living conditions. The womb, however, is not a padded cell. The embryo and fetus are highly sensitive to what happens outside their warm pool (Kwong *et al.* 2000, Walker *et al.* 2000, Winston and Hardy 2002). This is clear from Fleming's review (Chapter 4). The various and varying supply of foods shape their structures and mould their systems. They may affect gene expression by epigenetic mechanisms (see Whitelaw and Garrick, Chapter 5). The nutrients they receive do not merely supply the building blocks for growth; they establish metabolic and hormonal set-points which endure for a lifetime. These long-term effects are reviewed by Sloboda *et al.*, Cutfield *et al.* and Byrne and Phillips (Chapters 13, 14 and 19).

Maternal nutrition

Because, in Western communities, supplementation of the diets of pregnant women with protein, fat and carbohydrates has relatively small effects on birthweight, the view has formed that fetal development is little influenced by normal variations in maternal diet (Kramer 1993). This view neglects growing evidence from experimental studies and assisted reproductive technology that periconceptional nutrition establishes the trajectory of fetal growth and thereby sets the demand for nutrients in mid to late gestation (Stewart *et al.* 1980, Harding *et al.* 1992, Barker 1998, Kwong *et al.* 2000). The view also takes no account of a growing body of evidence that links the balance of protein and carbohydrate in the mother's diet, rather than the absolute amount, with blood-pressure levels and other risk factors in the offspring (Campbell *et al.* 1996, Roseboom *et al.* 2001a, Shiell *et al.* 2001). This is clearly relevant to developing countries (see Fall and Sachdev, Chapter 35). However, in Western countries also many fetuses remain poorly nourished, because the macronutrients delivered to them are unbalanced or essential micronutrients are lacking.

The fetus does not live solely on the mother's daily intake of food: that would be too dangerous a strategy. It also lives off stored nutrients and the turnover of protein and fat in the mother's tissues (James 1997). Maternal size and body composition account for up to 20 per cent of the variability in birthweight and placental weight (Catalano *et al.* 1998). The concept of maternal nutrition has to extend beyond the mother's food intake in pregnancy to include her body composition, metabolism and physiological response to pregnancy (see Chapter 8 for a review by Morton). Studies in Europe and India have shown that high maternal weight and adiposity are associated with coronary heart disease, insulin deficiency and type 2 diabetes in the offspring (Forsen *et al.* 1997, Fall *et al.* 1998, Shiell *et al.* 2000). A number of studies have shown that maternal thinness, as measured by low body mass index, is strongly associated with insulin resistance in the adult offspring (Ravelli *et al.* 1998, Mi *et al.* 2000, Shiell *et al.* 2000). In contrast, maternal thinness measured by low skinfold thickness is associated with raised blood pressure in the offspring (Margetts *et al.* 1991, Godfrey *et al.* 1994, Clark *et al.* 1998, Adair *et al.* 2001). These associations are largely independent of the baby's body size at birth. One of the known metabolic links between maternal body composition and birth size is protein synthesis. Women with a greater lean body mass have higher rates of protein synthesis in pregnancy. Around a quarter of the variability in birth length may be explained by variations in the mother's rates of protein synthesis (Duggleby and Jackson 2001). This is a further illustration of how what are regarded as normal biological variations have far-reaching effects on the health of the next generation.

Inconsistency of associations with placental size

Experiments in sheep have shown that maternal undernutrition in early pregnancy can exert major effects on the growth of the placenta, and thereby alter fetal development (Robinson *et al.* 1994). The effects produced depend on the nutritional status of the ewe in the periconceptional period. In ewes that were poorly nourished around the time of conception, low nutrient intakes in early pregnancy

reduced the size of the placenta. Conversely, in ewes well nourished around the time of conception, low intakes in early pregnancy resulted in increased placental size. Placental expansion may be an adaptation by the fetus to extract more nutrients from the mother. Seemingly it can only occur in previously well-nourished ewes.

There is evidence that high dietary intakes in early pregnancy can suppress placental growth in humans (Godfrey *et al.* 1996). Among women who delivered at term in Southampton, those with high dietary intakes of carbohydrate in early pregnancy had smaller placentas, particularly if this was combined with low intakes of dairy protein in late pregnancy. High intakes of simple carbohydrates, such as are found in soft drinks, had the strongest effects. These effects were independent of the mother's body size, social class and smoking, and resulted in alterations in the ratio of placental weight to birthweight. There is a U-shaped relation between this ratio and later hypertension and coronary heart disease (Barker *et al.* 1990, Martyn *et al.* 1996). Associations between the birthweight/placental-weight ratio and later disease are inconsistent in the literature. This has led to the conclusion that the placenta is unimportant in programming. The inconsistency may exist, however, because placental responses to maternal undernutrition vary according to the mother's periconceptional nutritional state. In some studies the ratio has provided some of the strongest markers of later hypertension and coronary heart disease ever documented. Nutritional effects on placental growth are, therefore, important, but little is known about them in humans.

Why disease

The last in this list of obstacles to acceptance of the developmental origins of chronic disease is the question why a baby, small but seemingly normal, should be at increased risk of later disease. To this there is both a general answer, and an increasing number of specific answers that are described in this book. The general answer is that the human baby, like other living things during their development, does not have sufficient resource to perfect every trait. The requirements for growth, body maintenance and reproduction have to be traded off against each other. Smaller babies, as a group, will have had a lesser allocation of energy and other resources, and the trade-offs and the costs they incur will be greater. They include, it seems, disease in later life.

Infant and child growth

In a number of studies it has been possible to examine both birth size and postnatal growth among children who later developed cardiovascular disease and type 2 diabetes (Forsen *et al.* 2000, 2004, Eriksson *et al.* 2001). Some of the most detailed information comes from the Helsinki cohort comprising 8760 men and women born during 1934–44. Each man and woman had on average 18 measurements of height and weight between birth and 12 years. Having been small at birth they tended to remain small during infancy. Among men, small size at 1 year of age predicted coronary heart disease independently of size at birth. Hence there appear to be at least two pathways of growth that lead to the disease: one begins with slow fetal growth, the other with slow infant growth.

A recent hypothesis predicts that 'a high nutrient intake, which promotes early growth, would adversely programme cardiovascular health' (Singhal and Lucas 2004). If true, this would have far-reaching consequences for infant care practices. There is, however, no support for the hypothesis in the Helsinki studies, which are able to examine postnatal growth in relation to disease outcomes rather than intermediary markers. At any stage of infancy, greater weight gain is associated with a lower risk of later disease. It is not until after 2 years of age that children who later develop coronary heart disease and type 2 diabetes begin to 'catch up' in weight and body mass index (Eriksson *et al.* 2003a, 2003b, Barker *et al.* 2005a).

When undernutrition during early development is followed by improved nutrition many animals and plants stage accelerated or 'compensatory' growth. Compensatory growth has costs, however, which in animals include reduced life span (Metcalfe and Monaghan 2001). We still know little about the processes by which, in humans, rapid childhood weight gain leads to later disease. In both sexes the risk of coronary heart disease is more closely related to the tempo of weight gain during childhood than to body size at any particular age. As D'Arcy Thompson wrote in 1917, 'To say that children of a given age vary in the rate at which they are growing would seem to be a more fundamental statement than that they vary in the size to which they have grown' (Thompson 1942). Both coronary heart disease and osteoporotic fracture are associated with slow linear growth in childhood (Cooper *et al.* 2001). It will therefore be necessary to distinguish the long-term biological effects of rapid weight gain and slow linear growth in childhood. An overarching question is the extent to which growth at any time is an expression of what has gone before rather than of environmental circumstances at the time. The theoretical implications of such ideas are developed by the editors in relation to wider concepts in evolutionary and developmental biology (Chapter 3).

Childhood markers of later chronic disease

Low birthweight, though a convenient marker in epidemiological studies, is an inadequate description of the phenotypic characteristics of a baby that determine its long-term health. The wartime famine in Holland produced lifelong insulin resistance in babies who were in utero at the time, with little alteration in birthweight (Ravelli *et al.* 1998). In babies, as in children, slowing of growth is a response to a poor environment, especially undernutrition, but the same birthweight can be attained by many different paths of fetal growth and each is likely to be accompanied by different long-term morphological and physiological consequences (Harding 2001). Nevertheless, birthweight provides a basis for estimating the magnitude of the effects of the fetal phase of development on later disease, though it is likely to underestimate them.

Table 37.2 Cumulative incidence (%) of hypertension according to birthweight and change in standard deviation score for body mass index between 3 and 11 years of age in 6424 men and women born 1934–44.

	Change in standard deviation score for body mass index 3 to 11 years	
	Decrease	Increase
Birthweight (kg)		
≤ 3.2	15.9 (1075)	21.3 (1080)
≤ 3.6	14.8 (1274)	19.4 (950)
> 3.6	12.0 (1190)	13.9 (855)

Source: Barker *et al.* (2002a).

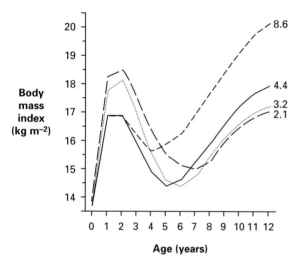

Figure 37.1 Cumulative incidence (%) of type 2 diabetes in a cohort of 8760 men and women born in Helsinki according to age at adiposity rebound. From Eriksson *et al.* (2003a).

Because the risk of cardiovascular disease is influenced both by small body size at birth and during infancy and by rapid weight gain in childhood, estimation of the risk of disease attributable to early development requires data on fetal, infant and childhood growth. Currently the Helsinki studies are the main source of information. If each man in the cohort had been in the highest third of ponderal index at birth, and each woman in the highest third of birth length, and if each man or woman had lowered

their standard deviation score for body mass index between age 3 and 11 years, the incidence of coronary heart disease would have been reduced by 40% in men and 63% in women (Barker *et al.* 2002a). Table 37.2 is based on 1036 people being treated for hypertension in the Helsinki cohort. Subjects are divided into six groups according to thirds of birthweight and whether their standard deviation score for body mass index decreased or increased between ages 3 and 11 years. Birthweight and change in score have independent effects. The highest cumulative incidence was among the people who had the lowest birthweight, but whose standard deviation score for body mass index increased.

The age at adiposity rebound is a strong predictor of later type 2 diabetes. After the age of 2 years the amount of fatness in young children, as measured by body mass index, decreases to a minimum around 6 years of age before increasing again – the so-called adiposity rebound. The age at adiposity rebound ranges from around 3 years to 8 years or more. Figure 37.1 shows the relation between age at adiposity rebound and the cumulative incidence of later type 2 diabetes, with a fourfold difference in incidence between people whose rebound occurred at 4 years or before, and those in whom it occurred at 7 years or later (Eriksson *et al.* 2003a). Early age at adiposity rebound is therefore a marker of increased incidence of type 2 diabetes in later life. That measurement of height and weight before the age of 10 years can predict, without taking into account any subsequent events, such large differences in incidence of type 2 diabetes indicates that there are strong biological effects. This observation has been replicated in a longitudinal study in Delhi, India (Bhargava *et al.* 2004). In both studies an early adiposity rebound was found to be associated with thinness at one year of age. It was not therefore the young child who was overweight who was at greater risk of type 2 diabetes, but the one who was thin but subsequently gained weight rapidly.

Such strong findings show that paths of growth can be used as childhood markers of later chronic disease risk in aetiological studies or targeted prevention. Other markers could include trajectories of

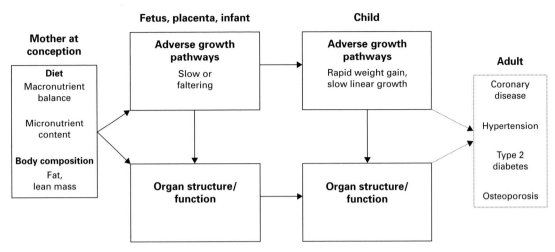

Figure 37.2 Framework linking maternal diet and body composition and pre- and postnatal growth to chronic disease in adult life.

fetal and placental growth, prenatal changes in organ structure recognisable by ultrasound or changes in placental gene expression. Figure 37.2 gives a simple framework linking pre- and postnatal growth to chronic disease in adult life.

Biological processes

This book gives insights into processes which may underlie the association between small body size at birth, rapid childhood weight gain and later disease. Evidence on two processes, renal development and body composition, is increasing especially rapidly, and offers explanations of why the combination of small body size at birth and during infancy, followed by rapid weight gain in childhood, leads to disease.

Renal development

People who were small at birth may have fewer cells in key organs, including the kidney. This may be part of a general reduction in cell numbers or a selective one: undernourished babies may divert blood flow away from one organ to protect another. There is now a body of evidence that the kidney plays an important role in programming hypertension. This is reviewed by Moritz *et al.* (Chapter 23), and the dis-

cussion is broadened to effects on fluid and electrolyte homeostasis by El-Haddad and Ross (Chapter 24). In animal models retarded fetal growth often leads to reduction in glomerular numbers (Merlet-Benichou *et al.* 1994, Langley-Evans *et al.* 1999, Bassan *et al.* 2000, Vehaskari *et al.* 2001, Woods *et al.* 2001). In humans fetal growth retardation has been shown to be associated with reduced nephron numbers (Hinchliffe *et al.* 1992), reduced renal volumes (Spencer *et al.* 2001) and fewer glomerulae with greater glomerular volumes (Manalich *et al.* 2000). A reduced number leads to increased blood flow through each glomerulus. Over time this hyperfiltration may lead to the development of glomerulosclerosis, which, combined with the loss of glomeruli that accompanies normal ageing, leads to accelerated age-related loss of glomeruli, and a self-perpetuating cycle of rising blood pressure and glomerular loss (Brenner and Chertow 1993). Rapid childhood weight gain may also lead to renal injury. High body mass is associated with increased excretory load, which induces hyperfiltration and creates intraglomerular changes that mimic those of reduced nephron numbers (Bagby 2004).

Evidence to support the development of self-perpetuating cycles comes from a study of elderly people in Helsinki, among whom the effect of

Table 37.3 Cumulative incidence (%) of hypertension according to birthweight and father's social class.

| | Father's social class | | | |
	Labourer	Lower middle class	Upper middle class	*p* for trend
Birthweight (g)				
≤3000	22.2	20.2	10.5	0.002
≤3500	18.8	15.2	10.6	<0.001
≤4000	14.5	12.5	10.3	0.04
>4000	11.1	15.6	15.7	0.11
p for trend	<0.001	0.05	0.79	

Source: Barker *et al.* (2002b).

birthweight on blood pressure was confined to those being treated for high blood pressure (Ylihärsilä *et al.* 2003). Despite their treatment, the blood pressures of those who had low birthweight were markedly higher. There was a more than 20 mm Hg difference in systolic pressure between those who weighed 2500 g (5.5 pounds) or less at birth and those who weighed 4000 g (8.8 pounds) or more. Among the normotensive subjects, birthweight was unrelated to blood pressure. An inference is that by the time they reached old age most of the people with lesions acquired in utero had developed clinical hypertension and that this was difficult to control. A study of 3236 Medicaid beneficiaries being treated for hypertension also suggests that hypertension is more difficult to control among patients who had low birthweight (Lackland *et al.* 2004).

Insulin resistance and body composition

Another process by which slow fetal growth may be linked to later disease is in the setting of hormones and metabolism. This may operate at a fundamental cellular level, for example in mitochondria (see McConnell, Chapter 6). An undernourished baby may establish a 'thrifty' way of handling food (Phillips 1996). Tissue resistance to the effects of insulin, which underlies type 2 diabetes and is associated with low birthweight, may be viewed as persistence of a fetal response by which glucose concentrations are maintained in the blood for the benefit of the brain, but at the expense of glucose transport into

the muscles and muscle growth. These processes are reviewed by Reusens *et al.*, Smith and Ozanne, and Symonds and Gardner (Chapters 16–18). Rapid childhood weight gain may lead to an unfavourable body composition. Babies that are small and thin at birth lack muscle, a deficiency which will persist as the critical period for muscle growth occurs in utero and there is little cell replication after birth (Widdowson *et al.* 1972). If they develop a high body mass during later childhood they may have a disproportionately high fat mass in relation to lean body mass, which will lead to insulin resistance. In this and other ways the epidemic of childhood fatness in western countries may be amplifying the effects of poor fetal and infant growth.

Pathways to disease

New studies increasingly suggest that the pathogenesis of cardiovascular disease, type 2 diabetes and osteoporosis depends on a series of interactions occurring at different stages of development. To begin with, the effects of the genes acquired at conception may be conditioned by the intrauterine environment. For example, the Pro12Pro polymorphism of the PPARγ gene has been shown to be associated with insulin resistance, but only among people who had below-average birthweight (Eriksson *et al.* 2002). A number of such gene interactions with birth size have been found, and many more are likely to be found in future (Dennison *et al.* 2001, Kajantie *et al.* 2004, Kubaszek *et al.* 2004). Such interactions would

Table 37.4 Hazard ratios (95% confidence intervals) for coronary heart disease in 3676 men according to ponderal index at birth (birthweight/length^3) and taxable income in adult life.

Household income in pounds sterling per year	Ponderal index at birth	
	≤26 kg m^{-3} (n = 1475)	>26 kg m^{-3} (n = 2154)
>£15,700	1.00	1.19 (0.65 to 2.19)
£15,700	1.54 (0.83 to 2.87)	1.42 (0.78 to 2.57)
£12,400	1.07 (0.51 to 2.22)	1.66 (0.90 to 3.07)
£10,700	2.07 (1.13 to 3.79)	1.44 (0.79 to 2.62)
≤£8,400	2.58 (1.45 to 4.60)	1.37 (0.75 to 2.51)
p for trend	<0.001	0.75

Source: Barker *et al.* (2001).

be predicted if chronic disease originates through developmental plasticity (West-Eberhard 1989).

Observations on animals show that the environment during development can permanently change not only the body's structure and function (see for example effects on the heart, reviewed by Thomburg in Chapter 20), but also its response to environmental influences encountered in later life (Bateson and Martin 1999). The effects of the intrauterine environment on later disease are conditioned not only by events at conception, but by childhood growth (Table 37.2) and by living conditions in childhood and adult life. Table 37.3 is based on the Helsinki cohort (Barker *et al.* 2002b). It shows how the effects of low birthweight on later hypertension are conditioned by living conditions in childhood, as indicated by the occupational status of the father. Among all the men and women, low birthweight was associated with an increased incidence of hypertension, as has been shown before. This association, however, was present only among those who were born into the poorer families, in which the father was a labourer or of lower middle class.

Table 37.4 shows how the effects of body size at birth are conditioned by the environment in adult life, as indicated by income (Barker *et al.* 2001). As expected from the known association between coronary heart disease and low socioeconomic sta-

tus, men who had a low taxable income had higher disease rates. This association, however, was confined to men who had had slow fetal growth and were thin at birth, defined by a ponderal index (birthweight/length^3) of less than 26 kg m^{-3}. Men who were not thin at birth were resilient to the effects of low income on coronary heart disease. One explanation of these findings emphasises the psychosocial consequences of a low position in the social hierarchy, as indicated by low income and social class, and suggests that perceptions of low social status and lack of success lead to changes in neuroendocrine pathways and hence to disease (Marmot and Wilkinson 2001). People who are small at birth are known to have persisting alterations in responses to stress, including raised serum cortisol concentrations (Phillips *et al.* 2000).

Table 37.5 shows how the effects of body size at birth can be conditioned both by childhood growth and by living conditions in adult life, indicated by occupation. In the Helsinki cohort hazard ratios for coronary heart disease rose progressively from 1.00 in men who worked as 'higher officials' to 2.15 (95% CI 1.59 to 2.91) in men who were labourers (Barker *et al.* 2002b). Similar associations with low occupational status have been found in many other studies. Among men with a low ponderal index this effect was apparent only in those who had experienced rapid childhood weight gain and increased their standard deviation score for body mass index between 2 and 11 years. The processes underlying this are unknown, but this illustrates a complex interaction between the effects of small size at birth and postnatal growth and the social environment.

It seems that the pathogenesis of cardiovascular disease and type 2 diabetes cannot be understood within a model in which risks associated with adverse influences at different stages of life add to each other. Rather, disease is the product of branching paths of development. The branchings are triggered by the environment. The pathways determine the vulnerability of each individual to what lies ahead. The pathway to coronary heart disease can originate either in slow fetal growth as a consequence of undernutrition, or in poor infant growth as a consequence

Table 37.5 Hazard ratios (95% confidence intervals) for coronary heart disease in men with a ponderal index at birth below 26 kg m⁻³, according to adult social class and changes in body mass index between 2 and 11 years.

Social class	Change in standard deviation score for body mass index between 2 and 11 years	
	Decrease	Increase
Higher official	0.89 (0.36 to 2.20)	1.00
Lower official	1.22 (0.48 to 3.09)	1.29 (0.53 to 3.18)
Self-employed	1.46 (0.32 to 6.65)	1.41 (0.39 to 5.13)
Labourer	1.68 (0.76 to 3.75)	3.43 (1.70 to 6.91)
p for trend	0.12	0.0001

Source: Barker *et al.* (2002b).

of poor living conditions. Thereafter the pathway is determined by rates of weight gain in childhood, by living conditions and, presumably, by other influences as yet undiscovered.

The effects of slow fetal growth and low birthweight, and the effects of postnatal development, depend on environmental influences and paths of development that precede and follow them. Low birthweight, or any other single influence, does not have 'an' effect that is best estimated by a pooled estimate from all published studies. As René Dubos (1960) wrote, 'the effects of the physical and social environments cannot be understood without knowledge of individual history.' Unravelling the causation of chronic disease, and hence the way to prevent it, will therefore require an understanding of biological heterogeneity. Small studies with well-defined phenotypes may contribute more than larger studies with poor phenotype data.

Sensitive periods

Different organs and systems have critical periods of development at different times during fetal life and infancy. These often coincide with periods of rapid cell replication, and during them the organ or system is sensitive to its environment. For most organs and systems they occur before birth. The famine in Holland began suddenly in November 1944 and ended six months later. Official rations fell to around 700 calories. The subsequent effect on people who were in utero at the time depended on the stage of gestation at which they were exposed to the famine (Roseboom *et al.* 2001b). People who were conceived during the famine now have raised serum cholesterol and raised rates of coronary heart disease. In contrast, those conceived before the famine but exposed to it in mid to late gestation are insulin-resistant and have impaired glucose tolerance. These differences seem likely to reflect sensitive periods of organs including the liver, heart and muscle occurring at different stages of fetal development. The effects of growth failure at different phases after birth also depend on its timing. Type 2 diabetes is associated with failure of linear growth between birth and 3 months, which may coincide with a sensitive period of development for the endocrine pancreas (Eriksson *et al.* 2003b). Coronary heart disease is associated with growth failure in late infancy, which may be one of the sensitive periods for cholesterol regulation by the liver.

Intergenerational effects

Experimental studies in animals have shown that undernutrition can have effects on reproductive performance which may persist for several generations (Drake and Walker 2004; see also Poston *et al.*, Chapter 21). Among rats fed a protein-deficient diet over 12 generations there was a progressive fall in fetal growth rates (Stewart *et al.* 1980). When restored to a normal diet it took three generations before growth and development were normalised. Strong evidence for major intergenerational effects in humans has come from studies showing that a woman's birthweight influences the birthweight of her offspring (Emanuel *et al.* 1992). A study in the UK showed that whereas low-birthweight mothers tended to have thin infants with a low ponderal index, the father's birthweight was unrelated to ponderal index at birth (Godfrey *et al.* 1997). The effect of maternal birthweight on thinness at birth is consistent with the hypothesis that in low-birthweight mothers the fetal supply line is compromised and unable to meet fetal nutrient demand. Intergenerational effects on disease processes have been demonstrated. For example, the blood pressures of a group of young adults were shown to be related to their mothers' birthweights independently of their own birthweights (Barker *et al.* 2000). We can expect many more such associations to be identified.

Wellbeing

This book shows that the list of adult diseases whose origins lie in early development has now extended beyond cardiovascular disease and type 2 diabetes. Studies of osteoporosis and sarcopenia are making especially rapid progress (Cooper *et al.* 2002; see also Chapters 29 and 30 from Cooper *et al.* and Oreffo and Roach). Underlying the associations between early growth and later disease, however, are processes which are likely to affect the wellbeing of people who are, from a medical viewpoint, healthy. People who were small at birth have heightened stress responses (Phillips *et al.* 2000), one manifestation of lifelong settings of hormones and metabolism that are established before birth. These settings affect reproductive physiology, as is well known in animals (Barraclough 1961). In Hertfordshire, men who were small at birth are less likely to marry, an observation confirmed in Sweden (Phillips *et al.* 2001). Around 20 per cent of men who weighed 2500 g or less at birth remained unmarried in middle age compared with only 5 per cent in men weighing 3500 g or more. This is not an effect of adult height: at any height, those who were smaller at birth were less likely to marry. It seems that restriction of growth before birth alters some aspect of partner selection – sexuality, socialisation, personality or emotional responses.

Women born after term tend to have altered gonadotrophin production and polycystic ovaries (Cresswell *et al.* 1997). A possible explanation is that the human fetus produces large amounts of androgens, which are converted to oestrogen by the placenta and pass to the maternal circulation. Placental failure associated with postmaturity could expose the fetal hypothalamus to increased concentrations of androgens or oestrogens and alter hypothalamic–pituitary set-points for release of luteinising hormone. Further evidence that a woman's reproductive fitness may be influenced in utero comes from studies of age at menarche. In a national sample of British girls, those who reached menarche at the youngest age had low birthweight but put on weight rapidly in childhood (Cooper *et al.* 1996). Similar findings came from a study of Filipino girls (Adair 2001). Again the suggested link between fetal growth and age at menarche is the setting of the pattern of gonadotrophin release. Pulsatile release of luteinising and follicle-stimulating hormone is initiated in utero, continues through infancy, and thereafter ceases until it resumes at puberty.

In the Hertfordshire study men and women who committed suicide, which is commonly the result of depression, had low weight gain in infancy (Barker *et al.* 1995). This could be due to adverse psychosocial influences in infancy, but there are no data on this. Another possibility is that depression is initiated by in utero programming of hormonal axes which influence growth in infancy and mood in later life. Patients with depression have been found to have abnormal secretion of growth hormone and abnormalities in the hypothalamic–adrenal and hypothalamic–thyroid axes (Checkley 1992). Growth in infancy has been shown to be linked to income in adult life. Irrespective of family circumstances men who were longer at 1 year of age earn more 50 years later (Barker *et al.* 2005b). Infancy may be a critical period for cognitive function and reduced brain growth, or reduced physical activity associated with recurrent minor illness may prejudice it. The effects of the early environment on later behaviour and cognitive function are reviewed in this volume by Landon *et al.* and Rees *et al.* (Chapters 27 and 28).

Conclusion

The demonstration that normal variations in fetal size at birth have implications for health throughout life has prompted the re-evaluation of fetal development described in this book. There is an urgent need to expand this area of research, and there are already indications that the concept of DOHaD applies to cancer (see Ekbom, Chapter 31), ageing or longevity (see Kirkwood, Chapter 32), lung development and asthma (see Harding *et al.* and Warner, Chapters 25 and 26), atheroma and lipid homeostasis (see Napoli *et al.*, Chapter 22, and Burdge and Clader, Chapter 11). There is now evidence that a range of environmental agents, including chemicals (see Heindel and Lawler, Chapter 7) and hypoxia (see Giussani, Chapter 12), can produce developmental effects on the offspring. Paradoxically, one hopes that this book will soon be out of date. The public health application of all this new knowledge now commands attention (see Chapters 33 and 34 by Forrester and Law and Baird). The ethical implications of such ideas are reviewed by Noble (Chapter 36). It is sometimes said that the first rule of public health is to do no harm. An alternative first rule might be not to stand idly by while bad things, which are remediable, are happening. There are already many reasons to encourage a varied and balanced diet among girls and young women, to protect the growth of babies after they are born, and to prevent rapid weight gain in childhood. This book strengthens the arguments for action.

REFERENCES

Adair, L. S. (2001). Size at birth predicts age at menarche. *Pediatrics*, **107**, E59.

Adair, L. S., Kuzawa, C. W. and Borja, J. (2001). Maternal energy stores and diet composition during pregnancy program adolescent blood pressure. *Circulation*, **104**, 1034–9.

Bagby, S. P. (2004). Obesity-initiated metabolic syndrome and the kidney: a recipe for chronic kidney disease? *J. Am. Soc. Nephrol.*, **15**, 2775–91.

Barker, D. J. P. (1998). *Mothers, Babies and Health in Later Life*. Edinburgh: Churchill Livingstone.

Barker, D. J. P. and Osmond, C. (1986). Infant mortality, childhood nutrition and ischaemic heart disease in England and Wales. *Lancet*, **1**, 1077–81.

Barker, D. J. P., Osmond, C., Winter, P. D., Margetts, B. and Simmonds, S. J. (1989). Weight in infancy and death from ischaemic heart disease. *Lancet*, **2**, 577–80.

Barker, D. J. P., Bull, A. R., Osmond, C. and Simmonds, S. J. (1990). Fetal and placental size and risk of hypertension in adult life. *BMJ*, **301**, 259–62.

Barker, D. J. P., Osmond, C., Rodin, I., Fall, C. H. D. and Winter, P. D. (1995). Low weight gain in infancy and suicide in adult life. *BMJ*, **311**, 1203.

Barker, D. J. P., Shiell, A. W., Barker, M. E. and Law, C. M. (2000). Growth in utero and blood pressure levels in the next generation. *J. Hypertens.*, **18**, 843–6.

Barker, D. J. P., Forsén, T., Uutela, A., Osmond, C. and Eriksson, J. G. (2001). Size at birth and resilience to the effects of poor living conditions in adult life: longitudinal study. *BMJ*, **323**, 1273–6.

Barker, D. J. P., Eriksson, J. G., Forsén, T. and Osmond, C. (2002a). Fetal origins of adult disease: strength of effects and biological basis. *Int. J. Epidemiol.*, **31**, 1235–9.

Barker, D. J. P., Forsén, T., Eriksson, J. G. and Osmond, C. (2002b). Growth and living conditions in childhood and hypertension in adult life: longitudinal study. *J. Hypertens.*, **20**, 1951–6.

Barker, D. J. P., Osmond, C., Forsen, T. J., Kajantie, E. and Eriksson, J. G. (2005a). Trajectories of growth among children who have coronary events as adults. *N. Engl. J. Med.*, **353**, 1802–9.

Barker, D. J. P., Eriksson, J. G., Forsen, T. and Osmond, C. (2005b). Infant growth and income 50 years later. *Arch. Dis. Child.*, **90**, 272–3.

Barraclough, C. A. (1961). Production of anovulatory, sterile rats by single injections of testosterone propionate. *Endocrinology*, **68**, 62–7.

Bassan, H., Trejo, L. L., Kariv, N. *et al.* (2000). Experimental intrauterine growth retardation alters renal development. *Pediatr. Nephrol.*, **15**, 192–5.

Bateson, P. and Martin, P. (1999). *Design for a Life: How Behaviour Develops*. London: Jonathan Cape.

Bhargava, S. K., Sachdev, H. S., Fall, C. H. D. *et al.* (2004). Relation of serial changes in childhood body mass index to impaired glucose tolerance in young adulthood. *N. Engl. J. Med.*, **350**, 865–75.

Brenner, B. M. and Chertow, G. M. (1993). Congenital oligonephropathy: an inborn cause of adult hypertension and progressive renal injury? *Curr. Opin. Nephrol. Hypertens.*, **2**, 691–5.

Brooks, A. A., Johnson, M. R., Steer, P. J., Pawson, M. E. and Abdalla, H. I. (1995). Birth weight: nature or nurture? *Early Hum. Dev.*, **42**, 29–35.

Campbell, D. M., Hall, M. H., Barker, D. J. P., Cross, J., Shiell, A. W. and Godfrey, K. M. (1996). Diet in pregnancy and the offspring's blood pressure 40 years later. *Br. J. Obstet. Gynaecol.*, **103**, 273–80.

Catalano, P. M., Thomas, A. J., Huston, L. P. and Fung, C. M. (1998). Effect of maternal metabolism on fetal growth and body composition. *Diabetes Care*, **21**, B85–90.

Checkley S. (1992). Neuroendocrinology. In *Handbook of Affective Disorders* (ed. E. S. Paykel, Edinburgh: Churchill Livingstone. pp. 255–66.

Clark, P. M., Atton, C., Law, C. M., Shiell, A., Godfrey, K. and Barker, D. J. P. (1998). Weight gain in pregnancy, triceps skinfold thickness and blood pressure in the offspring. *Obstet. Gynecol.*, **91**, 103–7.

Cooper, C., Kuh, D., Egger, P., Wadsworth, M. and Barker, D. (1996). Childhood growth and age at menarche. *Br. J. Obstet. Gynaecol.*, **103**, 814–17.

Cooper, C., Eriksson, J. G., Forsen, T., Osmond, C., Tuomilehto, J. and Barker, D. J. P. (2001). Maternal height, childhood growth and risk of hip fracture in later life: a longitudinal study. *Osteoporos. Int.*, **12**, 623–9.

Cooper, C., Javaid, M. K., Taylor, P., Walker-Bone, K., Dennison, E. and Arden, N. K. (2002). The fetal origins of osteoporotic fracture. *Calcif. Tissue Int.*, **70**, 391–4.

Cresswell, J. L., Barker, D. J. P., Osmond, C., Egger, P., Phillips, D. I. W. and Fraser, R. B. (1997). Fetal growth, length of gestation and polycystic ovaries in adult life. *Lancet*, **350**, 1131–5.

Dennison, E., Arden, N. K., Keen, R. W. *et al.* (2001). Birthweight, vitamin D receptor genotype and the programming of osteoporosis. *Paediatr. Perinat. Epidemiol.*, **15**, 211–19.

Drake, A. J. and Walker, B. R. (2004). The intergenerational effects of fetal programming: non-genomic mechanisms for the inheritance of low birth weight and cardiovascular risk. *J. Endocrinol.*, **180**, 1–16.

Dubos, R. (1960). *Mirage of Health*. London: Allen and Unwin.

Duggleby, S. L. and Jackson, A. A. (2001). Relationship of maternal protein turnover and lean body mass during pregnancy and birth length. *Clin. Sci.*, **101**, 65–72.

Ebrahim, S. and Davey, Smith G. (1997). Systematic review of randomized controlled trials of multiple risk factor interventions for preventing coronary heart disease. *BMJ*, **314**, 1666–74.

Emanuel, I., Filakti, H., Alberman, E. and Evans, S. J. W. (1992). Intergenerational studies of human birthweight from the 1958 birth cohort. I. Evidence for a multigenerational effect. *Br. J. Obstet. Gynaecol.*, **99**, 67–74.

Eriksson, J. G., Forsen, T., Tuomilehto, J., Osmond, C. and Barker, D. J. P. (2000). Fetal and childhood growth and hypertension in adult life. *Hypertension*, **36**, 790–4.

Eriksson, J. G., Forsen, T., Tuomilehto, J., Osmond, C. and Barker, D. J. P. (2001). Early growth and coronary heart disease in later life: longitudinal study. *BMJ*, **322**, 949–53.

Eriksson, J. G., Lindi, V., Uusitupa, M. *et al.* (2002). The effects of the Pro12Ala polymorphism of the peroxisome proliferator-activated receptor-γ2 gene on insulin sensitivity and insulin metabolism interact with size at birth. *Diabetes*, **51**, 2321–4.

Eriksson, J. G., Forsen, T., Tuomilehto, J., Osmond, C. and Barker, D. J. P. (2003a). Early adiposity rebound in childhood and risk of type 2 diabetes in adult life. *Diabetologia*, **46**, 190–4.

Eriksson, J. G., Forsén, T. J., Osmond, C. and Barker, D. J. P. (2003b). Pathways of infant and childhood growth that lead to type 2 diabetes. *Diabetes Care*, **26**, 3006–10.

Fall, C. H. D., Stein, C. E., Kumaran, K. *et al.* (1998). Size at birth, maternal weight, and type 2 diabetes in South India. *Diabet. Med.*, **15**, 220–7.

Forsen, T., Eriksson, J. G., Tuomilehto, J., Teramo, K., Osmond, C. and Barker, D. J. P. (1997). Mother's weight in pregnancy and coronary heart disease in a cohort of Finnish men: follow up study. *BMJ*, **315**, 837–40.

Forsen, T., Eriksson, J., Tuomilehto, J., Reunanen, A., Osmond, C. and Barker, D. (2000). The fetal and childhood growth of persons who develop type 2 diabetes. *Ann. Intern. Med.*, **133**, 176–182.

Forsen, T., Osmond, C., Eriksson, J. G. and Barker, D. J. P. (2004). Growth of girls who later develop coronary heart disease. *Heart*, **90**, 20–4.

Frankel, S., Elwood, P., Sweetnam, P., Yarnell, J. and Davey Smith, G. (1996). Birthweight, body mass index in middle age, and incident coronary heart disease. *Lancet*, **348**, 1478–80.

Godfrey, K., Robinson, S., Barker, D. J. P., Osmond, C. and Cox, V. (1996). Maternal nutrition in early and late pregnancy in relation to placental and fetal growth. *BMJ*, **312**, 410–14.

Godfrey, K. M., Forrester, T., Barker, D. J. P. *et al.* (1994). Maternal nutritional status in pregnancy and blood pressure in childhood. *Br. J. Obstet. Gynaecol.*, **101**, 398–403.

Godfrey, K. M., Barker, D. J. P., Robinson, S. and Osmond, C. (1997). Maternal birthweight and diet in pregnancy in relation to the infant's thinness at birth. *Br. J. Obstet. Gynaecol.*, **104**, 663–7.

Hales, C. N., Barker, D. J. P., Clark, P. M. S. *et al.* (1991). Fetal and infant growth and impaired glucose tolerance at age 64. *BMJ*, **303**, 1019–22.

Harding, J. (2001). The nutritional basis of the fetal origins of adult disease. *Int. J. Epidemiol.*, **30**, 15–23.

Harding, J., Liu, L., Evans, P., Oliver, M. and Gluckman, P. (1992). Intrauterine feeding of the growth retarded fetus: can we help? *Early Hum. Dev.*, **29**, 193–7.

Hinchliffe, S. A., Lynch, M. R., Sargent, P. H., Howard, C. V. and Van Velzen, D. (1992). The effect of intrauterine growth retardation on the development of renal nephrons. *Br. J. Obstet. Gynaecol.*, **99**, 296–301.

Huxley, R. R., Shiell, A. W. and Law, C. M. (2000). The role of size at birth and postnatal catch-up growth in determining systolic blood pressure: a systematic review of the literature. *J. Hypertens.*, **18**, 815–31.

James, W. P. T. (1997). Long-term fetal programming of body composition and longevity. *Nutr. Rev.*, **55**, S41–3.

Kajantie, E., Rautanen, A., Kere, J. *et al.* (2004). The effects of the ACE gene insertion/deletion polymorphism on glucose tolerance and insulin secretion in elderly people are modified by birth weight. *J. Clin. Endocrinol. Metab.*, **89**, 5738–41.

Kramer, M. S. (1993). Effects of energy and protein intakes on pregnancy outcome: an overview of the research evidence from controlled clinical trials. *Am. J. Clin. Nutr.*, **58**, 627–35.

Kubaszek, A., Markkanen, A., Eriksson, J. G. *et al.* (2004). The association of the K121Q polymorphism of the plasma cell glycoprotein-1 gene with type 2 diabetes and hypertension depends on size at birth. *J. Clin. Endocrinol. Metab.*, **89**, 2044–7.

Kwong, W. Y., Wild, A., Roberts, P., Willis, A. C. and Fleming, T. P. (2000). Maternal undernutrition during the preimplantation period of rat development causes blastocyst abnormalities and programming of postnatal hypertension. *Development*, **127**, 4195–202.

Lackland, D. T., Egan, B. M., Syddall, H. E. and Barker, D. J. P. (2002). Associations between birthweight and antihypertensive medication in black and white Americans. *Hypertension*, **39**, 179–83.

Langley-Evans, S. C., Welham, S. J. and Jackson, A. A. (1999). Fetal exposure to a maternal low protein diet impairs nephrogenesis and promotes hypertension in the rat. *Life Sci.*, **64**, 965–74.

Leon, D. A., Lithell, H. O., Vagero, D. *et al.* (1998). Reduced fetal growth rate and increased risk of death from ischaemic heart disease: cohort study of 15 000 Swedish men and women born 1915–29. *BMJ*, **317**, 241–5.

Lithell, H. O., McKeigue, P. M., Berglund, L., Mohsen, R., Lithell, U. B. and Leon, D. A. (1996). Relation of size at birth to non-insulin dependent diabetes and insulin concentrations in men aged 50–60 years. *BMJ*, **312**, 406–10.

Manalich, R., Reyes, L., Herrera, M., Melendi, C. and Fundora, I. (2000). Relationship between weight at birth and the number and size of renal glomeruli in humans: a histomorphometric study. *Kidney Int.*, **58**, 770–3.

Margetts, B. M., Rowland, M. G. M., Foord, F. A., Cruddas, A. M., Cole, T. J. and Barker, D. J. P. (1991). The relation of maternal weight to the blood pressures of Gambian children. *Int. J. Epidemiol.*, **20**, 938–43.

Marmot, M. and Wilkinson, R. G. (2001). Psychosocial and material pathways in the relation between income and health: a response to Lynch et al. *BMJ*, **322**, 1233–6.

Martyn, C. N., Barker, D. J. P. and Osmond, C. (1996). Mothers' pelvic size, fetal growth, and death from stroke and coronary heart disease in men in the UK. *Lancet*, **348**, 1264–8.

McCance, R. A. (1962). Food, growth and time. *Lancet*, **2**, 621–6.

McCance, D. R., Pettitt, D. J., Hanson, R. L., Jacobsson, L. T. H., Knowler, W. C. and Bennett, P. H. (1994). Birth weight and non-insulin dependent diabetes: thrifty genotype, thrifty phenotype, or surviving small baby genotype? *BMJ*, **308**, 942–5.

Merlet-Benichou, C., Gilbert, T., Muffat-Joly, M. and Lelievre-Pegorier, M. and Leroy, B. (1994). Intrauterine growth retardation leads to a permanent nephron deficit in the rat. *Pediatr. Nephrol.*, **8**, 175–80.

Metcalfe, N. B. and Monaghan, P. (2001). Compensation for a bad start: grow now, pay later? *Trends Ecol. Evol.*, **16**, 254–60.

Mi, J., Law, C. M., Zhang, K. L., Osmond, C., Stein, C. E. and Barker, D. J. P. (2000). Effects of infant birthweight and maternal body mass index in pregnancy on components of the insulin resistance syndrome in China. *Ann. Intern. Med.*, **132**, 253–60.

Osmond, C., Barker, D. J. P., Winter, P. D., Fall, C. H. D. and Simmonds, S. J. (1993). Early growth and death from cardiovascular disease in women. *BMJ*, **307**, 1519–24.

Phillips, D. I. W. (1996). Insulin resistance as a programmed response to fetal undernutrition. *Diabetologia*, **39**, 1119–22.

Phillips, D. I. W., Walker, B. R., Reynolds, R. M. *et al.* (2000). Low birth weight predicts elevated plasma cortisol concentrations in adults from 3 populations. *Hypertension*, **35**, 1301–6.

Phillips, D. I. W., Handelsman, D. J., Eriksson, J. G., Forsen, T. and Osmond, C. (2001). Prenatal growth and subsequent marital status: longitudinal study. *BMJ*, **322**, 771.

Ravelli, A. C. J., van der Meulen, J. H. P., Michels, R. P. J. *et al.* (1998). Glucose tolerance in adults after exposure to the Dutch famine. *Lancet*, **351**, 173–7.

Rich-Edwards, J. W., Stampfer, M. J., Manson, J. E. *et al.* (1997). Birth weight and risk of cardiovascular disease in a cohort of women followed up since 1976. *BMJ*, **315**, 396–400.

Rich-Edwards, J. W., Colditz, G. A., Stampfer, M. J. *et al.* (1999). Birthweight and the risk for type 2 diabetes mellitus in adult women. *Ann. Intern. Med.*, **130**, 278–84.

Robinson, J. S., Owens, J. A., de Barro, T., Lok, F. and Chidzanja, S. (1994). Maternal nutrition and fetal growth. In *Early Fetal Growth and Development* (ed. R. H. T. Ward,, S. K. Smith, and D. Donnai,). London: Royal College of Obstetricians and Gynaecologists, pp. 317–34.

Roseboom, T. J., van der Meulen, J. H. P. and van Montfrans, G. A. *et al.* (2001a). Maternal nutrition during gestation and blood pressure in later life. *J. Hypertens.*, **19**, 29–34.

Roseboom, T. J., van der Meulen, J. H. P., Ravelli, A. C., Osmond, C., Barker, D. J. P. and Bleker, O. P. (2001b). Effects of prenatal exposure to the Dutch famine on adult disease in later life: an overview. *Mol. Cell. Endocrinol.*, **185**, 93–8.

Shiell, A. W., Campbell, D. M., Hall, M. H. and Barker, D. J. P. (2000). Diet in late pregnancy and glucose-insulin metabolism of the offspring 40 years later. *Br. J. Obstet. Gynaecol.*, **107**, 890–5.

Shiell, A. W., Campbell-Brown, M., Haselden, S., Robinson, S., Godfrey, K. M. and Barker, D. J. P. (2001). High-meat, low-carbohydrate diet in pregnancy: relation to adult blood pressure in the offspring. *Hypertension*, **38**, 1282–8.

Singhal, A. and Lucas, A. (2004). Early origins of cardiovascular disease: is there a unifying hypothesis? *Lancet*, **363**, 1642–5.

Spencer, J., Wang, Z. and Hoy, W. (2001). Low birth weight and reduced renal volume in aboriginal children. *Am. J. Kidney Dis.*, **37**, 915–20.

Stein, C. E., Fall, C. H. D., Kumaran, K., Osmond, C., Cox, V. and Barker, D. J. P. (1996). Fetal growth and coronary heart disease in South India. *Lancet*, **348**, 1269–73.

Stewart, R. J. C., Sheppard, H., Preece, R. and Waterlow, J. C. (1980). The effect of rehabilitation at different stages of development of rats marginally malnourished for ten to twelve generations. *Br. J. Nutr.*, **43**, 403–12.

Thompson, D. W. (1942). *On Growth and Form*. Cambridge: Cambridge University Press.

Vehaskari, V. M., Aviles, D. H. and Manning, J. (2001). Prenatal programming of adult hypertension in the rat. *Kidney Int.*, **59**, 238–45.

Walker, S. K., Hartwick, K. M. and Robinson, J. S. (2000). Long-term effects on offspring of exposure to oocytes and embryos to chemical and physical agents. *Hum Reprod Update*, **6**, 564–7.

West-Eberhard, M. J. (1989). Phenotypic plasticity and the origins of diversity. *Ann. Rev. Ecol. Syst.*, **20**, 249–78.

Widdowson, E. M., Crabb, D. E. and Milner, R. D. G. (1972). Cellular development of some human organs before birth. *Arch. Dis. Child.*, **47**, 652–5.

Winston, R. M. L. and Hardy, K. (2002). Are we ignoring potential dangers of in vitro fertilization and related treatments? *Nat. Cell Biol.*, **2**, S14–18.

Woods, L. L., Ingelfinger, J. R., Nyengaard, J. R. and Rasch, R. (2001). Maternal protein restriction suppresses the newborn rennin–angiotensin system and programs adult hypertension in rats. *Pediatr. Res.*, **49**, 460–7.

Ylihärsilä, H., Eriksson, J. G., Forsén, T., Kajantie, E., Osmond, C. and Barker, D. J. P. (2003). Self-perpetuating effects of birth size on blood pressure levels in elderly people. *Hypertension*, **41**, 446–50.

Index